Supportive
Cancer
Care

The Complete Guide for Patients and Their Families

Ernest H. Rosenbaum, M.D.
& Isadora Rosenbaum, M.A.

Preface by Susan Molloy Hubbard, B.S., R.N., M.P.A.
Special Assistant for Communication, Office of the Director,
National Cancer Institute, National Institutes of Health

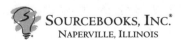
SOURCEBOOKS, INC.®
NAPERVILLE, ILLINOIS

Published by Sourcebooks, Inc.
P.O. Box 4410, Naperville, Illinois 60567-4410
(630) 961-3900
FAX: (630) 961-2168
www.sourcebooks.com

Library of Congress Cataloging-in-Publication Data

Rosenbaum, Ernest H.
Supportive cancer care: the complete guide for patients and their families / by Ernest H. Rosenbaum and Isadora Rosenbaum.
     p. cm.
   Includes bibliographical references and index.
   ISBN 1-57071-696-X (hardcover)—ISBN 1-57071-787-7 (pbk.)
1. Cancer—Popular works. I. Rosenbaum, Isadora R. II. Title.

RC263 .R6378 2001
616.99′4—dc21

00-066170

Printed and bound in the United States of America
DR 10 9 8 7 6 5 4 3 2 1

This book is dedicated to our mother, Dora Rosenbaum, who in spite of medical disabilities returned to active living, through her own determination and indomitable spirit. At age ninety-one she is a teacher and a pianist.

To Ida Friend, who because of her unshakable valor in facing her illness, and for her gift of love and kindness, will long be remembered by all who knew her.

To Joseph Friend, for his wisdom and commitment to the UCSF Comprehensive Cancer Care Program.

And to the Susan G. Koman Breast Cancer Foundation for their support of breast cancer patients, research, and quality of life.

Acknowledgments

We wish to give special thanks and recognition to our original editor, Mary Anne Stewart, for her dedication and invaluable creative efforts in developing and organizing the first edition of *A Comprehensive Guide for Cancer Patients and Their Families*; to the late David Bull, past president of the Bull Publishing Co. of Palo Alto, California, who published the 1980 edition; to Jane Gaspari-Somerville, who edited the 1980 edition with David Bull, and to James Bull, Bull Publishing Co., for permission to reprint excerpts from *Nutrition for the Cancer Patient* by Janet Ramstack, Ph.D., and Ernest H. Rosenbaum, M.D.

We wish to thank Ruth Chernia, who did extensive critical editing, revising, and updating on the second Canadian edition of *Cancer Supportive Care* (1998).

This third edition has extensive changes and major updates that were guided and edited by Eileen Pichersky. Her devotion and expertise in psychology has helped make this third edition all encompassing.

We wish to thank RoseAnn Kurshner, R.N., and Randy Mont-Reynaud, Ph.D., for their assistance and support in promoting the Cancer Supportive Care Program.

We wish to give thanks and recognition to our special editors Tina Anderson, Diane Behar, and Mary Heldman; Michael Glover (preliminary editing), Christopher Benz, M.D.; Gail Gordon; consultants Susan Claman, Francis Perkins, and Zoli Zlotogorski, Ph.D.; and typists Paula Chung and Diane McElhiney for their work on the second edition of *Cancer Supportive Care*.

Thank you to Mary Connell, June Fraps, Jason Gans, Ann Gossman, Brian Greenwald, Noah Kahn, Holly Miller, M.D., Fay Volk, Steven Heilig, Stephen Dobbs, Edmund Pellegrino, M.D., and Martin Diamond for their editing and general support for the section "Planning for the Future."

We wish to thank contributors to the 1980 edition: Stephanie Conger, R.N., B.A., R.A.; Diana Denker, R.N., M.S.; Lizabeth Light, B.A., R.S.N., B.N.; Joanne Meany-Handy, R.N., M.S.; Eileen Shepley, R.N., B.S.N., M.S.N.; Marie Smith, R.N., B.S.N.; Carol Stitt, R.N.; and Julie Williams, R.N., B.S.N.

We would also like to acknowledge the support of the Ernest H. Rosenbaum Cancer Research Fund at the Mount Zion Health Fund, San Francisco, California and the following pharmaceutical companies:

- Aventis Pharmaceutical
- Bristol-Myers Squibb Oncology
- Eli Lilly & Co.
- Ortho Biotec, Inc.
- Pharmacia Oncology
- Schering Oncology Biotech

Contents

Foreword

Alan Glassberg, M.D., Clinical Professor of Medicine, UCSF, Associate Director for Clinical Care, UCSF Comprehensive Cancer Center

The Rosenbaums have devoted much of their lives and an enormous amount of their boundless energies to the care, well-being, and comfort of cancer patients and their families. Their indefatigable and unending efforts on behalf of their patients are widely recognized and lauded.

This book is a distillation of the Rosenbaums' shared experience gained from years of constant study, communication, and practice of sound and compassionate care for cancer patients. It will give patients and families everywhere an opportunity to benefit from the knowledge and wisdom of these two exceptional caregivers.

This guide will take cancer patients and their families, caregivers, and advocates through the myriad of confusing and overlapping paths toward physical and emotional improvement and stability.

Readers will find orderly recommendations based on experience, good sense, and science. These recommendations are designed to help cancer patients either maximize their chances to recover fully, or at least lead lives filled with joy, dignity, serenity, and a sense of purpose. The guide also will be useful to care providers who have not been exposed to the challenging issues involved in helping cancer patients.

A look at the table of contents reveals the book's comprehensive scope. The authors and contributors understand the heavy emotional toll that cancer has on patients, friends, and family, just as they understand the debilitating physical toll it has on patients. They recognize and address the crucial role of an array of alternative therapies and complementary social, aesthetic, emotional, and physical services in improving a patient's prognosis and quality of life. The authors emphasize the importance of strong personal support from family and friends.

The guide includes medical information about cancer—its causes, diagnoses, and standard therapies. There is an exceptionally good chapter describing the elements of an honest and compassionate physician-patient relationship.

Most important, this book acknowledges the huge role that a cancer patient's own determination, positive attitudes, lifestyle, and sense of fulfillment can play in one's rehabilitation, quality of life, and—sometimes—full recovery, while recognizing the extreme anxiety—even terror—that a cancer diagnosis brings to all involved. Thus, this book devotes numerous chapters to topics such as personal coping, nutrition, exercise, sexuality, and the concept of one's will to live.

Finally, this book is realistic. It includes a final frank and informative section on life and death issues.

However, the bulk of the book is dedicated to living, not dying: to helping cancer patients concentrate on enhancing and cherishing the quality of their lives despite, and sometimes because of, their brush with this frequently life-threatening illness. To my knowledge, this is the only book that looks so comprehensively at the full spectrum of cancer patients' needs and the medical and other services and supports that are designed to meet those needs.

It has been my personal and professional privilege to be associated with the Rosenbaums and all the other contributors to this guide. They have taught me the expert and compassionate ways to care for patients who encounter challenges every day that most of us fear to ever face.

This book reflects the standards of care that all of us at the UCSF Comprehensive Cancer Center in San Francisco strive to implement every day with every patient and with the patient's family and friends.

Preface

Susan Molloy Hubbard, B.S., R.N., M.P.A., Special Assistant for Communication, Office of the Director, National Cancer Institute, National Institute of Health

When cancer strikes an individual, it strikes the whole family. Fear, turmoil, and loss of control are felt by all. The patient and his or her loved ones need a book like this to empower them with information so they can face the many challenges they will deal with during their cancer experience. This book provides a framework for cancer care that focuses on the full spectrum of physical, psychosocial, and spiritual support. Right from the start, it prescribes a team approach of shared decision making. It is chock full of wisdom gleaned from individuals who have committed their lives to learning about cancer and caring for individuals with a cancer diagnosis. It is an invaluable resource for any family facing the diagnosis of cancer, as well as every caregiver trying to provide the best cancer care possible.

Throughout the book there are a series of recurring refrains critical to shared decision making:

- Work in partnership with your physician and the other members of the health care team that have been assembled to help you. If you do not feel you are being allowed to actively participate in your care, say so. If the situation does not change after you voice your concern, carefully consider other options.
- Do your own research. Learn how to assess and obtain the care that you need and want. If a different choice is made by your health team, ask why.
- Share in every medical decision by telling your doctor what you are expecting and asking if your expectations are realistic. Affirm that you want only honest assessments of your options and any side effects that may accompany them—even when this request poses a challenge to your health care team.
- Discuss the potential adverse effects of any proposed plan of action and inquire about the availability of supportive services that may help you and those you love cope with what you may encounter—even if that support must come from a provider outside your health team. While information is not an answer, it is the tool that enables an enlightened patient, family, and/or significant other to participate in care in ways that optimize the health care team's ability to prescribe reasonable action.

At issue is responsibility and who has it. The answer is not simple and involves a complex interplay among all members of the health care team if an organized and comprehensive program of care is to be provided for each cancer patient. Again, that is why this book is so valuable. It is a road map that shows cancer patients and their loved ones how to have an intelligent and measured level of control with active participation of the health care team. Although informed and shared decision making may not always produce a cure, it will ensure that each patient's desires and values are given adequate consideration in the selection of a course of action.

Among the many issues carefully considered by the Rosenbaums are the nature of cancer and its management; the all-important unwritten and contractual relationship between a patient and a physician; and the critical components of a healthy rehabilitation and recovery. More than half of the book is devoted to mind and body issues that range from the will to live, stress, depression, and spirituality to nutrition, therapeutic massage, and sexuality. Almost a third of the book is focused on the medical and social support services, the financial aspects of cancer care, dealing with death and bereavement, and coping with a future without a loved one. Having lost my best friend to ovarian cancer last year, I can attest to the importance of these issues and the crying need for greater understanding and emphasis of these critical areas of comprehensive and high-quality cancer care.

However, the beauty of this book is its emphasis on physical, psychological, social, and spiritual health in the context of a life-threatening illness that can incapacitate and isolate people who are not taught how to mobilize their own resources. The book is a wellspring of perceptive advice and practical information about personal action, strength, health, hope, and recovery—and a font of astute wisdom.

A Patient's Point of View

Diane Behar (d.1998)

It has been a great privilege for me to contribute to the second edition of this exceptional book. In addition to my involvement as an editor, I come to this subject from a very personal perspective. Like many of you, I have been diagnosed with cancer. I have been living with this illness—in my case, breast cancer—for close to ten years and am all too familiar with the difficulties and challenges that many of you face each day as you deal with your condition, absorb new information, make decisions about your care, and continue to lead productive and meaningful lives.

As a long-term survivor, I know that a diagnosis of cancer is not a death sentence. Nor does it have to be a barrier to living a full and active life. Today, more than half of all cancer patients can be cured. And those of us who cannot be cured can look forward to the same life expectancy as people with other chronic diseases. And besides, tomorrow always brings the hope and possibility of a cure.

Learning that I had cancer was an unexpected wake-up call that has changed my world forever. It forced me to take a closer look at my life and to reevaluate my goals and priorities. It made me aware of the important role of good health care, proper nutrition, exercise, and relaxation in strengthening my immune system and prolonging my life. Most important, it has taught me to live life to the fullest, with a more positive outlook and a deeper appreciation for every precious moment while I am here.

At the same time, coping with a life-threatening disease is difficult and certainly not something that any of us would take on willingly. There are many times when dealing with the demands and dimensions of having cancer can be overwhelming, even with the love and support of family, friends, and a dedicated health care team. This is why it is so essential to have an overall program that can enable you to take the right steps toward finding suitable treatment, gain greater control over your situation, and, it is hoped, achieve full recovery.

This remarkable book can show you the way. Written by a team of experts who possess a rare combination of knowledge, sensitivity, and expertise, it offers you a comprehensive program that focuses on you as the total patient. It will provide you with a full range of tools and strategies to help you manage every aspect of your illness and to make the most of the resources and information available to you. The active participants are you, your family and friends, and your coordinated health care team.

As its name suggests, this book is comprehensive—and best of all, it is highly comprehensible. It is well organized and easy to read. It even has a glossary in the back for looking up scientific and medical terms. And whether you choose to read it from cover to cover (as I recommend you do) or to use it as a reference guide for focusing on those areas of special interest to you, you will find it to be an invaluable resource for making intelligent and informed decisions about your mental and physical well-being.

The first edition of this book made a difference in my life. I came away from reading it with more confidence and courage for facing my disease, and more determined than ever to forge ahead and not give up. I wish the same for each and every one of you with this updated edition, and hope that it will become a valuable partner in your road to recovery.

I send you my heartfelt wishes for renewed and continued health.

Introduction

Ernest H. Rosenbaum, M.D.
Isadora R. Rosenbaum, M.A.

This book was written especially for you, the patient. It also will be useful to members of your support team—your family, friends, health care providers, and other important people in your life. But remember, you are the most important person, and this book can provide you with valuable tools to help you meet the challenges of living with a serious illness and finding your true path to restored health.

Living with cancer has many different and difficult dimensions, and your needs go well beyond those of receiving basic medical care. Equally important are your psychological, social, and spiritual needs, which must also be addressed.

As the healing arts have become more and more specialized, the gap between all these needs has widened to a point where an artificial division now exists between the mind and body. Physicians and other medical practitioners focus primarily on the physical body, while clergy and mental health professionals work to heal the mind and spirit. But in order to heal you—the "whole" patient—an approach is needed that can bring all these important components together for your total care.

This book is designed to provide just that. It will point the way to an organized program of comprehensive rehabilitation to complement the standard forms of cancer therapy (surgery, radiation therapy, chemotherapy, and immunotherapy). It specifically examines psychosocial aspects, nutrition, exercise, sexuality, nursing, hospital issues, community services, medical economics, and end-of-life care.

This book presents programs of cancer care which involve the full participation of your physician, who is responsible for its supervision and implementation; your health care team—clergy, educators, nurses, dietitians, social workers, therapists (occupational, physical, and recreational); your family and friends; and—most important—you, the patient.

We feel that this total team approach offers the best form of therapy. To use less or only part of the team means that you are receiving only partial care. When you are an active participant in your medical care and rehabilitation, you maintain a sense of control over your disease and therapy. Only you can take responsibility for your state of mind, nutritional status, and physical fitness. The act of taking responsibility is, in itself, an important factor in promoting self-esteem, independence, and faith in your ability to cope. It is a crucial part of getting well.

When you are ill, you have one overriding goal: to get well as quickly as possible to return to an active, fulfilling life. A well-organized, structured program— coordinated by you, your family, and your health care team—can facilitate getting well faster and can make the difference between continued good health or illness and chronic disability. Many resources are available, though it can be difficult for you to take advantage of them when you are seriously ill. This book will help make your own healing program—and progress—that much easier and more manageable.

Efforts must be implemented to maintain the body's strength and to encourage endurance, courage, and hope. These can greatly enhance the effectiveness of medical therapy or support a comfort care program where efforts are made to relieve pain and suffering.

Thirty years ago, President Richard Nixon declared war on cancer when he signed the National Cancer Act, thereby expanding the National Cancer Institute's mission and the government's cancer research laboratories. Unfortunately, it has taken longer than projected to see the early results. Two recent major studies have confirmed that for the first time there has been a drop in the overall cancer mortality rate. The studies showed a turning point after decades of continuous rise, with a 6.5 percent rise in cancer mortality between 1971 and 1990. The largest mortality reductions have occurred from 1990 to 1997 in African-Americans. Their mortality rate has declined 5.6 percent compared with an 18.3 percent increase from 1971 to 1990. African-American men saw a drop of 8.1 percent; the rate declined 2.5 percent in African-American women. Among whites, the decline was 3.6 percent for men and 0.2 percent for women. Breast, colon, and prostate cancer mortality rates are now declining.

In 1996, Dr. Richard Klausner, director of the National Cancer Institute, said, "What we report today is not a cause for complacency, but just the opposite. It is a demand for increased commitment. We are on the eve of the twenty-fifth anniversary of the National Cancer Act, the legislation that made cancer research a high national priority. Now our nation's investment is paying off by saving lives."

The evidence shows that lifestyle changes that influence prevention, such as a 50 percent reduction in tobacco use, improved diet, less alcohol consumption, and more cancer screening (e.g., mammography, colonoscopy, and Pap smears), have made a difference. If this trend continues, there could be a 20 to 50 percent reduction in the overall cancer mortality rate in the next twenty years.

The goal of cancer treatment is to cure cancer or, if that is not possible, to control and slow the cancer growth so that the person can live as long as possible with a full quality of life. One of the goals of this book is to improve your quality of life no matter how much your cancer progresses or regresses. We do know that the better a person's physical status and the stronger their will to live, the better the chances for cancer control or cure are. Thus, a person can have a longer and better quality of life despite the presence, control, or growth of disease.

The Cancer Supportive Care Program

We have developed a free Cancer Supportive Care Program (CSCP) that was initially started at Mount Zion Hospital in San Francisco in 1975. In 1995, it was integrated into the Cancer Resource Center at UCSF/Mount Zion Hospital. The CSCP is now undergoing further development, promotion, research, and evaluation at the Complementary Medicine Clinic at Stanford University Medical Center in Stanford, California.

The purpose of the Cancer Supportive Care Program is to provide multidisciplinary information and services for cancer patients and their families and friends. Program curricula, videos, and implementation tools are free to any persons or institutions that may be interested in starting a similar program for their patients.

The Cancer Supportive Care Program supports patients and their families and friends who are actively participating with their teams of physicians, nurses, physical therapists, clergy, social workers, and counselors. The team approach empowers patients and their families and friends by providing the opportunity to select support services to meet their individual needs.

The act of taking responsibility is, in itself, an important factor in promoting patient self-esteem, independence, and ability to cope with illness. Taking

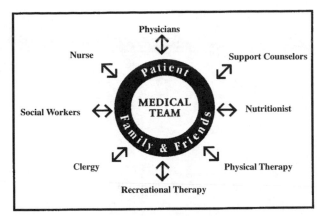

responsibility can make the difference between continued good health, or illness and chronic disability. Patient empowerment is a crucial part of getting well, surviving longer, and living a more fulfilling life.

When a person is given a diagnosis of cancer or experiences a progression of the disease, the choosing and coping with various treatments and side effects can be overwhelming. Many patients find it difficult to cope and may become depressed. Patients often do not know what to do next and can experience treatment as a dehumanizing process requiring them to grapple with therapeutic alternatives, six-syllable drug names, and treatment schedules. Many of these concerns are fed by the patient's belief in the myths of cancer rather than by knowledge of the facts. Patient education on various topics related to cancer helps to relieve this stress, promote wellness, and is an essential ingredient for patient care and survival.

The Approach of the CSCP

At the Cancer Supportive Care Program at the Stanford Complementary Medicine Clinic, there are weekly lecture series and/or workshops. To promote the general well-being of cancer patients and their families, individually scheduled lectures and discussion meetings occur on a weekly basis. Patients have an opportunity to ask questions, receive professional support, and learn ways to help themselves. For further information see our website at www.cancersupportivecare.com.

In addition to lectures, participatory workshops are offered. Workshops provide more practical, hands-on instruction about topics such as:

- regular exercise classes, tai chi, yoga, and qi gong
- nutritional hints, literature, and free consultations for coping with fatigue, nausea, and other therapy side effects

- free fifteen minute massage treatments
- ways to reduce chemotherapy toxicity
- controlling pain and using drugs optimally
- coping with anxiety and depression
- exercises in mindfulness meditation
- poetry and healing
- art and healing
- behavior modification treatment for insomnia
- advice on "end-of-life" care

Internet access, video programs, books, and literature on various cancer-related topics are available at the Complementary Medicine Clinic Library. The Stanford Health Library also provides educational materials and is broadcasting the weekly lectures on their website, www.med.stanford.edu.

In addition, the CSCP offers free videos, a program implementation guide, and a tool-kit to people or institutions interested in developing their own CSCP. More information is available on the CSCP website, www.cancersupportivecare.com or by contacting the Cancer Supportive Care Program at the Complementary Medicine Clinic, 1101 Welch Road, Suite A6, Stanford Hospital and Clinics,, Stanford, CA 94304, (650) 498-5566.

This program is being implemented in centers around the United States and abroad.

STANFORD COMPLEMENTARY MEDICINE CLINIC
CANCER SUPPORTIVE CARE PROGRAM
Introductory Four-Part Lecture Series

1) Overview and Internet Program
2) Psychosocial Needs
3) Supportive Strategies
4) Therapeutic Issues

Weekly Lecture Series and Workshops
(Examples)

- **Coping with Fatigue**
- **"Inner Fire" - The Will to Live**
- **Mind/Body Interactions**
- **Intimacy and Sexuality after Cancer**
- **Depression and Cancer**

Educational Modules On the Web
Internet-www.cancersupportivecare.com

1. Psychosocial Support	8. Sexuality and Intimacy
2. Nutrition Support	9. Lymphedema
3. Exercise and	10. "Diversion"--Art Creativity
Aids to Daily Living	11. Spirituality and Chaplaincy
4. Managing Fatigue	12. Planning for "End of Life" Care
5. Anemia	13. Pharmacologic Support Care
6. Pain control	14. 2nd Opinion
7. Sleep Problems	15. Web Tutorial

Additional Services
Video Programs • Books • Literature

Part I

Cancer: Diagnosis, Information, and Treatment

1

Understanding Cancer
What It Is and How It Is Treated

Ernest H. Rosenbaum, M.D.
Isadora R. Rosenbaum, M.A.
Britt-Marie Ljung, M.D.

Cancer Facts 2001

According to the *Cancer Facts and Figures 2001* from the American Cancer Society, in the year 2001, cancer will be responsible for about 25 percent of the deaths in the United States. Approximately 553,400 Americans will die of cancer—more than 1,500 a day—which makes cancer the No. 2 killer in the United States after heart disease. And by 2020, cancer is projected to exceed heart disease as the leading cause of death in the U.S.

The lifetime risk of developing cancer in the U.S. is one in two for men, and one in three for women. The ACS predicts that 1,268,000 men and women will be diagnosed with cancer and 553,400 will die this year. Prostrate cancer and lung/bronchial cancer are the two most common types of cancers in men. This year, approximately 31,500 men will die of prostrate cancer, although it is 90 to 100 percent curable if diagnosed and treated in its early stage. Lung cancer is the most deadly form of cancer in women, killing approximately 67,000 women. In the year 2001, approximately 193,700 women will be diagnosed with breast cancer and, of these cases, 40,000 will die.

Cancer is a very costly disease. According to the National Institutes of Health, the annual cost of cancer is about 180 billion dollars, more than 105 billion dollars of which are the costs of lost productivity. Approximately 60 billion dollars are spent annually on medical treatment, and cancer therapy for breast, lung, and prostrate cancer accounts for about 18 billion dollars of this figure.

Given such statistics, it is understandable that cancer is one of the most feared diseases. Yet, we are currently curing approximately 58 percent of cases, and the current relative five-year survival rate is about 60 percent for all types of cancer. Presently, there are ten million Americans alive who have had cancer; seven million more have lived five years after their treatments and are considered cured.

What Is Cancer?

Cancer manifests itself by tumor cell growth with invasion into normal tissues. Tumors are of two types: benign and malignant. The benign (noncancerous) tumor does not invade or destroy surrounding structures or tissues, but remains local. The malignant, or cancerous, type grows larger by cell division, invades the surrounding tissues (the lymphatic system or the bloodstream), and metastasizes (spreads) to distant areas of the body.

Malignant tumors are invasive and differ from normal cells in their number, structure, and chromosomes (composed of deoxyribonucleic acid, DNA). Cancer cells vary from slow-growing, low-grade malignancies to high-grade, more aggressive cancers. The grade of a tumor is classified by a pathologist after examining a tissue sample under a microscope.

Although we speak of cancer as one disease, it is not a single disease. There are more than two hundred different cancers, and they can originate in any cell or organ in the body. All cancers have one thing in common: malignant, uncontrolled, invasive growth of cells. When the word *cancer* is used in this book, it means any one of the many forms of cancers.

Sometimes a cancer is reported as "in situ." An in situ cancer is confined to one small area (localized) and is an early stage (precancerous) condition. If it is not treated or controlled, it may never grow, or it may grow and become invasive and malignant. A good example is an abnormal Pap smear with an in situ precancerous lesion that, if surgically removed (excised), may never recur.

Forms of Cancer

There are three basic forms of cancer, named for the body tissues where they originate:

- *Sarcomas* are found in fibrous or soft tissues (muscles, bone, or blood vessels).
- *Carcinomas* are found in the epithelium—cells that cover the body surface and line body organs (e.g., lung, breast, and colon).
- *Leukemias* and *lymphomas* are found in blood cells of the bone marrow or lymph node cells.

Period of Growth

With both malignant and nonmalignant tumors, there is usually a long latency period of from one to thirty years before a growing tumor is clinically demonstrable (can be felt on physical examination or detected by X-ray examination, isotopic scan, or chemical or immunology tests). It is believed that a normal cell requires multiple "hits," or injuries, over months or years by a carcinogen before cell mutation can occur, transforming a normal cell into a cancer cell.

Approximately thirty cell divisions must occur for cancer cells to reach a mass that is detectable on physical examination or by chest X ray (usually greater than one cubic centimeter, or one-third square inch).

Each form of cancer has its own growth rate and pattern of spread. Some cancers remain localized,

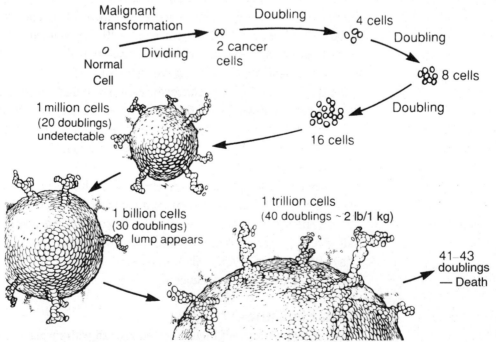

The malignant transformation of a normal cell and subsequent doublings. After twenty doublings (one million cancer cells) the cancer is still too small to detect. Source: Malin Dollinger, M.D., Ernest H. Rosenbaum, M.D., and Greg Cable. *Everyone's Guide to Cancer Therapy*, Third Edition. Kansas City, MO: Andrews McMeel Publishing, 1997

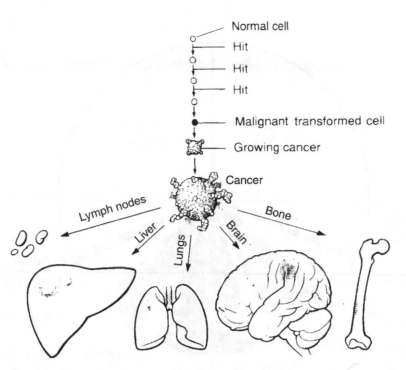

After two or more "hits," a transformed malignant cell grows into a lump we call cancer. Cells may eventually break off and spread (metastasize) via lymph vessels or blood vessels. Source: Malin Dollinger, M.D., Ernest H. Rosenbaum, M.D., and Greg Cable. *Everyone's Guide to Cancer Therapy*, Third Edition. Kansas City, MO: Andrews McMeel Publishing, 1997.

some cancers invade adjacent structures, and other cancers metastasize into the blood or lymphatic vessels, where they are carried through the body to a distant site(s).

Cancers in the abdomen or chest cavity are detected late because they have to grow to a size that will cause symptoms. For example, most cases of ovarian cancer remain "silent," or camouflaged, until they have progressed enough to create a distended and painful abdomen due to excessive buildup of abdominal fluid (ascites). Unfortunately, by that time this cancer is usually in an advanced stage.

Causes of Cancer

Because there are so many types of cancer, it is highly improbable that research will unearth a single cause or a single cure. Until we have more specific knowledge, we can only speculate about the causes and cures of cancer. It is impossible to refute some of the wilder speculations that frighten and confuse people. One such belief is that cancer is contagious or that you can get it from using aluminum cookware. There is no scientific evidence for these statements. Chapter 12, "Alternative and Complementary Therapies," helps to sort out probable from totally speculative ideas. Our knowledge of cancer is incomplete, but there is common agreement on some points.

External Factors

It is widely believed that most cancers develop from normal cells that have been injured by external factors known as carcinogens (e.g., drugs, radiation, smoking, and other environmental toxins). For example, smokers have a ten times greater risk of developing lung cancer than nonsmokers. It appears that environmental carcinogens, mainly cigarettes and alcohol, initiate more than 40 percent of cancers. Diet is responsible for about 33 percent of cancers. Occupation and geographic location also can be factors in the development of cancer.

Internal Factors

Internal factors that play a role in many cancers include hormones, infection, and stress. Data from animal and human experiments suggest that viruses also may play a role in causing cancer. So far only a few viruses—the Epstein-Barr virus (Burkitt's, lymphoma head and neck cancers), HTLV-1 (leukemia and lymphoma), and hepatitis virus (liver cancer)—have been shown to have a causal relationship to cancer in humans. Note that a positive test for the Epstein-Barr virus antibody, confirming past exposure to infectious mononucleosis, also can be found in healthy children and adults who never develop cancer. This demonstrates that other factors, such as perhaps

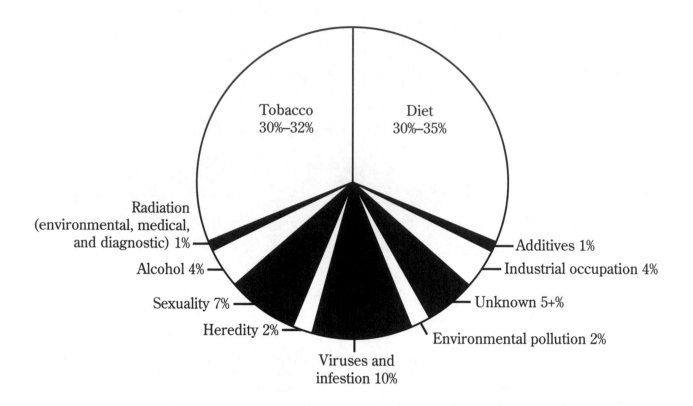

Cancer risk factors with approximate percentages in relation to influence on all cancers (statistical averages, male and female combined). Modified from Doll, R., and Peto, R. *The Causes of Cancer*, Oxford University Press; and Higginson, J.: "Cancer and Environment: Higginson Speaks Out," *Science 205*: 1363, 1979

a specific susceptibility, are required to develop cancer.

Age, sex, and race also can be factors in the development of cancer. In recent years, there has been much discussion of the role of the mind and stress in causing cancer. There is *no* evidence whatsoever that the mind is a major contributing factor in the development of cancer, although it may play a minor role in determining susceptibility or a modest role in accelerating cancer growth. (See Chapter 15, "Does Stress Cause Cancer?")

Our bodies have built-in defenses for destroying or containing cancer cells in their earlier stages. These include tumor-suppressor genes, parts of our immune system, and gene-repair mechanisms—about which researchers are only beginning to learn. Proper nutrition, exercise, and relaxation also may help to keep small, incipient cancers in check. If all these defenses prove inadequate, then the cancerous cells may replicate out of control and eventually spread.

The Diagnosis of Cancer

The best approach to beating cancer is prevention and early diagnosis. Early diagnosis is the prerequisite for cure. Unfortunately, physicians lack routine techniques for diagnosing cancer at its earliest inception, when the likelihood of its spread is minimal. The exceptions are the Pap smear for detecting cervical cancer, the colonoscopy examination to detect polyps and the colon sigmoidoscopy to remove them, mammography to detect breast cancer, and prostate digital rectal examination and prostate-specific antigen (PSA) blood test for prostate cancer detection.

"CAUTION": The seven danger signals, as listed in the American Cancer Society brochure "Listen to Your Body," are:

- Change in bowel or bladder habits
- A sore that does not heal
- Unusual bleeding or discharge
- Thickening or lump in breast or elsewhere
- Indigestion or difficulty in swallowing
- Obvious change in a wart or mole
- Nagging cough or hoarseness

Among those diseases for which early detection is especially important are breast, colon, and prostate cancers; melanoma; certain lung cancers; and leukemias.

Although new tests are becoming available, currently most cancers grow for months or years before they cause symptoms that lead to their detection by physical examination, X rays, CT (Computerized Axial Tomography) scans, MRI (Magnetic Resonance Imagining) scans, and the Positron Emission Test (PET). Additional tests include complete blood counts (CBC), serum chemistry profiles, blood cancer markers (CEA, CA-125, PSA, CA-19-9, or CA 27-29), and/or immunological tests. Bone and body isotope scans also are helpful in the evaluation of metastatic disease and for baselines to make future evaluations more accurate.

The Pathologic Evaluation

Britt-Marie Ljung, M.D.

The essential diagnostic test is a biopsy that is done by removing a small bit of tissue to see if it has the characteristic pattern and cell types that can determine the diagnosis of cancer. This examination is done by a pathologist who is an expert in the microscopic diagnosis that can separate normal cells from malignant cells. There are several types of biopsies. Initially, a fine needle aspiration (FNA) may determine if a mass or lump is benign or malignant. An FNA is accomplished by inserting a small needle into the tumor and removing a small amount of tissue for examination under a microscope. Other types of biopsies include a larger needle (core) biopsy, incisional biopsy (cutting out a small piece of the tumor for examination), or an excisional biopsy when the entire tumor is removed.

Often, the obvious symptoms a person can notice are ignored, despite the American Cancer Society's public education program and the public statements of many cancer specialists. Any delay allows cancer to spread and may preclude the chance for a cure.

2

Genetics and Cancer

Ernest H. Rosenbaum, M.D.
Isadora R. Rosenbaum, M.A.
Patricia T. Kelly, Ph.D.
David A. Foster, Ph.D.

Our knowledge of cancer is incomplete, but there is now common agreement that all cancers arise from abnormalities such as damaged, changed, or lost genes in a person's genetic material or DNA (deoxyribonucleic acid). A person who develops cancer has either inherited a changed gene from his or her parents (5 to 10 percent) or has experienced injury to or a loss of normal genes. It is believed that in some cancers and in some persons, both inherited and acquired genetic defects may be necessary before cancer can develop.

It should be emphasized that although all cancers are due to changes in a person's genes, *most* cancers are not hereditary. That means that most cancers are due to changes in the genes that occur after conception.

Genetic Predisposition

A hereditary predisposition (as reflected in a strong family history of cancer or having a positive test for a defective gene) may, in part, determine one's susceptibility to cancer. The most common forms of inherited cancers occur in the breast, colon, and prostate. However, these cancers also occur in the absence of any genetic predisposition. Not everyone who inherits a predisposition by family history or a positive defective gene test will develop cancers.

For example, a woman who has a first-degree relative (mother, sister, or daughter) who has breast cancer has twice the risk of developing breast cancer (100 percent increased risk) than a woman who does not have a family history of breast cancer. Women who have two close relatives with breast cancer have a higher risk of developing breast cancer during their lifetimes. Scientists are starting to uncover some of the specific inherited genetic defects that contribute to these and other cancers. At least two breast cancer genes have been found in the past few years; together these genes are thought to account for approximately 15–20 percent of all breast cancer cases that are inherited. Thus, approximately 90 percent of breast cancer cases are not caused by heredity. Genetic mutations can be inherited or can arise after birth from environmental and other causes, such as estrogen pills or shots.

In June 2000, doctors J. Craig Venter, Ph.D., and Francis Collins, Ph.D., released a report detailing the decoding of about 90 percent of the human genome. Their work eventually will lead to many new discoveries that will help solve the mysteries of why a disease occurs and to new and more effective treatments.

The following special contribution by Patricia T. Kelly, Ph.D., explains how genetic damage leads to the unregulated cell division that we call cancer. The contribution by David Foster, Ph.D., explains the genetics of cancer at the molecular level.

Genetic Changes and Cancer

Patricia T. Kelly, Ph.D.

In the last few years, scientists have learned much about the causes of cancer on the cellular level. It now appears that all cancers originate from changes in a person's genetic material, or DNA. DNA is present in almost every cell of a person's body. It orchestrates the production of the chemicals that cause our bodies to grow and develop.

Genes are composed of DNA and are located on chromosomes, which are long strings of chemicals resembling unclasped necklaces. You can think of the genes as multicolored beads on a necklace. Human beings have twenty-three pairs of these chromosomes. One of each pair is inherited from the father and one from the mother. With the exception of identical twins, triplets, etc., no two individuals' genes are exactly alike.

Only 5–10 percent of most cancers are thought to be due to strong hereditary factors. Actually, scientists think that only rare cancers—such as retinoblastoma (an eye cancer found in children) or familial polyposis colon cancer (a form of colon cancer)—can be brought about by changes in, or the loss of, a single gene or even a single pair of genes.

How could a change in only one of 30,000 or more genes result in the formation of a cancer cell? Those cancers that are *not* strongly hereditary appear to be brought about by a number of changes (mutations) that have accumulated in the genes of a single cell over time. All of the changes occur *after* conception in a somatic (non-egg or non-sperm) cell. Scientists have found that these changes can occur in different orders (sequences), which suggests that cancer cells arise when a sufficient number of regulatory mechanisms have

been compromised. For most cancers to occur, changes in or damage to several genes seem to be required.

Almost all cells in the body are thought to contain the full complement of genetic material—enough to make an entire human being. It already has been possible to grow a whole plant from just a single cell of a vegetable. Obviously, not all genes in all cells can be active at all times if the body is to function properly. For example, skin cells—which also contain the genes to make ear cells, eye lenses, and so on—must have a way to turn off all genes except those needed to produce and maintain skin. It is as though we have a piano in each cell, with specific keys blocked in different cell types, so that only the appropriate notes are played in any given type of cell.

Clearly, our bodies must have some method of regulating the appropriate activation of genes in the various tissues. Some of this regulatory activity appears to be brought about by gene pairs called tumor-suppressor genes that help to control cell division. These genes create chemicals that prevent cells from dividing at inappropriate times and that also can prevent other genes from making their usual product. If only one member of a suppressor gene pair is lost or damaged, the cell can rely on the undamaged member of the pair to maintain control. However, if both members of a gene pair are lost or damaged, the cell may lose its growth constraints and begin unregulated cell growth. When suppressor genes begin to divide in abnormal ways, over time more and more irregularities occur in the cell. It not only divides when it shouldn't, but it also doesn't die at the appropriate

(Continued from page 9)

time. It is this unregulated cell growth that we call cancer.

What about cancers which are due to strong hereditary factors? Here, it is important to remember that individuals normally inherit two copies of genes: one from their mother and one from their father. Hereditary cancers appear to be due to changes that occur in *both copies* of a very strong suppressor or gatekeeping gene. In many cases, if one member of a gene pair is lost or damaged during the change, the cell can continue to function normally because of the presence of the second healthy gene. However, if a second event should occur, bringing about the loss of the second member of the gene pair, cancer may occur.

Scientists have identified other ways in which cancer cells can develop. For example, some hereditary cancers appear to arise when changes (mutations) occur in genes that are responsible for repairing genetic damage. It seems that everyday living can damage a gene's chemicals, so some genes are responsible for fixing this damage shortly after it occurs. When mutations occur in the repair genes themselves, they are unable to perform their duties or to do them effectively. The result is that genetic damage can accumulate in a cell's genes, which, in turn, can lead a cell to become a cancer cell.

This improved understanding of the various ways in which cancer cells can develop is important because it will, in time, provide scientists with new ways of treating and even preventing cancer. For example, once scientists have found a suppressor gene, they can study the chemical that it makes and the role that chemical plays in helping to regulate the cell's processes. Then, even if a person has damage to a gene (either due to hereditary or nonhereditary factors) it will be possible to correct it by supplying the appropriate chemical that is needed to keep the cell in check. Or, it may be possible to provide chemicals to help repair genetic damage as it occurs. Then, even if the repair genes are not working, cancer cells will not be formed.

Scientists are also studying why cancer occurs at younger ages in some individuals and at older ages in others. The older a person is, the longer his or her cells have been dividing, and so the more likely it will be that a mistake or accident in cell division can occur.

No one single cause of cancer will ever be found, because cancer cells can occur whenever changes happen in a sufficient number of the numerous genes responsible for orderly cell growth and division. Environmental carcinogens, such as cigarette smoke, may also play a role in producing changes in the genes or in disrupting regular cell division. Individuals appear to differ in their sensitivities to environmental agents and the ability of these agents (pesticides, pollution, chemicals like Agent Orange, etc.) to damage their cells' genes. Those with increased hereditary susceptibility to cancer may be born with a change in, or loss of, a suppressor gene. In these people, only one more change in a strong or important gene could lead to the formation of cancer cells. In time, it may be possible to determine which environmental agents are most likely to cause harm to a particular individual so he or she can avoid them.

In the next few years, scientists expect to make great strides in determining which substances in the environment can produce harmful changes to the genes, leading to cancer. The next steps will be to reduce exposure to these substances and to learn how to help the cell repair any damage that occurs.

Molecular Genetic Pathways to Cancer

David A. Foster, Ph.D

Cancer is a complex disease caused by the uncontrolled proliferation of a single cell that has lost the ability to respond to the negative controls that normally restrict cell division. Natural selection has made sure that cancer is unlikely to occur during a normal life span, which varies substantially for different species. However, when life expectancy is increased, cancer incidence increases. Animals in the wild rarely get cancer, whereas cancer is common in animals maintained in zoos, where their life spans are frequently extended. Prior to this century, cancer was a relatively rare disease in humans. During the twentieth century, however, life expectancy for most human populations has nearly doubled. With increased longevity, there has been a corresponding increase in cancer incidence.

Cancer occurs when a single cell acquires a set of mutations to the genes that encode the proteins controlling cell proliferation. These mutations make it possible for a cell to divide in an environment where cell proliferation is highly restricted. We all acquire mutations in our genes during our lifetime, and with the increased life span of humans during the twentieth century, there has been a corresponding increase in the number of mutations that we acquire. As a result of increased longevity and genetic mutation, cancer has become responsible for 20 percent of all deaths in long-lived populations, such as those in the United States.

During the past two decades, enormous strides have been made in characterizing the genes that are mutated as a normal cell progresses to a cancer cell. There are several discrete steps that a cell must take in order to proliferate uncontrollably and migrate to other sites where the dividing cancer cell ultimately becomes lethal. Each of these steps involves a genetic mutation that overcomes a strict control that keeps cell proliferation under control. The following is a brief description of the control steps that must be overcome during tumor progression.

Cell division signals: A cell divides only when instructed. The instructions come from other cells, usually in the form of small molecules known as growth factors or hormones. These hormones function by binding to the surface of a cell that has a receptor for a specific hormone. The binding of the hormone to its receptor on the outside of the cell induces changes on the inside of the cell such that the cell responds in some specific way to the hormone. In the case of a cell division signal, the hormone binds to its receptor and this stimulates assembly of a "signaling machine." The signaling machine consists of enzymes that become activated as a consequence of the binding of the growth factor to its receptor. The best characterized mutations in cancer cells are in the genes that encode the components of this signaling machine. These mutations result in a constant signal to divide in the absence of the hormone. Numerous genes have been identified that, when they mutate in a specific way, cause a signal to be sent that instructs the cell to divide.

Tumor-suppressor genes: Mutations that cause cell division signals to be sent are, in general, not sufficient to stimulate cell division. Just prior to replicating the genetic material (DNA), there is a critical checkpoint that is guarded by a set of genes known as "tumor-suppressor genes." The tumor-suppressor genes encode proteins that prevent replication of the DNA and cell division, unless the cell is supposed to divide. For reasons that are not yet clear, tumor-suppressor genes have the capability to recognize when inappropriate cell division signals are being sent and prevent inappropriate cell division. The tumor-suppressor genes must therefore be neutralized in order for cell division to occur. Inactivating mutations to tumor-suppressor genes are essential for progression to a cancer cell.

Programmed cell suicide: In order to maintain a constant cell number in the body, cell

(Continued from page 11)

division must be matched by cell death. Our bodies have efficient means for ridding the body of unwanted cells. Unwanted cells commit a genetically programmed cell suicide and this suicide mechanism is emerging as a major defense against cancer. Introduction of a mutated gene from the signal machinery to a normal cell generally leads to cell suicide in the absence of another genetic change that suppresses a default cell suicide pathway. In order for a cell to become cancerous, it must overcome the cells' ability to commit suicide.

Immortality: Most of the cells in our body have a limited number of times they can divide. This is because each time a cell divides, it incompletely replicates the ends of the chromosome. Successive rounds of replication ultimately lead to a shortening of the chromosome so genes near the ends of the chromosomes are lost. Ultimately, chromosomal degradation results in a cell that is unable to function and cell death occurs. In this way, cells have a limited number of times that they can divide and are therefore protected from becoming cancerous. However, there is an enzyme known as telomerase that is able to replicate the ends of the chromosomes, thus preventing the chromosomes from shortening and the loss of needed genes. The presence of this enzyme is generally restricted to the germ (sperm and egg) cells, where it is critical that the entire complement of genetic material be protected for passage to succeeding generations. Cancer cells are somehow able to stimulate the telomerase gene to maintain the ends of the chromosomes to achieve the immortality needed to divide indefinitely and become fully cancerous.

Invasion and angiogenesis: Once a cell has attained the ability to divide in the absence of cell division signals, it still must gain the ability to migrate to foreign sites in the body and then stimulate the formation of blood vessels (a process called angiogenesis) that will provide the nourishment needed for developing a large tumor mass. A primary tumor must gain access to the blood stream in order to migrate or metastasize. This process involves digging through blood vessel walls. Cancer cells accomplish this by secreting enzymes that eat away the blood vessel wall so that the cancer cell can gain access to the circulatory system. Once a cancer cell has migrated to another site in the body and begun to proliferate, it must stimulate the formation of blood vessels if it is to grow, sometimes to a size that will be harmful to the invaded organ. Angiogenesis is initiated by secreting factors that stimulate the proliferation of cells that form blood vessel walls. Cancer cells must either secrete these factors themselves or stimulate other cells to do so.

Caretakers: Genetic mutations occur naturally during the replication of DNA during cell division. DNA can become chemically damaged by exposure to many compounds from diet and other sources. The ability to repair damaged DNA prior to replication is critical to preventing the mutations that contribute to cancer. DNA repair mechanisms are more efficient in species with longer life spans, indicating that DNA repair mechanisms have evolved in order to prevent cancer. Consistent with this hypothesis, individuals with inherited defects in DNA repair mechanisms have a greater risk for cancer. While defects in DNA repair do not contribute directly to uncontrolled cell proliferation or cancer, the inability to repair chemically damaged DNA dramatically accelerates the accumulation of genetic alterations in genes that control cell proliferation. Genetic mutation in genes necessary for DNA repair is one of the most common reasons for a genetic predisposition to cancer.

Tumor promotion: A cell that has acquired some, but not all, of the genetic changes to become fully cancerous can sometimes be stimulated to divide by an external stimuli. Compounds that stimulate the proliferation of partially cancerous cells are known as "tumor promoters." A well-known example of tumor promotion occurs in human breast cancer, where estrogen stimulates the proliferation of partially cancerous breast cells. In this situation, estrogen is acting as a tumor promoter to stimulate cell division. Cell division requires replication of DNA, which results in additional mutations. These additional mutations

(Continued from page 12)

will ultimately lead to a more malignant cell capable of dividing in the absence of the promoter. Compounds in diet and tobacco products that stimulate cell division and the replication of DNA, and—as a consequence—additional mutations, are likely the most significant causes of human cancer.

Understanding the genetic changes that occur as a normal cell progresses to a cancerous one reveals that there are many hurdles a cell must overcome to become a fully malignant tumor. These hurdles are overcome by the acquisition of several genetic mutations that: (1) activate a signaling machine, (2) inactivate tumor-suppressor genes, (3) overcome cell suicide programs, (4) attain immortality, (5) penetrate blood vessel walls, and (6) stimulate the production of blood vessels to provide nutrients. The genetic mutations that do all of the above can be accelerated by inherited defects in the ability to repair DNA or by tumor-promoting agents that stimulate excess cell proliferation.

In light of all the obstacles in the progression to cancer, it is somewhat surprising that as many as 40 percent of people in the United States will get the disease, and as many as 20 percent will die of cancer. However, if you consider that this number could be cut in half through avoidance of tobacco and changes in diet, the picture is not as bleak. During an average human life span, there are approximately 10^{16} (10 million billion) cell divisions that take place where the DNA is replicated and genetic changes are possible. In this regard, it is actually quite remarkable that as little as one in ten of us will acquire the set of genetic changes necessary for the formation of a fatal malignant cancer.

Cell proliferation leads to genetic changes and this is the basis for biological evolution. Natural selection has made sure that it is difficult for cells to become cancerous in species with long life spans where so much cell proliferation occurs. The process of progression to a malignant cancer is now beginning to be understood at the molecular and genetic level. This understanding has provided many new targets for therapeutic intervention. The several steps that a cell must take to become a cancer provide an equally large number of places for us to therapeutically intervene. The next generation of cancer research promises understanding of the molecular pathways to cancer so we can treat and eradicate this disease.

3

Patient-Physician Relationships
The Unwritten Contract

Ernest H. Rosenbaum, M.D.
Isadora R. Rosenbaum, M.A.

"The day I found out I had cancer was the worst day of my life."
—*Senator Hubert H. Humphrey*

Not every person who consults with a doctor about a perplexing ailment suspects or assumes that cancer is present; nor does every person who suspects that he or she has cancer actually have it. However, because my specialties are hematology (blood) and oncology (tumors), patients are referred to me by other doctors, and they usually are aware of the reason for the consultation. Some people are referred by their family physicians for a second or third opinion to confirm a diagnosis; others are referred by their internists, surgeons, or cancer specialists for further evaluation or to reassess a treatment program.

If a doctor is to treat a person for cancer, it is important to have a candid exchange of information during the initial meeting. Because new patients are always apprehensive, oncologists try to give them the basic facts about cancer and its treatment and ask them to describe their symptoms and some of the personal facts that are needed for their physician or consultant to provide the best treatment for each patient.

Information about cancer is readily available and useful to a person who will undergo treatment and live with the disease. Informed patients are more receptive to treatment, which improves their chances of successfully combating the disease. Moreover, the attitudes they acquire in these initial interviews may well affect the quality of life they are able to maintain for the duration of their illnesses.

Patients should be aware that they are entitled to all available information about testing, test results, and therapeutic procedures. In the United States, patients now read and sign in the presence of their doctors an "informed consent" form for special diagnostic procedures (such as angiograms) and specific treatments (such as surgery, radiotherapy, and experimental chemotherapy and immunotherapy). Each state has its own legal definition of informed consent. For example, in Massachusetts, California, and some other states, the law specifies that patients with breast cancer must be fully informed of all alternative forms of treatment.

Knowing that what I say may affect the patient's future, when I meet with a patient, I proceed slowly and carefully, ready to temper my approach as the person reveals how much he or she wants to know at that moment.

It is, after all, a patient's prerogative to determine how much he or she wants to hear. I, on the other hand, must be sure to provide an opportunity for a patient to find out everything he or she wants to know.

Many patients now bluntly ask, "Do I have cancer?" In such circumstances, I can be frank. But if a patient tells me to take over, that he or she does not wish to know the details of the disease or the treatments, I usually do not press the issue. Each person knows how he or she is best able to function. The only people who I believe *must* be informed are those who are financially responsible for others.

Whether our initial meeting takes place in the hospital or in the office, I prefer, whenever possible, to have the closest family members present during the explanation. This eliminates the need for repetition and reduces the possibility of misunderstanding. Sometimes, too, including loved ones lessens a patient's fear of abandonment and provides reassurance that the family is not concealing any facts. Together, the family and the patient can ask questions and consider problems that may arise, for, ideally, the long-term treatment of cancer involves the cooperation of the whole family.

During the initial explanation, patients can be helpful—and ultimately better informed—if they respond to leading questions such as "Do you have any questions about your diagnosis?" A doctor is not helped by a reply of "No," or "You're the doctor. You should know." As I mentioned, the doctor-patient relationship works best when both parties are responsive, as in the following dialogue:

Doctor: "What do you think is wrong?"

Patient: "I'm not sure."

Doctor: "Well, there are several possibilities. Acute infection or arthritic or systemic disease—or some other type of disease such as an ulcer or a malignancy. What do you think is causing your problem?"

Patient: "I really don't know. Can you tell me?" or "Do I have cancer?"

When the reply is "Yes, you have cancer," or "Yes, you have a tumor," the doctor should give a detailed explanation, repeating much of the basic information the patient may have received during the diagnostic procedures. The doctor should explain the type and extent of malignancy, although not necessarily all at one time, and it is most important to make the patient aware of the treatments that are available to combat the disease. I always explain that we will begin with the mode of therapy prescribed for this particular form and stage of cancer, but that there are other treatments that may be equally effective or provide a backup if the first one is not effective.

A lot of misunderstandings can result from the initial discussion of diagnosis and treatment. Patients are usually too stunned to think clearly and need time to assimilate the bad news. Often, they cannot respond to my final question, "Is there anything you don't understand about your problem?" They may have understood nothing of our conversation because they heard nothing after the word *cancer* was uttered.

Several years ago, a patient left my office after an extensive thirty-minute discussion of her cancer and was met at the office door by her cousin, who asked, "What did the doctor tell you?" Although only ninety seconds had elapsed since our talk, she replied, "I forgot." It was obvious that my explanation had fallen on deaf ears. She was still in a daze from the first few sentences of our conversation.

For this reason, I usually ask my patients if they would like to have a record of our initial conversations concerning diagnosis and treatment on a cassette tape. The patient, and whomever else (family member or friend) the patient wishes to have present for the explanation, can listen to the tape later at home in a less stressful environment. Someone who receives a diagnosis of cancer needs time to absorb the information, to reflect, and to plan.

The patient, family members, and friends may have misconceptions, fears, and anxieties that should be expressed. The tape helps to deal with these and enables those close to the patient to talk with him or her openly.

Also, patients and their families or friends may have left my office with different ideas about what has been said. By listening to the tape, they can clear up misunderstandings or decide on questions for the next visit. The cassette recording can also help maintain vital communication between the cancer patient and those close to him or her when the latter are unable to be present during a consultation. Some patients have sent the recording to concerned relatives in other parts of the country to keep them informed.

The presence of the tape recorder makes me more conscious of the need for clarity, and I therefore tend to present my explanations in a concise and organized manner. At the same time, the tape recorder tends to make patients more conscious of their right to ask questions and of their responsibility for exercising that right.

Whether or not patients exercise their option to use the tape, I encourage them to write down questions raised during our consultations. In effect, I ask them to make what I call a "shopping list" of all questions that occur to them about their form of cancer, future treatments, or anything else that worries them, no matter how unrelated or trivial it may seem to them. Such a list helps them to include worries that they might otherwise suppress or questions they think they might forget to ask me during our next talk. (The list of questions also makes the most efficient use of the often limited time of an office visit.)

Questions and concerns run the gamut, such as:

- Please explain the whole thing again. What is happening inside my body?
- If I lose my hair, will it grow back?
- Is there anything I can take if I get nausea from chemotherapy? I have to go to work every day.
- I've had no medical insurance since I left my job two months ago. I can't afford to be sick. Are there any sources of financial aid?
- Can I play tennis while having chemotherapy?
- I know this is going to take a lot out of me. What can I do to get the extra nutrition my body will need?
- I have to be able to do housework soon after I get home from the hospital. What can I do to keep my muscles strong while I'm hospitalized?
- I know cancer isn't catching but I can't quite rid myself of the notion. Is it really all right if I sleep with my partner?

Any facts that I can give patients that will relieve their worries will free them to devote their energies to self-care and living.

The Family and the Diagnosis

Occasionally, a family member takes me aside and requests that the patient not be told the diagnosis if it turns out to be cancer. My feeling is that any agreement concerning a patient should be between the patient and the physician. When someone comes to me for medical help, it is with that person that I make the "unwritten contract" for mutual candor and trust, although I welcome the support of family or friends.

Supposedly weak patients are usually stronger than anyone thinks and are quite capable of dealing openly with the cancer.

The reverse situation has also arisen. Patients have requested that their disease be kept a secret to protect a spouse or other family member. In these cases, I try to explain to the patient the therapeutic advantages of treating the family as a unit. For instance, a husband who joins his wife during an office visit will share her problems, know her fears and the routine of her therapy, and therefore be able to give invaluable support. I had one patient who always told me she felt great, but her husband sometimes interrupted, saying "That's not true. You felt nauseated last night." I could then prescribe an antinausea medicine.

Everyone has heard of instances when a family member and the patient each thought he or she was alone in knowing the truth. Generally, this protective attitude is self-defeating, not only because precious energy is expended, but also because the longer the facade is maintained, the greater the fear and anxiety are for both. Therefore, I try to bring the two together.

Sometimes the circumstances are even more difficult. I am occasionally brought in on a case in which the deception of a patient has been going on for some time. The family or the primary physician has decided not to tell the patient the truth, so the question arises as to the wisdom of intervening in an established relationship. My policy in such a case is that if a patient has no psychiatric problem, is not senile, and asks me directly, I explain the nature of the disease in as much detail as the patient wishes. If the patient shows no inclination to know about his or her illness, I tend to comply with the wishes of the family and the primary physician, even though such a policy has often brought unfortunate results.

This situation may occur when a patient and family observe certain cultural customs where in their part of the world a diagnosis of cancer is not given to the patient but is shared with the family. I feel the patient usually knows the diagnosis but takes part in this deception. Sometimes these patients do worse and lose their will to live when informed that they have cancer.

Planning Treatment

In accordance with the terms of the unwritten contract, I try not to make any medical decisions without taking into consideration the emotional needs of patients. The more I talk with a patient about his or her family, work, religious views, hobbies, moods, and general lifestyle, the more I learn what those needs are. At the same time, I have to tell a patient that our choice of therapy, or combination of therapy, will be limited at any given time by the patient's type of cancer and its stage of development. I describe the risks, side effects, and anticipated results of the most current therapies, so that there will be no unnecessary shocks in the future.

A therapy that is new to a patient must be given time to work so that the effects can be properly assessed. I try to explain to patients that when they buy a new car, they have no idea how well it is going to function until they have driven it for a few weeks or months. They then will know how it functions in gas mileage and economy, how often it needs repairs, and so on. This also applies to cancer therapy. Although the treatment differs for each type and stage of cancer, one must usually wait six to twelve weeks after a treatment has begun to assess the early results through laboratory tests, X rays, and scans.

Many people are concerned when changes are made in their therapeutic program, but a change does not always mean that the cancer has progressed or that a new problem has appeared. On the contrary, it is not uncommon to change from one mode of therapy to another, to alter the dosage and content of a therapy, or even to stop treatment for a short time. A change may be made because a therapy is not effective, a new concept of treatment has proved valid, or a new treatment shows promise. Sometimes an unrelated medical problem or the patient's desire necessitates a change in, or end of, a particular therapy.

Fortunately, there are alternative medical therapies for most forms of cancer. I was told by one of my patients that I sometimes sound like a sorcerer with a magical bag of tricks containing an indefinite number of therapies. Yet, it is amazing how often a person who has been successfully treated on a given program and has subsequently relapsed can achieve another remission with a change in therapy.

I am not saying that just because a person accepts treatment, success is guaranteed. We all know there are limits to the possibilities of therapy. But a patient will never know what might have happened unless he or she is willing to try another therapy, assume the risks, and undergo assessment of the results. This is the commonsense approach to the treatment of cancer.

Oncologists must know what is current and available in cancer therapy, as well as what may be forthcoming from cancer research, so that they can send their patients to specialized centers for treatment unavailable elsewhere. Nevertheless, despite assurances that they are receiving the most up-to-date and effective treatment known, some patients are so terrified that they will not accept standard therapy. This pattern is seen most frequently in patients who have been told that the available therapy for this disease will slow the rate of spread but holds little promise for cure. Unable to accept that fact, they spend much of their remaining lives running in desperation to distant clinics or other countries seeking a miracle cure.

Patients may also choose alternative treatment (See Chapter 12). One patient who came to me for consultation and therapy had traveled to Germany and Mexico with her husband because they had been unwilling to accept the therapy recommended at a major university cancer center in California. Instead, she took at least twenty types of vitamins, plus carrot juice, various enzymes, and Laetrile. I recommended certain alternative *medical* therapies to this couple, but they were unable to make a choice.

Finally, because valuable time was passing, I said to them, "There is no sense in my discussing this with you any further until you are willing to come to a decision. If you want me to decide for you, I'll be happy to do so. You have two choices at this time: surgery plus medical therapy—hormones and/or chemotherapy— or radiotherapy and chemotherapy. I've explained the pros and cons of both approaches, and although I have a preference, I am not absolutely certain which is the better treatment for you. That can be assessed only after a therapy has been tried and the results analyzed. If you don't wish to try either one because of your own fears, that's your business. As far as I'm concerned, I'll wait to hear from you." This may sound like a tough approach after my description of a reciprocal exchange between patient and physician, but a decision had to be made. Subsequently, it was made, and it resulted in a dramatic improvement with radiotherapy and chemotherapy.

Panic and flight are one type of response. There are other reactions—anger, frustration, depression—for which we must be watchful. Obviously, some problems are resolvable, whereas others are chronic, with no satisfactory solution. In the latter cases, I believe it is good medical practice to consult another physician. Second and third opinions are becoming increasingly acceptable to both patients and physicians because everyone realizes that no one has all the answers and that another point of view can be helpful—both psychologically and therapeutically.

No matter what a patient's anxieties may be, they should be brought to the attention of the doctor during regular office visits. Many of my patients use the "shopping list" that reminds them of the troubling thoughts and questions that have arisen since the first visit. Discussing them relieves many anxieties.

Anxiety may also be related to the ordinary pressures of life—fear of losing a job or a spouse, or a misunderstanding with a relative or a friend—and be compounded by having to cope with cancer.

One of my patients holds a responsible, demanding job that could be jeopardized by the limitations on her energy resulting from cancer and the therapy required. Her teenage children are always in trouble, and her husband is unable to help emotionally or even take care of the children when she is hospitalized. Because of these worries, she continued to be depressed even after she obtained a remission from anemia and advanced involvement of the liver and bone from breast cancer. However, because she shared her concerns with me, I was able to offer her extra emotional support. The nurses in the office and the nurses and social workers from the hospital are also available to chat or make a referral to such services as group therapy, family counseling, or home assistance programs.

I envisage the role of a physician as an adviser and a friend. In this capacity, I try to help patients plan new approaches with the aid of the medical team. This sometimes involves discussions of how a patient's illness or the knowledge of his or her eventual death is affecting each member of the family and circle of friends.

Sometimes, too, when making a will or arranging insurance or other personal affairs becomes an unwelcome acknowledgment that an illness is terminal, I try to encourage a patient to act for the protection of his or her family. I explain that most people spend their entire working lives planning for the protection and support of their family. They buy insurance and make a will years before illness or imminent death to assure that financial support will be available whenever it is needed (See Part V, "Planning for the Future").

Listening, talking, creating an atmosphere of openness and candor are the means by which an enduring, supportive relationship between the physician and the patient is developed. If a patient will share emotional, financial, and other concerns with his or her physician, unexpected and welcome interest and help may be forthcoming. What patients tell me guides me in each decision regarding the treatment of their cancer and their general well-being. I hope that what I tell them—the knowledge of their disease and its treatment, present and future—reduces their anxiety and frees them to direct their thoughts toward life. But to make such a relationship a reality, patients must have the wisdom to know their needs and be able to discuss them with their doctors.

Remissions and Relapses

A remission is the goal of every cancer patient. As with any other chronic disease, such as heart disease, arthritis, or kidney disease, a remission can vary in its duration and effect on a person's long-term health. A complete remission can mean a return to good health. A partial remission is a more limited medical response than a complete remission.

A person who gets some good news, such as being told of a partial remission, may feel better and enjoy a complete return to health even though a tumor remains. The reason he or she feels well is that the tumor has been significantly reduced. Even a small reduction in size can bring physical relief.

Some patients remain on therapy indefinitely in the hope of containing or eradicating their disease. Typically, physicians encourage them not only to remain on therapy but also to resume the activities of daily living—going to work, doing work around the house, participating in social events, and taking vacations—even if participation is limited while they are on therapy.

Completing a course of therapy is similar to graduating from high school or college. But, in spite of that first feeling of elation, life is not the same as it was before. No one can go through such an experience without suffering some trauma. Living with cancer affects, to a greater or lesser extent, one's emotional reactions and intellectual approach to life. Every new ache or pain, which we all experience daily and ignore, for the former cancer patient raises the fear of a recurrence. I have been through this myself. After surgery in 1980 for a chest tumor that proved to be a low-grade malignancy, I experienced new symptoms. Only a chest–X ray examination convinced me that the tumor had not recurred.

A recurrence for a person who has been in remission is devastating. But, just as when the cancer was first detected, a therapeutic approach will be planned with the goal of a new remission. Anxiety, fear, and depression will again dominate, but they will also be dealt with as they were before.

Most people who achieved a first remission and have a recurrence need only minimal encouragement to sustain their hope for a new round of treatment. Others are reluctant to continue. They may have found the side effects of surgery, radiotherapy, or chemotherapy—even when minimal—to be more than they can tolerate. For example, an executive who underwent four intensive courses of chemotherapy combined with immunotherapy was elated during a period of remission. I warned him his case would have

to be followed closely. Now another recurrence is suspected, and although an intensive program of chemotherapy might produce another remission, he insists that treatment be kept to a minimum. Of course, this decision is his prerogative.

When patients announce that they no longer wish to be treated, or wish to receive only minimal treatment, I try to convince them that a person with a recurrence may have another chance at remission. The potential is there. I believe it is a chance worth taking. The final decision is the patient's. There does, however, come a time when the value of treatment is less than the effort involved, and thus the goal should be to achieve the best possible quality of life.

The condition of every cancer patient, whether cured or in remission, should be closely monitored for years. Patients should also be well informed about the prospects for a recurrence. With this knowledge, they will be more likely to take the preventive measures that may save or prolong their lives.

A Patient's Bill of Rights

In recognition of the patient's human dignity, legal rights, and rights to information concerning one's medical care, the American Hospital Association has developed A Patient's Bill of Rights. The bill was first adopted by the AHA in 1973 and then revised in 1992. It has been approved by more than 75 percent of American hospitals.

The American Hospital Association adopted A Patient's Bill of Rights with the expectation that observance of these rights will contribute to more effective patient care and greater satisfaction for the patient, his or her physician, and the hospital organization. Further, the Association presents these rights in the expectation that they will be supported by the hospital on behalf of its patients, as an integral part of the healing process. It is recognized that a personal relationship between the physician and the patient is essential for the provision of proper medical care. The traditional physician-patient relationship takes on a new dimension when care is rendered within an organizational structure. Legal precedent has established that the institution itself also has a

responsibility to the patient. It is in recognition of these factors that these rights are affirmed.

The AHA encourages hospitals and clinics to simplify or translate the original document to better serve their communities. What follows is one such adaptation.

A Patient's Bill of Rights

A patient—or his or her designated surrogate or proxy decision maker—has the right to:

1. Exercise these rights without regard to sex or cultural; economic, educational, or religious background; or the source of payment for care.
2. Considerate and respectful care.
3. Knowledge of the name of the physician who has primary responsibility for coordinating the care and the names and professional relationship of other physicians and nonphysicians who will see the patient.
4. Receive information about the illness, the course of treatment, and prospects for recovery in terms that the patient can understand.

(Continued from page 19)

5. Receive as much information about any proposed treatment or procedure as the patient may need in order to give informed consent or to refuse this course of treatment. Except in emergencies, this information shall include a description of the procedure or treatment, the medically significant risks involved in this treatment, alternate courses of treatment or nontreatment and the risks involved in each, and the name of the person who will carry out the procedure or treatment.

6. Participate actively in decisions regarding medical care. To the extent permitted by law, this includes the right to refuse treatment.

7. Full consideration of privacy concerning the medical care program. Case discussion, consultation, examination, and treatment are confidential and should be conducted discreetly. The patient has the right to be advised as to the reason for the presence of any individual.

8. Confidential treatment of all communications and records pertaining to the care and the stay in the hospital. Written permission shall be obtained before the medical records can be made available to anyone not directly concerned in the care.

9. Reasonable responses to any reasonable requests made for service.

10. Leave the hospital even against the advice of physicians.

11. Reasonable continuity of care and to know in advance the time and location of appointment as well as the identity of persons providing the care.

12. Be advised if hospital/personal physician proposes to engage in or perform human experimentation affecting care or treatment. The patient has the right to refuse to participate in such research projects.

13. Be informed of continuing health care requirements following discharge from the hospital.

14. Examine and receive an explanation of the bill regardless of source of payment.

15. Know which hospital rules and policies apply to the patient's conduct while a patient.

16. To be informed of hospital policies and practices, including resources that are available for resolving disputes, grievances, and conflicts, and available payment methods.

4

CancerNet
Current, Credible, and Comprehensive Cancer Information

Susan Molloy Hubbard, B.S.,
R.N., M.P.A.,
Special Assistant
for Communication,
Office of the Director,
National Cancer Institute,
National Institutes of Health

The availability of accurate, credible information is essential for anyone making decisions about cancer care. Cancer patients, their families, and many of those who perceive themselves at risk of developing cancer face the arduous task of gathering and interpreting information they find or are given in order to make well-informed decisions about their care options. Cancer patients learn about their diagnosis and management options from many sources and, in today's health care environment, are more and more likely to ask health care providers sophisticated and pointed questions. Advances in computing technology, particularly the advent of the World Wide Web, have revolutionized access to information on health information.

When faced with the task of gathering cancer information either for one-self or for a family member, the Internet provides an instantaneous, inexpensive, and voluminous source of information. Valuable information resources are available on websites, email services, news and user groups, and online discussion groups for anyone seeking cancer information, whether the focus of the search is on treatment, prevention, screening, or support. An increasing number of cancer-oriented websites offer opportunities for individuals to tailor information to meet specific needs and/or preferences. The use of the Internet as a major resource for communicating medical information will continue to increase as interactive communication technologies become more sophisticated and the costs of electronic devices and Internet access decrease.

It should be noted, however, that almost anyone with a computer, an Internet connection, and the appropriate software can create a website. This fact has staggering implications for the amount and quality of the medical information available to consumers. It can be difficult to determine whether the information is current, accurate, and/or complete, unless the information provider clearly articulates the standards of quality that are being used for the inclusion of materials on the site and the criteria for linking to other websites. Users must prepare to take responsibility for making decisions about the value and applicability of the information—just as those using more traditional information sources do.

A search on the term "cancer" via any of the popular search engines will retrieve more than two thousand websites offering cancer information from one of the more than twenty thousand health-related websites. This plethora of health information often represents a mixed blessing. Information that is anecdotal, unreviewed, and undated can be found on many websites, email services, and news and user groups. In an article on the accuracy of medical information on the Web, an oncologist searching for information on Ewing's sarcoma found that half the online material was irrelevant and 6 percent contained major errors. Inaccuracy of information is not the only cause for concern. Some health-oriented sites hawk health care products or refer users to e-commerce partners and then take a cut of the sales. Others post information in an attempt to advance unproven approaches to disease management that are not medically or scientifically sound.

NCI's Information Services

For more than two decades, the National Cancer Institute (NCI) has worked to meet the challenge of assisting health professionals and the public to understand and effectively use medical information by providing current, high-quality information through a variety of communication tools. The primary information resources are PDQ, a comprehensive database of current, peerreviewed summaries of information on cancer care; and CANCERLIT, a comprehensive source of bibliographic citations on published cancer research.

PDQ first became available in 1984. It is unique in the fact that its content is developed based on systematic reviews of the medical literature and expert opinion. Five editorial boards composed of experts in the field synthesize information from the literature into concise, clear summaries that are updated on a regular basis. PDQ provides current information on cancer treatment, prevention, and detection; cancer genetics; complementary and alternative medicine; and the management of physical and psychosocial complications of cancer. It also contains up-to-date information on clinical trials designed to test new approaches to cancer prevention, detection, treatment, and support. Health care professionals, patients, and their families can use these materials as educational resources to promote understanding of the diagnosis and treatment options.

CANCERLIT is a bibliographic archival database containing more than 1.5 million citations and abstracts of published research in cancer biology, etiology, screening, prevention, and treatment published from 1963 to the present from more than four thousand different sources. It is updated monthly and provides a comprehensive, up-to-date resource of cancer literature. Preformulated search "digests" for more than ninety clinical topics are also available.

PDQ and CANCERLIT are updated on a monthly basis, which ensures that users are provided with more current information than can be provided by most hard-copy publications. Both databases are distributed at CancerNet [cancernet.nci.nih.gov], an Internet website that provides point-and-click access to many of NCI's information resources. Over the past several years, CancerNet has become the primary mechanism for disseminating PDQ and CANCERLIT information. The CancerNet website also contains a growing number of NCI publications, a glossary of medical terms, and links to other cancer information websites.

Cancer Information Summaries

PDQ and CancerNet contain cancer information on the treatment of adult and pediatric cancers, cancer prevention and detection, coping with cancer, cancer genetics, and a growing number of nontraditional approaches to cancer prevention, treatment, symptom control, and coping. The cancer information summaries in PDQ and CancerNet are dynamic and may be updated as frequently as every month. On average in 1999, 15 percent of the summaries were revised each month. Approximately 90 percent of the changes were revisions of the summaries. About 30 percent of the summaries underwent substantial revisions. All licensees are required to ensure that the information a user prints contains a date so that it is clear to the user when the information was retrieved from the database.

PDQ and CancerNet contain treatment information on all of the major types of cancer in children and adults. Treatment options are provided for all major types of cancer—more than ninety different types— and information on a growing number of rare cancers is being added. For each major type of cancer, there is an overview summarizing current information on *prognosis* (chance of recovery), *staging* (extent of spread), *histopathology* (tumor cell type), and *state-of-the-art* (effective or standard) *treatment options* by important parameters (such as stage, histology, and/or anatomic location). Treatment summaries are available in two formats: fully-referenced technical statements written to meet the information needs of health care professionals and less technical summaries written in lay language that contain references to resources developed for cancer patients. Cancer specialists write both formats with input from experts around the country, and they are available in both English and Spanish. Each section of the technical statements contain references to the findings of cancer research that have been published in the medical literature.

Because treatment for a patient with a cancer that has not spread from its site of origin is often quite different from the treatment for a patient whose tumor has spread to other organs (metastasized), PDQ and CancerNet generally recommend treatments by the stage of disease (extent of spread). In certain cancers, other factors—such as the location of the tumor or the type of cells that have become cancerous—can be more important in the selection of treatment. In such situations, PDQ and CancerNet recommend treatment options by those factors. When there is no effective standard therapy, PDQ and CancerNet recommend that health care professionals and their patients consider clinical trials that are evaluating new approaches to treatment.

PDQ and CancerNet also include information on approaches to the early detection of breast, cervical, colorectal, endometrial, gastric, liver, lung, oral, ovarian, prostate, skin, and testicular cancer, as well as neuroblastoma. Each summary is evidence based and provides information on the efficacy of screening, both as a means of accomplishing the early detection of cancer in asymptomatic individuals and in reducing mortality.

PDQ and CancerNet also contain information on current approaches to the prevention of breast, cervical, colorectal, endometrial, gastric, lung, oral, ovarian, prostate, and skin cancer. These summaries provide information on factors that increase or decrease cancer risk and on the latest methods of cancer prevention. Similar in format to the PDQ information on approaches to early detection, these summaries also contain information on the strength of evidence supporting benefit.

PDQ and CancerNet also contain information on research on cancer genetics as it relates to cancer prevention, detection, and treatment strategies. An overview of cancer genetics and the genetics of breast, ovarian, and colorectal cancer are currently available, as is a list of familial cancer genes, policy statements on genetic testing for cancer, and a dictionary of genetic terms. Summaries on the genetics of prostate cancer and the elements of cancer risk assessment and counseling are in preparation.

A directory of approximately three hundred health professionals of various disciplines provides information on health professionals who provide services related to cancer genetics that include cancer risk assessment, genetic counseling, and genetic susceptibility testing. Each person listed must be licensed, certified, or eligible for board certification in her or his profession, have specific training in cancer genetics, and be affiliated with an interdisciplinary team with substantial expertise in cancer genetics. They must also be members of one of the professional organizations listed on the application, and be willing to accept referrals.

PDQ and CancerNet have summaries on issues that relate to coping with the side effects of cancer treatment, complications caused by cancer, and the psychosocial sequelae of cancer detection and treatment. The summaries also deal with survivorship issues.

In collaboration with the National Institute of Health's National Center for Complementary and Alternative Medicine (NCCAM), the NCI is also preparing evidence-based summaries on nontraditional approaches to cancer prevention, treatment, symptom control, and coping. An advisory board composed of oncologists and members of the complementary and alternative medicine community review the summaries to ensure that they are up-to-date, informative, and well balanced.

Clinical Trials

New approaches to detect, prevent, and treat cancer must be proven safe and effective before they can be made widely available. PDQ and CancerNet contain more than 1,700 summaries of organized clinical research programs, called clinical trials, that are open or approved for patient accrual. Each clinical trial is designed to answer specific research questions and to find new and better ways to help cancer patients and those at risk of developing cancer.

There are many kinds of clinical trials. They range from studies of new methods to prevent, detect, diagnose, control, and treat cancer to studies on cancer genetics, the psychological impact of cancer, symptom control, quality of life issues, and nontraditional approaches to cancer prevention, treatment, symptom control, and coping.

All of the clinical trials supported by the NCI are listed. Clinical trials being performed with other sources of support can be voluntarily submitted by the physicians performing them, following approval by cancer specialists on a clinical trial review board. The NCI encourages physicians to submit their clinical trials on cancer to PDQ/CancerNet.

New treatments often use surgery, radiation therapy, chemotherapy, and/or biological therapy alone or in combination with one another. The clinical trials in PDQ and CancerNet are classified by:

- research goal (prevention, screening, or treatment, for example)
- primary tumor type (breast cancer, for example)
- modality or type of treatment (surgery, radiotherapy, or chemotherapy, for example)
- accrual status (open, closed, or approved but not yet active)
- study phase (Phase I, II, III, or adjuvant trial)
- specific drugs or biological substances
- sponsorship (NCI-sponsored, or pharmaceutical or other organizational support)

Clinical trial summaries give detailed information on the objectives of the study, the patient entry criteria (medical requirements), and details about the treatment regimen, including dosages and schedules. In addition, each clinical trial provides the names, addresses, and phone numbers of the physicians performing the study. Information on clinical trials is updated monthly.

Short, consumer-oriented summaries have been created for all active clinical trials since 1996. These single-paragraph summaries contain information on the purpose of the trial, the rationale for the study, the study phase, the treatment modality, and some of the key entry criteria that explains the basic rationale and design of the trial. Such information helps patients easily search for clinical trials for which they might be eligible. Special links in the text of the summary enable patients to use their computer's mouse to click on words to look up the definitions of unfamiliar medical terms in a glossary. Each summary also provides the names and phone numbers of the physicians perform-

ing the study. Each summary is hyperlinked to the technical version of the trial summary—where the patient can find more detailed information of the intervention under evaluation and more details on the entry criteria.

Users may search CancerNet to identify clinical trials by a specific type and stage of cancer, treatment modality, drug or biological compound, phase of investigation, sponsorship, and geographic location. PDQ and CancerNet contain the latest information on clinical trials being offered anywhere in the United States and also include information on studies being conducted in Canada and in many European and other foreign countries. Information in the summaries can help individuals who want to participate in a clinical trial enroll in one that is suitable for them.

The Phases of a Clinical Trial

Clinical trials are designed to determine if a new approach to prevention, early detection, treatment, or support is more effective than an existing standard of care. For example, a clinical trial might compare a standard surgical procedure with a more conservative surgical procedure followed by chemotherapy to determine if the less radical operation can produce more cures without the disfigurement caused by the standard operation. Because many standard treatments are first shown to be effective in clinical trials, trials represent the scientific foundation for building new and better management approaches. Trials are designed to take advantage of what has worked in the past and to improve on this foundation.

Clinical trials are carried out in steps called phases. Each phase depends on, and builds on, information from an earlier phase. Patients may be eligible for studies in different phases, depending on their general condition and the type and stage of their cancer.

Phase I Trials. The purpose of a Phase I treatment study is to find the best way to give a new treatment and to discover how much of it can be given safely. The new treatment is given to a small number of patients, and physicians watch carefully for any harmful side effects. The treatment has already been well tested in laboratory and animal studies, but the side effects in humans are not completely predictable. For this reason, Phase I studies may involve significant risks and are offered only to patients whose cancer has spread and who would not be helped by other known treatments. Side effects are carefully assessed and recorded. Patients are also observed closely for anticancer effects by repeated measurement of the cancer sites present at the beginning of the trial. If those sites shrink appreciably, the patient is said to have responded to the treatment. Phase I trials of new approaches to early detection and cancer prevention also address safety.

Phase II Trials. These studies determine the effect of a research treatment on various types of cancer. Usually, groups of thirty to forty patients with one type of cancer—breast cancer that has become resistant to standard therapy, for example—receive a Phase II treatment. Side effects are assessed and, because more people receive the treatment than in Phase I, there is more chance to observe less common side effects. Patients are closely observed for anticancer effects, and response rates are determined. If at least one fifth of the patients respond, the treatment is judged active against their tumor type. A treatment that shows activity against cancer in this phase moves to Phase III. Phase II trials of new approaches to early detection and cancer prevention also address efficacy.

Phase III Trials. Trials in this phase require large numbers of patients—some trials enroll thousands—who are divided into groups. One group, called the "control" group, receives an accepted standard treatment. Another group receives the new therapy. In this way, the response rate, duration of response, and impact on survival can be compared directly. All patients in Phase III trials are monitored closely for side effects, and treatment is discontinued if the side effects are too severe. Phase III trials of new approaches to early detection and cancer prevention also are comparative studies.

Adjuvant Trials. These are conducted to determine if an additional therapy—the adjuvant therapy—will improve the chance for cures in patients at risk for recurrence after surgical removal of all visible disease. At one time, the standard therapy for breast cancer was surgery alone. Adjuvant trials of chemotherapy in women with breast cancer, in which one group received surgery and the other received surgery plus chemotherapy, showed that surgery plus chemotherapy is better than surgery alone. Surgery plus chemotherapy is now the standard therapy for many women with breast cancer.

Taking Part in a Clinical Trial

Clinical trials offer patients the most up-to-date care available. Patients who take part in clinical trials have the first opportunity to benefit from new research and can make a very important contribution to medical science. The medical requirements for taking part in a trial depend on many factors. Patients who want to know more about clinical trials should talk with their physicians and ask them to print out the summary in PDQ on the design of clinical trials.

Patients should learn as much as they can about the various trials before deciding whether or nor to participate. A cancer specialist is often the best person to counsel a patient about the selection of a standard treatment option or a clinical trial. A patient should ask questions about a clinical trial before deciding whether to participate in it. Some of the questions to ask include:

- What is the purpose of the study?
- What does the study involve? What kinds of tests and treatments are done and how are they done?
- What is likely to happen in my case with or without this new research treatment?
- What are my other choices and their advantages and disadvantages? Are there standard treatments for my case and how does the study compare with them?
- How could the study affect my daily life?
- What side effects could I expect from the study?
- How long will the study last? Will it require an extra time commitment on my part?
- Will I have to be hospitalized? If so, how often and for how long?
- Will I have any costs? Will the treatment be free?
- If I were harmed as a result of the research, to what treatment would I be entitled?
- What type of long-term followup care is part of the study?

CancerTrials

Since April of 1998, NCI has provided additional contextual information on clinical trials on its CancerTrials website http://cancertrials.nci.nih.gov. CancerTrials was established to raise awareness about clinical trials and to address some of the perceived barriers to participation in trials. The information contained on CancerTrials falls into the following categories:

- a framework for understanding what clinical trials are and deciding about participation
- information about clinical research grouped by type of cancer (which features hypertext links to the cancer information summaries on CancerNet)
- information on how to find trials (which features a hyperlink to the CancerNet clinical trials search form)
- news and features highlighting topics under clinical investigation and trial results
- resources for researchers, including a library of downloadable resources for clinical investigators that include templates, guidelines, and policy documents.

Quality Control

The NCI has always had a formal review process for the inclusion of content in its databases and information services. All of the information undergoes review by broadly based editorial boards composed of experts who assure that the information is accurate, current, and of high quality.

NCI staff also have established a formal process for ensuring that its CancerNet website only provides hypertext links to websites that have accurate, useful, and current information. Other medical information providers have begun to recognize the need to take responsibility for ensuring that patients are not exposed to bogus and potentially harmful cancer information by utilizing criteria for selecting information they disseminate. To help users determine what websites are credible, the Health on the Net (HON) foundation (www.hon.ch) has established criteria for evaluating websites. The principles embodied in these criteria have been widely adopted by credible health-related websites.

Privacy

As "profiling" of users becomes a more common feature of interactive health communication, understanding a site's position on the confidentiality of personal information is becoming increasingly important. Users should determine what personally identifiable information is collected from them by the website; how the information will be used; with whom the information may be shared; what choices they have regarding the collection, use, and distribution of the information; the kind of security procedures that are in place to protect the loss, misuse, or alteration of information; and how they can correct any inaccuracies in the information.

Access to PDQ, CancerNet, and CANCERLIT

Over the past several years, the CancerNet website has become NCI's primary dissemination vehicle for PDQ and CANCERLIT data. At the end of 1999, monthly user statistics documented more than fifteen million "hits" (four million page views) and nearly 500,000 user sessions per month. In addition to its own distribution outlet, the staff manages a licensing program that allows for use of the databases by a variety of commercial and nonprofit distributors. Through a trademark license, these distributors deliver PDQ and CANCERLIT data to worldwide audiences through a variety of media.

The mechanisms fall into two general categories: (1) online time-sharing systems with dial-up and/or Internet access; and (2) "local" implementations in which the database resides on a computer, CD-ROM, kiosk, or local area network. CANCERLIT is also available online through a variety of commercial database vendors as an online or CD-ROM product. The program, started in 1982 with one agreement, has grown to seventy-two agreements (thirty-nine for PDQ, fifteen for CANCERLIT, and eighteen for CancerMail), and continues to grow. All new requests to license are reviewed and evaluated on the following criteria:

- Does the organization share NCI's goal of disseminating/sharing cancer information?
- What is the impact of the organization's efforts?
- Would licensing the information to the organization enable NCI to reach a larger and/or new audience?
- Is the organization willing and able to update the information monthly and provide ICIC with user feedback and statistics?

Licensing efforts include partnerships with vendors that produce websites and public kiosks with credible health information, as well as those that are developing health information "portal" sites.

CancerFax. The NCI disseminates PDQ data in English and Spanish through its CancerFax service, which enables those without computers to obtain access to cancer treatment information with a fax machine. Users dial the CancerFax telephone number (301-402-5874) from the telephone handset on their fax machine, request a contents list, enter a code number from the CancerFax contents list for the desired information, and follow the voice prompts to receive a faxed image of any of the information that is available through the CancerNet Mail Service. The service is available twenty-four hours a day and there is no cost to the user other than the telephone call. In addition, CancerFax provides current information on the NCI's scientific journals, its patient education materials, and commercial vendors that distribute PDQ.

CancerMail. The NCI also makes information from PDQ's cancer information files available through the CancerNet Mail Service, an electronic service that enables computer users to obtain access to any of PDQ's physician and patient treatment statements, supportive care statements, screening and prevention statements, bibliographic data, or news articles via the Internet twenty-four hours a day, seven days a week. Users of the CancerNet Mail Service send an electronic mail message containing the appropriate code to the NCI computer and receive the desired information in English or Spanish. To obtain a CancerNet Mail Service contents list, send an email message to cancernet@icicc.nci.nih.gov and include the word "help" in the subject line of the message.

The CIS—NCI's Cancer Information Service. One of the problems faced by those responsible for disseminating health care information is how to make it easily accessible to people without direct access to the technology. The Cancer Information Service (CIS) is an NCI-supported nationwide network of fourteen regional offices located at thirty-four sites in the United States, Puerto Rico, and the U.S. Virgin Islands. Through its toll-free telephone service (1-800-4-CANCER), certified information specialists trained by the NCI use a variety of printed and computerized resources to provide accurate, up-to-date information on cancer.

In 1999, the CIS responded to more than 890,000 calls from patients, family members, health professionals, and the general public. More than 300,000 inquiries came over the Internet and 17 percent of callers reported that they got the toll-free number from the Internet.

The CIS staff members conduct customized searches of PDQ and CancerNet and make more than one hundred thousand referrals to clinical trials each year. Staff members also interpret research findings,

explain diagnostic and treatment information, inform callers about emerging areas of science such as hereditary risk, clarify media stories about scientific discoveries, and provide smoking-cessation counseling.

The CIS makes available nearly six hundred publications and materials on a range of topics, including treatment information and research studies, specific types of cancer, community services, screening tests and exams, adopting healthier behavior, coping with cancer, and cancer risk. Some of the materials are in Spanish. A Web-based publication ordering service is also available.

The CIS serves as a health communications laboratory through an NCI-funded research consortium. CIS staff is involved in studies that test and identify the most effective ways to communicate health information in order to help people adopt healthier behaviors. These studies have evaluated types of information messages provided, the manner in which they were delivered, how often messages should be communicated to affect health behaviors, and the value of tailoring messages to an individual's particular perspective. The CIS intends to apply the strengths of the telephone service to the Internet and plans to provide real-time interactions over the Web.

PDQ/CancerNet Redesign

In 1998, NCI embarked on an initiative to restructure the system to take full advantage of advances in computing technology. A formal, two-day meeting was held in 1998 to identify requirements for the new system. This meeting provided an opportunity for more than 190 patients, advocates, clinical investigators, practicing oncologists, oncology nurses, librarians, health educators, social workers, and other health professionals; experts in medical and consumer informatics; and representatives from the pharmaceutical and insurance industry to advise NCI on what should be included in the new system. Participants in the meeting provided specific input on the range of content; ease of navigation; user interface issues; the use of current and emerging technologies as well as barriers to access; and operational, marketing, and evaluation issues. Their recommendations were used to develop the specifications for a more robust and flexible system that can accommodate interactive communication with multimedia data and provide advanced concept search capabilities.

An integral part of the redesign was the prospective gathering of data on the information needs of the full spectrum of current and potential users. An online questionnaire provided input from more than six hundred individuals; 37 percent were accessing the old site for the first time, 23 percent were looking for information on a specific cancer, and 11 percent were seeking clinical trial information. Following this, direct interviews were conducted with current and potential users to define their information requirements.

Based on this feedback, the first prototypes, focusing on the top information layers, were constructed and then subjected to repeated evaluations with current and potential users to see if their needs were being served by the prototype. Volunteers from a variety of backgrounds were recruited to search for information on the prototype in response to a series of specific questions. While they attempted to find the information that was required to answer the questions, the volunteers were prompted to "think out loud" so their thought processes could be captured and recorded on videotape.

This exercise was used to identify flaws in the layout of information hierarchy, menu structure, and navigational elements. These usability tests conclusively documented that users find information in multiple ways. As a result, the new design has multiple pathways linking to the same page to raise the probability that the user will find needed information. In November of 1999, ICIC launched the first version of the redesigned CancerNet website. One of the things ICIC was most proud of was the fact that the new site was built with user input at every stage of development. Major enhancements include:

- a new interface that makes site navigation easy
- cancer-specific pages that provide ready access to all of the information on the site about that cancer
- powerful, new search capabilities
- a network of hyperlinks between PDQ summaries, clinical trials, and CANCERLIT citations
- a guide for first-time visitors with hyperlinks to the information described in the user guide
- a site map and a dictionary of more than 1,200 medical terms
- an expanded list of links to other cancer-related websites
- a publication locator where users can view, download and/or order NCI publications

Updates on new enhancements, new content, search tools, and other changes are featured in a "What's New" area. This area also will be used to highlight feedback from users, enable them to automatically receive updates on enhancements to CancerNet; and sign up for the CancerNet listserv. Feedback from this area and interactive usability testing will continue to drive the development of CancerNet.

Acknowledgment

The information in PDQ and CancerNet is developed, maintained, and disseminated by the staff at the International Cancer Information Center. The staff includes content and technical specialists whose goal is to ensure that PDQ is of high quality and easily accessible to health professionals, patients, and the public. The authors gratefully acknowledge the work of these people. We also are indebted to the many courageous patients and families whose participation in clinical research has led to advancements in cancer screening, prevention, treatment, and support.

Health on the Net (HON) Criteria for Site Evaluation

Adapted from www.hon.ch/honcode/conduct.html

Authorship: Authors and contributors, their affiliations, and relevant credentials are provided. Medical/health professionals give medical/health advice.

Attribution: References and sources for content are clearly listed with copyright information. The site supports claims with clear references to scientific research results and/or published articles.

Disclosure: The site has a clear statement about the funding for the site; website "ownership" should be prominently and fully disclosed, including any sponsorship, advertising, underwriting, etc.

Currency: Dates of posting and updates are indicated. The last update date is clearly displayed. The site's pages display the email address of the webmaster or a link to it on all of the pages.

Linkage site: There is an accurate description of the linkage site's content, size, and location. The site and the sites that it links to respect the legal requirements of medical information and privacy that apply. The information from other sources with an HTML link is valid and regularly updated.

Other unique or innovative features: In addition, other variables that might be useful, such as interactive or tailored sites, surveys, search options, etc., are included to make it a more user-friendly site.

Peer-reviewed process: Reveals if there is an editorial board and/or a review process for what is included.

5

Cancer Therapy

Ernest H. Rosenbaum, M.D.
Isadora R. Rosenbaum, M.A.
Lawrence Margolis, M.D.
T. Stanley Meyler, M.D.
Daphne Haas-Kogan, M.D.
Margaret Hawn, R.N.
Christopher Benz, M.D.
John Park, M.D.

"The desire to take medicine is perhaps the greatest feature which distinguishes man from animals."

—*Sir William Osler, M.D.*

Surgery, radiation therapy, and chemotherapy are the three mainstays of cancer treatment. For certain cancers, hormonal therapy is also useful. Using one or a combination of these treatments, physicians are able to effect a definitive cure (five to ten years free of cancer) in about 50–58 percent of all cancers. (The cure rate for some types of cancer is much higher and for others much lower than this average.) It is important to note, however, that although treatment fails to cure approximately 50 percent of those who have cancer, it is rare that vigorous treatment does not benefit the patient.

Biological therapy such as immunotherapy and gene therapy—including antibodies and vaccines to improve the efficiency of the immune system—is a new and fourth kind of therapy. Immunotherapy, once considered experimental, has entered some treatment programs as a standard therapy for many cancers.

Even in cases when it is obvious from the outset that a cure is unlikely or impossible, appropriate therapy, including palliative therapy (comfort), can assure a chronic cancer patient freedom from pain and many months or years of a relatively normal life. A person may even live a normal life span and eventually die of an unrelated cause.

Over the past seventy-five years, many improvements have been made in the early detection, diagnosis, and treatment of cancer. Improvement in the five-year survival rate has increased from 20 percent in 1930 to more than 50 percent in 2000. Yet it is surprising how often one encounters a negative attitude toward the treatment of cancer, not only among patients and the public but even within the medical community. This attitude could be summed up as: "If it cannot be cured, why bother treating it?" It seems strange that such thinking persists in a society in which the treatment of other incurable diseases (heart disease, kidney failure, and diabetes, to name just three) is readily accepted.

Sometimes people refuse treatment for their disease because they have heard frightening stories about the side effects of treatment and are more afraid of the treatment itself than they are of the cancer. These fears are largely unwarranted, especially today when side effects are better controlled with improved antinausea drugs, such as Kytril, Zofran, Anzemet, Compazine, and Marinol. Bleeding and infections also are better controlled, and pain and suffering can be reduced, alleviated, or even prevented.

There are four types of responses to cancer treatment. They are graded by changes detected by physical examination, laboratory tests, X rays, and scans:

1. Complete response (CR): a 95–99 percent reduction in cancer as measured by tests and/or scans.
2. Partial response (PR): a greater than 50 percent reduction of the cancer as measured by X rays and/or scans.
3. Stable response (SR): the tumor, with treatment, either remains the same size or shrinks by no more than 50 percent.
4. No response (NR): the tumor grows despite various treatments and treatment is considered a failure.

Surgery

Surgery offers the ideal primary approach to cancer. If you can "cut it out" without major functional impairment, and if there is no residual disease, a person may be considered cured. A surgical excision is appropriate when the cancer is localized and does not involve vital structures. For example, a normal life can be achieved after the removal of a kidney or part of a lung because the remaining organ can provide enough function to sustain a normal life.

In some cases, a fine needle aspiration (FNA) biopsy is performed before surgery. A fine needle aspiration involves inserting a thin needle into a tumor to obtain a specimen that can be analyzed by a pathologist. A biopsy is a small, surgically removed specimen (part of the tumor). The specimen is sent to a pathologist for a "frozen section" examination. The pathologist immediately reports the findings to the surgeon. If the tumor contains no malignant cells, the surgeon can perform a conservative, or limited, operation to remove the entire suspicious mass. If the tumor does contain malignant cells, the surgeon can immediately perform a more extensive cancer operation designed to eliminate all traces of the malignancy.

A surgeon often is able to remove all visible evidence of the cancer in the hope of effecting a cure. However, depending on the type and stage of the tumor, cancer may recur in a percentage of cases either adjacent to its original location or at some distant site (metastasis), such as the liver, lungs, brain, or bone. This is one of the hallmarks of cancer—its tendency to metastasize (spread) before the parent tumor is diagnosed and removed. This characteristic constitutes the single most important problem in the management of malignant diseases. It is the reason for having close medical follow-up after treatment and for the necessity of follow-up examinations several months or even years after an operation to be certain that a cure has been achieved.

If the tumor cannot be completely removed or if there is a risk of recurrence, adjuvant (additional) therapy may be considered, using radiation, chemotherapy, immunotherapy, or all three to reduce the risk of a recurrence.

Radiation Therapy

Radiation therapy can damage or kill cells by injuring the DNA chromosomes of the cancer cell. Normal, healthy cells that surround the tumor, and are also struck by the radiation, can recover from the damage. Certain tumors, such as cancer of the cervix and Hodgkin's disease, may be cured by radiation therapy. Hope for many cancer patients not cured by surgery may lie in this treatment. It is not the last resort, as many people think, but is a practical method of killing cancer cells, restricting cancer growth, controlling pain, or reducing a tumor to a size where surgery is more practical.

The most likely candidate for radiation therapy is the patient with localized cancer. But even when the tumor has spread, radiation still may be used because it can reduce a cancer mass that may be causing an organ obstruction, causing pain, or presenting a risk for a bone fracture.

By damaging the cells' DNA, radiation therapy usually renders the cells incapable of further growth or cell division. In radiation therapy, a beam of X rays or gamma rays (from cobalt, linear acceleration, or radium) is aimed directly at the tumor from an X-ray machine. Newer, still experimental techniques use heavy particles—pi-mesons (pions) and neutrons—to treat cancers that are less sensitive to conventional radiation.

For each patient, the area to be treated is carefully outlined with a color skin marker. This colored outline remains on the skin throughout the course of therapy.

The staff radiotherapist maps out the area of the tumor mass to be treated. The normal tissues surrounding the tumor receive careful consideration to protect them. A lead mold is made, customized for each patient so that during radiotherapy the beams will strike only the tumor. A dosimetrist, a specialist who calculates the dose of radiation to be given, usually does this work. During radiotherapy, the mold is placed above the patient on a special tray attached to the radiation machine. Nevertheless, it is impossible to totally avoid some damage to normal cells that lie in the path of the radiation beam. To minimize this problem, as well as to obtain the most efficient results, normal tissues are shielded as much as possible, and the recommended radiation dose is spread out over a period of time.

The complex mathematical calculations for the radiation dose appropriate for each patient (dosimetry) consider the tumor and the tolerance of the surrounding tissues in the area to be treated, as well as the anticipated side effects. These calculations are based on CT (computerized tomography) scans and other sophisticated roentgenographic techniques.

The development of high-energy radiation delivery machines has markedly reduced damage to surrounding normal cells. Most major medical centers now have a full range of megavoltage equipment ranging from cobalt to linear accelerators. The radiotherapist will select the most appropriate machine to treat the tumor and spare normal tissues, taking into account the type and location of the tumor.

A patient does not feel any pain or discomfort while receiving radiation therapy. Undergoing treatment is like having a chest X ray, with the difference being that in radiation therapy the X-ray machine is left on for several minutes to give a higher dose of radiation. In contrast, chest X rays take only a few seconds and deliver a minute dose of radiation.

Side effects may occur as a result of damage to normal tissues. These side effects are discussed in Chapter 7, "Side Effects of Cancer Therapy." New, more sophisticated equipment and safety techniques have lessened or eliminated some of these side effects (particularly skin irritation, nausea, vomiting, and diarrhea) for many patients. Fortunately, radiation therapy is usually limited to one to six weeks and few of the side effects are permanent.

Sometimes radiation is administered internally, directly into the cancer. IORT (intraoperative radiation therapy) and brachytherapy (implanting radioactive seeds or needles into a tumor or implanting catheters to be loaded with radioactive substances for the delivery of sharply localized doses of radiation) are two forms of internally administered radiotherapy. They can spare surrounding tissues from significantly higher radiation exposure. These procedures are usually carried out in an operating room under anesthesia. The tubes or needles are allowed to remain in the tumor for a calculated number of hours or days, allowing the tumor to be treated with a high dose of radiation. This radiation treatment also can be used in conjunction with external-beam radiation to concentrate the dose to the local area.

Certain tumors—such as cancer of the cervix, breast, and prostate—may be cured by radiation therapy. Many cancers not eliminated by surgery may be successfully treated with radiation. Radiation therapy is often given in conjunction with other cancer treatments. For example, after surgery a dose of radiation may be given as a preventive measure to sterilize microscopic tumor cells that may have been left behind when the bulk of the cancer was removed.

Chemotherapy often is used before (neoadjunctive) or during (concurrent) radiation therapy, with drugs such as Adriamycin, 5-fluorouracil (5-FU), and Platinol or Taxol, which are radiosensitizers, to enhance the effects of radiation therapy. The combination of these therapies is often more effective in controlling certain cancers, but also may have more side effects. These side effects can be reduced or minimized by monitoring and adjusting the doses of the chemotherapy and radiation therapy. (See Chapter 27, "Nutrition Problems: Causes and Solutions" for hints on reducing drug side effects.)

Chemotherapy

Chemotherapy uses drugs that attack and may destroy cancer cells. Chemotherapy is generally reserved for systemic or invasive cancers that have spread to other parts of the body through the lymphatic or blood system, and for cases where surgery and radiation therapy are no longer effective. More recently, chemotherapy has been used as an adjunct to surgical treatment (the primary treatment) to destroy small amounts of undetectable cancer.

Chemotherapy has a bad reputation. Some of this reputation is deserved, but some of it is not. Not all of the drugs produce serious side effects, and, today, many patients have minimal toxic reactions. There is no publicity about the person who comes to the office or clinic, sticks out an arm, takes chemotherapy shots for breast or ovarian cancer, and then goes home or to work and functions fairly well. Often, these people don't talk about their disease or therapy, so what is heard is often from the minority of people who suffer severe side effects from chemotherapy.

Most people can tolerate chemotherapy, some patients have moderate-to-severe reactions, and a few cannot tolerate this therapy at all. Fortunately, there are many ways to reduce the side effects, many of which are discussed in Chapter 8, "Side Effects of Chemotherapy."

Chemotherapy is used to treat more advanced or metastatic cancer. It was originally used only in cases where surgery and radiation therapy were no longer effective, but now it is also used as an extra safeguard after surgical removal of a tumor that has a high risk of recurring. For example, chemotherapy may be administered soon after surgery for breast cancer (when cancer cells have been found in adjacent lymph nodes). See "Adjuvant Chemotherapy" on page 34.

In a few diseases, such as Burkitt's lymphoma, choriocarcinoma, acute leukemia, ovarian cancer, testicular cancer, and some cases of advanced Hodgkin's disease, the judicious and aggressive use of chemotherapy—with or without radiation therapy—may bring about a remission or cure.

Like healthy cells, cancer cells are involved in a continuous process of alternately resting and dividing (the cell cycle). This is the process of cell division, when a cell makes two daughter cells. Unlike healthy cells, cancer cells divide in an uncontrollable manner. Chemotherapy takes advantage of the way cells multiply by dividing.

Approximately sixty chemotherapeutic drugs are currently available, although only about thirty of these are used in the majority of cancers. The chemotherapeutic agents are cellular poisons classified as cell-cycle-specific (targeted at dividing cells), noncell-cycle-specific (aimed at resting or nondividing cells), or miscellaneous. These classifications refer to the stage at which the particular chemotherapeutic agent is effective. There are several classes of drugs that act by various means to injure the cell and prevent growth by inhibiting cell division. Chemotherapeutic agents are frequently used in combination to increase their effectiveness and to prevent drug resistance by cells.

Because many cancer cells are killed more easily during the process of division than when they are resting, the cell-cycle-specific class of drugs (the antimetabolites) is used to attack those cancer cells while they are dividing. The noncell-cycle-specific class of drugs (the alkylating or mustard group) tends to attack the DNA of all the cells in a tumor, whether they are resting or dividing. These drugs are generally used to reduce the tumor mass. Then the remaining tumor cells (many of which were inactive before the drug was administered) may become active and start dividing, at which time a cell-cycle-specific drug can be given. These two classes of drugs are often used sequentially or in combination to obtain the maximum effect.

We are constantly devising more effective chemotherapy to use the most effective method and frequency of administering drugs, find better combinations of these drugs, and develop new drugs.

Making the Decision to Take Chemotherapy

The decision to take chemotherapy is a personal decision based on information, personal philosophy, and accurate medical advice. Many who accept therapy despite poor odds are making a decision to choose to fight. The benefits can be few, marginal, or major. Desperate patients with advanced disease are often willing to accept chemotherapy in hopes of even a small chance to live.

More than 50 percent of cancer patients are eligible for chemotherapy and will receive it. New research has shown that breast cancer patients who are at increased risk for recurrence can significantly increase survival time or delay recurrence by using chemotherapy. This is also true for Hodgkin's disease, lymphomas, testicular cancer, ovarian cancer, and leukemias that respond well to treatment.

Despite years of research and increased knowledge on how best to administer chemotherapy and reduce side effects, the cost of therapy continues to escalate and quality of life is often threatened.

To help you make a decision about whether to take chemotherapy, ask your health care provider the following questions:

1. Will therapy be effective in controlling or curing my cancer?

2. Will therapy increase my life span?

3. What are the chances that the disease will recur if I don't accept chemotherapy? What can I expect will happen?

4. Is my cancer early or advanced? Does this make a difference in choosing a chemotherapy program?

5. Should I be enrolled in a research protocol? What are the advantages?

6. How will success (response) to chemotherapy be measured? (A 70 percent response rate means that 70 percent of treated persons will have a reduction in tumor size or bulk, reflecting a significant improvement for a certain time.)

7. What are the side effects of therapy? How will side effects be modified or controlled? Are there long-term side effects? How will they be modified or controlled?

8. Will my chemotherapy program relieve pain, pressure, or other symptoms of cancer, even if it will not prolong my life?

9. May I talk to a patient who has been treated with this chemotherapy program?

10. Where will chemotherapy be given and who will give it?

Hormonal Therapy

Hormonal therapy attempts to reduce or control a tumor by the administration of hormones (either orally or by injection) or by the removal of organs that produce hormones (ovaries, testicles, adrenal glands, or the pituitary gland). The goal is to reduce the body's production of, or to block the action of, hormones that promote the growth of certain types of tumors. Cancers of the prostate and breast, and occasionally kidney and ovarian cancer, have been controlled or significantly reduced by hormonal therapy. The mechanisms are still only partly understood, but the role of hormonal-receptor proteins is a key element.

Hormone receptors are special proteins on the surface of both normal and cancer cells that "lock on" to particular hormones manufactured by the body and transport them into the cell. The prevalence and types of hormonal receptors on the cancer cells removed in surgery are important in predicting whether a cancer will respond to hormonal therapy. Tests for hormone receptors are a part of the pathologist's examination of the surgically removed tissue. When a specific receptor is absent, it is considered "negative." Negative

receptors are associated with an increased risk of recurrence.

As an example, breast cancers are generally tested for both estrogen and progesterone receptors. A sufficient presence of one or both of these receptors indicates that these hormones stimulate the growth of the tumor cells. If a breast tumor is estrogen- and/or progesterone-negative, there is an increased risk of recurrence. When the tumor is receptor-positive, there is a higher likelihood that treatment with a hormone, such as Tamoxifen, Arimedex, Aromasin, or Femora, that counteracts the effects of those hormones will reduce the rate of recurrence.

Adjuvant Chemotherapy

Adjuvant chemotherapy is additional chemotherapy administered to patients who have a high risk of recurrence of their cancer. Adjuvant therapy reduces this risk and is administered after the primary treatment; the primary treatment could be surgery or radiation therapy. The goal of adjuvant chemotherapy is to eliminate undetectable microscopic cells that may have traveled to other parts of the body. Adjuvant therapy also reduces the risk of metastases. If this treatment does not lead to a cure, it usually will prolong the interval before a recurrence.

The most commonly used adjuvant chemotherapy program is for treating breast cancer, especially in the following four conditions:

- cancer cells have been found in the lymph nodes during surgery;
- the tumor is large, indicating a possibility of metastasis;
- aggressive, high grade pathology; or
- the tumor has negative hormone receptors (see "Hormonal Therapy" in this chapter) or a positive Her-2/neu breast cancer gene test.

Adjuvant therapy for breast cancer is usually administered for three to nine months.

Neoadjuvant Chemotherapy

Neoadjuvant chemotherapy refers to the use of drugs as the primary therapy before surgery or radiotherapy. Its goal is to reduce the size of a large tumor. With initially large tumors, such as large breast or head and neck cancers, surgery and radiotherapy can be more successful after the tumors have been shrunk by neoadjuvant chemotherapy treatments. The use of chemotherapy before other treatments also may help to reduce the incidence of metastatic disease.

Bone Marrow Transplantation

A bone marrow transplant is a supportive therapy that uses very high-dose chemotherapy as a means of curing cancer or delaying its growth in patients with metastatic disease. High-dose chemotherapy can be toxic enough to deplete the bone marrow (where white blood cells, red blood cells, and platelets are made). To help the bone marrow to recover, healthy bone marrow—from a relative or other person who is a blood (HLA) match (allogeneic donor), or from the patient's own previously donated bone marrow or peripheral venous blood (autologous stem cell donation)—is transplanted into the patient after the high-dose chemotherapy has been administered.

Additional support is needed with this procedure. This consists of regular blood and platelet transfusions, antibiotics for infections, and nutritional support. Recent results of high-dose therapy with bone marrow transplant have not significantly increased survival rates for high-risk breast cancer or metastatic breast cancer patients. More time is needed to determine whether the results signify a cure in a small number of cases or a delay in disease recurrence. Bone marrow transplantation is discussed in detail in Chapter 6, "Survivor's Guide to Bone Marrow Transplantation."

Administering and Monitoring Chemotherapy

If your doctor prescribes chemotherapy that needs to be given intravenously (IV), your oncology nurse will be the person to administer the medication. There are many things you can do to make the infusion experience easier. Communicating your fears, anxieties, and expectations with your nurse is very important. In order for your nurse to make this experience tolerable, he or she needs to know the following:

- Have you had any previous experience with receiving IVs?
- Do you have any needle phobias?
- Have you ever fainted or felt lightheaded during or after receiving an injection?
- Have you been told your veins "roll" or "collapse"?
- Do you have any particular injection sites you prefer?

Answers to all these questions will help the oncology nurse tailor your treatment.

If you are very anxious or are very fearful about receiving IVs, often times anxiety-reducing activities can help, such as:

- listening to soothing music
- closing your eyes
- holding a loved-one's hand
- smelling a pleasant fragrance, such as lavender or lemon oil
- looking at a colorful magazine
- reading an engrossing book
- listening to books-on-tape
- bringing a "comfort object" from home, such as a blanket or pillow

Some offices even provide televisions with VCRs. Ask your medical office what is available to you so you can take something that will be distracting to you.

Receiving Chemotherapy

Receiving intravenous chemotherapy should not be a painful experience. Having a needle inserted may provide initial discomfort, but this should subside after the needle is taped down. Some chemotherapy agents can be irritating as they are infused. Be sure to let your oncology nurse know if you have any discomfort. If it is not contraindicated, diluting the solution or slowing the infusion rate can help decrease discomfort. Patients often report a cold feeling radiating from the needle insertion site. This is simply the solution infusing into your veins. Solutions tend to be room temperature and subsequently feel cold as they infuse into your warmer body. This cold feeling usually subsides after a few minutes. If you find this bothersome, a warm towel wrapped around the site can bring relief.

Many chemotherapy agents are infused over a long period of time—an hour or more. Other chemotherapy agents are manually pushed into the vein using a syringe. There is a class of chemotherapy medications called "vesicants" that, if they leak outside of the vein, can cause burning of the surrounding tissues. Be sure to ask your nurse if you are receiving "vesicant" chemotherapy. If so, always immediately report any burning, stinging, redness, or swelling you may notice at the needle insertion site.

During the time it takes for you to receive your chemotherapy, you may have your vital signs (blood pressure, pulse, temperature) checked. This is just an assessment made by the nurse to be sure everything is stable. After your chemotherapy infusion is finished, the nurse removes the needle and places a bandage on the site. You will need to monitor the site for the next few days for any signs of inflammation or infection. Blood counts are done at specific intervals to observe the normal lowering of blood counts, to help judge future doses of chemotherapy, and to watch for low blood counts (see Chapter 8, "Side Effects of Chemotherapy").

Vascular Access Devices

There are ways to access the venous system other than putting a needle directly into a vein. Some patients have very small veins or have had chemotherapy in the past, making it very difficult to place a needle. Your oncology nurse or doctor may recommend a Venous Access Device (VAD). These devices come in many different forms. Some are external catheters that are placed in a major vein and then exit the body, usually in the upper chest area. This looks like a clear or white tube exiting the body. Blood can be drawn out of and infusions given directly into this tube. The tube remains in place for the duration of your therapy (the one to six weeks of chemotherapy, for example).

External catheters require daily maintenance, which is usually performed by the patient or caregiver. This includes daily dressing changes, cleaning of the skin around the catheter exit site and flushing heparin or sterile saline through the catheter. It also is a good idea to keep the site dry at all times. The site needs to be examined daily for redness, drainage, or swelling. Any of these findings must be reported immediately to your doctor.

Another type of VAD is placed under the skin. These are referred to as "medi-ports" or "portacaths." These are usually placed under the skin in the chest area and look like an inch-and-a-half bump under the skin. While a needle is required to access the device, it usually takes only one quick stick and is less uncomfortable than regular daily injections. Implanted devices must be flushed with sterile saline and heparin every four weeks when not in use. Your oncology nurse will do this.

VADs allow the patient with small or scarred veins to receive chemotherapy and other supportive infusions as well as to give blood samples with a minimum of discomfort. Like any foreign device placed in the body, VADs carry the risk of infection and blood clot formation. Your doctor and oncology nurse will discuss with you in detail the advantages and disadvantages should a VAD become a choice for you.

Hyperthermia

Hyperthermia, the use of heat in the treatment of cancer, has been practiced periodically for four thousand years. Since 1900, there has been mounting evidence that tumor cells can be killed by heating tumors to $108°F$ $(42–43°C)$ for a short time.

Hyperthermia works because cancer cells are more sensitive to heat than normal cells. Additionally, most tumors have poor circulation (blood supply), which means that they tend to retain heat and cannot eliminate it as well as normal cells.

The heat is often delivered by a radio frequency that can heat internally without damaging the skin. Local tumors and many metastatic tumors can be treated in this way. After treatment, the dead tumor cells (known as tumor necrosis) are replaced by scar tissue. The use of radiation therapy or chemotherapy concurrently with hyperthermia may enhance the anticancer therapeutic effect.

Although still considered experimental, hyperthermia may join surgery, radiation therapy, chemotherapy, and immunotherapy to become a fifth modality of cancer treatment. Further improvements in methods of application, combined with appropriate combinations of chemotherapy and/or radiation therapy, are needed.

Immunotherapy

John W. Park, M.D.
Christopher C. Benz, M.D.

The concept of immunotherapy is based on the body's natural defense system, which protects us against a variety of diseases. Although we are less aware of it, the immune system also works to aid

(Continued from page 36)

our recovery from many illnesses.

For many years, physicians believed that the immune system was effective only in combating infectious diseases caused by such invading agents as bacteria and viruses. More recently, we have learned that the immune system may play a central role in protecting the body against cancer and in combating cancer that has already developed. This latter role is not well understood, but there is evidence that in many cancer patients the immune system slows down the growth and spread of tumors. The body's ability to develop an immune reaction to tumors may help determine which patients are cured of cancer using conventional therapies, including surgery, radiation, and drugs.

One immediate goal of research in cancer immunology is the development of methods to harness and enhance the body's natural tendency to defend itself against malignant tumors. Immunotherapy represents a new and powerful weapon in the arsenal of anticancer treatments.

Immunotherapy seems to offer great promise as a new dimension in cancer treatment, but it is still very much in its infancy. Immunotherapies involving certain cytokines and antibodies have now become part of standard cancer treatment. Other examples of immunotherapy remain experimental. Although many clinical trials of new forms of immunotherapy are in progress, an enormous amount of research remains to be done before the findings can be widely applied.

Immunotherapy of cancer began about one hundred years ago when Dr. William Coley, at the Sloan-Kettering Institute, showed that he could control the growth of some cancers and cure a few advanced cancers with injections of a mixed vaccine of streptococcal and staphylococcal bacteria known as Coley's toxin. The tuberculosis vaccine, Bacillus Calmette-Guérin (BCG), developed in 1922, is known to stimulate the immune system and is now used to treat bladder cancers.

Many years of research have finally produced the first successful examples of immunotherapies for cancer. Sometimes referred to as biological response modifiers or as biological therapies, these new treatments—such as interferons and other cytokines, monoclonal antibodies, and vaccine therapies—have generated renewed interest and research activity in immunology.

Interferons and Other Cytokines

Interferons belong to a group of proteins known as cytokines. They are produced naturally by white blood cells in the body (or in the laboratory) in response to infection, inflammation, or stimulation. They have been used as a treatment for certain viral diseases, including hepatitis B.

Interferon-alpha was one of the first cytokines to show an antitumor effect, and it is able to slow tumor growth directly, as well as help to activate the immune system. Interferon-alpha has been approved by the FDA and is now commonly used for the treatment of a number of cancers, including multiple myeloma, chronic myelogenous leukemia, hairy cell leukemia, and malignant melanoma. Interferon-beta and interferon-gamma are other types of interferons that have been investigated.

Other cytokines with antitumor activity include the interleukins (e.g., IL-2) and tumor necrosis factor. IL-2 is frequently used to treat kidney cancer and melanoma.

Some of the problems with these cytokines, including many of the interferons and interleukins, are their side effects, which include malaise and flu-like syndromes. When given at a high dose, the side effects can be greatly magnified.

Monoclonal Antibodies

Another important biological therapy involves antibodies against cancer cells or cancer-associated targets. Monoclonal antibodies are artificial antibodies against a particular target (the "antigen") and are produced in the laboratory. The original method involved hybridoma cells (a fusion of two different types of cells) that acted as factories of antibody production. A major advance in this field was the ability to convert these antibodies, which originally were made from mouse hybridomas, to "humanized" antibodies that more closely resemble our natural

(Continued from page 37)

antibodies. Even newer techniques can be used to generate human antibodies from genetically engineered mice or bacteria containing human antibody genes. Monoclonal antibodies have been widely used in scientific studies of cancer, as well as in cancer diagnosis.

As therapy for cancer, monoclonal antibodies can be injected into patients to seek out the cancer cells, potentially leading to disruption of cancer cell activities or to enhancement of the immune response against the cancer. This strategy has been of great interest since the original invention of monoclonal antibodies in the 1970s. After many years of clinical testing, researchers have proven that improved monoclonal antibodies can be used effectively to help treat certain cancers. An antibody called rituximab (Rituxan) can be useful in the treatment of non-Hodgkin's lymphoma, while trastuzumab (Herceptin) is useful against certain breast cancers. Other new monoclonal antibodies are undergoing active testing.

Researchers also are studying ways of linking cytotoxic drugs, toxins, or radioisotopes to monoclonal antibodies to enhance their effectiveness against cancer cells. In this case, the antibodies would function as a targeted delivery mechanism; the result would be like a "guided missile," capable of seeking out a specific target—a cancer cell.

Cancer Vaccines

As described above, biological therapy or immunotherapy is now considered a fourth modality of cancer treatment, and examples such as interferon and monoclonal antibodies have become part of standard cancer treatment. Many types of immunotherapy, such as cancer vaccines, remain experimental. Experimental therapies in general are also discussed in the next section.

Vaccines have revolutionized public health by preventing the development of many important infectious diseases, including polio, small pox, and diphtheria. It has been much more difficult to develop effective vaccines to prevent cancer, or to treat patients who already have cancer. Attempts

to develop such cancer vaccines, despite many decades of experimental work, have yet to yield proven results. In spite of this, a notable increase in interest has been generated by recent advances in the areas of immunology and cancer biology, which have led to more sophisticated and promising vaccine strategies than those previously available. Cancer vaccines typically consist of a source of cancer-associated material (antigen), along with other components, to further stimulate the immune response against the antigen. The challenge has been to find better antigens, as well as to package the antigen in such a way as to enhance the patient's immune system to fight cancer cells that have the antigen.

Increasingly, cancer vaccines have been shown to be capable of improving the immune response against particular antigens. The result of this immunologic effect is not always sufficient to reverse the progression of cancer. However, cancer vaccines have been generally well tolerated, and they may provide useful anticancer effects in some situations. For example, in malignant lymphoma, a number of laboratory studies have indicated that vaccination using lymphoma-associated proteins called "idiotype" can stimulate the immune systems of mice sufficiently to help them resist the development of lymphomas.

In clinical trials, idiotype vaccines continue to be tested, and have been associated with indications of clinical benefit in some lymphoma patients. In malignant melanoma, a wide variety of vaccine strategies have been introduced into clinical trials, and some have been found to stimulate the immune response against the cancer.

Cancer vaccines continue to be evaluated in these diseases as well as most other cancer types. The many new strategies for vaccine construction and immune stimulation may lead to the emergence of clinically useful cancer vaccines. An example of one exciting new approach being tested in melanoma and other cancers is the use of dendritic cell vaccines. Dendritic cells help to "turn on" the immune response.

Experimental Cancer Therapies

Physicians and other scientists are constantly developing new and experimental therapeutic approaches to cancer. Unique combinations of the three standard anticancer therapies of surgery, radiation, and chemotherapy (known as multimodality therapy) and new forms of immunotherapy are examples of recent innovations.

Experimental approaches to cancer treatment undergo lengthy testing in the laboratory and in animals before being introduced into human medicine. But we cannot conclude that human reactions will be the same as those from animal experiments. There comes a moment of truth when an experimental treatment is accepted for trial with cancer patients (called a clinical trial). Patients participating in experimental treatments are always given a detailed explanation of the reasons why their doctors feel that an experimental treatment is justified in their cases. There is an unwritten law that an unproven experimental therapy is never used on any patient for whom there remains a tried and effective nonexperimental treatment. Experimental therapy is used only when there is a reasonable basis for believing that the outcome will be superior to that from conventional therapy.

Clinical Trials

Depending on the type and stage of your cancer, your doctor might recommend a new treatment that has not yet been proved effective. The word *investigational* might come up. *Experimental* is a term that might also be used. If the standard treatment options available to you are not likely to be effective, your doctor might suggest that you take part in a clinical trial.

All these terms might make you feel more than a little anxious. They shouldn't. Investigational treatments that are being given a clinical trial are used only under very stringent conditions. These clinical trials wouldn't be used at all if there weren't some hope they would be more effective than more conventional treatments.

What a Clinical Trial Is

Advances in cancer treatment usually come about because of some clever idea or concept for a new therapy proposed by a cancer research physician. After a new anticancer drug has been found to be effective against one or more experimental tumor systems in the lab, it is tested in rats or other small animals to find out what dosage might be both effective and reasonably safe for humans. The treatment is eventually tested in a large number of patients (clinical trial) to find out two things: Is it effective? And, is it as good as or better than conventional treatments? The treatment's safety is also investigated through testing for adverse effects.

It takes several hundred and sometimes several thousand patients to prove quickly and reliably whether a new treatment will work and is worthwhile. It is almost impossible to conduct a trial in any single hospital or cancer center. The concept of cooperative clinical trials, involving multiple clinical settings and doctors, was developed for just this reason. The rules and procedures for clinical trials are standardized and quite specific.

The Clinical Protocol

A clinical trial consists of an exact written description of a treatment program that is called the clinical protocol. This is formulated and written with great care. Not only do the researchers need to be sure that the trial will answer the two main questions about effectiveness, but they also must safeguard the rights of the patients being treated. The risks involved must be minimized and disclosed to all participants. The clinical protocol (plan) outlines the criteria for patients who might participate in the trial. It also describes what tests will be done and how the researchers will determine whether a tumor is responding. Systems for monitoring the patient and checking for any adverse effects will be detailed. Also, there will be provisions for "informed consent" and for the patient's right to drop out of the trial at any time.

Who Approves the Trial?

A committee made up of physicians and nonphysicians who are unconnected with the study must approve the clinical trial. The members of this committee certify that the patients' rights are protected, that the trial is reasonable and logical, and that the study will answer the questions it is designed to answer. The same committee reviews the ongoing progress of the trial and its results. The Cancer Therapy Branch of the National Cancer Institute also keeps watch on these investigational studies.

The Importance of Clinical Trials

Almost every advance in cancer treatment over the past twenty years has come about because of clinical trials. In fact, just about every chemotherapy drug and radiation treatment now considered standard therapy was first given in a clinical Phase I trial. These treatments were given to patients who were willing to be in the forefront of advances in medical knowledge.

For example, the willingness of thousands of women to participate in clinical trials by the National Surgical Adjuvant Breast Project (NSABP) has resulted in answers to extremely important treatment questions. These trials have formed the basis for adjuvant chemotherapy in breast cancer patients with a high risk for recurrence even though no apparent tumor is left after surgery. This treatment has saved many lives.

The Three Phases of Clinical Trials

Whether for surgery, chemotherapy, radiotherapy, or biological therapy, clinical trials are always conducted in three phases.

Phase I. About twenty human patients are treated with the same drug. There is no assurance or certainty that a significant tumor response will occur, although, again, every single anticancer drug now useful in therapy was initially a Phase I agent. During this phase, various dosage levels are tried.

Patients selected for these trials are almost always in cancer research centers and have already received all known effective anticancer therapy. After the proposed treatment is explained to them, they must volunteer to receive the new treatment. There is, therefore, no moral objection to giving this new treatment. Since there is "nothing to lose," it is hoped that a specific new agent and/or dosage may prove effective.

This phase is completed when no unusual problems or toxic effects have been found and the dose necessary to produce a biologic effect has been determined. The study can then move to the next phase.

Phase II. In this phase, ten to twenty patients are treated, each having one of the various types of tumors known to be responsive to chemotherapy. These might include lymphomas, breast cancer, or colon cancer. Because these tumor types are known to be responsive, the patients will be those who have already received all standard forms of chemotherapy that seem reasonable; therefore, participation in a Phase II trial

does not deprive anyone of any therapy already proven to be effective. If a significant number of patients with each type of tumor respond to the therapy, the trial moves to the next phase.

Phase III. In this phase, the number of participants is increased greatly, and the new drug therapy is compared with standard treatment to see if there is an improvement in the response or if the same response rate is achieved but with fewer toxic side effects. Usually, there is a control group that receives the chemotherapy already proven to be effective.

A therapy tested in a drug-related clinical trial does not necessarily involve a drug not already in clinical use. A new treatment or therapy often consists of standard drugs used in a new combination or a new sequence, in new dosages, or even administered in a new way. If a new drug is involved, and the Phase III trial is successful, the National Cancer Institute will approve the drug for general use. Eventually, the new therapy might become the standard treatment.

Clinical Trials and the "Approved" Uses of Drugs

When using anticancer chemicals, it is important for both you and your doctor to be aware of how the pharmaceutical industry works. Once drug companies have fulfilled the lengthy and complex testing and the drawn-out legal procedures required to market a new drug, they tend not to devote a lot of effort to discovering new uses for that drug. They more or less delegate this responsibility to the cancer physicians conducting clinical trials.

Every drug comes with an official "package insert" detailing what dosage to use for what illness. This information is also listed in the *Physician's Desk Reference*. These summaries usually contain only the information "passed" by the government's approval agencies. Why this is important is that many drug programs in standard use for cancer are not listed as "approved." Such drugs are used because experience with patients has shown them to be effective. About half of the current uses of anticancer drugs in the United States and Canada are for indications and schedules that are not given in the official inserts.

Because the inserts do not necessarily reflect the most up-to-date cancer research, the current standard use of these drugs, or even their optimum use, your doctor should not be restricted to the usage on the printed drug-listing materials. In fact, the appropriate use of anticancer drugs may be for indications not listed in such official sources.

This is another reason why an oncologist can be a useful member of your health care team. Cancer physicians are up-to-date on the most recent research findings and important advances in treatment even though that information may not appear in the drug-related literature.

Unproven Treatments

Living with cancer creates a state of uncertainty, insecurity, and fear that at times is unendurable. It is understandable that anxiety can reach so high a level that a person is willing to try an unproven method of treatment that has been publicized in the press as a "miracle cure." Among those who resort to these therapies are people who are receiving good medical support as well as those who are not. Neither a high level of education nor the ability to reason will deter the desperate patient.

A person who has cancer wants a cure. When standard therapy cannot guarantee a cure, that person may go to any length to obtain a treatment that has not been sanctioned by any reputable doctor, researcher, or government agency. No one wants to die without exhausting every possible means of a cure, and a patient is often encouraged by well-meaning friends and family members who have no knowledge of proper and proven cancer treatment.

Depression and panic can make a patient prey to any speculator who claims to have a cure for cancer. So can being told that there is no further conventional therapy that offers a reasonable chance of improving one's health.

Some quack practitioners may sincerely believe their methods are effective; others are just capitalizing on other people's misfortunes. In any event, false cancer cures cost American patients more than $3 billion a year. Furthermore, some quack cures can be extremely dangerous or may lead to death.

The clinical course of cancer is highly variable. A remission or a cure can occur without a patient's having received conventional medical treatment, although this is very rare. (Medical literature documents these cases.) However, if this happy event should coincide with or follow treatment by an unproven therapy, the patient will invariably credit that treatment with the improvement.

Whenever newspaper and magazine articles on "miracle cures" appear, physicians are bombarded with questions about these unorthodox methods of treatment. "What about diet?" "What about megavitamin therapy?" "What about that new drug that is only available abroad?" Physicians can only reply that in their experience and the experience of other practitioners, these methods have not proved to be of any benefit to cancer patients.

Unfortunately, the press and the public have given enormous attention to the rare successes of unproven treatments, without mentioning the thousands of failures of these unproven treatments reported by physicians in medical journals. Those tragic cases of failure are due not only to worthless therapies, but often to the general poor medical management that accompanies these treatments.

Some patients supplement conventional treatment with megadoses of vitamins, Laetrile (a drug derived from apricot pits), macrobiotic diets, herb supplements, coffee enemas, and other unorthodox methods. Although most doctors neither approve nor condone the use of these methods, they do not reject such patients for medical therapy, and, if required, some will provide them with medical literature on the useless treatment. A physician can tell them about cases of poisoning and even of death from taking Laetrile, but should not try to argue with them. It is their choice, and a physician should accept the compromise as long as they also take conventional medical therapy (see Chapter 12, "Alternative and Complementary Medicine.")

Over decades of practice, we have yet to see a single positive result from unorthodox treatment, but we have seen hundreds of patients with progressive advancing cancers who first tried a quack therapy. Sometimes, we were able to reverse the process after beginning traditional therapy, but many of these patients lost their chance for a cure by initially opting for a quack therapy.

The Federal Pure Food, Drug, and Cosmetic Act stipulates that a producer of a new drug (or treatment method) must prove not only that it is safe but also effective if it is to be licensed for public use. The act also provides for strict controls over investigational and experimental drugs and the sale of prescription drugs.

Unless a drug is approved by the FDA, it cannot legally be distributed through interstate commerce. It is a federal crime, reinforced by our postal laws, to advertise or ship such products. Many states prohibit the distribution and sale of unlicensed drugs and methods within the state, but until more states reinforce the federal legislation, unproved treatments will continue to be promoted and sold.

In the states that have not passed their own laws, ways have been found to circumvent the federal ban against false claims in advertising. The FDA has published booklets, such as "The Big Quack Attack: Medical Devices," that describe various methods of quackery and tell consumers how to register complaints about practitioners of these methods.

The Office of Alternative Medicine was established in 1992 as a part of the National Institute of Health. Its mission is to evaluate the merits of complementary and alternative methods to cure or relieve symptoms of cancer and other illness. This is an important step in the effort to clarify the role of complementary and alternative treatments for cancer (see Chapter 12).

Considering the fear, insecurity, frustration, and ignorance of the average patient or family, the readiness to believe in promised cures is understandable. The best way to fight quackery is by providing knowledge, understanding, and communication.

6

Survivor's Guide to Bone Marrow Transplantation

Keren Stronach, M. Ph.

Michael C. Dohan, M.D.

A bone marrow transplant is similar to a blood transfusion. In a bone marrow transplant, high dose chemotherapy and, in some cases, radiation, is used to destroy cancerous or diseased cells in the body. In accomplishing this goal, the treatment also destroys a person's bone marrow, the site where blood cells are produced. In order to restore the ability to make blood cells, a person must be given healthy marrow to replace the marrow that was destroyed.

The bone marrow transplant procedure was originally developed in the late 1960s to treat cancers and diseases of the bone marrow. The idea was to destroy the diseased bone marrow with chemotherapy and radiation and then to replace it with a donor's healthy marrow. Since then, the procedure has been refined and expanded to treat many other conditions, including cancers and diseases that do not involve the bone marrow. In the last few years, for example, bone marrow transplants have sometimes been used to treat ovarian and testicular cancer. In these cases, when the bone marrow is healthy, a person does not need to receive marrow from a donor. Instead, the patient's own marrow is harvested before the chemotherapy or radiation and that marrow is later used for the transplant procedure. The type of transplant a patient has depends on whether the patient's bone marrow or that of a donor is used. Before undergoing transplantation, it is also important to look into some of the new and promising treatments that are under investigation.

One new development, which at the time of this writing is reserved only for the elderly and those who are not eligible for transplantation, involves administering only very low dose radiation to the patient before transplant. Patients undergoing this type of transplant have far fewer side effects and do not experience the typical hair loss, mouth sores, and other symptoms that are characteristic of conventional transplants. This new procedure is called a nonmyeloablative stem-cell transplant; it also is referred to as a mini-transplant. If further study proves promising, this type of mini-transplant may become more widely available. In some cases, progress is also being made in the treatment of specific diseases that do not involve bone marrow transplantation. For example, the drug STI 571, which at this time is in clinical trials, shows promise in inducing remissions in people with chronic myelogenous leukemia. If it proves to be an effective alternative, some people may be able to avoid the transplant altogether.

Autologous Transplant

In an autologous transplant, a person has his or her own healthy bone marrow cells removed and stored until the time of the transplant. Chemotherapy and, in some cases, radiation is then administered to destroy any remaining diseased cells in the body. This treatment also destroys the bone marrow. The marrow cells that were removed and stored before the treatment are returned to the patient at the time of the transplant to replace the bone marrow that was destroyed.

Usually, autologous transplants are done when the bone marrow is healthy and the disease lies elsewhere in the body. In some instances, however, autologous transplants are done even when the bone marrow is diseased. When this is the case, the bone marrow that is removed may be treated, or purged, to clear out cancer cells. Currently bone marrow transplant (BMT) centers across the country use different methods to purge marrow. It will be up to you and your physician to decide how your marrow will be treated if it needs to be purged.

Allogeneic Transplant

When a person cannot be his or her own donor and the marrow needs to be taken from someone else, the transplant is called an *allogeneic transplant*. If the donor is a relative, the transplant is called a related allogeneic transplant. If it is from an unrelated donor, it is referred to as an unrelated allogeneic transplant. To find a donor, you will need to have your blood tested and typed so that it can be compared and matched to blood samples of potential donors. This is done through a test called the human leukocyte antigen (HLA) test that examines certain antigens or proteins on the surface of your white blood cells. These antigens serve as a kind of "fingerprint" and play an important role in the body's ability to distinguish between "self" and "other." Three pairs of antigens, known as HLA-A, HLA-B, and HLA-DR, are considered most important in determining the degree of fit between you and your donor. If you match your donor on these important sites, there is a good chance that

your new marrow will recognize you as "self" and will function effectively in your body. If you do not match your donor on these sites, the donor's marrow may recognize certain organs or tissues in your body as foreign and may attack them. This is called *graft versus host disease* (GVHD). The more closely matched you are to your donor, the less likely you are to get GVHD.

Syngeneic Transplant

In a syngeneic transplant, the donor is an identical twin and the new marrow will be genetically identical to the bone marrow that will be destroyed by the chemotherapy and/or radiation.

Hospitalization

The length of time you will spend in the hospital will depend in part on the type of transplant that you have and the hospital where you are receiving your care. Today, many autologous and some allogeneic transplants are done on an outpatient basis. In some cases, however, autologous transplants may require a two- or three-week hospital stay and allogeneic transplants may require a hospital stay of three to five weeks—or longer, depending on your condition and the specific procedures followed at your transplant center.

What Is Bone Marrow?

Bone marrow is the spongy center of your bones where blood is produced. It is also the home of your immune system. Bone marrow contains the parent cells, called *stem cells*, that later mature into white blood cells (infection fighting cells), red blood cells (oxygen carrying cells), and platelets (which aid in blood clotting). The numbers of your blood cells will be closely monitored throughout the transplant process. As your transplanted marrow begins to produce blood cells, your blood counts will begin to rise, and you will begin to regain your immunity, strength, and energy.

White blood cells, or *leukocytes*, are cells that fight infection; they comprise an important part of your immune system. When your white blood cell count is low, you are at greatest risk for infection. During the transplant, your white blood cell count will be carefully monitored. *Neutrophils* are a common type of white blood cells that play an important role in fighting infection by bacteria and yeast. During the transplant, your medical team will be closely monitoring your neutrophil count, which is also referred to as your ANC (Absolute Neutrophil Count).

Red blood cells, or *erythrocytes*, are cells that carry oxygen from the lungs to the rest of the body. The oxygen is carried in the red blood cell on a molecule called hemoglobin. During the transplant, your hemoglobin levels will be monitored to determine when you will need a red blood cell transfusion.

Platelets are essential in the process of clotting, thus preventing excess bleeding and bruising. When your platelet count is low, your risk of bleeding is high. Your platelets will therefore also be monitored to assess your risk of bleeding and to determine when a platelet transfusion is needed.

Stem cells in the bone marrow produce blood cells. Stem cells are destroyed by the chemotherapy and/or radiation treatment. In order for you to produce blood cells after chemotherapy or radiation treatment, stem cells—taken either from you or your donor—will be given to you during a transplant.

Methods of Stem Cell Collection

Stem cells, which are produced in the bone marrow, can be collected by a variety of methods. Traditionally, stem cells were collected from a large bone, such as the hipbone. In this procedure, known as a bone marrow harvest, a needle is inserted into a large bone and stem cells are removed directly from the bone. In the last few years, peripheral stem cell transplants have become more common. In this case, the patient or donor donates stem cells that are collected from the circulated blood stream instead of from the bone. In some cases, stem cells are collected from the placenta and the umbilical cord of a newborn baby. This is known as an umbilical cord blood transplant. Interestingly, this type of cord blood transplant poses a lower risk of graft-versus-host disease (GVHD) than when stem cells are collected from the bone or the peripheral blood.

Preparing for the Transplant

Once the very difficult decision to undergo a transplant has been made, there are several important steps that can be taken to prepare for the experience. On an emotional level, preparing for a transplant may entail spending time with friends and family. Or you may take time to be alone and to be in touch with your feelings regarding the transplant. On a physical level, prepara-tion may include eating a healthful diet, getting good dental care, and maintaining an exercise routine. On a practical level, it may mean choosing a transplant center, organizing caregiving arrangements, and obtaining items for the hospital stay.

Emotional Preparation

Facing the prospect of a transplant can be devastat-ing—evoking feelings of dread, panic, and helpless-ness. Coming to grips with the idea that you may have a life-threatening disease while simultaneously dealing with a tremendous volume of information and new medical jargon can be mind numbing. As you face the transplant and the most serious questions of life, it is common to feel overwhelmed by emotions. During this time, you are likely to experience feelings of anxi-ety, self pity, and self-blame. These feelings are a nor-mal part of the process. It is also normal to feel betrayed by your body, and feel anger and jealousy towards others who do not have to face the same ordeals that you face. At times, you may find that your feelings undergo intense fluctuations, alternating between hope, anticipation, and fear.

Another reaction you may have is that of denial. You may find yourself responding to the situation by becoming emotionally numb and very task oriented. As you go through various emotional responses, be understanding and gentle with yourself. You are facing some of the most difficult choices and most stressful conditions you will ever face, and therefore must not inflict extra stress upon yourself.

The transplant also may be seen as a new lease on life, and as such, a source of great solace and hope, as well as a great challenge to be overcome. Radical swings in emotions and moods, as well as periods of relative calm, are all part of the common ways of react-ing to the transplant.

How you choose to cope with the prospective trans-plant depends on how you perceive it, and on your feel-ings, personality, and own individual way of coping. Your three choices of coping are to (1) take a highly active stance in the process and actively research all medical and alternative options, (2) hand over control to others, or (3) do some combination of the two. Your mind will lead you to the plan of action that will work best for you.

In the following sections, you will find suggestions and strategies that others have found useful. Hopefully, you will find some suggestions that will be of benefit to you.

Express Your Emotions

If you are experiencing great anxiety or fear, give yourself permission to express these emotions so that you can process them. Choose to express your emotions to the people who are meaningful to you and who can be supportive. If certain people are unhelpful, don't feel guilty about avoiding them and focusing on your own needs. Seeing a professional therapist, particularly one who has had experience in counseling people with life-threatening diseases, can be very helpful in helping you deal with your emotions.

Contact a BMT Survivor

Contacting someone who has undergone a transplant can be very helpful and calming. This can be done through the National Bone Marrow Transplant Link, where you can leave a message requesting to speak to a BMT survivor who has been in a situation similar to your own. A peer volunteer who has undergone a transplant will usually return your call within the next few days and discuss their experience with you. Another possibility is to ask a member of your medical team or your social worker to put you in touch with someone who has undergone a transplant. If you have a computer and a modem, an effective way to get in touch with many transplant survivors is by signing on to a computer mailing list that specializes in bone marrow transplants or certain kinds of cancer.

Explore Books and Tapes

Books describing the experiences of others with cancer can be particularly helpful, as can many of the "self-help" books about coping and relaxation. Some survivors find that certain self-help books make them feel responsible for causing their diseases. In reading these books, remember that you are not in any way to blame for your condition. Cancer is caused by complex reasons having to do with the environment and genetic, social, and individual factors. Cancer can strike anyone. If a book you are reading makes you feel upset, put it down. You are not obligated to read a book just because a well-meaning friend has recommended it to you. You may even consider asking a friend to read and summarize the main points of a book or article for you.

Reduce Stress

During this stressful time, it might be helpful to think of ways that you can reduce superfluous stress in your life. Although you may not be able to avoid some of the factors that are producing stress, such as your diagnosis of cancer, there may be ways to cope with your stress. Establishing a clear set of priorities and letting go of less important obligations can reduce the amount of pressure that you feel. Some people find it useful to make a list of the factors contributing to stress and examine ways to reduce the pressures. One suggestion is to allocate tasks to family and friends who want to help. Some friends may be willing, for example, to help you gather information about different transplant centers or to help you find books and tapes about visualization or some other topic of interest.

Often, people around you will not know how to help and will be grateful to you for providing them with concrete suggestions. Many of those who feel close to you are likely to feel helpless in the face of your diagnosis and impending transplant. By giving them concrete suggestions of things they can do, you may not only be helping yourself, but helping them as well. For some people, continuing with their normal routine is the most effective way of reducing stress.

Practice Relaxation Techniques

Practicing stress reduction techniques that feel nurturing; muscle relaxation, meditation, hypnosis, or imagery may be helpful to you. Some people find that these techniques reduce their level of anxiety and are helpful in combating depression, as well as in lowering their level of discomfort and pain.

Get in Touch with Your Spirituality

Spirituality can also be an important source of comfort during this period. Many patients report that prayer and/or meditation can be a source of support and psychological well-being.

Participate in Activities You Enjoy

Reducing stress can also be done by incorporating activities that you find relaxing, healing, and fun. Finding creative outlets for one's feelings or creative ways to feed feelings of hope also can be an effective way of coping with emotions and reducing stress. Some people find that it is helpful to write in a journal, or to express themselves through painting or dance.

Take Care of Loose Ends

Taking care of loose ends and putting one's affairs in order does not necessarily signify an anticipated negative outcome. Sometimes, by dealing with difficult issues that may come up in the event of one's death, it is possible to put these issues aside and focus on more positive things. Some people have found that they need to put their financial affairs in order and take care of lingering interpersonal issues before fully focusing on the issues of treatment and recovery. This also may be a time to cancel student loans or to arrange for Social Security Disability so as to reduce financial pressures after the transplant. At this time, you also may wish to keep a notebook handy to record important information and phone numbers, particularly since, during times of upheaval, it may be more difficult to keep everything in mind.

Don't Take People's Reactions Personally

People who are close to you may be undergoing a lot of emotional turmoil themselves as a result of your diagnosis. They may feel helpless and panicked and may not know how to reach out and communicate. You may feel abandoned at times or feel very angry with loved ones for not comprehending your needs. These emotions are understandable and normal. However, it may be useful to remember that everyone involved may need some extra understanding and compassion during this difficult period. In some cases, friends or family members may withdraw, not because they don't care, but because they are too overwhelmed by their own feelings of fear, helplessness, and uncertainty as to how to treat you. If you do get some unexpected reactions from loved ones, remember that their reactions probably have a lot to do with their own internal turmoil.

Seek Medical Information

Seeking medical information can sometimes reduce fear and help people regain a sense of control. This can be done through library research, by talking to doctors and former transplant patients, by visiting transplant centers, and by calling different cancer organizations that have knowledgeable people who can respond to your questions and concerns.

In seeking out information, remember that it is always appropriate to seek a second or even third opinion. When, where, and how your bone marrow transplant is done may prove to be the most important decision of your life, and you should seek a number of medical opinions.

When consulting a physician, don't hesitate to ask for information a second or third time. Having a close friend or family member attend doctor's meetings with you can be useful, as it will allow you to review the information with someone else and to confirm that you understood the information correctly. Making a tape recording of the medical meetings also can be helpful to you.

Take Time for Yourself

Often, in times of stress, people become forgetful or experience mood swings. In this difficult period, take time to extend understanding and compassion to yourself. Give yourself permission to change your mind, to take things one day at a time, to pamper yourself, and to be sad. By taking the time to reevaluate and to make changes in your life, you may find that some of the best parts of your life may be expanding during the time when you are facing the worst trauma of your life. Allow yourself to think deeply about who you are and what matters to you so that you can prioritize your life and expand those areas that are most meaningful to you. Try as much as possible not to give up hope. As Michael Lerner wrote in *Choices in Healing*, "Give yourself permission to hope, even in the face of all the statistics that physicians may present to you. Statistics are only statistics. They are not you. There is no such thing as false hope." This does not mean that you need to be positive all the time. You are still entitled to "bad" days.

Physical Preparation

Exercise

Many people undertake some kind of regular exercise routine to improve their physical conditioning in preparation for the transplant. The extent and the rigor of the exercise you choose will depend in part on your normal activity level and physical condition at the time of diagnosis. Some people will be able to exercise vigorously whereas others may take on very moderate exercise routines involving just short walks or stretches in bed. Ideally, you should find some kind of exercise you enjoy. Joining a gym or finding friends who enjoy similar physical activities may be helpful. In addition to conferring physical benefits, exercise may be a helpful way to channel stress and promote general well-being.

If your medical condition does not allow you to undertake a rigorous exercise routine, be aware that many people enter the transplant in poor physical shape and do extremely well. To the extent that exercise is an option for you, consider doing some mode of exercise suited to your medical condition.

Nutrition

Eating a healthy diet and meeting your basic nutritional needs is important prior to transplant. Intuitively, we all know that a well-nourished body fights infection, aids healing, and deals with the demands of very aggressive treatment protocols better than a poorly nourished one does. It is beyond the scope of this chapter to discuss in detail the different alternative nutritional therapies. If you are considering an alternative diet, do some research to ensure that it provides all the necessary nutrients. Unless you are severely obese, it is not advisable to undergo rapid weight loss immediately prior to cancer therapy.

Generally, the guidelines for maintaining good health, as recommended by the National Academy of Sciences and the American Cancer Society, are as follows:

- Reduce dietary fats to less than 30 percent of total caloric intake.
- Eat plenty of fresh fruits and vegetables daily, particularly citrus fruits, green leafy vegetables, and carotene-rich vegetables such as carrots and squash.
- Increase intake of certain fibers such as wheat bran.
- Consume alcohol in moderation, if at all, and completely refrain from smoking.
- Maintain your weight within normal range.
- Minimize your consumption of salt-cured, pickled, and smoked foods.
- Cut out your consumption of red meat—protein alternatives include seafood, skinless poultry, legumes, tofu, and low-fat dairy products.

Dental Care

Good dental care prior to transplant is an essential part of your overall preparation for transplant. Healthy gums and teeth can eliminate potential infections and some of the painful mouth sores that may develop during transplant recovery. Meticulous mouth care prior to and during transplant can also confer protection against infections by limiting the number of open sores in the mouth. Taking care of lingering gum and tooth problems is important. It is strongly advised that you refrain from any routine dental care for some time after your transplant, until your immune system is strong and fully functional again.

To have your mouth in the best shape possible before the transplant, you will need to adopt good personal oral hygiene. This may entail regular flossing and brushing, as well as utilizing antiseptic mouth rinses. Before taking on a rigorous dental regimen of your own, however, it is a good idea to consult your dentist, to review the correct way to floss and brush your teeth, and to request a recommendation for a good toothbrush and mouth rinse.

Fertility

People undergoing treatment with total body irradiation and some forms of chemotherapy have a high risk of becoming infertile. If you are considering having children after the transplant, you may consider undergoing fertility treatment prior to the transplant. For males, sperm banking is a possibility. This entails contacting a sperm bank in your area and freezing and storing sperm for use after the transplant. For women, unfortunately, the situation is more complicated as they cannot simply freeze their eggs. Women, however, can freeze their fertilized eggs. In this process, women undergo hormonal treatment to induce ovulation. Once the eggs mature, they are surgically removed, fertilized with donor sperm (partner's or other chosen donor) in a test tube, and then frozen for later implantation. Because the procedure is time consuming, it should be undertaken well before the transplant date. Before undertaking this procedure, women should make sure that their medical condition allows for the procedures involved.

Another new and still experimental option for women is to freeze one of their ovaries or a portion of it prior to transplant and to have it reimplanted post-transplant. The advantage to this procedure is that women who do this may be able to regain ovarian function post-transplant and thus avoid the risks associated with early menopause. Another advantage to this procedure is that there is no need for fertilization of the eggs and the procedure is cheaper than embryo storage. There is also a small possibility that women undergoing this procedure may regain their fertility. At the time of this writing, only a handful of women have had their ovaries stored, and none have had them reimplanted. In animal studies, mice and sheep that had their ovaries reimplanted regained not only ovarian function but also, in some rare cases, fertility—giving birth to healthy offspring. For more information about fertility clinics, please see Part VI, "Resources" for information about fertility treatment.

Practical Preparations
Choosing a Center

There are distinct advantages to having the transplant at a large, experienced center with an excellent track record. If you have such a center close to home, the choice of where to do the transplant will be easy. If, however, this is not the case and there is no center near your home, or it has a poor track record or has performed fewer than five transplants of the kind you need, the choice may be more difficult.

Undergoing a transplant at a large BMT center with a good track record and a great deal of experience provides you with a sense of security that the physicians and staff will be able to handle unexpected complications, should they arise. Bigger centers may, in some cases, also have the advantage of having access to large blood banks that can cater to the needs of transplant patients. Large blood banks, for example, are more likely to set aside CMV-negative blood products. This may be important as CMV-negative blood products reduce the risk of CMV infection. However, large research centers may have the disadvantage of being more impersonal than small centers.

Having the transplant in a BMT center near your home allows you to be close to family and friends and, therefore, to have a strong support system on hand. You will also save on travel expenses and will not have to deal with the hassle of moving to an unfamiliar place. Your life and the life of your caregiver will be less disrupted, and you may have the advantage of already being familiar with some of the doctors and staff.

Calling the National Marrow Donor Program (800-526-7809) to get a listing of BMT centers is an excellent way to get initial information about different BMT centers. The NMDP guide contains phone numbers and addresses of most transplant centers, information

about the number and type of transplants performed at each center, and some statistics about the survival rates of individual centers.

In looking at these statistics, you should be aware that the general statistics often include all categories of age groups and illnesses and, thus, may be inapplicable to you. In order to compare survival rates of different BMT units, you need to ask directly about the survival rate for your age group, your illness, and the type of transplant you will undergo. Getting this information may be a difficult and frustrating process, as some centers are reluctant to disclose this information. Because gathering this information can be stressful, you may consider recruiting friends or your doctor to help you with this task.

Signing on to bone marrow transplant information bulletin boards or newsgroups on the Internet can be another useful way to get information. Many transplant survivors read these boards daily, answer questions, and share information about their experiences. To find out how to contact these groups, please see the section on BMT in Part VI, "Resources."

Calling up different centers to ask questions can provide useful information and give you a better sense of the transplant center and its atmosphere. Questions you may wish to ask include the following:

1. How many transplants has the center done for people with my specific condition? (Ideally, you should undergo a transplant at a center that has done at least five transplants of the type that you need).
2. Will I have the same staff treating me throughout the transplant? (Many BMT centers have the doctors and the physicians' assistants rotate on a monthly basis.)
3. Will the transplant be done on an outpatient basis, and, if so, what kind of support and information will be provided on caregiving in the home?
4. Will I be allowed to walk in the halls or will I be confined to my room? (Some centers allow patients to walk around the unit, whereas others do not.)
5. Will I have access to exercise machines or a physical therapist?
6. Will I have access to a social worker or counselor during the transplant?
7. Can the hospital accommodate my dietary needs? Can I ask for food at any time of the day

or do I have to order it a day in advance? Am I allowed to eat raw fruits and vegetables? (Having a flexible eating schedule can be helpful as you may be nauseated and may not want to eat during conventional mealtimes).

8. How many years experience does the average nurse have in the BMT unit?

9. How experienced are the physicians at the center and are there specialists available to handle complications should they arise?

10. Is there a support group for patients and/or their families?

11. What is the survival rate for patients with my condition in my age group undergoing my type of transplant?

12. How does the staff feel about patients putting up "Do Not Disturb" or "Please Knock" signs on the door?

13. Could someone who has undergone a transplant at the center contact me to tell me about his or her experience?

14. What is the visitor policy? How flexible is it? (Having your caregiver stay at the hospital with you overnight can be very comforting and make your stay easier to handle.)

15. What living arrangements can be made for me and my family if I need to move away from my home to the transplant center? What are the average living expenses for the areas around the transplant center?

16. Can the center provide any assistance to defray some of the family's expenses?

17. Does the center have a long-term follow-up department that is easily accessible and will respond to questions once I leave the transplant center? (This is particularly important if your oncologist in your area of residence has very little experience with BMTs.)

18. People undergoing a transplant from an unrelated donor should also inquire whether the center has a donor search coordinator and a quality tissue-typing facility.

Visiting the transplant center before the transplant to familiarize yourself with the transplant setting and some of the staff is often comforting. While you are there, you might inquire if you can speak to patients undergoing transplants at the center to get their impressions, feedback, and tips.

If you need to travel to your transplant center, you may save money by contacting companies that provide discounts for medically necessary travel. Most of the major national cancer organizations will have information about these companies. Often, airlines will provide discounted fares for patients and their caregivers on their way to treatments. Other organizations, such as the Leukemia and Lymphoma Society and Cancer Care, may reimburse you for travel expenses to and from medical centers.

Caregiving Arrangements

During the transplant, you will need at least one family member or friend who can provide you with emotional and physical support. This person is often referred to as a caregiver. In many cases, it will only be possible for you to have one caregiver with you. If this is the case, you may consider arranging occasional visits by other family members or friends who can provide additional support during weekends, so that the caregiving task does not fall on just one person.

Even though many people successfully make it through the transplant with only one caregiver or, in some cases, alone, having two or more caregivers is a real plus. When there are two or more caregivers, each one can have time to rest and can return to their caregiving activities more refreshed. Having more than one caregiver is also helpful as it allows you to share your feelings and experiences with more than one person. Because caregivers often experience a high degree of anxiety, sharing the responsibility of caring for you can serve to alleviate some of the tension. Finally, having more than one caregiver provides a safeguard in the event that a caregiver gets sick and is unable to be on the ward.

If you are planning to undergo the transplant at home or only expect to be in the hospital for a brief period, it will be helpful to arrange for someone to care for your pet for the first one hundred days after your transplant. During that time, your immune system is compromised and you should not be exposed to bacteria from indoor animals, or the uncertain weather you face when caring for outdoor animals. It also is important to make sure that there will be someone to help with housecleaning at regular intervals after the transplant until you can resume such activities. Getting family and friends to help or having paid help can make this period easier for you.

What to Take to the Hospital or Have at Home

Whether you are having the transplant in the hospital or not, it is important to have items around you that help bring your spirits up or that you might find helpful when you have less energy than usual. The following list of items was compiled by patients:

- Answering machine—Having an answering machine is extremely useful as it allows you to screen calls while resting. It also enables you to leave a daily message with an update of your condition for concerned friends and relatives who call.
- An extra phone for caregivers and guests—During the time that your blood cell counts are low and you are vulnerable to infection, it is advisable to use your own phone and have guests use a separate one. In this way you are secure in the knowledge that the phone you are using is always sterile and clean.
- Address book and telephone numbers.
- Favorite pictures and photographs to make the room feel comfortable and familiar.
- Comfortable shirts and sweat pants—It is good to get materials that can be easily washed and put in the dryer. Also make sure to bring some warm overshirts that open down the front as it is fairly common to feel cold during the period of immunosuppression, even when the environment is warm. Front-closure shirts will provide easy access to your central line or VAD, a small flexible tube in your chest that will be used to administer blood products and medications and to check your vital signs.
- Front buttoning pajamas, rather than nightgowns, as they allow you more modesty and provide easier access to your VAD.
- Comfortable walking shoes or slippers.
- Many pairs of warm, comfortable socks.
- Portable computer to communicate with relatives, friends, or work associates. Check with your transplant center to see if portable computers are permitted in the hospital room.
- Art materials (paints, needlework, knitting).
- Puzzles and games (scrabble, backgammon, crossword puzzles).
- Hats, scarves, wigs, or turbans—Even if you end up loving your bald head, it is nice to have some cozy warm covering.
- Something to make you laugh, such as a funny book or wig.
- Tape deck with music or relaxation tapes you enjoy. Have earphones so you can listen anytime without disturbing others.
- Good books or magazines—Books that can be read aloud by a caregiver are fun. Magazines and poetry books are also good options as they can be read at various intervals and do not require much concentration or long-term memory.
- A notebook to jot down your feelings and experiences.
- Paper, cards, and pens to write letters. Remember the stamps!
- A musical instrument for those who like to play music.
- A camera or video camera.

The Transplant Process

Regardless of whether you do the transplant as an inpatient or an outpatient, embarking on this journey may bring up many strong emotions. How long you will be immunocompromised or in the hospital will vary depending on the type of transplant you will be undergoing and on your overall physical condition. If you will be having an autologous transplant, you might do the whole procedure on an outpatient basis or experience a relatively short patient stay. If you are undergoing a transplant from a donor, you can generally expect to stay in the hospital for three to five weeks, and you will need to stay in the area of the transplant center for up to three months.

The Hospital Environment

In the following section, you will find a description of a typical day at one of the larger transplant centers. The specific times and the details of the routine at your hospital will probably vary from the one described here, but the main point to note is that the days at a hospital are often full of activity. People will be coming in and out of your room throughout the day to check on you, to check medical equipment, and to clean the room. When your energy level is low, interacting with the various members of the hospital staff that come in and out of your room and keeping up with your personal hygiene and exercise can take up a lot of your time and energy. Nevertheless, it is a good idea to have things that you enjoy available for the periods when you are alone and have time and energy to spare.

A Typical Hospital Day (Schedules Will Vary Depending on Patient's Condition and Medical Regimen.)

4–6 A.M.—A nurse enters the room to draw daily, routine blood tests.

7 A.M.—A nurse aid checks daily weight.

8 A.M.—A nurse comes in to take vital signs (every four hours).

8:30 A.M.—Doctors and their coterie of residents and students enter the room for daily rounds.

9 A.M.—Breakfast.

11 A.M.–3 P.M. (Items not in order)

A person from the housekeeping staff cleans the room.

A nurse aid or nurse changes the bed.

A physician's assistant comes by to review your general medical condition.

Various people from the hospital staff come in to replenish the medical supplies in the room and check the status of the medical equipment.

A nurse comes in at various intervals to administer medication and blood products and to check vital signs.

Lunch.

4 P.M.—Vital signs are taken and medications replenished.

6 P.M.—Dinner.

8–8:30 P.M.—Bedtime preparations.

Midnight—Vital signs are taken

12:00–6 A.M.—Various medications are administered throughout the night. Chest X rays and other tests are administered as needed.

Organizing a daily schedule of activities can be helpful. In addition to keeping you occupied, a daily schedule can motivate you to keep up important daily activities, such as exercising and personal hygiene. During the day, you will also have the opportunity to watch movies, walk around the halls, visit with guests, and rest. If the hospital schedule clashes with your desired schedule, discuss your preferences with a nurse to see if you can be accommodated.

Steps Through the Transplant

The Medical Evaluation

Upon your arrival at the transplant center, you will often undergo a general medical evaluation involving a physical exam and some lab and diagnostic tests to make sure it is safe to go ahead with the transplant and to provide a baseline for future comparison. These tests may include eye and dental exams, heart and lung studies, a bone marrow aspiration, a spinal tap, a chest X ray, and other tests. In certain instances, these tests may reveal certain underlying problems that need to be taken care of prior to proceeding with the transplant.

Signing Consent Forms

During this period, you will be required to sign one or more consent forms for the bone marrow transplant procedure, and also for research procedures if you are doing your transplant at a research center. The consent form is a legal document that protects the hospital from medical liability in case of complications. Be forewarned: the consent form often lists some of the most frightening and unsavory complications that may arise from the transplant, even those that may be quite rare.

Central Line

Before your transplant, you will have a small, flexible plastic tube inserted into the large vein above the heart. This is called a central line, central venous catheter, or Hickman catheter. The central line is a highly useful device that allows blood samples to be withdrawn and drugs and blood products to be given painlessly. The procedure for installing the central line generally requires local anesthesia. For many patients this is a relatively simple and painless procedure, whereas others find it more painful.

Bone Marrow or Stem Cell Collection— Autologous Transplant Patients

If you are having an autologous transplant, you will be your own donor and will have your own stem cells or bone marrow collected. If you are getting marrow from a donor, your donor will undergo the stem cell or bone marrow collection.

Your bone marrow contains a high concentration of stem cells—the cells that give rise to all the cells that make up your blood. A small number of these stem cells also are released into the blood stream. Stem cells can, therefore, be collected either directly from the bone marrow or they can be obtained from the blood stream.

Bone Marrow Harvest

If stem cells are collected from your bone marrow, you will have to undergo a surgical procedure in which a needle is inserted several times into the hipbone. Marrow rich in stem cells will be withdrawn and stored until the time of the transplant. During the time of the harvest surgery, you will be anesthetized and will not feel any pain, although the area of the surgery may be sore for a few days following the procedure.

Peripheral Stem Cell Collection

Stem cells can also be collected from the blood stream. The stem cells in your blood are called peripheral blood stem cells. Like stem cells inside your bone marrow, peripheral blood stem cells are able to make red blood cells, white blood cells, and platelets. Because your blood steam only has a small number of stem cells, you will need to take a drug, such as G-CSF, to increase the number of stem cells in your blood. Once there are enough of them, they will be collected by a process called apheresis. In this process, blood will be withdrawn from your central line, then circulated through a cell separator. The stem cells will be removed and stored until the time of your transplant, and your blood will be transfused back to you.

This process takes between three to four hours a day. Generally, one to three days of apheresis are required to obtain an adequate number of stem cells for transplant.

Patients generally experience little, if any, discomfort during the apheresis procedure. Others experience numbness or tingling in their fingertips or toes, hand or leg cramps, lightheadedness, dizziness, or chills. All of these are easily corrected.

Conditioning (Radiation and/or Chemotherapy Treatment)

The next stage of the transplant is conditioning treatment (also called preparative regimen), which will involve several days of chemotherapy with or without total body irradiation (TBI). The type and amount of chemotherapy and/or radiation you will receive depends upon your particular disease and the type of transplant you are having. Regardless of your exact treatment protocol, the goal of the conditioning treatment is to destroy all the cancerous or diseased cells.

The chemotherapy is often given through your central line, or in some cases orally. Generally, you will not feel anything during the administration of chemotherapy, but you will experience the side effects later. The same is true for radiation treatment, which is painless during the time of administration.

The effects of the conditioning treatment range from mild to severe. Common symptoms resulting from chemotherapy and radiation include nausea, vomiting, diarrhea, hair loss, fatigue, loss of appetite, and mouth sores. Some people develop all of these conditions after chemotherapy, whereas others only develop only a small subset of them.

The conditioning treatment also may irritate the bladder and cause bleeding. Bladder irritation can be prevented by taking a medication such as Mesna or by inserting a Foley catheter though your urinary tract into your bladder and flushing out the bladder.

The Transplant

The day of the transplant is an exciting day that offers a new chance at life. The procedure itself is surprisingly simple. A bag of bone marrow or peripheral stem cells is infused over the course of several hours through your central line, just like any other blood product or medication. Once the new marrow enters your blood stream, the stem cells migrate into your bones where they begin to reproduce, allowing you to once again produce your own healthy blood. This process is called engraftment.

Engraftment

Engraftment occurs when the newly infused cells begin to reproduce within your body. Often, the first sign of engraftment is a rising white blood cell count. If you have had a peripheral stem cell transplant, engraftment will usually occur within the first two weeks after transplant. If you have had a transplant with stem cells taken directly from the bone marrow, engraftment will usually take between two to four weeks. If you are someone who engrafts late, the waiting period can be trying and anxiety producing.

Throughout this period, your white blood cell count will be monitored carefully to check for signs of engraftment. Particular attention will be paid to your neutrophil count, also referred to as ANC (Absolute Neutrophil Count). Neutrophils, as mentioned earlier, are a common type of white blood cell that play an important role in fighting infection caused by bacteria and yeast.

Many patients like to keep close track of their blood counts and keep a calendar in their room to mark off the days until engraftment. Celebrating the day of your engraftment with loved ones can be a good way to bring cheer into this difficult period. Your rising white blood cell count indicates that your new marrow is starting to take hold. Once your white blood cell count is above a certain level and you are free of infection and other complications, you can leave the hospital.

Physical Effects of the Transplant Process

The transplant process is characterized by tremendous change. In response to the chemotherapy, radiation, and medications, your body will undergo many trans-formations. The changes will affect how you look, your energy level, and your strength—as well as the functioning of different organs in your body.

Throughout the process, your blood counts and health status will be monitored carefully. Your weight will be checked daily and your vital signs—tempera-ture, blood pressure, and pulse—will be checked every few hours. Often, you will be given a diary to record the fluids and food you take in by mouth and your output in the form of urine, vomit, and stool. This close monitoring of your condition is necessary to ensure that any changes in your health status are detected and, if necessary, treated as early as possible.

Nausea

Nausea is a very common side effect that can range from moderate nausea for several days to severe nausea over the course of several weeks or even months. Fortunately there are some very effective medications for nausea. Some nausea medications may make you sleepy or cause hallucinations. If this is the case, or your medications are not reducing the nausea effec-tively, make sure to explore different medication options with your medical staff. You also may try relax-ation or meditation to decrease nausea.

Tips to Reduce Nausea:
- Wear loose-fitting, comfortable clothes.
- Avoid overly sweet or greasy foods, as they may increase your discomfort.
- Eat salty, dry foods like crackers.
- Find ways to distract yourself with activities you enjoy.
- Practice relaxation and deep-breathing techniques.

- Eat and drink small quantities throughout the day.
- Eat and drink slowly so that only small amounts of food enter your stomach at one time.
- Rest in a chair after eating and keep your head elevated.
- Avoid eating very hot or very cold foods.
- Take antinausea medication regularly before the onset of nausea—prevention is key.
- Avoid foods and smells you find unappealing.
- Refrain from eating your favorite foods during the period you are most nauseated as you may Develop an aversion to these foods later on.
- Eating ginger may settle your stomach and relieve your nausea.

Mouth Sores

The conditioning regimens of chemotherapy and radi-ation often cause the tissues inside your mouth to become thinner and more delicate, leading to irritation and ulceration. In some cases, the whole digestive tract may become irritated and painful. The extent of irrita-tion will depend in large part on the type of treatment you receive and on your own unique reaction to the treatment. If you do experience pain, physicians who specialize in pain management may be available to help you cope with it, while psychologists and psychiatrists may help you cope with stress. As always, make sure to make your needs known. It is also helpful to keep in mind that the pain is transient and will subside once you engraft and have a better functioning immune system.

Energy Depletion

The transplant procedure will tend to make you feel weak. Don't be surprised if you can only accomplish a limited number of activities during the day. Simple tasks like reading or writing a letter may seem very taxing at times. Be patient with yourself. You will regain your energy, but it will take time.

Body Image

Coping with a changing body is an integral part of the bone marrow transplant. You may begin the transplant with lots of hair on your head and may then lose most or all of it. Some people lose their eyebrows and eye-lashes, whereas others don't. If you take certain immunosuppressive drugs, your face, abdomen, hands, and feet may become swollen and round for some time. Weight can fluctuate during the transplant.

Although many people experience weight loss during the transplant, others gain weight due to water retention and bloating.

As you go through the transplant process, other changes may take place. Once your hair starts coming back in, it may be a different texture or color than it was before. Medications such as Cyclosporine, which is commonly used to treat graft-versus-host disease (GVHD), may cause additional hair growth. After your initial bald state, you may find that your hair, eyebrows, and eyelashes are thicker than ever. Some patients may grow additional body and facial hair.

As you go through these transformations, remember to have a sense of humor. Suggestions by previous patients include getting a funny haircut before your hair falls out, buying hats or wigs you like, marveling at the changes, remembering to laugh at yourself, and keeping in mind that the changes are almost always temporary. Adjusting to a new and perpetually changing self may be difficult, but it is helpful to remember that it is part of the necessary process you must undergo in order to recover and regain your health.

Other Physical Changes

Other changes people experience include restlessness and difficulty sleeping, drowsiness, inability to concentrate, trembling hands, loss of memory, hemorrhoids, diarrhea, and difficulty eating. Keep in mind that not everyone goes through these changes. However, it is useful to hear what others have been through, and to know that despite even the most difficult circumstances, people make it through, recover, and return to normal, active lives after a transplant.

Graft-Versus-Host Disease (GVHD)—Allogeneic Transplant Patients

As your white count rises, you may experience graft-versus-host disease (GVHD). Graft-versus-host disease occurs when the white blood cells produced by your donor's transplanted marrow do not recognize your organs and tissues as "self." This happens because there are some genetic differences between you and your donor. Because of these differences, if your immune system identifies cells as foreign, the system will attack them. Patients getting an autologous transplant or getting a transplant from an identical twin do not get graft-versus-host disease. About half of the patients receiving a transplant from a related donor will

develop some form of GVHD. Your chances of getting GVHD are even higher if your donor is unrelated.

GVHD manifests itself in two forms: acute GVHD, which develops in the first three months after the transplant, and chronic GVHD, which develops any time after that. Acute GVHD primarily affects the skin, the digestive tract, and the liver; it can cause symptoms ranging from mild skin rashes that come and go to stomach pains, nausea, cramping of the intestines, and diarrhea. In more serious cases, GVHD can affect major body organs and can be life threatening. Acute GVHD may resolve itself with treatment or, in some cases, it merges with the onset of chronic GVHD.

The effects of chronic GVHD include dry eyes, dry mouth, skin and joint problems, or problems with organs such as the liver or lungs. The severity of GVHD varies dramatically from patient to patient, as does its time of onset and its duration.

A variety of methods are used to reduce the incidence of GVHD. Many patients receive immunosuppressive drugs such as Cyclosporine and/or Prednisone. These drugs weaken your immune system, thus reducing the severity of the attack on your organs. Unfortunately, however, they also increase your susceptibility to infections and prolong the period of immunosuppression. These drugs also may affect one's emotional and mental state. While on these drugs, some patients experience drug-induced depression, confusion, anxiety, roller coaster–like mood swings, and exaggerated feelings of anger or excitement. It is helpful to keep in mind that these effects are temporary and that many people never experience these side effects.

Some BMT centers reduce the incidence of GVHD through the use of T-cell depletion. In this procedure, some or all of the T-cells of the donor's marrow are removed, thus limiting the ability of the new immune system to orchestrate an attack on the host (the patient).

Coping Emotionally

For some, going through the transplant is extremely difficult emotionally, whereas others find it easier than they expected. Some people are relatively alert and active during the transplant treatment, whereas others suffer greatly. Losing one's independence and privacy, experiencing physical discomfort, and adapting to physical and emotional changes can be extremely tiring. In some cases, the medications you will take may affect your mood. Some patients find that while going through the transplant they lash out at the people who are closest and dearest to them. Dealing with a changed status and new role in the family may be difficult. You may find that other people are suddenly too protective or, in other cases, not as understanding as you wish. Taking it one day at a time and remembering to be gentle with yourself and others is helpful. As always, doing things you enjoy can be an effective way of reducing stress during this period. Suggestions for activities include: listening to relaxation and visualization tapes; talking to other patients; getting gentle massages; or sharing feelings with friends, family, or a counselor.

Make Your Needs Known—Be Assertive

Generally, the medical staff and your loved ones will want you to feel as comfortable as possible and will try to accommodate your specific needs and preferences. Make sure to articulate your preferences and needs to those around you. Things that may seem obvious to you may not be obvious to others. Let people know what you would like: what kind of food, what kind of schedule, and what kind of care. Ask what your options are, and find out what services are available to you.

It is not uncommon for the members of your medical team and other staff members to neglect to tell you about various services and options that are available to you. If you are interested in a certain service that was not mentioned, ask if it can be made available. Remember, it never hurts to ask.

If you like your privacy respected, put a sign on your door requesting that people knock before entering. Or, if there are certain hours that you would prefer to be alone or with family, see if the medical schedule can be arranged to accommodate you. If you would like to have your spouse or parent stay the night in your hospital room, request a bed for them or buy a small folding camping bed and bring it to the hospital room. If having an overnight guest in the room is not allowed, see whether an exception can be made in your case.

The key is to communicate with your doctors and nurses! If there is some aspect of your care that you are not satisfied with, make this known, either by speaking directly to a member of your medical team or to the person in charge, or by asking your caregiver to express your concerns. Communicating with others about your needs is the first step in having them addressed.

Maintain a Sense of Humor

Laughter and a good attitude can be powerful sources of support and healing. Clearly, if you are not feeling well, this can be quite a challenge. To the extent possible, try to incorporate some fun into your days. Rent some funny movies or ask friends and family to send you videos of themselves. If you like to dance, turn up the music in your room and dance a jig or two. Try to incorporate a few things you enjoy into your day. Remember, every day on this earth is incredibly precious, and we all owe it to ourselves to make the most of this gift of life.

Caring for Yourself While You're Still in the Hospital

Following the conditioning treatment and the transplant, your immune system will be compromised and, thus, you will be at risk for infections. In order to minimize risk of infection, good hygiene, mouth care, and exercise are all recommended.

Good Hygiene

One of the important ways to minimize infections is to require that all visitors entering your hospital room or your house wash their hands thoroughly. As a patient, you also should wash your hands regularly throughout the day, before meals, before taking your pills, and after using the bathroom. Daily bathing or showering is also highly recommended, as it will help to reduce skin bacteria.

Dental Care

One of the best things you can do for yourself to reduce discomfort and infections during the transplant is to take meticulous care of your mouth. By maintaining good oral hygiene during the transplant, you are likely to prevent or reduce oral infection and bleeding gums.

Remember, optimal mouth care entails frequent mouth rinses throughout the day. You also should brush your teeth regularly with a soft nylon bristle toothbrush; if the regular toothbrush hurts, use a sponge tooth brush. While brushing, thoroughly rinse your mouth several times to remove bacteria and debris. Brush or rinse your mouth after taking any food; this will help minimize infection and pain. If you are good at flossing and are able to do so without injuring your gums, continue to do so.

Exercise

On days when you are weak and sick, it will be particularly tempting to curl up in bed and not move. However, exercising and moving is your ticket to doing many of the things you will want to do when you are discharged. Exercising regularly will mean that you have more energy to carry out daily activities, and it also is likely to lower your risk of injury from falling or twisting an ankle. You do not need to be in great shape to exercise. Many exercises and stretches can even be done in bed.

The benefits of exercise are manifold:

- Exercising promotes good circulation and encourages the continued normal functioning of your body.
- Exercise prevents or minimizes muscle atrophy from prolonged bed rest and steroid treatment.
- Exercise is associated with improved nutritional status as it promotes protein assimilation and decreases body fat.
- Exercising and deep breathing help prevent the accumulation of fluids in the lungs, which often can lead to pneumonia.
- Exercise is known to combat depression and promote feelings of well-being, as well as to enhance physical comfort.
- Exercise facilitates cardiac function and blood circulation.

During your time at the hospital, and also as an outpatient, you may have visits from a physical therapist who will work with you on maintaining your overall strength and endurance, as well as working on particularly important things like ankle strength and chest expansion. If you feel you need more information on exercises and stretches, make your needs known and have a physical therapist visit you more often.

Nutrition

Often, the treatment will affect one's appetite and ability to eat and digest food. Eating may be difficult for some people because of changes in taste and smell, nausea, general dryness of the mouth, or difficulty swallowing. If you are having difficulty eating, you will be fed intravenously through your central line so that your basic caloric and nutritional needs will be met. Good nutrition is particularly important post-transplant as your body will require additional calories, protein, vitamins, and minerals to heal and recover.

Eating Tips

Although your nutritional requirements can be met through intravenous feeding, it is highly recommended that you try to continue eating, at least small amounts, throughout the period of the transplant. By eating and keeping your digestive tract active, the digestive and absorptive functions of your digestive tract will be better maintained, thus making it easier for you to eat post-transplant. During this period, your dietitian can serve as an important resource in helping you find ways to meet your nutritional needs.

A helpful suggestion is to begin increasing your oral intake with small meals and snacks every few hours. Nutritious beverages are often well tolerated and can be an excellent source of vitamins, minerals, and calories.

In order to aid digestion and prevent heartburn, eat and drink slowly. Sitting up, rather than lying down, after meals can also help. If you are not experiencing much nausea, light exercise such as walking can promote digestion and may help you feel more comfortable.

Although there are no specific rules about which foods to eat, many patients find that moist, bland, low-fat soups, casseroles, or noodle dishes are relatively easy to digest compared to fried foods, meats, and some raw fruits and vegetables. The best rule of thumb is to eat the foods that are most appealing to you. If there are particular foods you crave that are not on the hospital menu, see if they can be made available for you.

Finally, in order to reduce the probability of food-borne illness, you and any caregiver who is helping feed you should wash your hands prior to eating meals and follow the food safety guidelines that are recommended by your dietitian.

Caring for Yourself at Home

If you have been an inpatient in the hospital during the period of your transplant, you may be surprised to find the transition from the hospital to home more difficult than you expected. Whereas in the hospital everything was taken care of for you, in the home environment you have the responsibility of caring for yourself and the pressures of the everyday world. Reacclimating to the world that you used to function in can be frustrating, particularly because you might not be able immediately to do all that you did in the past.

Outpatient Care Post-Transplant

In the first few months following the transplant, you are likely to visit the outpatient clinic several times a week—or in some cases every day—for blood draws, physical exams, intermittent blood or platelet transfusions, or for tests such as throat, urine, and stool cultures to screen for infections. Depending on your protocol, you also may undergo periodic X rays, bone marrow aspirations, lumbar punctures, or other procedures. This intensive follow-up care is necessary to monitor your progress and to treat complications should they arise. As the weeks and months progress and your condition stabilizes, your visits will become less frequent.

Readmission and Setbacks

Returning to the inpatient department of the hospital for treatment post-transplant is very common and is part of the recovery process. Although returning to the hospital or contracting an infection is discouraging, it is important to recognize that recovery is a bumpy road and that many patients experience small complications and may need to be readmitted for short periods of time to manage symptoms that cannot be safely treated in the outpatient department. Returning to the hospital for short stays is often just one of the many steps involved in the recovery process.

Guidelines Post-Transplant Care

During the period immediately following hospitalization, you will be vulnerable to infections and will need to take extra precautions. The time of immunosuppression varies from person to person and depends upon the type of transplant and the amount of immunosuppressant drugs being taken.

People who have had autologous transplants tend to be least immunocompromised, because they do not need to take immunosuppressants to combat GVHD. As a result, they are less vulnerable to infections than recipients of transplants from donors. Because of this, autologous transplant recipients only have to follow the guidelines for the one or two months post-transplant. People who have undergone a transplant from a donor,

however, should follow the guidelines more strictly and for a longer period. Because every patient's condition is different, your physician will determine how long you should follow the guidelines. In general, the time period will range from a few months to a year or more, depending on the type of transplant and your condition.

Coping with all the restrictions post-transplant requires a lot of energy and effort. Although living with these recommended precautions can be challenging, maintaining good hygiene is a very important part of regaining your health and avoiding infection during the period of immunosuppression.

In the months following the transplant, it is helpful to remember that these restrictions are temporary. In the course of a lifetime, six months or a year of avoiding certain foods or certain places is a minor sacrifice.

Hand Washing

Following the transplant, you should wash your hands frequently during the day, as hand contact is by far the most common way of contracting infections. Touching doorknobs or other objects and then touching one's mouth, nose, or eyes transmits many bacteria and viruses. Frequent hand washing is the best protection against infection and should be done regularly before eating meals, taking medications, and after using the toilet. Ideally, everyone who comes into contact with you should wash their hands frequently to minimize the risk of transmitting infectious microorganisms to you. Some patients recommend instituting a "hand-washing policy" in the house, and requiring that everyone wash their hands upon entering, so as to minimize the risk of transmitting infection.

Personal Hygiene

After the transplant, personal hygiene is of paramount importance. Make sure to bath daily, using soap and shampoo. Often, your skin post-transplant will be dry and sensitive. If this is the case, frequent applications of body lotion can be helpful. Using a milder soap can also reduce dryness and irritation. As part of general hygiene, towels and clothing should be changed daily. You should avoid sharing towels and washcloths.

Contact with People

In order to restrict potential exposure to bacteria and other infection-causing agents, it is generally recommended that you restrict touching or hugging to a few special people with whom you have frequent contact. It is also important to avoid settings in which you are likely to come into contact with sick people. In particular, you should avoid kindergarten and school settings because children are more likely to be sick than adults. Because the transplant can destroy previous immunity to diseases, it is also important to avoid contact with babies or adults that have been vaccinated with live viruses such as polio within the last thirty days. Although you do not have to avoid public spaces altogether, I also recommend avoiding crowded spaces such as movie theaters and restaurants during peak hours, crowded elevators, and auditoriums.

If someone living with you gets sick, check with your medical provider to determine how much risk the infectious person poses to you and what is the best course of action. It is likely that the sick individual will be advised to move elsewhere temporarily until he or she is no longer infectious. If that is not possible, arrange to have the person stay away from you as much as possible and avoid sharing household items with that person.

If you choose to eat at restaurants, make sure to choose ones that have a reputation for cleanliness and that serve fresh foods. In the period that you are immunocompromised, don't hesitate to ask when foods were prepared and to ask that foods be prepared fresh especially for you. Many restaurants will accommodate you.

Hygiene in Your Home

Your living quarters post-transplant should be kept clean. Again, there are no hard and fast rules as to the degree of cleanliness you should maintain. The recommendations vary according to the type of transplant you have had and your degree of immunosuppression. In any case, the amount of dust, mold, and fungus in the house should be kept to an absolute minimum, as these have the potential to transmit infection. Depending on the amount of dust and dirt in your house, the house should be cleaned once a week or every few days. The bathroom and eating areas should be cleaned most often, and cleaning sponges should be replaced weekly with new ones. You may also consider having the refrigerator cleaned prior to stocking it so that it is free of mold spores, which can get into your food. Using a cleaner with antibacterial disinfectant

properties such as Lysol or bleach is recommended. Do not, however, expect the antibacterial agent to take the place of a good, thorough cleaning. Use a damp cloth to clean and dust because feather dusters stir up dust and disperse it through the air. Allocate cleaning tasks to family members and/or, if you have the financial resources to do so, hire someone else to do the housework.

Plants and Pets

As part of the general cleanliness and hygiene requirements, it is recommended that you avoid keeping fresh plants and flowers in your home as the organisms that grow in dirt, water, and plants can cause infections. In general, you should avoid handling plants in the first few months following the transplant. Obviously, you also should avoid contact with soil, lawn waste, or compost. Thus, refrain from gardening or sitting on grass, logs, or dirt. This restriction should not prevent you, however, from enjoying the outdoors. If you wish to sit outside, have a clean cover to sit on.

In general, it is recommended that you limit your contact with animals and household pets during the first one hundred days post-transplant. During this time, you should not clean up after your pets or touch any human or animal excrement. It is particularly important to avoid cat litter boxes and birdcages. You should check with your physician to determine the extent of contact you may have with your pets.

Construction Sites

Avoid construction sites as they often have upturned earth, old wooden beams, or other materials that may expose you to dust or fungus. If you are aware of a construction site in your neighborhood, consider walking upwind from it or going around the block to avoid it. If you are driving by, roll up your windows.

Exposure to the Sun

The effects of radiation, chemotherapy, and certain drugs may increase your skin's sensitivity to sunlight. During the first year post-transplant, stay out of the sun as much as possible and apply a sunscreen with a sun protection factor (SPF) of twenty-five or more when going outdoors, even on overcast days. On sunny days, wear protective coverings such as hats, sunglasses, pants, and long-sleeved shirts for at least a year post-transplant.

Swimming

Avoid swimming in lakes or untreated water until your immune system has reconstituted itself. If you have had an autologous transplant, the restriction applies for several months. Check with your physician before resuming swimming activities.

Food Safety

Until your immune system rebuilds itself, you will be at a greater risk for developing food-related infections. Thus, in the period following the transplant, it is extremely important to follow food-safety guidelines.

Although the food guidelines may vary slightly from center to center, in general eat only those foods that have been freshly prepared in a clean environment and which have not been sitting out for any length of time.

Smoking/Alcohol/Drugs

Your risk for lung damage post-transplant will considerably increase. It is, therefore recommended that you avoid smoking before, during, and after your transplant. You should also avoid secondhand smoke.

The damaging side effects of alcohol are also greatest post-transplant. For this reason, you should avoid

Food Safety Guidelines

Adapted from Food Safety Guidelines from the Fred Hutchinson Cancer Research Center.

Grocery Shopping

- Do not buy items that are past their "sell by" dates. Do not buy items that you cannot consume by their "use by" dates.
- Do not buy or use any bulging, damaged, or deeply dented cans.
- Make sure frozen foods feel solid and that refrigerated foods are cold.
- Do not buy cracked or unrefrigerated eggs.
- Store groceries promptly after shopping.
- Do not buy bulk foods that cannot be washed from self-service bins.

Food Preparation

- Prepare food on surfaces that have been thoroughly washed in hot soapy water.
- Clean cutting boards in a solution of ten parts water mixed with one part household bleach, then rinse with hot water.
- Use separate cutting boards for cooked foods and raw foods.
- Do not use raw, unpasteurized eggs in uncooked foods, because raw eggs are the perfect medium for the growth of bacteria such as salmonella.
- Discard eggs, egg mixtures, or prepared egg dishes left at room temperature for more than an hour.

- Wash the tops of cans and the can opener before use.
- All meats should be cooked until well done and should have no remaining pink color.
- Do not leave hot food to cool off before refrigerating; place it in the refrigerator immediately after finishing your meal (divide large amounts of hot food into small, shallow containers for quick cooling in the refrigerator).
- Do not eat perishable foods that have been left out of the refrigerator for more than two hours.
- Do not eat foods that have been sitting in the refrigerator for more than three days (to help keep track of this, date them when you open them); it is helpful to refrigerate only the amount of food that you will eat in two or three days and freeze the rest.
- Thaw meats and fish in the refrigerator.
- Throw away food that has any mold on it.
- Never taste foods that look or smell strange.
- Wash and rinse fruits and vegetables thoroughly before eating them.

Foods to Avoid

The following foods often carry infection-causing organisms. Discuss your personal food-safety guidelines thoroughly with your dietitian or

(Continued from page 60)

medical provider and modify or add to this list:

- unpackaged foods being offered as samples in grocery stores
- food at potluck meals where you don't know how food was prepared
- food from sidewalk vendors, delicatessens, smorgasbords, buffets, and salad bars
- soft serve ice cream, milk shakes, and frozen yogurt from yogurt machines
- sushi, raw fish, and smoked fish
- raw eggs, dressings containing raw eggs, mayonnaise-based foods, custards, or other dishes that may contain raw eggs
- unpasteurized fruit and vegetable juices
- all raw vegetable sprouts, including but not limited to alfalfa, radish, and broccoli sprouts, as well as mung beans
- raw fruits and vegetables that are not fresh or that have not been well washed before serving
- well water, unless it has been tested recently and found to be safe
- unpasteurized honey, milk, cheese, and yogurt
- unrefrigerated cream
- raw (unroasted) nuts or nuts in the shell
- aged cheeses such as sharp cheddar cheese
- moldy cheeses such as Brie and blue cheese

Nontraditional nutrition supplements such as herbal preparations should be avoided as they may contain toxic impurities or infection-causing fungi, yeast, molds, or bacteria. These can be life threatening for a person with a weakened immune system. Unsupervised, high-dose vitamin/mineral supplements should also be avoided, as they may interfere with various medications or may be harmful to major organs, especially the liver and kidneys.

alcohol for the first six months post-transplant. If you are still taking medications six months post-transplant, do not drink alcohol until you have discussed the matter with your physician.

Do not take any over-the-counter medications without consulting your BMT doctor or clinical nurse specialist.

Work/School

Avoid work and school for at least three to six months after an autologous BMT. The time you need to take off depends on the kind of work you do and the degree of fatigue caused by your work. A computer consultant working at home, for example, may be able to return to work much earlier than an elementary school teacher. Give yourself time to take care of yourself and fully recover. You deserve it!

Sexual Activity

Generally, sexual activity is considered safe as long as both you and your partner are healthy, practice good personal hygiene, and have no sexually transmittable diseases. Before resuming sexual activity, however, talk with a member of your transplant team to see if there are any restrictions that pertain to your particular case.

Some transplant centers recommend using a condom post-transplant, whereas others maintain that a condom is not necessary if you are in a mutually monogamous relationship and neither of you is suspected of having a sexually transmittable disease. If one of you has a sexually transmittable disease, it is recommended that you refrain from sexual activity, as a condom may not provide a sufficient barrier during the time of immunosuppression. Some BMT centers recommend refraining from unprotected oral-genital sex during the time of immunosuppression whereas others maintain that it is safe as long as oral hygiene is good and there are no oral lesions, genital lesions, or mucositis. Anal sex should be avoided until platelets have stabilized at a level above thirty-five thousand, and there is no evidence of diarrhea, anal lesions, bleeding, or hemorrhoids.

The extent to which the transplant affects one's sexual life varies dramatically from individual to individual. Some people resume an active and highly satisfying sexual life shortly after transplant, whereas others find that their sexual life is greatly disrupted.

Changes in body image or sexual desire post-transplant can disrupt previous behavior patterns or lead to insecurities about starting new relationships. Often, the physical toll of the transplant and the resulting side effects, such as nausea and lower energy levels, may reduce the desire for sexual activity. In other cases, worry or depression or nervousness about one's ability to "perform" and to be sexually attractive post-transplant may result in loss of desire.

If your sexual drive post-transplant is reduced, it is important to explore other ways of intimacy such as touching, holding hands, hugging, and kissing. At this time, communicating with your partner is key to modifying your sexual routine in a way that will meet both your needs for love and intimacy. Recognizing that your partner may share your feelings of concern about resuming an active sexual life is a good starting point for discussion. Once you begin sharing your feelings, you may find that your partner has been holding back because of apprehension about appearing to be overeager, insensitive, or of hurting you physically in some way.

One suggestion to reduce nervousness when you first resume intimate physical contact is to set certain limits on sexual activity. You and your partner, for example, may choose to devote an evening to all-over body touching, where each partner takes a turn touching and being touched. If this feels comfortable, then you can try adding some genital touching during the next session. If lack of sexual desire persists, androgens, which are sometimes referred to as "male hormones," can be taken by either men or women to increase sexual energy.

For patients who are not in a relationship, finding a partner and resuming sexual activity post-transplant may provoke a great deal of anxiety. Although the sad reality is that some potential lovers may reject you because of infertility or because you have had cancer, try not to limit yourself by not dating at all. After all, anyone—with or without cancer—can get rejected for a multitude of reasons. Although you may avoid rejection by not dating, you may also miss the opportunity to build a happy and rewarding relationship.

Women and Sexuality

Sexuality after a bone marrow transplant can also be affected by early menopause which can result from chemotherapy and radiation treatment. The symptoms of early menopause may include hot flashes, vaginal dryness and tightness, as well as mood shifts and irritability. Not all women become menopausal. In some rare cases, women have regained ovarian function

post-transplant, and in even rarer instances, women have also regained fertility and given birth to healthy babies.

For the majority of women who experience early menopause, hormone replacement therapy is effective in alleviating many of the symptoms. It also is useful in reducing some of the risks associated with early menopause, such as osteoporosis (weakening of the bones) and coronary heart disease. For women who have had breast cancer, however, hormone replacement therapy is not an option, as it may increase the chance of recurrence.

Women who cannot or choose not to use hormone replacement therapy may choose to use estrogen creams applied directly to the vagina. Such creams can be effective in improving vaginal dryness without having systemic effects.

Women who experience vaginal dryness post-transplant may also find the use of a water-soluble lubricating jelly helpful.

Exercise

Regular exercise is an important part of the recovery process. By improving your stamina, muscle tone, and muscle strength, you not only will feel better physically but also emotionally. Exercise can help counteract problems such as stiff joints, breathing problems, poor appetite, and psychological lows. Seeing improvement in your physical state can be a real boost, particularly when you are adjusting to the stresses and difficulties of returning to a normal lifestyle.

It may be difficult at first to initiate an exercise routine if your energy level is low and you are not feeling well. A good way to begin exercising is to take walks outside or to visit the outpatient physical therapy department in your hospital, where a physical therapist can work with you in selecting appropriate exercises and building your strength and stamina. You also may be able to get your doctor to write you a prescription to buy an exercise machine such as a stationary bicycle. If this is the case, your insurance may cover a portion or all of the cost of the purchase. A doctor's prescription may also save you from paying sales tax on the purchase.

Physical exercise is particularly important if you are taking Prednisone. Prednisone may cause muscle wasting and weakness; regular exercise can be instrumental in maintaining muscle mass and strength.

When taking Prednisone, however, choose low-impact exercises to minimize stress on your joints because Prednisone can also cause joint damage.

When exercising, pay attention to the messages your body gives you. You should challenge yourself, but you should stop or slow down if you are experiencing pain. On a scale of very light to very arduous, an optimal level of exercise is one that you would rank as moderately hard. The best way to regain strength is through regular exercise, suited to your level of physical conditioning, that builds slowly to progressively higher levels of activity.

Nutrition

After the transplant, your body will require many nutrients to regain strength and to recuperate. Your nutritional requirements will vary, depending on your medical condition, the type of transplant you had, and the medications you are on. Your nutritional needs post-transplant may increase, requiring you to take mineral and vitamin supplements. During this period, it is important to consult a dietitian about food choices to ensure that your nutritional needs are met.

If you are nauseated and find eating and drinking difficult, it is helpful to eat and drink small amounts throughout the day rather than eating three large meals. Make sure to have a wide variety of healthy, appealing snacks at hand for the times that you do feel hungry. Eating in a pleasant setting or having an attractive food arrangement also may facilitate eating. You may need to increase your fluid intake to prevent dehydration and to help flush the drugs and their residues from your bladder and kidneys.

Physical Changes Post-Transplant

There is considerable variation among bone marrow transplant survivors in physical, psychological, and social functioning post-transplant. Some patients recover fully, returning to their old activity level several months after the transplant. For others, the recovery period is slow, and they never return to old levels of vigor and health. The difficulty of the recovery process is often closely tied to the degree of physical difficulties post-transplant. Having repeated infections or chronic episodes of graft-versus-host disease can contribute to stress and difficulty in returning to normal activities. Some of the potential problems that survivors may experience include fatigue, decreased strength, muscle cramps, difficulty concentrating, memory problems, sleep disturbances, numbness in hands and feet, cataracts, skin and joint problems, dry eyes or mouth, frequent infections, and kidney or other organ dysfunction. Keep in mind when reading this list that not everyone experiences these problems. Generally these problems resolve themselves with time and most people return to productive and fulfilling lives post-transplant.

Some of the physical and mental changes post-transplant also may occur as a side effect of some of the drugs. Many of the drugs taken post-transplant can affect organ function, immune function, physical appearance, and psychological well-being. Knowing that many of the changes are temporary can be helpful for everyone involved.

Emotional Adjustment Post-Transplant

Going through a bone marrow transplant changes us in many ways, requiring us to reevaluate many aspects of our lives. Give yourself time to deal with the emotional impact of the transplant. Often, people expect you to be over the experience in a month or two. In reality, however, the process may take much longer. Recovering from the transplant entails not only a physical process but requires a mental shift from seeing yourself as sick to seeing yourself as healthy.

Some people experience recurring memories of the transplant, which conjure up feelings of vulnerability, anxiety, or depression. You may find yourself going over the decisions you made, questioning the reasons for the transplant, and reliving the difficult times you had. Fear of relapse or complications is also common.

If these fears cause a major disruption in your life or cause sleep disturbances, consider seeking some kind of outside help. Often, speaking to a professional therapist or to members of a support group can help you put the experience in perspective and move on. Keeping in touch with someone who went through a transplant at the same time as you can be particularly helpful, as it can allow you to compare notes, exchange information, and reduce your sense of isolation. Do not, however, expect your recovery experiences to be identical.

The transplant may have a strong positive impact on your emotional well-being. Many people find that they emerge from the experience strengthened, more resilient, better focused, and better prepared for the challenges of life.

Changes in Self-Esteem

Making it through the transplant is a heroic accomplishment. However, many people, upon emerging from the experience, tend to compare their performance to their previous levels of activity or to the activity levels of their friends and colleagues. The inability to accomplish as much as before or to be self-supporting may dash one's self-esteem. As you begin the recovery process, set realistic goals for yourself and adapt your activities to your energy level instead of berating yourself for not being able to do more. Respect your need for rest and relaxation. In the months following the transplant, both family members and the patient have to readjust to the new role and new capacities of the patient.

Changes in Family Ties and Relationships

The transplant experience can also result in changed relationships among family members. Often these changes bring families closer, but, in some cases, the changes in roles exacerbate tensions and lead to additional strains.

Friendships may also change or take on new meaning as you reflect on the people who were supportive of you during the transplant and those who were not. Some friendships will be enhanced and enriched, whereas others may dissolve under the pressures of the transplant.

Recommendations for Coping during Recovery

Although it is difficult to know ahead of time how the transition period from the hospital to the outpatient phase will be for you, keep in mind that recovery is a long-term process that does not always proceed in a smooth linear fashion.

Celebrate Landmarks

Often during the ups and downs of recovery, it is difficult to see the bigger picture and to appreciate how far you have come. Celebrating special dates, such as your six-month or one-year anniversary, may serve as an important reminder of your progress. Another way to mark your progress is to give yourself a special treat at the end of a designated period.

Beyond the Transplant

Regardless of how long or how difficult the transplant process is for you, it is important to remember that most people return to a normal and active lifestyle post-transplant. Survivors often report that the quality of their lives post-transplant is similar to or better than before the transplant. Others have some lingering effects, but do not experience significant deterioration in quality of life. A small number of people suffer from more significant handicaps resulting in the need to change their professions or to cease working altogether.

Although the transplant process affects people differently, everyone, without exception, is changed as a result of the experience. Through the transplant, people are forced to look at themselves, their lives, and their priorities. Those who undergo a transplant will inevitably suffer losses, but they also will gain new strengths and insights. By becoming aware of the frailty of life, we all uncover many treasures and learn to live our lives more fully. It is my hope that by reading this chapter, you will be better able to face the road ahead. I wish you all a safe journey.

On Being a Patient:
Reflections on a Bone Marrow Transplant

Michael C. Dohan, M.D.

I am sixty-three years old and have been living with chronic lymphocytic leukemia for more than seven years. Two years ago, progression of symptoms and a worsening hematologic profile despite chemotherapy forced me to make an important personal decision regarding whether or not to receive a bone marrow transplant. As a physician, I knew that transplants for chronic lymphocytic leukemia were controversial and not based on rigorous, controlled studies. It would be risky and difficult, but there was still so much I wanted to do, including living long enough to play an important role in my grandchildren's lives. I chose to go ahead.

After ten months of chemotherapy, my response was good enough for me to qualify for an autologous transplant. At first I rejoiced, but joy was replaced by anxiety and doubt. Many of those around me—including my physicians, friends, and family—assumed that I, as a physician, had more insight into the proposed therapy than I actually did, heightening the isolation of my decision.

In December 1998, I was admitted overnight for the bone marrow harvest, and the following day I was readmitted to the transplantation service. My room was small and had a special air lock to prevent hospital-borne infections. My wife and any other visitors had to wash and put on a mask and gloves to enter the room. I could leave the room and wander in a tiny hallway only if I put on a mask and gloves. At first, I did not realize how physically and emotionally isolating this space would become.

My therapy started immediately with a double-lumen Hickman catheter. Many of the staff addressed me as "doctor," which made me feel special. Initially, I played the role by checking the doses of medications, but quickly I found playing doctor-patient to be a struggle. As much as my professional life in medicine had been about control, I

needed to let go and trust someone else to care for me. I remembered an editorial that Dr. Franz Ingelfinger had written in *The New England Journal of Medicine* many years ago about his battle with cancer, relaying how difficult it was to stop being a consultant in his own case, and how much inner peace he achieved when he finally found a doctor he could trust to treat him as a patient. I needed to do that, too.

Radiation therapy started on the third day. I lay on a trampoline with an X-ray machine above and below me. I quickly learned to time the sessions by counting the clicks of the machines. Every five minutes the machines seemed to shut down briefly and then start up again with a whirring sound. There was nothing physically painful about the radiation, but the sessions were lonely, and the clicking of the machine seemed like the ticking of a bomb. The radiotherapist had assured me that I would receive a lethal dose—as was therapeutically necessary—and so lethality was always very much on my mind during my trips to therapy. I became weaker and more aware of my feelings of isolation and helplessness. I thought about the survivors of Hiroshima and Nagasaki who had no one waiting in the wings to give them bone marrow back. I wondered what might happen if something went wrong with my harvested marrow and there was none to give back. The progressive and extreme physical and mental weakness accompanied by constant nausea left me with a desire to withdraw from the world. I wished at times that I could just say, *"STOP! No more therapy!"* But I never said a word to anyone.

As I reflect back, I find my inability to share my terror with anyone an enigma. Admitting my feelings of terror would have made it harder to deny the reality and to remain a dispassionate physician who believed in the science of this therapy. During those days, I just wanted to lie in bed with the

(Continued from page 65)

blankets over my head and disappear. I did not know how I would survive. But I did force myself to get out of bed and walk every day and, on a few days, even to ride an exercise bicycle. After these adventures, I would nearly collapse from exhaustion. When I looked up at my intravenous lines, two going constantly, with smaller bags awaiting their turn—I couldn't believe that I was at the other end. I thought of the sick patients in the intensive care unit I had cared for so often with multiple lines going. Now I was on the receiving end of this life-sustaining device, and it was frightening. I wondered whether my patients ever had the same reaction, or whether they found the intravenous bags reassuring.

On the day after the last radiation treatment, my team of doctors, along with several nurses and my wife, gathered around me and, in a twenty-minute ceremony, infused my previously purged bone marrow. Now began the wait for engraftment.

With the intravenous therapy, I urinated constantly, day and night. One night I slept too soundly and was incontinent of urine. Embarrassed, I changed my surgical scrubs and sheets myself and didn't tell the nurse until the morning; at that time, she assured me that many patients experience this. The radiation therapy caused severe diarrhea and, later on, so too did the antibiotics. On one particular night, I was incontinent of feces; I rang for the nurse, feeling my last bit of dignity slip away.

As my leukocyte count started to climb, I hung onto every day, hoping it might be the day I'd get to go home. As the day of discharge approached, my nausea intensified and I developed dry heaves. My nurse correctly attributed this to anxiety. That tiny room, which at times seemed like a cell, was, along with the support staff, more important to me than I realized.

On returning home, I decided not to talk to anyone about my experience in the hospital. The few times I attempted to talk about it, I cried. I was totally surprised at how intense my reaction was. When the doctor had warned me that I might have trouble sleeping at home, it seemed preposterous, since nearly all I did in the hospital was sleep. But it was true. I couldn't sleep, despite taking a variety of sleeping pills, and the nausea was worse than ever. I suspected that I was suffering from post-traumatic stress disorder and decided that I had to talk about all I had been through. My wife and I set up an appointment with a psychiatric social worker. The first meeting was difficult; I cried more than I talked. As a child, I had always been fearful of going to the doctor, and perhaps part of my decision to go into medicine was an effort to master that fear. Now all of that was turned upside down. I was no longer the healer but an utterly helpless patient. That night, I had the first decent sleep since coming home.

On reflection, it's hard to understand why my experience was so difficult and why it had such a severe emotional impact on me. Was it simply because I had never been so sick before? Was it the experience of being brought so close to death, with a last-minute rescue? Was it the utter helplessness of both the mental and physical situations? Was it some effect specific to the therapy? Did having a physician's perspective make all of this more difficult?

It was probably all these, and more. What I seem to remember now, months later, was my sense of extreme helplessness, and my inability to muster the strength to fight it. Visitors were most helpful by just being there. Conversation was difficult, and there was little I wanted to do, except to occasionally listen to music. Everything was out of my hands. There was nothing I could do to assure a successful outcome, nothing I could do to make myself feel better, nothing I could do to get back into the world. I just had to wait, and hope. As a doctor, I had always taken pride in caring for others, and, even though I might not always have succeeded in making my patients better, I was the one in charge. I also was accustomed to feeling in charge of my own health—pursuing athletics and a "healthy" lifestyle with vigor. This experience attacked that sense of control so completely that even now, some emotional fragility remains.

Six months after completing therapy, I resumed my practice part time and felt I had

(Continued from page 66)

rejoined the living. As I returned to my traditional role as physician, I found I had gained new insights into the doctor-patient relationship. My patients welcomed me back and looked to me for support and help. I, in turn, drew comfort from their trust and regained much mental strength from returning to the role of healer.

Nine months after transplantation, I visited the unit. The haunting memories made it difficult to go back, but I wanted to thank the staff and show them the success their efforts had achieved. I was surprised at how accessible that unit was. When I went home after the transplantation, it had seemed such a long journey, when in reality it was only a few steps from the elevator. It was good to see the staff. I visited with a young woman going through a similar transplantation. Although a rush of emotion returned, it was not as raw, and I felt I could react appropriately as a patient, doctor, and supporter. It was helpful for both of us.

Much has been written about the impersonalization of modern medical care. The trust we place in our caregivers remains an essential component in recovering from illness. My own physician and other providers were with me every step of the way, and their support has been enormously important—important enough that I trusted them to kill me, and then bring me back to life.

Reprinted with permission from *Annals of Internal Medicine,* April 4, 2000, Volume 132, Number 7, pages 589-590

7

Side Effects of Cancer Therapy
Causes and Treatments

Ernest H. Rosenbaum, M.D.
Isadora R. Rosenbaum, M.A.
Robert J. Ignoffo, Pharm.D.
Larry Mintz, M.D.
Chris Wilhite

It is virtually impossible to attack cancer cells without affecting normal tissues as well. The normal cells in the body also are dividing, and those that divide the fastest are more susceptible to damage. Fast-dividing normal cells are found in the lining of the digestive tract, in the hair follicles, and in the bone marrow that makes blood cells. Chemotherapy and radiation therapy may damage normal tissues. The type of treatment and the tissues involved determine the kind of side effect.

For example, hair loss may result from radiation to the head. Loss of taste and problems in swallowing also can occur with radiation to the head and neck. Nausea, vomiting, and diarrhea are often the result of radiation passing through the gastrointestinal tract on the way to the targeted tumor. The skin may become red, itchy, and dry.

Damage to cells from chemotherapeutic agents leads to side effects such as hair loss, nausea, vomiting, and lowered blood counts. Each drug has its own side effects. Fortunately, these side effects are not permanent. Nutrition and medications can be used to help reduce the common side effects of chemotherapy and radiation therapy, such as loss of appetite, weight loss, nausea, vomiting, diarrhea, and constipation. Information on reducing these side effects is found in Chapter 8, "Side Effects of Chemotherapy" and Chapter 27, "Nutrition Problems: Causes and Solutions."

Many people have heard frightening stories about side effects. Such stories can create more fear of therapy than of cancer; but such fears are largely unwarranted. Through today's sophisticated diagnostic and therapeutic techniques, side effects can be reduced, alleviated, or prevented altogether. New drugs have been developed that can prevent nausea and vomiting or decrease the toxicity of chemotherapy drugs.

Tolerance to a particular drug or combination of drugs varies with each patient. Psychological support from family, friends, and the medical team is important. We do not like to overemphasize the possibility of side effects, because we believe that anxiety about discomfort has produced, in some of our patients, stronger reactions than they might have had without the warning. Conversely, we are convinced that other patients experience fewer side effects because of their attitude toward chemotherapy. At one time, the philosophy of medical therapy was that a medicine had to make you sick. There does not appear to be a direct correlation between the degree of discomfort from drug treatment and the degree of its medical effectiveness. The most toxic therapy may be ineffective; favorable results may be obtained with therapies having minimal side effects.

Anemia

Anemia is defined as "a pathologic deficiency in the oxygen-carrying material of the red blood cells (RBC) and hemoglobin." It is a common problem for cancer patients and is often a result of the therapies used to keep tumors at bay.

Anemia is associated with fatigue—a feeling of weakness or diminished physical and mental capacity unrelieved by rest. Additional symptoms include headaches, dizziness, chest pains, shortness of breath, nausea, and depression.

Causes of Anemia

- Blood loss: excessive bleeding such as hemorrhages or abnormally heavy menstrual bleeding (iron deficiency).
- Nutritional deficiency: lack of B_{12}/folic acid.
- Chronic illness: inflammatory diseases, arthritis, kidney or liver failure, and chronic infections such as AIDS. Bone marrow may have decreased production.
- Cancer therapy: surgery, radiotherapy, chemotherapy, and/or immunotherapy.
- The breakdown or destruction of red blood cells (hemolysis).
- Decreased erythropoietin (EPO) production or impaired bone marrow response to EPO.

Low Red Blood Count (Anemia)

Your doctors will periodically monitor all of your blood counts. One of the blood counts is of the red blood cells. Cancer and its treatment with chemotherapy or radiation can depress the number of red blood cells to a low level and eventually produce tiredness, lack of energy, and anemia. A normal value of red blood cells produces a hematocrit of nearly 40 percent or a hemoglobin of fourteen to fifteen gm/DL. Symptoms of anemia appear when the hematocrit falls, especially below thirty, or the hemoglobin is low. If you have severe

symptoms of anemia, you may be prescribed a red-blood-cell transfusion. A trend toward anemia may be prevented with the early initiation of a weekly injection of epoetin alfa (Procrit or Epogen). The usual therapy for anemia is outlined below.

Treatment of Anemias

The successful treatment of anemia depends on identifying and treating the underlying cause: blood loss, bone marrow infiltration, chronic illness, inflammation, hemolysis, or decreased response to erythropoietin. Through laboratory test results and a physical examination, a physician can usually determine the cause of your anemia and identify the best approach to treating it. This may include:

1. Nutritional supplements—iron, B-12 or folic acid
2. Treatment of infections and inflammations
3. Transfusions: Providing red-blood-cell transfusions for bleeding and severe chronic anemias. Red-blood-cell transfusions are the old main stay that offer the quickest relief for anemias. However, there are risks associated with transfusions, including:
   - allergic reactions
   - transmissions of infectious agents—hepatitis, HIV, and Human Leukemia Virus (HTLV)
     The risks of such transmissions are:
     - hepatitis B virus: 1 in 63,000
     - HIV (AIDS) risk: 1 in 675,000
     - HIV 2: < 1 in 10,000,000
     - HTLV: 1 in 641,000. The viral risks of blood transfusions have recently been reduced due to a more accurate blood test called NAT (Nucleic Acid Test). This tests specifically for evidence of HIV and hepatitis C virus (HCV).
   - immune suppression
   - iron overload from multiple transfusions (usually over 25–50 units of red cells)
4. Administration of erythropoietin injections (Procrit or Epogen)

Erythropoietin

Erythropoietin is a hormone produced by the kidneys (90 percent) and liver (10 percent) in response to anemia or low blood-oxygen levels. Erythropoietin selectively stimulates early red blood cell (erythroid) in the bone marrow to increase bone marrow activity.

This, in turn, will help deliver more oxygen to the tissues and resolve some symptoms of weakness and fatigue.

A weakened bone marrow due to cancer infiltration (marrow replacement), lymphoma, or leukemia may lead to low erythropoetin levels. These patients may respond to epoitin alfa (laboratory-produced erythropoetin) therapy. Patients who cannot produce adequate erythropoietin due to liver or kidney disease may also be helped by epoitin alfa injections, 30,000–40,000 u weekly.

The side effects of this treatment must be considered. They include: hypertension, iron deficiency, occasional minor allergies, edema (tissue swelling from water retention), and/or frequent bowel movements (diarrhea). It can cause growth of some tumors, especially myeloid tumors (increase in bone marrow cells).

Summary of Cancer-Related Anemias

- Anemia is common in cancer and contributes greatly to patient fatigue and reduced quality of life.
- Your doctor can help you to assess and correct the underlying cause of anemia.
- Red-blood-cell transfusions provide immediate short-term relief.

Laboratory-produced erythropoietin (Procrit or Epogen) can increase hemoglobin levels, reduce the need for transfusions, and improve quality of life.

Transfusions

When chemotherapy drugs damage the bone marrow, red-blood-cell, platelet, and/or white-blood-cell transfusions can be given. The need for red cell transfusions is determined by the blood cell count (hemoglobin), which is monitored frequently during treatment. Usually, the bone marrow returns to normal about ten to twenty days after receiving chemotherapy.

Other Medications to Stimulate Bone Marrow Production of White Blood Cells and Platelets

Medications such as Neupogen (G-CSF, or granulocyte-colony stimulating factor), which help to increase production of white blood cells, and Procrit and Epogen (Erythropoietin), which help increase production of red blood cells, will help the patient to tolerate further chemotherapy. Neumega (oprelvekin) is a growth factor to promote platelet production in conjunction with chemotherapy

Low White Blood Counts (Neutropenia)

In the process of destroying cancer cells, chemotherapy also can cause damage to other rapidly dividing cells, such as the bone marrow cells. Bone marrow is responsible for producing red blood cells (RBCs), white blood cells (WBCs), and platelets. The reduced activity of the bone marrow is named myelosuppression. Blood components will decrease after chemotherapy, but at different speeds. White blood cells will be affected more rapidly, because they have the shortest life span of the three.

White blood cells are the soldiers defending the human body against infections, so a low number is associated with increased infections because many have died in the battle. Your doctor will track the number of white blood cells (counts) throughout your cancer treatments. White blood cells will reach their lowest number ten to fourteen days after the end of chemotherapy. The lowest number is also known as the nadir. White blood cells usually will recover within three to four weeks; exceptions are for some drugs that can cause a slower increase and a longer recovery, such as the nitrosoureas or mitomycin C.

There are two methods of measuring your number of cells. The first one is by counting the total number of white blood cells, which is preferably over $3,000/mm^3$. The other method is to calculate the Absolute Neutrophil Count (ANC), which should be more than $1,500/mm^3$ to reduce the risk of infections. If the white-blood-cell count or ANC does not come back fast enough, your doctor may decide to delay the next cycle of chemotherapy until your blood count is sufficient.

In order to speed up the recovery and the activity of your white blood cells, drugs that act as "colony-stimulating factors" (CSFs) can be administered. Two colony-stimulating factors are used in the United States to increase the white-blood-cell count, G-CSF (Neupogen) and GM-CSF (Leukine). They are given according to the weight of the patient and the level of bone marrow recovery. G-CSF is given by subcutaneous injection (under the skin) every day for about one week after chemotherapy. Patients experiencing bone pain (usually in the sternum or hips) may take pain-relieving medication such as acetaminophen or a nonsteroidal analgesic (ibuprofen, Motrin, naproxen, Aleve) if necessary.

Colony-Stimulating Factors (CSFs)

G-CSF (Filgastrim, Neupogen)	5mcg/kg/day SQ for 7 to 10 days rounded to: 300 mcg if < 75kg 480 mcg if >75 kg Until ANC>1,000	Nausea, fever, bone pain	$$$$
GM-CSF (Sargramostim, Leukine)	250 mcg/m² SQ or IV for 7 to 14 days	Fever, flushing, hypotension, rigors, bone pain.	$$$$

$= inexpensive $$$$=very expensive

Low Platelet Counts (Thrombocytopenia)

Your doctors will periodically monitor all of your blood counts. One blood count is of the platelets. A normal value ranges from 150,000 to 300,000 per ml (milliliter) of blood. Low blood counts, including a low platelet count, can occasionally occur after receiving a lot of chemotherapy or radiation therapy. Thrombocytopenia, a very low platelet count (less than 20,000 per ml of blood) can result in bleeding from the nose, gums, urinary tract, or gastrointestinal tract. The usual time for a low platelet count to occur is ten to twenty-one days after chemotherapy, but any bleeding at any time should be reported immediately to your doctors. In order to reduce the risk of bleeding during chemotherapy, it is best to avoid drugs that can affect the functioning of platelets. Such drugs include aspirin, ibuprofen (Advil), and naproxen (Aleve). If your platelet level is very low, your doctor may prescribe a platelet transfusion. In patients who have a low trend to thrombocytopenia, a drug called Neumega may be prescribed to prevent further fall in their platelet counts.

Hot Flashes (Menopause-like Symptoms), Flushing

Hot flashes can be a troubling symptom in women who have undergone antiestrogen therapy (tamoxifen) or in men who have been given androgen deprivation therapies (Lupron or Goserelin or orchiectomy). Drugs that may be effective for hot flashes are megestrol acetate, Megace, venlafaxine, Effexor, metoclopramide, and vitamin E. (See table on page 72)

High Calcium Level (Hypercalcemia)

Occasionally, cancer can spread to the bones and cause an increased calcium release in the blood stream. Most patients can eliminate the overflow of calcium, but 10 to 20 percent of cancer patients cannot and will experience a calcium level greater than the normal 10.5mg/dl level; this is known as hypercalcemia (high calcium level). Some cancer, such as breast cancer, can cause a higher incidence of hypercalcemia.

A high calcium level is a serious situation and can cause tiredness, confusion, decreased appetite, increased urination, bone pain, cardiac problems, and convulsions. Your doctor may prescribe some drugs (biphosphonates) to stabilize the bones and prevent hypercalcemia. Pamidronate (Aredia) is the preferred drug for treating hypercalcemia, although etidronate (Didronel) is also used. Other measures include a lot of fluid (usually a saline solution) along with a diuretic (Lasix).

Neuropathy from Chemotherapy

Chemotherapy can have adverse effects on the nervous system. Vincristine, for example, can cause autonomic deficiency, causing constipation. Cisplatin, paclitaxel (Taxol) and vincristine can cause numbness, tingling, and pain in extremities. These drugs also can cause difficulty in fine motor skills and, in severe cases, impair walking abilities. These side effects normally disappear after chemotherapy ends, but may take several months to do so. Some drugs can be given to alleviate the symptoms, such as pyridoxine, gabapentin, or Neurontin, but results vary.

Bladder or Urinary Toxicity from Chemotherapy

Two chemotherapy drugs are associated with toxic side effects to the bladder and ureter. Both cyclophosphamide and ifosfamide can irritate the bladder and ureter leading to a condition called cystitis, which can occur in up to 10 percent of patients receiving intermittent or chronic low-dose cyclophosphamide

Drugs to Treat Hot Flashes

Megestrol Acetate (Megace)	20 mg orally twice daily	weight gain, vaginal bleeding, chills	$$ beneficial effects may require 2 to 3 weeks of treatment
Venlafaxine (Effexor)	25 mg orally twice daily	In this low dose regimen: after 4 weeks, sweating (38%), fatigue (8%), dry mouth (19%), trouble sleeping (8%)	$$$ about 60% of patients respond after 4 weeks of therapy
Metoclopramide (Reglan)	20 mg orally three times daily.	sedation, jitteriness, diarrhea.	$$ less well studied than Megace or Effexor
Vitamin E	800 units orally daily	blurred vision, dizziness, flu, nausea, and headaches are signs of an overdose	$ less well studied

$= inexpensive $$$$=very expensive

and 40 percent receiving cyclophosphamide in a high-dose bone marrow transplant program. Cystitis is manifested as urinary burning or bleeding after several cycles of chemotherapy.

Prevention of cystitis is achieved through frequent voiding and vigorous hydration. A patient receiving either of these drugs will be instructed on a method to prevent cystitis from becoming a problem. Adequate fluids, either taken orally or intravenously, dilute the urine such that the offending metabolites of these drugs will not damage the lining of the bladder or ureters. For ifosfamide, a uroprotectant drug called Mesna will be given concurrently with good hydration. Treatment of hemorrhagic cystitis may require bladder irrigation with saline or formalin.

Hypersensitivity Reactions from Chemotherapy

Chemotherapy can cause some types of allergic reactions, better classified as hypersensitivity reactions (HSR). With proper premedication, less than 3 percent of patients have such reactions. Severe HSRs include shortness of breath, wheezing, hives and itching, and low blood pressure, which typically occur within minutes after treatment, usually after the first or second dose. Chemotherepy drugs which can lead to severe HSRs include paclitaxel (Taxol), docetaxel (Taxotere), etoposide (VP-16) and bleomycin. Most reactions resolve completely after stopping treatment and occasionally after treatment with diphenhydramine, fluids, dexamethasone, and occasionally ephinephrine. After resolution of the symptoms, the drug may be restarted at a slower infusion rate and gradually increased with premedications. HSRs from bleomycin can occur from the first dose on, especially in patients with lymphoma. These reactions manifest as chills, fever, shortness of breath, low blood pressure, or wheezing. The drug should be stopped and the reaction treated with dexamethasone, diphenhydramine, and epinephrine (if necessary). A test dose of 0.5–1 units should be given to all patients prior to the first dose of bleomycin.

Dermatologic Reactions from Chemotherapy

Chemotherapy can cause several skin reactions. Vesicant drugs (nitrogen mustard, vincristine, etoposide, doxorubicin, and others) can blister skin and also

Drugs to Treat Hypercalcimia

Pamidronate (Aredia)	60 to 90 mg IV every month	fever, bone pain	$$
Etidronate (Didronel)	depending on calcium levels	fever, bone pain	$$

$= inexpensive $$$$=very expensive

The Impact of Cancer Therapy on Male Fertility

Disease	Regimen	% Low Sperm Count
Hodgkin's Disease	MOPP	85%
Hodgkin's Disease	Cisplatin, vinblastine, bleomycin	0%
Testes Cancer	MOPP	14–28%
Sarcoma	Doxorubicin + Cyclophosphamide	65%

The Impact of Cancer Therapy on Female Fertility

Disease	Regimen	% Amenorrhea
Ovarian Cancer	Cisplatin, Vincristine, methotrexate, etoposide, actinomycin D	6%
Breast Cancer	CMF	85%
Breast Cancer	Cyclophosphamide	83%
Breast Cancer	FU	9%
Hodgkin's Disease	MOPP	24%
Hodgkin's Disease	COPP	57%
Hodgkin's Disease	ABVD	0%

Tables are modified from M. Perry; *Chemotherapy Source Book*, Second Edition; Williams and Wilkins; 1997, pp. 813-832.

produce local skin reactions when injected, but precautions and antidotes can minimize these reactions. Liposomal doxirubicin (DOXIL) can also cause skin reactions. Specific drugs (bleomycin, paclitaxel) have the potential of causing allergic reactions. This reaction can be minimized with adequate antiallergic medications taken before chemotherapy. Patients receiving tretinoin can experience redness, dryness, itching, and increased sensitivity to sunlight; they should take adequate precautions. Finally, the hand-foot syndrome is characterized by painful redness, irritation, and fissuration of the hands and soles caused by fluorouracil and capecitabine. Treatment of this syndrome is mainly support and moisturizing of the affected regions with creams and emollients.

Fertility Effects of Chemotherapy

Today, many young patients are cured of cancer after receiving chemotherapy. However, alterations in gonadal (reproductive) function are now known to be a common complication of cancer chemotherapy. Women may experience premature gonadal failure, menopause, sterility, and even osteoporosis (from estrogen deprivation). Men may have low sperm counts and infertility. Other issues concerning cancer survivors are risks of complications of pregnancy, birth defects, and malignancy in their offspring.

Although many questions remain to be answered, your doctors will provide counseling and use the newest strategies to prevent gonadal complications from chemotherapy. One approach is to use alternative hormonal therapies or the preservation of sperm or eggs for future use.

Chemotherapy (especially cyclophosphamide) given to boys before puberty has resulted in 1 percent gonadal dysfunction; when given during puberty it has resulted in 67 percent gonadal dysfunction. MOPP chemotherapy used in Hodgkin's therapy inhibits virtually 100 percent of sperm function in men. Gonadal damage after puberty is usually assessed by analyzing the seminal fluid. The effects of various chemotherapy regimens on male spermatogenesis are shown in the table below. It appears that the major drugs that cause gonadal dysfunction are the alkylating agents such as cyclophosphamide, thiotepa, nitrogen mustard, and chlorambucil.

For patients in whom fertility is spared, the outcome of pregnancies has not shown a higher incidence of congenital anomalies, spontaneous abortion, or neonatal mortality. There are fewer studies of men surviving cancer who then become fathers. In men with germ cell tumors, there has not been an excess of congenital anomalies and chromosomal abnormalities in their offspring. In addition, there is no difference in growth maturation. In pregnancy, fetal exposure to multidrug chemotherapy has been associated with minimal risk when chemotherapy was after the first trimester.

Cardiac (Heart) Toxicity from Chemotherapy

Some chemotherapy drugs, such as doxorubicin, epirubicin, and daunorubicin, or radiation therapy to the chest can cause adverse reactions on the heart. The effects (cardiac congestion, decreased exercise tolerance) are generally seen with prolonged treatment, but can also occur faster. Your doctor may record an echo of your heart before and during your treatment. In case of damage to the heart, the drug may be stopped or modified. One other medication, Dexrazoxane (Zinecard) can be given to minimize the

effects of chemotherapy on the heart muscle. Another way to decrease the adverse effect of chemotherapy is to give doxorubicin in a liposomal format.

Hair Loss

Losing your hair (alopecia) can be an upsetting experience. It is one of the most visible side effects of cancer treatment. The amount of hair loss varies from hair thinning to baldness. You may find it helpful to have your partner, a close friend, or a relative with you when you talk to your doctor about hair loss.

Chemotherapy stops cell division of the more active cells in the body, including those of the bone marrow, the gastrointestinal lining, and the scalp. About 85–90 percent of hair cells are in the growth phase at any one time and therefore can be affected by drugs. Many drugs, including bleomycin, Cytoxan, Adriamycin, etoposide (VP-16), vincristine, Velban, 5-fluorouracil, methotrexate, and Taxol, can cause partial or total hair loss.

Scalp tourniquets and ice caps have been used with limited success, especially with drugs that remain in the circulatory system for many minutes or hours. However, because these methods reduce the delivery of drugs to the scalp, cancer cells in the scalp are not treated and the cancer could recur locally.

Hair loss usually occurs about two to three weeks after the beginning of treatment. Hair may come out in large clumps. Hair regrowth usually begins about four to eight weeks after chemotherapy ends, and sometimes hair begins to grow back during treatment. The new hair may change color or texture.

How to Care for Your Hair

Gently shampoo to avoid drying out the hair and scalp. Avoid over-brushing or over-combing. Gently use a wide-tooth comb or a vent-style hairbrush to avoid pressure or damage to the hair roots. Also avoid heat-generating hair appliances such as dryers, hot rollers, and curling irons. Use styling aids such as sprays, mousses, and gels to give the appearance of fullness and volume.

Although many patients avoid permanents and coloring, no relationship between hair loss and perms or coloring is proven. You might want to avoid permanents and hair coloring early in chemotherapy because if hair loss occurs, you have wasted your money.

Reduce Your Risk of Infection

Larry Mintz, M.D.

During chemotherapy or radiation therapy, there may be a decrease in your blood counts—white blood cells, red blood cells, and platelets. Neutropenia is the term used to describe a lack of special white blood cells called neutrophils or polys, which are blood cells that fight infections caused by bacteria, fungi, and viruses. Therefore, patients with neutropenia are more susceptible to serious infections. When the absolute neutrophil count (ANC) is less than 1,000 cells/mm^2, the risk for an infection is greater. When the ANC falls below 500, and especially below 200, the risk becomes extremely great, so that any fever, chills, or other signs of possible infection must be evaluated by your nurse or doctor immediately.

Tips for Reducing Your Risk of Infection

- Hand washing is the No. 1 priority. You should wash your hands before meals, on awakening, and after using the toilet. All visitors should wash their hands when they arrive.
- Get adequate sleep.
- Eat frequent meals with high amounts of calories and protein (make an appointment with a dietitian if you need guidelines). For more specific recommendations, see Chapter 26, "Nutrition for The Cancer Patient," and the special diet for neutropenia included in Chapter 28, "Modified Diets."
- Avoid raw fruits and vegetables unless they have an intact skin or peel that will be removed before eating.
- Avoid foods that are rough, hard, very hot, or difficult to chew as they might cause injury to your gums or oral mucous membranes.
- Bar visitors who have a cold, sore throat, or some other infection.
- Limit your guests to short visits so you have time for adequate rest.
- Do not use rectal thermometers. Rectal examinations, suppositories, and enemas should also be avoided.
- Avoid constipation. (See Chapter 8, "Side Effects of Chemotherapy.)
- Monitor fever (temperature above 100°F) three times a day or when you feel hot.
- Drink plenty of fluids (six to eight glasses a day—more if you have a fever).
- Report any sores, infections, or new symptoms to your nurse or doctor. These include hot or flushed skin, fever, shaking, chills, rapid heart rate, cough, cloudy urine, skin infections, rashes, or ulcers.
- Avoid contact with stagnant water. Common sources are denture cups, soap dishes, and flower vases. Make sure the water in humidifiers, irrigation containers, and respiratory equipment is discarded and replaced with fresh water daily.
- Use a soft-bristle toothbrush to protect your fragile gums.
- Shower or bathe daily, using soap.
- Use skin creams and emollients (skin barrier creams) to avoid dryness.
- Massage skin daily.
- Use an electric razor to avoid skin cuts.
- Use a special pressure-relief mattress to prevent skin breakdown or pressure sores and ulcers. Change position frequently when sitting or when lying in bed.
- Keep skin around the anus clean and dry. Use special creams as needed to reduce the risk of perirectal infections.
- Treat hemorrhoids with sitz baths and special medicated creams.
- Report any mental changes to your nurse or physician. These include headaches, irritability, restlessness, mental confusion, a change in mental status, sleepiness, or a decrease in level of consciousness.
- Maintain a list of the drugs you are taking—especially antibiotics.

Wigs and Turbans

Chris Wilhite

Wigs can boost your morale, improve your appearance, and improve your self-confidence. Purchase a wig before you start treatment so that a good match to your natural hair color and texture can be found. Synthetic wigs are less expensive than natural hair wigs and are easier to clean and style. Wig care includes soaking the wig in a mild soap or cleaning solution (such as Woolite), drying it in a towel, and then keeping it on a wig-form so it can be styled and brushed. A purchased wig can be styled and shaped to fit your personality and may be individualized. Wig prescriptions are usually covered by health insurance. Some synthetic wigs can cost about $200.

How To "Look Good Feel Better"

There is a national program called The Look Good Feel Better Cosmetic Program, sponsored by The Cosmetic, Toiletry, and Fragrance Association Foundation and the American Cancer Society. It provides an opportunity to improve your appearance.

If you are a woman getting cancer treatment, you may find that certain physical changes are especially hard to bear. Your personal appearance directly affects your self-image and your psychological well-being.

Look Good Feel Better (LGFB) is a free, nationwide public service program designed to teach you—through practical, hands-on experience—the beauty techniques that will help improve your appearance during chemotherapy and radiation treatments.

So, while your medical treatment helps heal the inside of your body, the Look Good Feel Better program helps you renew your self-esteem by enhancing your "outside" appearance. It encourages you to pay attention to yourself during a time of dramatic physical changes

These free programs provide:

- patient education—through group or individual sessions—by volunteer cosmetologists and beauty advisers
- complimentary makeup kits for everyone participating in a group program (Look Good Feel Better is "product neutral" and does not promote any specific cosmetic product line or manufacturer.)
- free program materials such as videos and patient information pamphlets

The Look Good Feel Better program is administered nationwide by the ACS and is designed to meet the needs of local communities. All volunteers for the program are trained and certified

For more information, or to find out about programs in your area, call your local or state division of the American Cancer Society, or call 1 (800) 395-LOOK.

Adapted from *Everyone's Guide to Cancer Therapy*, Fourth Edition, by Dollinger, Rosenbaum, Tempero, and Mulvihill, 2001.

8

Side Effects of Chemotherapy

Robert Ignoffo, Pharm.D.
Bernadette Festa, M.S., R.D.
Ernest H. Rosenbaum, M.D.
Isadora R. Rosenbaum, M.A.

Chemotherapy Drugs and Their Potential Side Effects

Chemotherapy involves giving drugs (chemicals) to kill cancer cells. The goal of chemotherapy is to control, reduce, or cure a cancer. Unfortunately, when cancer cells are killed, normal cells can be injured, resulting in side effects. In addition to nausea, anemia, low white blood cell counts, vomiting, pain, or diarrhea, additional side effects include psychological side effects, cognitive defects, taste changes, mouth or esophageal mucositis (irritation of the lining), and fatigue. The side effects can cause mild to severe debilitation, affect your desire to get well, or reduce your will to live. By knowing the side effects of chemotherapy drugs, you can reduce or control many side effects with the help of your doctor.

Adrenocorticosteroids (Prednisone, cortisone, dexamethasone)
Adverse Reactions: mood changes, hypertension (high blood pressure), edema (fluid and salt retention), headaches, sleeplessness, vertigo, psychiatric problems, muscle weakness (low potassium), osteoporosis, increased hair growth, cataracts, malaise, and increased infections.

Side Effects That May Affect Nutrition: nausea and vomiting, altered taste and smell, loss of appetite, stomach or esophageal inflammation or ulcers, ulcerated mouth and throat (mucositis), diabetes, pancreatitis, dehydration, electrolyte imbalance, increased appetite, and protein breakdown (catabolism).

Food-Drug Interactions: consume some food in the morning to help initiate the body's normal hormone production time. Take medication one hour before or two hours after breakfast, or when fasting. Antacids and antiulcer drugs (Tagamet, Zantac, Pepcid, and Prilosec) can help reduce heartburn, upset stomach, or ulcers.

Bicalutamide (Casodex)
Adverse Reactions: hot flashes, breast pain, breast enlargement in men, hepatitis (rare).

Side Effects That May Affect Nutrition: nausea and vomiting, diarrhea, constipation, and flatulence.

Bleomycin (Blenoxane)

Adverse Reactions: pulmonary dysfunction, faintness, confusion, sweating, wheezing, coughing, shortness of breath, skin darkening, rash, and fluid retention in fingers.

Side Effects That May Affect Nutrition: loss of appetite, nausea and vomiting, sore mouth or throat (mucositis), and weight loss.

Food-Drug Interactions: none known; avoid excessive doses of vitamin C.

Busulfan (Myleran)

Adverse Reactions: low blood counts, skin pigmentation, male breast enlargement, loss of menstrual periods, coughing, fever, bruising, confusion, dizziness, and malaise.

Side Effects That May Affect Nutrition: loss of appetite, nausea and vomiting, diarrhea, dry mouth, and elevated uric acid (hyperuricemia).

Food-Drug Interactions: full meals may reduce drug absorption. Take one hour before or two to three hours after a meal. Take with a small amount of starchy food, such as bread or crackers, that will help clear the stomach quickly and not interfere with absorption.

Carboplatin (Paraplatin)

Adverse Reactions: low blood counts, hearing loss, neuropathy, numbness and tingling in hands and feet.

Side Effects That May Affect Nutrition: loss of appetite, nausea and vomiting, diarrhea, constipation, sore mouth or throat (mucositis), altered taste and smell, and high uric acid levels (hyperuricemia).

Food-Drug Interactions: none known.

Chlorambucil (Leukeran)

Adverse Reactions: low blood counts, rash, hair loss, pulmonary fibrosis, low sperm count, secondary leukemia (rare), fever, cough, chills, sore throat, joint pains, shortness of breath, fluid retention in legs, and skin bleeding.

Side Effects That May Affect Nutrition: nausea and vomiting, high uric acid (hyperuricemia).

Food-Drug Interactions: full meals may reduce drug absorption. Take an hour before or two hours after a meal. Take with a small amount of starchy food, such as bread or crackers, that will help empty the stomach and not interfere with drug absorption.

Cisplatin (Platinol)

Adverse Reactions: low blood counts, hearing loss, loss of feeling in hands and tingling of fingers and toes, muscular weakness, facial swelling, fast heartbeat, wheezing, fever, chills, sore throat, joint pains, swelling of feet and legs, blurred vision, and bleeding and bruising. Drinking more fluids and salt intake may reduce kidney insufficiency.

Side Effects That May Affect Nutrition: loss of taste, distorted taste, nausea and vomiting, loss of appetite, sore mouth or throat (mucositis), electrolyte imbalance, and high uric acid (hyperuricemia).

Food-Drug Interactions: none known.

Cyclophosphamide (Cytoxan, Neosar)

Adverse Reactions: low blood counts, bladder scarring and bleeding, loss of menstrual periods, decreased sperm count, lung scarring (fibrosis), respiratory insufficiency, skin pigmentation, hair loss, and liver toxicity.

Side Effects That May Affect Nutrition: lactose intolerance, loss of appetite, nausea and vomiting, sore mouth and throat (mucositis), diarrhea, high uric acid (hyperuricemia), bleeding and ulceration of the gastrointestinal tract, and altered sense of taste.

Food-Drug Interactions: decreased absorption when taken orally if you have stomach inflammation. Do not take with a full meal. Take one hour before or two to three hours after meals. Take with a small amount of a starchy snack such as bread or crackers that will help clear the stomach and will not interfere with absorption.

Cytarabine/Cytosine Arabinoside (ara-C, Cytosar)

Adverse Reactions: low blood counts, bleeding, bruising, confusion, and disorientation.

Side Effects That May Affect Nutrition: lactose intolerance, loss of appetite, nausea and vomiting, sore mouth and throat (mucositis), loss of taste, and loss of smell.

Food-Drug Interactions: none known.

Dacarbazine (DTIC, Imidazole Carboxamide)

Adverse Reactions: fever, chills, sore throat, mouth sores, and bleeding and bruising. Sun exposure one or two days after taking the drug can produce facial flushing and light-headedness.

Side Effects That May Affect Nutrition: lactose intolerance, loss of appetite, nausea and vomiting, sore mouth or throat (mucositis), and high uric acid (hyperuricemia).

Food-Drug Interactions: none known.

Docetaxel (Taxotere)

Adverse Reactions: low blood counts, flushing, hypertension, itching, sweating, hair loss, rash, phlebitis, and peripheral neuropathy.

Side Effects That May Affect Nutrition: nausea and vomiting (usually mild to moderate), mouth sores (mucositis), and diarrhea.

Food-Drug Interactions: none known.

Doxorubicin (Adriamycin) and Liposomal Doxorubicin (Doxil)

Adverse Reactions: low blood counts, potential heart damage and risk of congestive heart failure, and hair loss. Urine may be orange or red on first day after chemotherapy.

Side Effects That May Affect Nutrition: nausea and vomiting, loss of appetite, loss of taste, sore throat and mouth (mucositis), diarrhea, and iron loss.

Food-Drug Interactions: none known. Vitamin C may improve action of Adriamycin.

Etoposide (VP-16, VePesid)

Adverse Reactions: low blood counts, wheezing (rare), fever, chills, sore throat and mouth, bruising, numbness and tingling in toes and fingers, shortness of breath, rapid heart rate, and weakness.

Side Effects That May Affect Nutrition: loss of appetite, altered taste and smell, nausea and vomiting, sore throat and mouth (mucositis), diarrhea, protein loss, and loss of fluids and electrolytes

Food-Drug Interactions: full meals may reduce absorption when drug is taken orally. Take one hour before or two to three hours after meals. Take with a small amount of a starchy food, such as bread or crackers, that will help to clear the stomach and will not interfere with absorption.

5-Fluorouracil (5-FU, Adrucil) and Floxuridine (FUDR)

Adverse Reactions: low blood counts (rare), hair loss (frequent, but usually mild), skin hyperpigmentation (age spots), rash, loss of coordination and confusion (rare), headache (rare), cough, shortness of breath, fever, nasal and skin dryness, nose bleeds, bruising, and sun sensitivity.

Side Effects That May Affect Nutrition: loss of appetite, nausea and vomiting, sore throat and mouth (mucositis), bleeding and ulceration of the gastrointestinal tract, bile salt losses, bitter taste, diarrhea, niacin deficiency, and thiamin deficiency.

Food-Drug Interactions: none known.

Flutamide (Eulexin)

Adverse Reactions: hot flashes, loss of libido, impotence, and male breast enlargement.

Side Effects That May Affect Nutrition: loss of appetite, nausea and vomiting, diarrhea. Note: about 12 percent of patients have diarrhea often associated with lactose intolerance. Taking flutamide with Lactaid or a lactase supplement may prevent diarrhea.

Food-Drug Interactions: none known.

Gemcitabine (Gemzar)

Adverse Reactions: low blood counts, skin rashes, and flu-like symptoms.

Side Effects That May Affect Nutrition: loss of appetite, nausea and vomiting, diarrhea, and sore mouth (mucositis).

Food-Drug Interactions: none known.

Goserelin (Zoladex)

Adverse Reactions: common side effects include hot flashes, breast tenderness and enlargement in men, and breast pain. Infrequent side effects include fluid retention, worsening bone pain from tumor flare reaction, vaginal spotting or breakthrough bleeding, and hepatitis with increased hepatic enzymes (rare).

Side Effects That May Affect Nutrition: nausea, vomiting, diarrhea, constipation, and flatulence (all infrequent).

Hydroxyurea (Hydrea)

Adverse Reactions: low blood counts, fever, chills, sore throat, bruising, hallucinations, headaches, joint pains, and swelling of the feet and lower legs.

Side Effects That May Affect Nutrition: loss of appetite, nausea and vomiting, sore mouth (mucositis), diarrhea, constipation, and high uric acid (hyperuricemia).

Food-Drug Interactions: full meals and stomach

inflammation may delay absorption. Take one hour before or two to three hours after meals. If taken on an empty stomach, it may cause nausea. A small, starchy snack such as crackers or bread will help clear the stomach and does not interfere with absorption.

Ifosfamide (Ifex)
Adverse Reactions: low blood counts, urotoxicity with bladder/urine bleeding (reduced with a uroprotector, such as Mesna), hair loss, central nervous system toxicity (dizziness, sleepiness, confusion, depression, hallucinations, disorientation, and cranial/head nerve dysfunction), painful urination, cardiotoxicity, and allergic reactions.

Side Effects That May Affect Nutrition: loss of appetite, nausea and vomiting, and altered taste.

Food-Drug Interactions: none known.

Interferon-alpha (Intron A, Roferon-A)
Adverse Reactions: flu-like syndrome with fatigue, fever, chills, muscular pain and headache; also dizziness, rashes, dry skin, decreased mental status, visual and sleep disturbances, hypertension, chest pain, arrhythmia, palpitations, skin bleeding, night sweats, itching, conjunctivitis, and irritation at the site of injection.

Side Effects That May Affect Nutrition: flu-like syndrome, loss of appetite, weight loss, nausea and vomiting, diarrhea, dry mouth, and altered taste and smell.

Food-Drug Interactions: none known.

Irinotecan (Camptosar, CPT-11)
Adverse Reactions: low blood counts, hair loss, skin rash, and liver enzyme elevation.

Side Effects That May Affect Nutrition: nausea, vomiting, diarrhea (can be severe, starting about six days after chemotherapy), and mouth sores (mucositis).

Food-Drug Interactions: none known.

Leucovorin (Leucovorin Calcium, Wellcovorin)
Adverse Reactions: allergic reactions.

Side Effects That May Affect Nutrition: nausea and vomiting (rare).

Food-Drug Interactions: large amounts of folic acid may counteract the antiepileptic effect of phenobarbital, Dilantin, and primidone, increasing the frequency of seizures, especially in susceptible children. Leucovorin increases the toxicity of 5-fluorouracil.

Melphalan (Alkeran)
Adverse Reactions: low blood counts, increased risk of secondary leukemia, fever, chills, bruising, joint and stomach pains, and swelling of the feet and lower extremities

Side Effects That May Affect Nutrition: nausea and vomiting, sore mouth and throat (mucositis), and high uric acid (hyperuricemia).

Food-Drug Interactions: full meals and stomach inflammation may delay absorption. Do not take with a full or fatty meal; take one hour before or two to three hours after your meal. Nausea is common when this drug is taken on an empty stomach; take with some crackers or bread.

Methotrexate (Folex, Methotrexate, Mexate)
Adverse Reactions: low blood counts, sunlight sensitivity, and elevated liver enzyme. Toxicity can be reversed by the use of folinic acid (leucovorin factor). Do not take vitamin supplements for one to two days before taking methotrexate.

Side Effects That May Affect Nutrition: loss of appetite, nausea and vomiting, diarrhea, bleeding and ulceration of the gastrointestinal tract, lactose intolerance, loss of taste, protein loss, and fat-soluble vitamin loss.

Food-Drug Interactions: food containing high amounts of salicylates should be avoided one to two days before and after methotrexate (plums, gums, mints, jelly beans, root beer, apple, cherry and blueberry turnovers, and breakfast squares). Avoid drugs that can increase methotrexate toxicity, such as aspirin, sulfa, penicillin, and nonsteroidal anti-inflammatories (ibuprofen, naproxyn).

Mitomycin-C (Mutamycin)
Adverse Reactions: low blood counts, hair loss, long-term pulmonary toxicity, and kidney failure.

Side Effects That May Affect Nutrition: loss of appetite, nausea and vomiting, diarrhea, sore mouth and throat (mucositis), and loss of protein, fluids, and electrolytes.

Mitoxantrone (Novantrone)
Adverse Reactions: low blood pressure, itching, rash, hair loss (rare), shortness of breath, low blood counts, cardiac toxicity (congestive heart failure, arrhythmia, chest pain; risk increases in patients who have

previously taken doxorubicin or daunomycin).

Side Effects That May Affect Nutrition: nausea and vomiting, diarrhea, sore mouth and throat (mucositis), bleeding and ulceration of gastrointestinal tract, and high uric acid (hyperuricemia).

Food-Drug Interactions: none known.

Nilutamide (Nilandron)

Adverse Reactions: interstitial pneumonia (rare), visual disturbances, abnormal light adaptation, hepatitis with increased hepatic enzymes (rare), and alcohol intolerance (rare).

Side Effects That May Affect Nutrition: nausea, constipation, and diarrhea (rare).

Paclitaxel (Taxol)

Adverse Reactions: low blood counts, numbness in the hands and feet, and hypersensitivity reaction.

Side Effects That May Affect Nutrition: nausea and vomiting, loss of appetite.

Food-Drug Interactions: none known. Vitamin C may improve action of Taxol.

Procarbazine (Matulane)

Adverse Reactions: lowered white blood cell and platelet counts, headaches, dizziness, fever, abdominal or back pain, muscle and joint pains, shortness of breath, tiredness, weakness, and weight loss (rare).

Side Effects That May Affect Nutrition: loss of appetite, nausea and vomiting, diarrhea, constipation, altered taste and smell, dry mouth, swallowing difficulties, iron loss, vitamin B_6 loss, and protein loss.

Food-Drug Interactions: procarbazine can elevate norepinephrine and serotonin in the nervous system, increasing the risk of reaction with certain food substances such as tyramine, which can cause a "pressor effect" characterized by transient high blood pressure, headache, palpitations, nausea and vomiting, and (rarely) cerebral hemorrhage.

Foods high in tyramine include ripened cheese (especially cheddar), wines (especially Chianti), broad beans, bananas, and fermented milk products like yogurt.

Antidepressants like the monoamine oxidase (MAO) inhibitor elevate serotonin and norepinephrine levels in the nervous system. This can cause transient hypertension headaches, palpitations, and nausea and vomiting. Concurrent use of barbiturates, antihista-mines, narcotics, hypotensive agents, and phenothiazines with procarbazine may cause central nervous system effects. Avoid alcoholic beverages and hidden sources of alcohol such as sauces and desserts.

Tamoxifen (Nolvadex)

Adverse Reactions: hot flashes, menstrual irregularities, vaginal irritation (discharge, dryness, and occasionally bleeding), and leg cramps.

Side Effects That May Affect Nutrition: loss of appetite, altered senses of taste and smell, nausea and vomiting, fluid retention in legs, and weight gain.

Food-Drug Interactions: to promote absorption, take pill one hour before or two hours after a meal. If taken on an empty stomach, nausea or upset stomach may occur. Take with a small amount of starch.

Thiotepa (Thioplex)

Adverse Reactions: dizziness, headaches, hives, and bronchospasm. Rare side effects are amenorrhea, loss of fertility, irritability, and bladder bleeding.

Side Effects That May Affect Nutrition: loss of appetite, nausea, and vomiting.

Food-Drug Interactions: none known.

Topotecan (Hycamtin)

Adverse Reactions: low blood counts.

Side Effects That May Affect Nutrition: diarrhea, loss of appetite, nausea and vomiting, and mouth sores (mucositis).

Food-Drug Interactions: none known.

Vinblastine (Velban)

Adverse Reactions: low blood counts (lowest between seven and ten days after therapy), tingling in hands and feet, and jaw pain.

Side Effects That May Affect Nutrition: loss of appetite, nausea and vomiting, mouth sores (mucositis), abdominal discomfort, and constipation.

Food-Drug Interactions: none known.

Vincristine (Oncovin, Vincasar)

Adverse Reactions: nervous system damage (sensory impairment, loss of deep tendon reflexes, and nerve pain), skin irritation, and hair loss. Rare side effects include abdominal pain and intestinal obstruction, decreased blood sodium, and seizures.

Side Effects That May Affect Nutrition: nausea and

vomiting, constipation, abdominal discomfort, mouth sores and ulcers (rare), dry mouth, altered taste and smell, and high uric acid (hyperuricemia).

Food-Drug Interactions: none known.

Vinorelbine (Navelbine)

Adverse Reactions: decreased white blood cells, ane-mia, hair loss, vein irritation, numbness in hands and feet (rare), jaw pain (rare), and acute shortness of breath.

Side Effects That May Affect Nutrition: nausea, vomiting, and constipation.

Food-Drug Interactions: food decreases the oral absorption of vinorelbine by 20 percent.

9

Pain Control

Wendye Robbins, M.D.
Ernest H. Rosenbaum, M.D.
Isadora R. Rosenbaum, M.A.

"Pain is an even more terrible lord of mankind than even death itself."

—*Albert Schweitzer*

Ask any group of cancer patients to describe their greatest fear. The chances are that they will say, "Pain and suffering—not death." This is not an unreasonable response. Pain is terrifying and debilitating. It can lead to depression, loss of appetite, fitful sleep, irritability, and feelings of isolation. Those reactions, in turn, can strain relations with family and friends, and even erode the will to live.

Pain can occur at any time in the course of dealing with some forms of cancer—during treatment that leads to remission or cure as well as in the terminal phase. However, 90–95 percent of most pain problems can be controlled, according to the Committee on Pain of the World Health Organization (WHO). Yet many cancer patients still are not receiving adequate pain relief. Why?

Among the obstacles to giving and receiving appropriate pain medication are widespread misunderstanding about the effects of opioids, poor communication between patients and caregivers, and a need for increased awareness—among patients and caregivers alike—of the causes and ramifications of different types of pain. In developing individually tailored pain relief programs, patients and caregivers also need to ensure that they are well informed about the various pain-relief options through frequent consultation with pain specialists and given clarification about the many myths that surround the use of opiods.

Common Misunderstandings about the Use of Opioids for Pain Control

Opioids are drugs originally derived from the poppy plant. Although morphine is the best-known member of this class, many similar molecules (including oxycodone, hydromorphone, fentanyl, hydrocodone, and methadone) have been synthesized to produce effects similar to those of morphine. Unfortunately, many people adhere to certain myths about the use of opioids for pain control. Because of their belief in the misconceptions of these myths, many people take insufficient doses of opiods or refuse to take them at all.

Five Myths about Opioids

Myth 1: Opioids should only be administered as a last resort to the gravely ill or those near death. Not true! Opioids are highly effective at any time in the disease process when severe pain calls for strong medication.

Myth 2: The use of opioids for pain leads to addiction. Addiction is a compulsive need to take a substance despite a known risk of harm. Opioids used for pain control do not function in this manner. Patients do not become drug-crazed or switch to street drugs; and they do not misuse prescribed medications. However, patients can become physically dependent on opioids if they take them over a long period of time. When people achieve a cure of their cancer through therapy, they can then reduce their opioid intake slowly to avoid withdrawal symptoms.

Myth 3: People who take opioid medications develop a tolerance for them, leading to a need for increasingly larger doses. Tolerance, if it occurs at all, does not develop suddenly. If it does occur, it is true that physicians will respond by increasing the dose; however, when administered correctly, opioid medications are safe even at very high doses.

Myth 4: Opioids are dangerous because they make it harder for terminally ill patients to breathe. Morphine and other opioid drugs are not dangerous respiratory depressants in patients with advanced cancer and pain. Tolerance to the respiratory-depressant effects of these drugs usually develops before tolerance to their pain-relieving effects. Other drugs—such as sedatives and anti-anxiety agents—present a greater risk of respiratory depression than opioids.

Myth 5: Patients should take opioids by injection because they are poorly absorbed when taken orally. Most opioids are absorbed very well when taken orally. However, because a fair amount of an oral dose is lost to nontarget body tissues, oral doses are usually three times larger than those given intravenously or intramuscularly.

Communication between Patients and Caregivers

Good communication between patients and caregivers is essential to achieving optimal pain relief, and the failure to achieve it can lie with either or both parties. Patients' attitudes are a melange of their past and current experience with pain, cultural and religious teachings, the attitudes of family and friends, and their own personal values and coping mechanisms. As a result of one or more of these influences, many people feel they should be able to tolerate pain and are therefore ashamed to discuss the extent of their suffering with their physicians. Not wanting to be perceived as weak, they fail to receive adequate pain relief.

Another reason for poor communication between patients and caregivers is that pain has its own vocabulary, making it difficult for many people to accurately describe its quality, texture, and intensity. Is it sharp? Dull? Electric? Sporadic? Insistent? Moreover, the memory of pain is inexact. Between attacks of pain, people tend to forget about the level of intensity and other specifics. To compound the problem, some caregivers may not be sufficiently experienced at eliciting such crucial information from their patients.

For example, pain can be somatic (originating in the tissue, bones, or organs) or neuropathic (resulting from damage to, or pressure on, nerves)—or a combination of the two. Somatic pain is often described as "achy, dull, and localized" when it results from a broken bone associated with tumor involvement, or as "crampy and diffuse" when it results from an obstruction in the intestinal or urinary tract.

Neuropathic pain, on the other hand, is usually described as "sharp, burning, electrical, shooting, or buzzing." These sensations typically occur in areas served by the injured nerves, which can be either in peripheral nerves or the central nervous system. Such an injury can be caused by the direct spread of a tumor. For example, a colon cancer patient may have pain in the pelvis, where the nerves to the legs or pelvic structures reside. Pain also can be caused by pressure on nerves, as when spinal tumors pinch or press on nerves leading to the arms or legs. Other types of neuropathic dysfunction include hypersensitivity of the skin; an exaggerated, painful response to nerve stimuli (even a simple touch); and occasionally motor changes such as weakness or atrophy of an affected muscle group. Surgery, various chemotherapeutic drugs, and radiation treatment also can produce temporary side effects of somatic and/or neuropathic pain or discomfort.

Progressive Pain Relief Measures

In recommending palliative measures for pain, physicians use guidelines set forth by the World Health Organization (WHO), which include standard treatments for mild, moderate, and severe pain—sometimes given with adjuvant medications. For those who fail to benefit from these standard procedures, physicians can try one or more means of direct intervention. And, to augment all of these options, patients also can experiment with any of several methodologies that enlist the mind and emotions in reducing the stress that exacerbates pain.

World Health Organization Guidelines

An expert committee convened by WHO's Cancer Unit developed a "pain ladder" on a scale of one to ten to aid physicians in assessing the source, quality, and intensity of pain and determining the most appropriate relief measures. The goal is to keep the pain down to a level of less than four through continual reassessment of the cause of the problem and the effectiveness of the means of control. "Effectiveness" requires that a balance be maintained between the administration of any necessary increases in the strength of a medication and the production of toxic side effects, such as delirium, confusion, constipation, nausea or vomiting, allergies, or skin rashes.

Primary Pain Relief Measures

The following medications are recommended for different levels of pain, as determined by the pain ladder scale:

Mild pain: nonnarcotic medications, such as aspirin, acetaminophen (Tylenol), or other aspirin-like drugs—known as nonsteroidal anti-inflammatory drugs (NSAIDs).

Moderate pain: a combination of NSAIDs and weak narcotics, such as codeine, hydrocodone (Vicodin or Lortab), Percocet, Percodan, or propyxphene (Darvon).

Severe pain: strong opioids, such as morphine, Demerol, Dilaudid, fentanyl (Duragesic patches), or methadone in combination with an NSAID.

Adjuvant Medications

When the above medications do not achieve the desired results, the WHO guidelines suggest using an adjuvant (added) medication with either an opioid or nonopioid medication, as appropriate. In cases of mild-to-moderate pain where increased or more frequent doses of aspirin, Tylenol (with or without codeine), or ibuprofen have not succeeded, adjuvant medication can sometimes make the difference. Similarly, for pain that is not responsive to opioids, doctors have found that adjuvant medications such as steroids, anticonvulsant and antidepressant medications, antihistamines, and sedatives have been successful, even though they are not usually labeled for relief of pain. A few examples of adjuvant medications are given below.

Steroids, used in association with COX2 inhibitors such as Vioxx or Celebrex (selective anti-inflammatories) and opioids or other pain medications, can reduce pain. Steroids also can also counteract the loss of appetite and decrease the nausea that often accompanies chemotherapy and help patients with metastases to the bone, spine, brain, and liver by reducing swelling and pain.

Two tricyclic antidepressants, amitriptylene (Elavil) and nortriptylene (Pamelor), can help reduce pain with hepatic and bone metastases, and decrease the severity of headaches from cancer.

Some selective serotonin re-uptake inhibitors (SSRIs), such as Effexor, which help control depression as well as pain, are replacing the tricyclics. SSRIs have fewer side effects than the tricyclics and can help counteract the sedative effects of opioids.

Anticonvulsants such as carbamazepine (Tegretol), phenytoin (Dilantin), and gabapentin (Neurontin) also can also play a role in pain relief. Carbamazepine can be helpful to patients with diabetic neuropathy or cancer neuritis; and 100 mg of gabapentin three times a day will not only ease pain but can help restore normal sleep patterns, even for those on anti-inflammatory agents and physical modalities, such as heat, ultrasound, or massage.

The benzodiazepines—diazepam (Valium) and lorazepam (Ativan)—decrease anxiety.

Radiation is also used for control of local pain, especially bone pain. In low doses, it can provide excellent palliative care for many lesions by shrinking them. Often, five to eight treatments are all that are needed to achieve quick and—for many people—prolonged effects.

Other Pain Relief Options

For the 5–10 percent of patients who do not receive adequate pain control under WHO's guidelines, there are other options. By means of direct intervention, pain specialists can prevent pain stimuli from reaching the central nervous system. Such interventions include the implementation of nerve blocks with a local anesthetic

(Novocaine or Xylocaine) or with nerve-destroying agents; the use of alternative delivery systems, such as the administration of opioids and other drugs subcutaneously or into the spine; or the use of a local spinal anesthetic. Transcutaneous electrical nerve stimulation (TENS) is also effective, as is ultrasonic stimulation.

Many people find that the ancient arts of acupuncture and acupressure, or the application of heat and cold compresses, can relieve pain. Exercise helps maintain strength and flexibility, which actually changes muscle cells so they are less sensitive to pain.

Harnessing the Mind and Emotions to Aid in Pain Relief

Anxiety, fear, and loneliness increase stress and heighten the experience of pain. Therefore, any means by which patients can limit the power of these emotions also decreases the amount of drugs required for pain control. Biofeedback, psychotherapy, family counseling, and listening to music have helped many people.

Biofeedback teaches patients how to manipulate unconscious bodily processes, such as heartbeats or brain waves, to gain ascendancy over the negative effects of stress.

Psychotherapy can provide patients with a sounding board, as well as insight into—and tools for dealing with—depression, anger, and fear.

Family counseling (with a professional counselor or a member of the clergy) allows patients and family members to talk openly about the tensions of living with cancer.

Listening to music not only provides relaxation and raises spirits, but it has proven to have an analgesic (painkilling) effect twice that of a plain background sound.

Summary

To achieve optimum pain control, patients need to be able to articulate the quality and intensity of their pain, and to understand that doctors are not mind readers. Caregivers need to sharpen their assesment skills. Both patients and caregivers need to stay abreast of available treatments, their side effects, and their appropriate uses. Finally, successful pain control requires an individually tailored program of appropriate drugs, auxillary or alternate therapies, and stress-reduction techniques—consistently monitored and reevaluated by all concerned.

10

Cancer-Related Fatigue

Barbara F. Piper, D.N.Sc., R.N.,
A.O.C.N., F.A.A.N.
Pat Kramer, M.S.N., R.N., A.O.C.N.

What Is Cancer-Related Fatigue?

Cancer-related fatigue is the most common and distressing side effect of cancer and its treatments. Fatigue associated with cancer treatments (known as cancer treatment–related fatigue) occurs in approximately 70–100 percent of cancer patients receiving anticancer therapies such as surgery, chemotherapy, radiation therapy, biological response modifier therapy (biotherapy), hormonal therapy, and bone marrow or peripheral stem cell transplants. When therapies are combined (i.e., combination or multimodal therapy), the incidence and severity of fatigue may be increased. Cancer-related fatigue may be more prevalent and severe in patients who have more extensive disease or who have metastatic or recurrent disease. It is reported to be a continuing problem for many cancer survivors, as well. They no longer receive therapy but still experience unusual fatigue; and they have not been able to return to their prediagnosis or baseline energy levels, months or years following treatment cessation.

Fatigue—like pain—is a very subjective experience. This means that the best person to describe the fatigue is the individual who is actually experiencing it. Patients have described their fatigue as a sense of overwhelming or unusual whole-body tiredness not easily relieved by a good night's sleep or by rest. Other words commonly used by patients to describe their fatigue include being weary; having no energy; feeling worn-out, drained, listless, and exhausted; being "bone-tired"; feeling heavy; or feeling like they're standing in "wet cement."

Research has shown that this fatigue, which is a side effect of cancer or its treatment, is very different from the universal sensation of tiredness that everyone has experienced. Cancer-related fatigue has been defined as an unusually persistent subjective sense of tiredness that interferes with usual functioning. Over time, this unusual sense of fatigue can lead to a decline in physical functioning and a diminished quality of life. As a consequence, it can negatively affect every aspect of someone's quality of life—their sense of personal well-being, their ability to work or perform daily activities, their ability to socialize with family and friends, and their ability to maintain hope and enjoy life.

As fatigue begins to change what cancer patients can do for themselves, family members and caregivers often begin to assume many of the roles previously performed by the patient. These increased role demands can lead to fatigue in family members and caregivers and may contribute further to the social isolation that is often experienced by patients and their families.

Patients who have been asked to describe their fatigue in research studies uniformly state that fatigue is the most frequent and distressing symptom they have experienced with cancer and its therapies. It is more distressing than the symptoms of pain, nausea, or vomiting. Despite this, fatigue remains an underreported, underdiagnosed, and undertreated symptom. Why is this?

There are several communication barriers that may exist between patients and healthcare providers that contribute to this problem. For example, patients may not want to "bother" the healthcare provider with complaints of fatigue, as patients may assume that they should just "learn to live with it," that nothing can be done, and that it is a natural consequence of their treatment or disease. Patients may become worried that their treatment may be stopped or their dosages reduced if they report their fatigue to their providers. Last, patients themselves may not be completely aware of just how much their functioning has been negatively affected by their fatigue, so they can't report it to their providers. Often family members and caregivers may be more cognizant of these changes than is the patient.

From the healthcare provider's standpoint, there are communication barriers as well. The provider may not question the patient about the presence or absence of fatigue because the provider may not recognize that it is a problem for the patient. The provider may believe that pain is the most prevalent and distressing symptom that needs to be assessed and so may neglect to assess fatigue. In addition, fatigue is still not being included routinely on documentation or medical record forms that can serve as reminders to the provider that it needs to be addressed at each and every patient encounter or visit. Last, providers may not be comfortable in bringing up the subject of fatigue themselves, particularly if they are unsure of what is causing the fatigue or how to treat it.

Despite these barriers, it is important to recognize that patients and family members are not powerless against fatigue. Research into cancer-related fatigue is beginning to identify several effective therapies that can manage and dissipate fatigue when it does occur. Patients also have shared strategies and tips that they have found work to combat their fatigue. Many of these patient-initiated strategies—such as conserving energy—are now beginning to undergo testing in clinical trials. The goal of this chapter is to provide the most current information about fatigue and to discuss assessment and management strategies that patients and families can use to deal with this distressing side effect of cancer treatment.

What Causes Fatigue?

No one knows exactly why people with cancer experience this unusual sense of tiredness that leads to decreased functioning. It is known, however, that a number of factors may work individually or in combination with each other to cause fatigue.

The Disease Itself

Cancer itself can contribute to fatigue both through its direct and indirect effects on the body. Cancer can directly affect various organ systems, particularly when breast or colon cancer invades the liver, or when ovarian or colon cancer causes a bowel obstruction that results in pain, nausea, and/or vomiting. Cancer can contribute to fatigue through its indirect effects on slowing the metabolism, and possibly through the release of substances such as cytokines may contribute to fatigue. Cytokines are natural cell products or proteins, such as the interferons and interleukins, that are normally released by white blood cells, lymphocytes, and macrophages in response to infection or inflammation. These cytokines carry messages that regulate other cells of the immune and neuroendocrine systems. In high amounts, these cytokines can be toxic and can lead to persistent fatigue, disturbances in metabolism, loss of appetite, and weight loss.

Because cancer is a chronic disease, anemia is quite common. This "anemia of chronic disease" can lead to a decreased number of red blood cells and a decrease in the oxygen-carrying capacity of the blood. This, too, can cause fatigue. As the disease responds to treatment, fatigue may improve.

Metabolic Changes

Changes in metabolism or energy production, and the lack of available nutrients, may cause fatigue in cancer patients. In these instances, a referral to a dietician or nutritionist knowledgeable about cancer can help. Changes in metabolism can result from:

- The tumor itself. A tumor may make the body function in an overactive or hypermetabolic state. Tumor cells compete for nutrients, often at the expense of the normal cells' growth and metabolism. The result is weight loss, lack of appetite, and fatigue.
- Increased demands on the patient's body. With cancer treatment, much of the body's available energy supply is claimed to heal surgical incisions or to replace healthy cells damaged in treatment. This increased demand for energy may exceed the supply of available energy stores and nutrients. This can lead to weight loss, fatigue, and depletion of energy reserves. Thus, if the individual already is feeling drained and exhausted just attempting to meet the body's basic metabolic needs, there is no extra energy available for the individual to expend elsewhere.
- Impaired or inadequate nutrition. Insufficient nutrition can contribute to fatigue, particularly in circumstances where a hypermetabolic state exists, or energy demands exceed energy supplies.

Toxic Waste

As cancer cells die in response to treatment, the body tries to rid itself of toxic waste products from cell metabolism and breakdown. If these waste products are not excreted, there can be an accumulation of toxic metabolic waste. This is why hydration (drinking eight to ten eight-ounce glasses of water per day) often is recommended.

Cancer Treatments

Cancer treatments can contribute to fatigue. Through clinical research, different patterns associated with specific forms of treatment are beginning to emerge. Despite the patterns previously exhibited by other patients, it is important to remember that every patient has an individual experience. Being forewarned about these anticipated patterns of fatigue could help the patient report initial symptoms of fatigue before it becomes too severe.

Surgery. Fatigue in cancer patients undergoing surgery has not been well studied. Anxiety and worry about the possible diagnosis and fears about surgery itself can produce fatigue preoperatively, as can the type and number of diagnostic tests required. Pain, disruption in sleep, anesthesia, medications, lack of adequate nutrition, and the increased energy needed for healing wounds can contribute to fatigue postoperatively. Symptoms of fatigue can continue for some patients, depending on the type and extent of the surgery, for as long as three or more months following surgery.

Chemotherapy. Chemotherapy is associated with fatigue in approximately 80–96 percent of cancer patients. Typically, the most severe fatigue occurs during the twenty-four to seventy-two hours immediately following chemotherapy administration, although this pattern may vary with the type of agent used and the way in which it is administered (e.g., orally or intravenously, by IV push, or by twenty-four-hour continuous infusion). Fatigue during this time is thought to be due primarily to the antinausea and vomiting medications that are prescribed, and the acute inflammatory cellular effects triggered by the chemotherapy. The person may go to bed feeling "fine" and wake up the next morning feeling as though he or she has been run over by a truck. This can be a very frightening experience, particularly for the individual who has not been forewarned. Over the next several days and/or weeks, the person's levels of fatigue and energy will usually begin to improve. This pattern repeats itself with subsequent chemotherapy cycles, although each cycle may vary somewhat.

In women with early stage breast cancer receiving Adriamycin-Cytoxan–containing regimens, fatigue may gradually become worse during the third treatment cycle. This is thought to be due to the gradually accumulating decreases in daytime activity patterns and increased disruptions in nighttime sleeping patterns observed in these women. In addition, certain chemotherapy drugs such as vincristine or vinblastine can be associated with increased levels of fatigue because of their effects on nerves (neurotoxicity). Other drugs, such as cisplatin, can affect the kidneys and interfere with the production of a hormone produced by the kidneys called erythropoietin. This hormone stimulates red blood cell production, and anemia can result if its production is affected. Cisplatin can produce low magnesium levels and this can cause fatigue.

Radiation Therapy. Radiation therapy is associated with fatigue in 50–100 percent of patients. The pattern of fatigue in radiation therapy is strikingly different than that noted in chemotherapy patients. Patients usually begin to notice an ever-increasing level of fatigue by the end of week two, or the beginning of week three, of treatment. Severity of fatigue may gradually increase as the weeks of radiation therapy continue. Fatigue may peak and plateau during the fourth to sixth week of treatment in some patients or may continue to rise until the end of treatment in others. It is important to recognize that as this fatigue increases over time, patients may feel worse rather than better, and may begin to worry unnecessarily that the treatment isn't working or that their cancer isn't responding to treatment. Fatigue associated with radiation therapy has been known to continue in some patients for one to three months, or longer, following treatment cessation.

Biotherapy (e.g., interferon, interleukin). These treatments are associated with significant fatigue, because they are external cytokines that produce side effects comparable to when internal cytokines are released within the body in response to infection or inflammation. Fatigue associated with biotherapy gradually increases over the course and duration of treatment (cumulative fatigue) and gradually gets worse as the total dose of the biological response modifier increases. Changes in treatment dosages or schedules may become necessary because of this fatigue.

Transplants. Fatigue has not been well studied in patients receiving bone marrow or stem cell transplants. In the few studies that have been done, patients describe the fatigue that they experience during transplant as being more severe than the fatigue experienced during other forms of cancer therapy.

Hormonal Therapies. Very few studies have addressed fatigue in hormonally treated cancer patients, although it has been reported to be experienced by patients on Tamoxifen and on other hormone therapies. Changes in hormone levels can occur in both men and women as a result of cancer treatment and hormone therapies. Hot flashes in these instances can be common in both genders and can disrupt sleep and cause fatigue.

Combination Therapies. When cancer therapies are combined, such as when surgery is combined with radiation therapy and/or chemotherapy, fatigue may increase, both in terms of the number of patients affected and its severity.

Complications and Side Effects

Complications of the disease and its treatments can cause fatigue. For example, electrolyte or chemical imbalances can occur that can cause fatigue. Dehydration, infection, and anemia are associated with fatigue. Research has shown that as the actual number and/or intensity of symptoms other than fatigue increase, so too does the frequency and intensity of fatigue increase. Symptoms that frequently "cluster" or occur with fatigue include insomnia (difficulty falling asleep and staying asleep, and premature awakening) and pain. Other symptoms, such as nausea or vomiting, shortness of breath, or difficulty breathing (dyspnea), can cause fatigue. Treatment directed toward treating these symptoms may result in decreased fatigue.

Anemia. Anemia is a frequent side effect of cancer treatment and has been shown to contribute directly to fatigue. Anemia occurs when there is a shortage of red blood cells (RBCs) produced by the body (shown as a decrease in the hematocrit level) or a decrease in the oxygen-carrying capacity of the blood (shown as a decrease in the hemoglobin level).

Red blood cells carry oxygen on the hemoglobin molecule of the red blood cell from the lungs to other tissues and organs in the body. When there are not enough red blood cells or the hemoglobin is too low to transport this needed oxygen, symptoms such as fatigue, weakness, dizziness, shortness of breath, chest pain, and decreased ability to perform activities or exercise can result. Anemia that results from chemotherapy or from the "anemia of chronic disease" can be treated with medication (Procrit or Epogen) in most instances. In clinical trials, when anemia was corrected with this medication, patients reported improvements in energy and activity levels and quality of life. Treatment should be started before anemia becomes too severe. Research suggests that treatment should be initiated when hemoglobin levels are between 10–11g/dl. The goal of treatment is to achieve and maintain a hemoglobin of approximately 12g/dl. Iron supplementation may be prescribed while patients are receiving this medication. Blood transfusions also can treat anemia, but they are indicated most often only as a temporary emergency measure when severe anemia needs immediate correction.

Immobility and Inactivity. Immobility, prolonged bed rest, unnecessary inactivity, and too much rest all can contribute to fatigue by causing decreased muscle strength and endurance. Muscles that are not exercised lose their ability to use oxygen efficiently, so more effort and more oxygen are required for the same amount of work performed by conditioned muscles. This is one of the reasons why exercise is often prescribed for patients and family members.

Insomnia. Difficulty falling asleep and staying asleep, and premature awakenings (insomnia) can cause fatigue. This can lead to increased sleepiness, increased daytime napping, and even more fatigue. Using relaxation techniques, sleep aids, and/or sleep medications may help to promote sleep and decrease fatigue.

Emotional Distress. Fear, anxiety, worry, and depression (emotional distress) can contribute to insomnia, create an increased energy demand, and contribute to fatigue.

Other Illnesses or Comorbidities. Research has shown that as the number of illnesses other than cancer increase in cancer patients, so too can fatigue. Such comorbidities might include hypertension (high blood pressure), low thyroid levels, and other illnesses. Often, the health care provider can reevaluate the current status and treatment of these comorbidities in order to decrease fatigue.

Concurrent Medications. Many over-the-counter and prescription medications can contribute to fatigue. Health care providers often can suggest changes in these medications and/or their dosages, which can have a positive effect on reducing fatigue.

Summary

The best way to manage fatigue is always to treat the underlying cause(s) of fatigue. Unfortunately, because of the number of factors that can be involved alone or in combination with one another, it may take some time to diagnose what the primary cause is and to determine the best form of treatment. In most cancer patients, fatigue is commonly associated with one of the following five factors: pain, insomnia, emotional distress, anemia, and low thyroid levels. Treatment directed toward alleviating these factors, if present, should be tried first and may relieve fatigue.

If, on the other hand, none of these five factors is present and the patient has fatigue, a further medical work-up is needed to determine the underlying cause. While medical science still has a lot to learn about what the underlying mechanisms are that cause fatigue in cancer patients, it is now known that fatigue should not be considered an inevitable part of the cancer experience that must be endured by patients and family members. Even when it is not possible to completely eliminate fatigue, medical treatments and lifestyle changes can help decrease the intensity of fatigue and minimize its negative quality of life effects.

Hints on How to Personally Manage Fatigue

View Fatigue as a Very Important Symptom to Report

Fatigue has been called the "sixth vital sign" (following temperature, pulse, respiration, blood pressure, and pain) by some health care providers because of its importance in functioning, quality of life, and disease. You need to view fatigue as being this important to you, too, and discuss it with your doctor and nurse, even if you have to be the first one to bring up the subject.

Explain how the fatigue feels to you and how it affects your ability to do the things that you want to do. The more attention you bring to fatigue, the more likely it will be evaluated by your provider within the context of your individual circumstances and be managed with appropriate treatment, referrals, and recommendations.

If you are not experiencing fatigue currently, or if it is at a mild level and is not interfering with your activities, that's great! Keep it up, but remember to report it right away if it should either increase in severity or if it begins to become a problem for you.

If you experience moderate or severe fatigue, however, (four or more on a ten-point fatigue scale), or if it is beginning to interfere with your activities, make sure your doctor or nurse knows about this promptly so that a more complete fatigue assessment and determination of what may be causing your fatigue can be performed.

Remember that managing fatigue requires a team effort. This means that you, your family, and your health care provider(s) must work *together* to communicate better about fatigue and determine the effectiveness of the treatment(s) prescribed so that your fatigue doesn't go underreported, underdiagnosed, or undertreated.

Maintain Some Form of Daily Exercise

Frequently, when patients complain of fatigue, they are told to rest more by well-intentioned friends and health care providers. Unfortunately, too much rest and inactivity can contribute to an ever-increasing downward spiral of decreased activity, increased fatigue, weakness, and loss of muscle tone.

Exercise can promote more efficient use of oxygen and production of energy. It can tone and strengthen muscles; improve strength, endurance, and stamina; and promote feelings of well-being. Talk to your physician, nurse, or physical therapist as to what form of exercise may be right and safe for you.

Try to adhere to some form of individually tailored exercise program approved by your health care provider. Walking is an activity that most patients can do. It is aerobic (i.e., uses and generates oxygen) and when performed three to five times per week has shown to decrease fatigue and emotional distress, decrease symptoms such as nausea and insomnia, and stabilize weight gain in women with early stage breast cancer for whom weight gain may be a problem.

Light exercise such as stretching, yoga, or tai chi also may help you feel more energetic.

Avoid exercise if you have a fever, have low blood counts, or have disease in your bones that might increase your risk for disease-related fractures. In such cases, consult with your health care provider.

If you should experience increased fatigue the following day after exercising, it may indicate that you have overdone your exercise, or that something else is going on that may need to be evaluated by your health care provider.

Use Your Energy Wisely

Learn to use your energy wisely. At times when your energy is limited, you must decide how you will use your available energy. Think about your energy stores as a "bank." You need to make deposits and withdrawals over the course of the day and over the week to insure a balance between activity and rest and energy conservation, restoration, and expenditure.

Keep a diary for one week to identify the time of day and the time of week when you have the most fatigue or have the most energy. Plan your activities accordingly.

Plan each day and prioritize what needs to be done. Make a list of the activities that you want to do. Schedule these activities ahead of time and according to when you have learned you will have the most energy to do them and still avoid becoming unusually tired.

Set realistic goals and avoid overloading yourself. Listen to your body. Try to find a good balance between activity and rest. Too much activity or too much rest can increase fatigue. Balance is essential.

Select those activities that are most important for you to do and that give you the most pleasure. Give yourself permission to do these activities first. For all other activities, delegate them to others or let them go.

Learn to feel less guilty about restructuring your life to do those things that are most important and pleasurable for you. Begin to cultivate the fine art of delegation as this may enable others to feel as though they are able to be of more help to you rather than perceive it as a burden.

Plan adequate rest periods between activities so that you can recover your energy before undertaking more activities. This is called "pacing" your activities. Research has shown that taking several short rest periods works better than taking one long rest period.

If you are continuing to work, talk to your employer about flexible schedules or modified responsibilities. Know your rights as an employee.

Apply Energy Conservation Techniques in Your Daily Activities

Organize your chores to promote efficiency and minimize unnecessary steps. For example, plan your day to limit the number of times you need to walk upstairs. Make grocery or shopping lists to minimize unnecessary walking and consider having someone deliver them to your home. Sit when preparing foods or getting dressed. Have someone drive you door-to-door if needed.

Use equipment aids that decrease unnecessary energy expenditure. For example, use electric carts available in supermarkets and retail stores; use ramps rather than stairs; use grooming and bathing aids (long-handled sponges or hairbrushes); and use wheeled walkers, canes, or electric wheelchairs, if needed, so that you have the energy to expend on other, more important activities. For meals, use frozen or prepackaged foods, and prepare double portions and freeze half for future use. Simplify cooking whenever possible.

Report Other Symptoms Promptly

As symptoms other than fatigue can be experienced and can make fatigue worse if left untreated, be sure to report these symptoms to your health care provider so that they can be properly assessed and managed. These symptoms might include pain, nausea, vomiting, diarrhea, constipation, shortness of breath, and weakness.

Your health care provider may initiate referrals to other health team members to better control your symptoms and to individually tailor your exercise program. These referrals might include consultations with a clinical pharmacist to decide on the most effective medication and its dosage; a physical therapist for range-of-motion and strength training; an occupational therapist for energy conservation; a dietician for nutritional support; and a medical social worker, psychologist, or psychiatrist for psychological counseling; plus support groups and information about other forms of support.

Maintain Adequate Nutrition and Hydration

Drink at least eight to ten eight-ounce glasses of liquids a day to maintain adequate hydration and to facilitate elimination of waste products.

Eat a nutritious and balanced diet that includes adequate amounts of calories, proteins, fats, vitamins, and complex carbohydrates (grains and vegetables) to give you more sustained sources of energy to meet the increased energy demands on your body. Consult with a dietitian to learn how to maximize your nutritional intake.

Maintain an Effective Sleep Pattern

Sleep often can be disrupted as you begin to cope with your cancer diagnosis, and as you go through and recover from your treatment(s). It's important that you adhere to or reestablish usual bedtime rituals that may help you fall asleep quickly, enable you to stay asleep, and avoid unusual early morning awakenings.

Sleep research has shown that consistently going to bed and awakening at the same time of day, and using your bed primarily for sleeping rather than for other activities, such as reading or eating, all contribute to promoting a good quality of sleep.

Sleep-enhancing aids and sleep medications may be helpful at certain times during your illness and treatment. Talk to your health care provider(s) if you are not sleeping well.

Take Care of Yourself Emotionally as Well as Physically

Coping with cancer and cancer treatments can be difficult, especially when fatigue becomes part of that experience. Joining a cancer support group can provide you with the kind of support that only people who are going through a similar experience can provide. A support group also can widen your social support network and enable you to learn tips for managing fatigue and other side effects. Research has shown that for women with breast cancer, consistently attending a support group over a period of time has resulted in less fatigue. Ask your provider or medical social worker to recommend a support group in your community.

Ask about resources, such as complementary medicine approaches, that can help to decrease stress and promote feelings of well being. Art, music, meditation, visual imagery, deep breathing, biofeedback, and light massage are just a few examples of strategies that other patients have said help to reduce stress.

Empower yourself through education. Ask questions. Take advantage of resources that are free and easily available (American Cancer Society, National Cancer Institute, Oncology Nursing Society's National Cancer Fatigue Awareness Day Materials & Resources, etc.).

Use Distraction and Energy-Restoring Activities

Use distraction techniques to focus on things other than fatigue, disease, or your treatment. Listen to music, visit with friends, watch television, go to the movies, and enjoy walks in the natural environment.

Focus on "restorative" activities that can improve or restore your emotional energy. These activities might involve a change in your routine to avoid boredom and doing things that catch your interest easily and are pleasurable to do. Research has shown that doing something that involves the natural environment— such as observing the trees changing colors in the fall; watching fish swim in an aquarium; being near water; or doing something creative such as drawing, writing, or pursuing a hobby—can reduce the symptoms of mental fatigue, such as difficulty in concentrating or directing attention, that many patients experience.

Contract with yourself to do these types of activities three times a week for at least thirty minutes at a time. Remember that your mind, heart, and spirit need exercising, too!

Final Tips:

- Learn as much as you can about fatigue to help yourself.
- Learn to recognize symptoms of fatigue.
- Report your fatigue to your health care providers.
- Ask for ideas to manage fatigue.
- Try these suggestions and let your health care providers know what works and what doesn't.

Resources on the Internet

- www.cancersupportivecare.com
- www.cancerfatigue.org
- www.cancercareinc.org
- cancernet.nci.hih.gov
- www.cancerhopenetwork.org
- oncolink.upenn.edu
- www.nccn.org

11

Lymphedema

John P. Cooko, M.D., Ph.D.
Andrzej Szuba, M.D.

Lymphedema is a swelling caused by a buildup of fluid (lymph) in the soft tissues of the limbs. It rarely occurs in other parts of the body (head, trunk). This buildup often occurs after surgical removal of lymph nodes, after radiotherapy to lymph nodes (because of blockage of the lymphatic system), and sometimes after chemotherapy. It occurs often after infections and sometimes may occur without an identified cause. In rare cases, lymphedema may be caused by a genetic abnormality (mutation) and multiple family members may be affected. Gaps in our understanding of lymphedema have limited treatment of it, but recent advances in genetic studies and imaging—X rays, scans, ultrasound, lymphoscintigraphy—as well as insights gained from physiologic studies, hold promise of a more definitive therapy.

Lymphedema is usually a chronic problem and it may be permanent. Where cancer is involved, lymphedema is most often seen after breast surgery and/or radiotherapy (15–30 percent of women after breast cancer treatment may develop lymphedema), however it may occur in connection with almost any other malignancy (like malignant melanoma; ovarian, cervical, testicular, or prostate cancer; and others). In lymphedema related to cancer treatment, it is surgical lymph-node dissection and radiotherapy that causes damage to the lymphatic system.

Chronic lymphedema may result in minor swelling and discomfort. Occasionally, it leads to a grave disability and disfigurement. If you have had surgery and/or radiation therapy for cancer, you might be at risk of lymphedema. To prevent lymphedema you should:

- avoid limb injuries, especially cuts and bruises;
- keep your skin lubricated with creams or oils;
- protect your fingers—for example, wear gloves to avoid injury when gardening or doing manual work;
- avoid cutting your cuticles and use extra care when cutting your nails;
- shave the affect limb with an electric razor rather than a blade;
- avoid the use of blood pressure cuffs on or injections in a limb with lymphedema;

- take care of cuts or injuries to the limbs immediately and see your physicians if you have any questions; and
- avoid heavy lifting.

Emotional problems associated with lymphedema are not uncommon and are often neglected by physicians. The need to address the psychological aspects of long-term disfigurement, especially with adolescent patients, cannot be overemphasized. In discussing these issues with the patient, the physicians should be realistic about the possibility of progression, but also should emphasize the patient's ability to modify the course of lymphedema by careful attention to the details of the medical program.

Some patients become sedentary in response to uncomfortable or heavy sensations in the affected limb. Reduced physical activity at work and at home leads to apathy and malaise; these can be avoided by encouraging physical activity with proper support hose. Regular exercise appears to reduce lymphedema as long as elastic support hose (or hydrostatic pressure) is applied. Swimming is a particularly good activity because the surrounding hydrostatic pressure of the water means compressive support isn't needed.

Elastic support hose should be fitted to the patient's limb after the edema has been reduced as much as possible by compression and elevation. This is important, because the stocking does not reduce the size of the leg but only maintains the circumference to which it is fitted.

Decongestive lymphatic therapy is a proven and safe technique to reduce lymphatic swelling. It consists of manual lymphatic massage, compressive bandaging, and decongestive exercises. It usually takes several days to achieve significant reduction in volume. After edema is sufficiently reduced, the arm or leg is fitted for a compressive garment that should be used daily. Self-applied manual lymphatic massage is also recommended for better control of lymphedema. Pneumatic compression pumps might be used in conjunction with or separately from massage to reduce, or at least maintain, arm or leg volume.

To maintain the reduction of limb volume, patients have to wear compressive garments. This is particularly important during airplane flights and exercises. Self-applied massage is also recommended. Many patients benefit from use of pneumatic compression pumps or other devices like the Reid sleeve.

The affected limb is more prone to infections (cellulitis). Infection may begin suddenly and progress rapidly. Oral antibiotics usually can cure such an infection, but in severe cases, hospitalization for IV antibiotics might be necessary.

The following precautions will help you to avoid infections if you have lymphedema:

- Keep your skin meticulously clean and moisturize daily using skin creams (e.g., Eucerin.).
- Avoid injuries, cuts, and animal scratches.
- Clean small wounds with warm soapy water and apply antibiotic ointment under your bandage.
- Contact your physician if you notice redness, pain, or increased swelling.
- Avoid wearing jewelry on affected arm or leg.
- Avoid heavy lifting.
- Use an electric razor rather than a blade for shaving the affected limb.

Decongestive Lymphatic Therapy

Special physiotherapy is an effective way to treat extremity lymphedema. Several variants of this treatment have been developed in different centers. Vodder, Foldi, and Casley-Smith are among the pioneers of physiotherapy treatments for lymphedema; their schools provide training for physiotherapists around the world. Principles of physiotherapy for lymphedema were outlined in the *Consensus Document* of the International Society of Lymphology. Physiotherapy treatment of lymphedema has four key elements: (1) manual lymphatic drainage—a special type of light massage that stimulates function of the lymphatic system and increases lymphatic flow; (2) compressive bandaging—multilayered wrapping with low-stretch bandages that provide gradient compression of the arm or leg; (3) decongestive exercises—special exercises designed to alleviate edema; and (4) meticulous skin care—to avoid skin infections.

Typical treatment starts with manual lymphatic massage (usually twenty to sixty minutes). Massage is first applied to the opposite quadrant of the trunk, then to the root of the affected extremity, and finally to the distal part of the limb. Multilayer compressive bandaging follows the massage. Low-stretch bandages are applied to the whole extremity, including fingers and/or toes. Proper wrapping of bandages provides gradual compression, with the highest pressure applied distally, and a lower pressure applied at the root of the limb. The pressure from bandages should not be too high, because there is a small risk of arterial or nerve compression.

Decongestive exercises are specially designed to help evacuate lymphatic fluid. Exercises are performed with bandages or with the compression garment worn. Bandages are worn overnight until the next session of massage. It is important to use proper low-stretch bandages for wrapping. *High-stretch bandages (like ACE wraps) are inappropriate for treatment of lymphedema and pose more risks (like worsening of edema or compromising circulation in arm or leg).* Meticulous skin care is necessary to prevent skin breaks and subsequent infections.

Massage sessions are performed once or twice daily for a period sufficient to maximally reduce edema of the limb. This may vary between one to six, or more, weeks. At the time of therapy, patients and/or their families are taught techniques of massage self-care, which includes self-applied lymphatic massage, bandaging, and exercises. After acute decongestive lymphatic therapy, patients are fitted for gradient, compressive garments, which should be worn daily.

Decongestive lymphatic therapy (decongestive physiotherapy, complex decongestive therapy, or manual lymphatic therapy) is a proven and effective way to treat lymphedema, with a reported edema reduction of 40–90 percent, after intensive treatment.

12

Alternative and Complementary Therapies
Acupuncture, Biofeedback, and Hypnosis

Barrie R. Cassileth, Ph.D.
Brenda Golianu, M.D.
Ian E. Wickramasekera, Ph.D.
David Spiegel, M.D.

A striking characteristic of "alternative" medicine throughout the twentieth century is its inconsistency. During the early decades of the century, all-purpose health tonics and a variety of "cancer cures" were widely available, sold from town to town in horse-drawn wagons, in stores, and through newspaper ads. "Energy" cancer cures, reflecting the growing capability and interest in radio waves, predominated during the 1920s. Competing mainstream therapies for cancer at the time included surgery, which had been used to remove tumors for many centuries, and radiation therapy, which had been discovered around the turn of the century. When chemotherapy was first developed following World War II, popular alternatives included Koch's Glyoxylide and then Hoxsey's Cancer Cure. Dr. Ivy's Krebiozen predominated during the 1960s, and Laetrile achieved prominence in the 1970s.

These popular, unproved therapies were given many names, including "unorthodox," "questionable," and "fraudulent." They were attacked as quackery, said to be doing more harm than good, and seen as robbing people of their money in exchange for worthless potions.

During the next decade, a new collection of unconventional approaches emerged. A return to the nineteenth century emphasis on self-care occurred in the form of an angry backlash against an increasingly technologic, specialized, and proficient medical system. Although medicine cured more illnesses than ever, the system was said to be impersonal, and focused on disease rather than on the patient. It was criticized for lacking a "holistic" emphasis (treating the whole person), and for failing to care for the individual as a social and spiritual being. This movement occurred for medicine in general, including specialties such as oncology.

Starting gradually around this time, unproved or unorthodox medicine took on a different and broader meaning. It incorporated not only regimens and therapies promoted outside of mainstream medicine but also many approaches concerned with people's emotional and spiritual life. The resurgence of self-care meant that folk remedies and the family's favorite home treatments belonged under the newly popular umbrella term "alternative," along with the old unproved, unorthodox methods and the soothing efforts aimed at the person behind the disease.

The Confusion of Terminology

The space under the "alternative" umbrella became crowded, filled as it was with a large collection of disparate healing products and techniques. "Alternative medicine" also became home to the views of new, as well as existing, extremist groups. These individuals and organizations claimed and continue to believe that a conspiracy-ridden medical establishment deliberately withholds "cures," which they defined as the treatments they offered commercially, despite the absence of scientific evidence that they work. The reason is economic, they say: if major serious illnesses such as cancer were abolished, the medical establishment, the National Institutes of Health, the American Cancer Society, and all the other groups involved in medical care would be out of business.

On several grounds—including the fact that health care professionals and advocates are no more immune to cancer and other serious illnesses than are other members of the general public—that contention seems far from rational or believable. Nonetheless, it persists as a no-longer-covert theme among radical believers.

At the other extreme of the continuum of therapies under the "alternative" umbrella, we see an assortment of approaches and techniques aimed not at curing a major disease but at reducing symptoms and enhancing quality of life. These techniques are used to sustain good health, as well as to lessen the symptoms of serious illness. These include spiritual, psychological, social, and physical approaches, as well as remedies contained in bottles or capsules. They are typically called complementary therapies in Europe and other parts of the world. In North America, we still use the term *alternative*, or sometimes *alternative and complementary*.

These general terms are unfortunate, because they mask crucial differences among very varied approaches: helpful, noninvasive therapies; unproven, harmful treatments; useless time- and money-wasters; and foolish and fraudulent methods. It is virtually impossible to judge whether one approves of alternative therapies without asking, "Which ones?"

To bring some clarity to this dissimilar collection of therapeutic techniques, it is helpful to look at the promoted purpose of a method and, thereby, separate "alternative" from "complementary" therapies. The former category includes treatments recommended for use instead of mainstream care. These therapies are literally sold as "alternatives" to conventional medicine.

Complementary therapies, in contrast and as the term literally implies, serve a supplementary role. Complementary therapies accompany mainstream treatment or are used as part of wellness and health-maintenance programs. They include regimens that are part of preventive medicine and supportive care. In distinction to alternatives, they tend to be noninvasive, inexpensive, and widely helpful.

Admittedly, this is a simplistic and imperfect differentiation. How and when a remedy is applied, as much as what the remedy is, can categorize it as complementary and appropriate or as alternative and potentially dangerous. Thus, some therapies would be considered "alternative" under a particular circumstance and "complementary" under another. Aromatherapy is an example of how a single regimen can be either alternative or complementary, depending on how it is promoted or used. As a soothing fragrance in the bath or during massage, aromatherapy can be pleasant and calming. However, some books and advocates claim that aromatherapy can cure disease, and its use for that alternative purpose could be harmful by delaying needed standard medical treatment. In other examples, a relaxation program known to lower anxiety becomes alternative when it is applied to cure disease rather than used as an adjunct to conventional medical treatment. Mainstream chemotherapy drugs become alternative when used in dosages that exceed or fail to meet accepted standards.

Current Acceptance of Complementary Therapies

The idea of separating alternative from complementary medicine, despite its occasional drawbacks, is generally useful. Further, the apparent change of attitude among patients, the public, doctors, and other health care providers toward the use of unconventional methods is due in large measure to the inclusion of complementary therapies under the "alternative" title. When reference is made to "alternative" approaches, frequently the therapy under discussion is actually "complementary."

The growing acceptance of complementary therapies today is evidenced in many ways, including the broad availability of information to the general public through every means of communication, including the Internet. Complementary and alternative medicine

(CAM) therapies represent an international phenomenon. They abound not only in North America, but also in Europe, Australia, and Asia.

Unconventional medicine has made unprecedented inroads into the major institutions of mainstream medicine: medical schools, academic medical research centers, peer-reviewed medical literature, insurance companies coverage, and federal government research. Many countries and institutions have developed research centers for alternative medicine.

In 1992, the United States Congress mandated the creation of the National Institutes of Health Office of Alternative Medicine (OAM). In 1998, Congress elevated the Office of Alternative Medicine to a center, the National Center for Complementary and Alternative Medicine (NCCAM), and expanded its budget and mandate. Congress increased funding for the NCCAM in 2000 to $68.4 million.

NCCAM is charged to conduct basic and clinical research, research training, and disseminate health information. Its mandate also includes the goal of identifying, investigating, and validating CAM treatments, diagnostic and prevention modalities, and disciplines and systems. NCCAM currently supports a broad-based collection of clinical and basic science-research activities, research training, and educational programs.

The NCCAM collaborates on research projects with many institutes at the National Institutes of Health, including the National Cancer Institute (NCI). Recently, the NCI developed its own office of complementary and alternative medicine. Both the creation of the NCI program and its collaboration with NCCAM enable more and better CAM research to be conducted on cancer. These are extremely important steps forward, because some promising CAM therapies now will be carefully studied in a scientific fashion.

The OAM performs two roles in furthering research on alternative and complementary therapies. First, it records and maintains interest in the numerous alternative medicine research projects funded over the years by the National Institutes of Health (NIH). Current support from the seventeen institutes of the NIH totals more than $13 million. The National Institute of Drug Abuse and the National Heart, Lung, and Blood Institute, spend more on alternative and complementary therapy research than each of the other health institutes.

Second, the OAM funds research under its own auspices, usually in conjunction with a relevant insti-

tute. To date, OAM has funded forty-two pilot studies for approximately $30,000 each. Seven of the funded pilot studies concerned cancer. Because these were pilot studies, results did not provide definitive data. They simply indicated which of the projects seemed promising and worthy of more careful investigation. The OAM also has funded eleven university-based centers where research in alternative and complementary medicine takes place. Each center focuses on a specific problem or disease, such as pain, women's health, cancer, or AIDS. Research results are not yet available from the centers.

The National Library of Medicine (NLM) represents another example of greater federal acceptance of unconventional medicine. A meeting of NLM staff and OAM council members increased researchers' access to articles about complementary medicine. In 1995, the NLM expanded its number of key words and included additional journals related to alternative and complementary practices. The NLM now contains more than sixty thousand citations for articles about alternative and complementary therapies.

Numerous medical schools and hospitals have developed programs or departments for the study of complementary therapies. It is estimated that at least half of all medical schools in the United States offer courses on alternative and complementary medicine. Many others provide occasional lectures or ongoing, informal programs.

The First Annual International Congress on Alternative and Complementary Medicine in the United States was held in 1995. In addition, dozens of meetings are held throughout the United States on specific approaches, such as homeopathy, herbal medicine, Ayur Veda, and spirituality. Medical doctors and others attend and speak at these conferences, which cover virtually every type of nonstandard treatment.

Journals and books devoted to alternative and complementary medicine intended for health professionals or the public abound. Many are proponent-driven rather than objective, and therefore cannot necessarily be accepted at face value. This major drawback lies behind the emergence of a journal in England and another in the United States that take a scientific look at this field, evaluating the quality of research and trying to differentiate between therapies that are worthwhile and those that are useless or little more than quackery.

In another example of mainstream acceptance of complementary medicine, some insurance companies now offer plans that reimburse practitioners of complementary therapies, such as chiropractors, acupuncturists, and massage therapists. These plans often are met with great public interest. The AlternaPath pilot program of Blue Cross gave subscribers access to acupuncturist, naturopaths, and homeopaths; it quickly was fully subscribed when first offered on a pilot basis. (Acupuncture is a good example of a former alternative therapy that, for researched problems such as pain and substance abuse, is now widely accepted in mainstream medicine.)

A further sign of acceptance of complementary medicine is the behavior of physicians. More than 60 percent of physicians in one survey were willing to refer their patients to alternative practitioners; primary care physicians were most likely to do so. Many complementary therapy practitioners are physicians; a 1984 study found that 51 percent were medical doctors. They tended to be family practitioners, generalists, and psychiatrists almost exclusively. A similar situation seems to exist today.

Alternative Cancer Therapies Popular Today

To bring structure to the wide and quickly changing universe of alternative therapies, complementary and alternative practices may be grouped into the seven categories summarized below.

Diet and Nutrition

Anticancer diets and nutritional supplements represent enduring alternative cancer treatments. Many alternative cancer clinics include special diets as part of their overall treatments. Up to 61 percent of British cancer patients use unconventional diets. It is true that the consumption of fruits, vegetables, and fiber, and avoidance of excessive dietary fat can reduce cancer risk. However, alternative anticancer diets go further, with proponents often claiming that a certain diet can cure cancer. Extending claims beyond what is supported by research is a hallmark of many alternative treatments. Although healthy diets are important in preventing some cancers, no diet has ever been shown to cure cancer or extend remissions.

Today's most popular dietary cancer cure is probably macrobiotics. The popularity of the macrobiotic diet can be traced to the efforts of Michio Kushi, a tireless proponent. Once nutritionally deficient, the macrobiotic diet has since been enhanced and now derives 50–60 percent of its calories from whole grains, 25–30 percent from vegetables, and the remainder from beans, seaweed, and soups. The diet avoids meat and certain vegetables and promotes soybean consumption. Miso, a product made with fermented soybeans, is claimed to be the crucial ingredient of the macrobiotic diet "cure."

Soy is an important aspect of the Asian diet, which is known to reduce the incidence of breast, prostate, and other cancers. Whether soy and soy products have a beneficial effect on patients following a cancer diagnosis is not known. This important issue is under study in a national oncology cooperative group.

In addition, soy products help relieve hot flashes and other discomforts associated with menopause. They do so through the same mechanism as hormone replacement therapy, because soy, like hormone replacement therapy, contains phytoestrogens (plant estrogens). Whether women with breast cancer can use soy products and other plants containing phytoestrogens remains very much in debate. Some experts feel that the more mild plant-based estrogens could be helpful against the symptoms of chemotherapy-induced menopause, but others fear that the estrogens in soy and other plants might encourage tumor growth. This is, of course, a very serious possibility. Until more data are collected and oncologists understand the effects of soy-type products in women with breast cancer, it is best to avoid soy without first talking with your oncologist.

Mind-Body Techniques

The notion that we can influence health with our minds resonates well within the individualism of U.S. culture. Mind-body medicine is extremely popular in the United States. Some mind-body interventions have moved from the realm of the unconventional into mainstream medicine. This category includes prayer. Good documentation also exists for the effectiveness of meditation, biofeedback, and yoga in stress reduction and the control of particular physiologic reactions.

Some proponents argue that patients can use mental attributes and mind-body work to prevent or cure cancer. This belief also has great appeal. It ascribes to the patient almost complete control over the course of illness and suggests that the will of the individual or mental toughness can overcome malignancy. Studies suggesting that mental factors or prayer influences the course of cancer are widely publicized, although they may involve small numbers of patients or remain unreplicated. Examples include a 1989 *Lancet* article showing that women with breast cancer who attended weekly support group sessions had double the survival time of women who did not attend. (A replication of this study has been under way for almost a decade, but no results have been reported.)

Another well-known example is the San Francisco intercessory prayer study, a prospective, randomized, double-blind study of 393 patients, one-half of whom were randomly selected to be prayed for by people at a distance. Results were significant, suggesting that intercessory prayer had beneficial therapeutic effects, although there were no differences in length of hospital stay whether patients were prayed for or not.

Attending to the psychological health of cancer patients is a fundamental component of good cancer care. Support groups, good doctor-patient relationships, and the emotional and instrumental help of family and friends are vital. The idea that patients can influence the course of their diseases through mental or emotional concentration, however, is not backed up by controlled studies and can evoke feelings of guilt and inadequacy when diseases continue to advance despite patients' spiritual or mental efforts.

Bioelectromagnetics

Bioelectromagnetics is the study of living organisms and their interactions with electromagnetic fields. Bioelectromagnetic therapies use the low-frequency portion of the electromagnetic spectrum. Proponents claim that magnetic fields penetrate the body and heal damaged tissues, including cancers. Wolfgang Ludwig, Sc.D., Ph.D., director of the Institute of Biophysics in Horb, Germany, asserts that magnetic fields can cure a wide variety of ailments, including malignant diseases. However, no peer-reviewed publications support any cancer-related claims regarding bioelectromagnetics.

Traditional and Folk Remedies

This category includes ancient systems of healing that often are based on concepts of human physiology different from those accepted by modern Western science. Two of the most popular healing systems are traditional Chinese medicine and India's Ayur Veda, popularized by bestselling author Deepak Chopra, M.D.

Traditional Chinese medicine is distinguished by its focus on *chi*, the life force said to flow through energy channels known as meridians. Traditional Chinese medicine relies on exercise techniques such as qi gong and tai chi to strengthen and balance *chi*. Traditional Chinese medicine also uses acupuncture, acupressure, and a full arsenal of herbal concoctions, with remedies for most ailments, including cancer. Chinese herbal teas, philosophy, and relaxation techniques are soothing and appealing to many patients with cancer who use them as complementary therapies. Many studies are under way to evaluate the benefits of Chinese herbal remedies.

The term Ayur Veda comes from the Sanskrit words *ayur* (life) and *veda* (knowledge). Ayur Veda's five-thousand-year-old healing techniques are based on the classification of people into one of three predominant body types. There are specific remedies for disease and regimens to promote health for each body type. Ayur Veda has a strong mind-body component, stressing the need to keep consciousness in balance. It uses techniques such as yoga and meditation to do so. Approximately ten Ayur Veda clinics in North America served an estimated twenty-five thousand patients over the past ten years. The number of cancer patients among them is not documented.

Pharmacologic and Biologic Treatments

This class of treatments remains highly controversial. Pharmacologic treatments typically are invasive and costly, and their proponents tend to encourage patients to try them and ignore or delay mainstream therapy.

A well-known pharmacologic therapy today is antineoplastons, developed by Stanislaw Burzynski, M.D., Ph.D., and available at his clinic in Houston, Texas. Clinical evidence evaluated under the National Cancer Institutes of both the United States and Canada failed to support the potential worth of this regimen; and a laboratory investigation by a respected scientist concluded that antineoplastons do not even exist.

Public interest remains high, elevated perhaps by publicity received not only from television appearances by Dr. Burzynski and his patients but also from the headline-producing indictment of Burzynski in late 1995 following a U.S. Postal Service and FDA raid of his Houston clinic. Dr. Burzynski recently initiated a plan to obtain follow-up information on his patients and maintain data on their progress. Such information has not been available previously and will be welcomed.

Immunoaugmentative therapy (IAT) was developed by the late Lawrence Burton, Ph.D., and offered in his clinic in the Bahamas. Burton's therapy is based on balancing four protein components in the blood. This injected therapy, as with antineoplastons, relies on strengthening the patient's immune system, although there has been no evidence to support those beliefs. According to proponent literature, Burton claimed that IAT was particularly effective in treating mesothelioma. Documentation of IAT's efficacy remains anecdotal. The clinic has continued to operate since Burton's death, but it seems to have declined in popularity, possibly because of the rise of other alternatives, such as shark cartilage.

A 1992 book by I. William Lane, Ph.D., *Sharks Don't Get Cancer*, spurred interest in shark cartilage as a cancer therapy. Such interest was continued by a television special that displayed apparent remissions in patients with advanced cancer treated with shark cartilage in Cuba. The televised outcome was strongly disputed by oncologists in the United States. Shark cartilage advocates base their therapy on the discovery, by Harvard's Judah Folkman, M.D., of a cartilage-based protein that inhibits angiogenesis, the creation of new blood vessels. (Tumors require a vigorous blood supply to thrive.)

According to mainstream scientists, however, the molecules of active ingredients in the "food supplement" shark cartilage sold at health food stores are too large to be absorbed. They decompose into inert ingredients and are simply excreted. Despite lack of positive evidence, shark cartilage pills and suppositories are widely publicized (for arthritis as well as cancer cures) and are available in health food stores throughout the United States. Bovine cartilage also is under study for its potential anticancer properties. Although finding a way to kill cancer cells by cutting off their blood supply remains a major research focus, there is little scientific hope that shark or bovine cartilage will be helpful.

Another biologic remedy, Cancell, is especially popular in the Midwestern United States and in Florida. Proponents claim that it returns cancer cells to a "primitive state" from which the cells are digested and rendered inert. FDA laboratory studies revealed that Cancell is composed of common chemicals, including nitric acid, sodium sulfite, potassium hydroxide, sulfuric acid, and catechol. The FDA found no basis for claims of Cancell's effectiveness against cancer.

Popular metabolic therapies are readily available in Tijuana, Mexico, and elsewhere in North America. One of the best-known Tijuana centers is the Gerson clinic, where treatment is based on the notion that toxic products of cancer cells accumulate in the liver, leading to liver failure and death. Gerson's treatment aims to counteract liver damage with low-salt, low-fat, high-potassium diets, and coffee enemas. The hills around Tijuana are dotted with similar cancer clinics, each offering its own version of metabolic treatment.

Manual Healing Methods

Manual healing includes a variety of touch and manipulation techniques. Osteopathic and chiropractic doctors were among the earliest groups to use manual methods. Hands-on massage is a useful adjunctive technique for cancer patients and others for its stress-reducing benefits.

One of the most popular manual-healing methods in North America is therapeutic touch, which, despite its name, involves no direct contact. In therapeutic touch, healers move their hands a few inches above a patient's body to remove "blockages" to the patient's energy field. Developed by a nursing professor emeritus at New York University, therapeutic touch is taught at most U.S. nursing schools. Although numerous critics in mainstream medicine deride its fundamental premises, the therapeutic touch is widely practiced and usually appreciated by patients. It is likely that psychological benefits are achieved by a caregiver's presence and concern.

Herbal Medicine

Herbal remedies typically are part of traditional and folk healing with long histories of use. Some form of herbal medicine is found in all areas of the world. Although many herbal remedies claim to have anticancer effects, only a few have gained substantial popularity as cancer therapies.

Essiac is one of the most popular herbal cancer alternatives in North America. It was popularized by a Canadian nurse, Rene Caisse (Essiac is Caisse spelled backwards), but developed earlier by a native Canadian healer. Essiac comprises four herbs:

burdock, turkey rhubarb, sorrel, and slippery elm. Research at the National Cancer Institute and the Memorial Sloan-Kettering Cancer Center in New York has found that it has no anticancer effect. It is illegal to distribute Essiac in Canada, although under a special arrangement Canadian patients may receive if from a supplier in Ontario. A problem with Essiac is that Caisse never revealed its formula; consequently, several competing firms sell different versions, each claiming to have the true formula. It is widely available in U.S. health food stores.

Combinations of Chinese herbs to treat cancer have been used for hundreds of years. Herbal combinations are still used by some people who do not have access to modern therapies, and some herbal remedies are used in Asia along with modern mainstream cancer care. Chinese herbal remedies, particularly teas, are prized for the comfort patients feel they bring.

Iscador, a derivative of mistletoe, is a popular cancer remedy in Europe, where it has been used as a folk treatment for centuries. Iscador is available in many mainstream European cancer clinics. European governments fund ongoing studies of Iscador's effectiveness against cancer, but no definitive data support proponents' claims.

The FDA does not examine herbal remedies for safety and effectiveness, and most have not been formally tested for side effects. There have been recent reports in the medical literature of severe liver and kidney damage from a limited number of herbal remedies, including chaparral tea. These reports underscore the fact that "natural" products are not necessarily safe or harmless.

The Prevalence of Complementary or Alternative Medicine

Complementary therapies are popular with the public, with better-educated people using them more often than others. A national telephone survey found that 34 percent of Americans visited alternative practitioners in 1990, spending $13.7 billion on these visits. Americans made more visits to alternative practitioners (425 million) than to primary care physicians (388 million).

A 1993 survey of 1,539 U.S. adults showed that about one-third of the public was using complementary or alternative medicine (CAM). Two surveys were published in 1997. One indicated CAM use in 50 per-

cent of 113 family practice patients. The other found similar results with an even larger survey: 42 percent of 1,500 members of the general public used CAM. In 1999, a survey of more than 24,000 people found 8 percent use of CAM.

These rates, as well as those from all CAM studies conducted in the U.S. and internationally, vary from less than 10 percent to more than 50 percent. The variation is most certainly due to differing understandings and definitions of CAM. Surveys do not always define CAM, or they may define it so broadly that everything we do to help ourselves when illness strikes is included in the figure.

The majority of physicians who practice alternative medicine are family practitioners or psychiatrists; very few oncologists or other medical specialists do so. Most oncologists are not familiar with the alternative and complementary therapies used by many of their patients.

CAM and Cancer Patients

A small minority of cancer patients uses alternative therapies, although it appears that many more patients adopt therapies such as massage, acupuncture, or herbal teas for strictly complementary purposes. It is vital that you, the patient, and your family feel comfortable talking with your oncologist about alternative and complementary therapies. You can teach your oncologist about complementary methods and learn together what can be done in addition to mainstream treatment and following completion of mainstream treatment.

The possible harms, benefits, and interactions of therapies require evaluation. Physicians also need to understand patients' motives for using alternative or complementary therapies. Inadequate pain management, for example, which remains a problem in cancer treatment, may be helped by nonsedating techniques such as acupuncture.

Access to psychosocial support services can be essential for many families and patients in improving quality of life, and psychosocial support services should be a routine component of cancer care. Providing such access also should help in counteracting the perception that alternative practitioners have cornered the market on caring and concern for patients as people.

One of the most difficult situations arises in terminal illness when some patients make last-ditch efforts to find a cure. These patients are most susceptible to quackery. They also risk emotional distress, false hope, and wasted money. In addition to failing to experience the promised "cures," patients are not likely to find enhanced quality of life. The combination of good communication between oncologist and patient and assiduous use of appropriate complementary therapies should reduce patients' frustrations and dissatisfactions with oncologic medicine and encourage them to continue conventional care. The soothing attention of complementary practices, including psychosocial care, along with the technologic expertise of oncology practice is a merger that can greatly enhance patients' quality of life and satisfaction with care.

Growing Interest and Acceptance

The substantial interest in alternative and complementary cancer therapies appears to stem from several sources. The sheer number, as well as content, of mainstream and alternative therapy magazine articles, books, media reports, patient reports, and so on suggest that the public is frustrated with establishment medicine's inability to treat many cancers effectively. The public is distressed by the absence of substantial treatment gains for the major cancers despite the decades and billions of dollars spent fighting this collection of diseases.

Chemotherapy and its side effects have become increasingly intolerable to a public focused on the appeal of natural products and wanting, as we all do, gentler as well as more effective substitutes for standard cancer treatments. Public distrust and dissatisfaction with establishment medicine and related institutions remain. The FDA is seen not as protective but as obstructive. The pharmaceutical industry is viewed as intent on maintaining prohibitive pricing, hindering access to promising products even for dying patients, and, despite commercial efforts to display a contrary image, ignoring natural products in favor of high-technology, high-priced drugs.

In many respects, CAM cancer therapies represent the antithesis of the perceived values and actions described above. Patients are simultaneously drawn away from mainstream medicine and toward competing types of care. A major reason for today's public and professional interest in complementary therapies is dissatisfaction with what is perceived as the technologic and impersonal nature of modern medicine.

Patients complain about insensitive, limited, and hurried interactions with oncologists in every setting, from small suburban hospitals to top-notch comprehensive cancer centers.

Patients complain that frequently provisions are not made to relieve the anticipated side effects of chemotherapy, and sometimes patients are not even told to expect these effects. Patients often feel helpless and ignored. Many fail to understand why oncology medicine does not include the nontoxic complementary techniques that control pain, reduce stress, and alleviate symptoms that are standard in other countries. The United States is approximately two years behind most European countries in establishing government-level offices of complementary medicine and in offering complementary therapies to augment mainstream cancer care.

Practitioners who provide alternative and complementary therapies are viewed as more caring, as treating the whole person, and as providing more emotionally satisfying, communicative relationships. Typically, they are able to spend more time talking with their patients than conventional physicians do. This is especially true today in the U.S. under managed care. For this reason, conventional physicians often are termed disinterested and "reductionistic," focused only on the disease, whereas practitioners outside of the mainstream are considered "holistic," concerned with the whole person. Some patients seek alternative care for its more egalitarian approach, for better practitioner-patient relationships, or for enhanced opportunities to make therapeutic decisions and play a major role in their own health care.

One can only hope that a more balanced position will emerge for alternative and complementary medicine, one that avoids irrationality and acceptance of therapies on the basis of anecdotal reports, rejects attacks against science, and accepts only methodologically sound research. Optimally, a balance can be forged between the science and technology of cancer medicine and the comfort that the best of complementary medicine can bring.

Complementary Therapies to Ease Cancer Treatment and Follow-Up Care

Alternative and Complementary Treatments for Cancer, a new publication from the American Cancer Society, along with information on the ACS website and publications such as those listed in Part VI, detail the complimentary and alternative therapies that help relieve symptoms and enhance quality of life for cancer patients.

Important interventions, such as individual and group therapy, are not included in the list below because they are considered mainstream, as opposed to complementary, therapies.

The complementary therapies listed below have been studied, primarily in Europe, and found to be effective for the purposes noted. They are inexpensive and easily accessible. Most of these remedies can be prepared or administered by the patient or a family member. Because some herbal and other ingested remedies may interact with prescription medications, it is important to discuss with your oncologist any therapy that you take on your own.

For Anxiety and Stress:
- Acupressure
- Aromatherapy
- Meditation/relaxation techniques
- Therapeutic massage
- Valerian tea
- Yoga

For Colds and Flu:
- Garlic
- Echinacea
- Eucalyptus or peppermint oil
- Ginger
- Iceland moss and plantain tea
- Watercress tea
- Zinc lozenges

For Constipation:
- Cascara or buckthorne bark
- Plantago seed
- Pureed rhubarb
- Water and fiber

For Depression:
- Hypericum or St. John's wort
- Light therapy
- Meditation
- Tai chi

For Headaches:
- Acupressure
- Evening primrose tea, sunflower seeds
- Garlic and onions
- Feverfew tea
- Progressive relaxation or massage

For Indigestion:
- Peppermint or chamomile tea

For Muscle Aches:
- Capsicum cream
- Hydrotherapy
- Massage
- Volatile mustard oil

For Nausea:
- Acupressure
- Cinnamon or peppermint tea
- Ginger

For Chronic Pain:
- Acupuncture
- Biofeedback
- Various herbs
- Hypnotherapy
- Massage

For Sleep Problems:
- Lavender oil-scented bath
- Lemon balm herb tea
- Chamomile tea
- Massage
- Meditation
- Other herbal teas

Acupuncture and Cancer Care

Brenda Golianu, M.D.

Acupuncture is an excellent complementary treatment that is easily integrated into the traditional care of the cancer patient. Acupuncture has been practiced in China for more than two thousand years. In the United States, acupuncture has been around for more than one hundred years. It has an excellent record of safety. The Federal Drug Administration approved the acupuncture needle as a medical device in 1997. Also in 1997, a consensus panel of the National Institute of Health analyzed the current scientific evidence for the efficacy of acupuncture. The National Institute of Health panel produced a consensus document endorsing the use of acupuncture for nausea, vomiting, and chronic pain.

Traditional Chinese medical theory teaches that acupuncture enhances the circulation of chi or vital energy. Chi flows in channels called *meridians*. Illness is associated with the obstruction or stagnation of chi. Acupuncture points are places on the body's surface where chi is more readily accessible for manipulation. Placement of needles unblocks "stuck" chi and facilitates homeostasis (balance). Diagnosis is based on a patient's history, and a physical examination including pulse, tongue, and abdominal palpation. A pattern of illness is identified and an individualized treatment plan is created. Acupuncture is an integral part of the Oriental Medicine tradition, which includes meditation, breathing exercises, herbal remedies, a proper diet, and exercise.

In the treatment of the cancer patient, acupuncture can be very helpful in ameliorating the adverse effects of chemotherapy and radiation therapy, including nausea and vomiting, weight loss, fatigue, and painful neuropathy, and in facilitating recovery after completion of treatment. It has relatively few side effects, and these side effects are very rare. Potential side effects include the risk of local infection or bleeding. Very rarely, pneumothorax can occur.

Practically, acupuncture involves placement of very tiny needles in the body, frequently in the distal extremities. The needles are left in place for fifteen to twenty minutes and gently manipulated at times. Mild electrical stimulation can be used. The needles also may be warmed with an herbal substance called *artemisia vulgaris*, or moxa. It is not uncommon to feel a mild aching sensation; however the needles are not painful.

One can expect nothing or mild improvement in symptoms after the first treatment. Usually, treatments are cumulative. Symptom relief will usually last a little longer each time. Often, pain medications can be reduced or discontinued over time. Once a new baseline is established, the frequency of visits is reduced. Acupuncture is extremely helpful in the care of cancer patients in that it does not involve additional medications. It can be easily integrated into the clinical care of cancer patients at any stage of diagnosis and treatment.

During the first visit, goals of treatment are established. At the fifth visit, these goals are revisited and treatment is altered if necessary. Usually, five to ten treatments are performed. Patients often report a sense of well-being and improved stamina after treatment. In part, this feeling may be related to endorphin release that is known to occur with acupuncture stimulation. However, other effects, for example, improved PO intake and improved mobility, are not attributable to endorphin production.

Much remains to be understood about the mechanism of action of acupuncture. Traditional explanations about endorphins and other neurotransmitters may be involved. Imaging techniques such as functional Magnetic Resonance Imaging (MRI) document increased activity in the cerebral cortex during therapeutic acupuncture stimulation. This is not present during sham acupuncture stimulation.

(Continued from page 107)

To begin acupuncture treatment, one should first consult one's treating physician. A referral can then be generated. Many conventional insurance plans and health maintenance organizations reimburse acupuncture treatment payments.

A full workup of one's symptoms should be performed prior to initiating acupuncture. Acupuncture should not be used instead of conventional treatment, but rather alongside it. Most commonly, acupuncture is utilized after all other treatments have failed. However, in certain settings it may be appropriate earlier in the treatment algorithm. For example, in the treatment of chronic pain, patients are sometimes reluctant to start long-term pain medications such as opiates or tricyclic antidepressants for pain symptoms. A trial of acupuncture may be appropriate for such individuals. Acupuncture also has a role in preventive medicine and in helping to rebuild the immune system. The traditional recommendation is that patients who are elderly, have frequent infections, or are otherwise compromised, undergo a "tune-up" treatment at the change of the seasons. Whether these types of applications will turn out to be effective only time and appropriate,

randomized double-blinded trials will tell. However, the risk of such a course of action is quite low.

In the areas of pain and control of nausea and vomiting, there are already several well-done studies that document the efficacy of acupuncture treatments over medication alone.

Acupuncture does not work for all patients. Perhaps 20 percent of patients will have no significant changes in their symptoms. Others will show a gradual response, eventually moving to a new baseline in their condition. Some, perhaps 10–15 percent, will have a spectacular improvement. Some percentage of patients will have complete resolution of their symptoms. Others will be able to better manage their remaining symptoms.

The best way to understand acupuncture is to try it. You can ask your physician about reputable acupuncturists in your area. Practitioners may be either Licensed Acupuncturists, or M.D. Acupuncturists. A list of local Licensed Acupuncturists is available through the Licensing Board for Acupuncture, present in most states. The Medical Academy of Acupuncture maintains a list of M.D. Acupuncturists who are accepting new patient referrals.

Biofeedback as an Adjunct to the Management of Cancer

Ian E. Wickramasekera, Ph.D.

Biofeedback is a learning and training procedure that enables a person to, within biological limits, alter physiological and bioelectrical events occurring within his or her body. For example, people can learn to reduce muscle tension (EMG), alter heart rate and blood pressure, warm their hands, and change the electrical activity of specific brain waves (e.g., increase EEG waves like alpha). Reducing muscle tension and warming cold hands can reduce or abolish tension or migraine headaches and reduce the symptoms of primary Raynaud's disease. Decreasing heart rate and blood pressure can help patients with cardiovascular diseases and moderate hypertension. Increasing EEG alpha waves can reduce anxiety and fears. Generally, biofeedback can turn off the "stress" (also called the "fight or flight" response).

When a diagnosis of cancer is made, and when the patient is told that he or she has to submit to painful or unpleasant medical tests and therapies that have uncertain outcomes, fear and sometimes despair are provoked in the person. Because the disease and the uncertainty of therapy are both a threat to the well-being of the person and a threat to the survival of their body, the traumatic news about the diagnosis, the subsequent tests, and the therapies can trigger the "fight or flight" or stress response. These tests and treatments go on for several weeks or months. The patient's body and mind goes to sleep feeling threatened and wakes up in the morning feeling threatened. This can go on for several months or even years. In other words, the body and mind have few opportunities to return to the prediagnosis level of peace and feeling of invulnerability.

Chronic activation of the stress response is known to be unhealthy and a suppressor of the body's immune system. Our immune system is our primary instrument of defense against tumors, viruses, and infections. Biofeedback can be used to turn off the "stress response" and its immunosuppressive effects. Biofeedback can prepare the patient to better cope with the tests and therapies required to treat their cancer and help reduce the anxiety and the nausea and vomiting that is associated with some cancer therapies.

The three essential features of biofeedback training are: (1) continuous and accurate monitoring of the physiological response to be altered (e.g., heart rate, blood pressure, muscle tension, or hand emperature); (2) immediate feedback to the subject of even small changes in the biological response to be altered; (3) motivation to alter the response. Some of the biological responses in animals and humans that have been altered to date include EEG responses (alpha and theta), blood pressure, heart rate, muscle tension, salivation, urine formation, gastric motility, blood flow, and skin temperature. It is through learning and conditioning that people appear to produce these basic biological changes in their bodies.

In the process of learning self-control of biological responses, it appears that certain reliable positive psychological changes occur in mood and motivation in the trainee. Some of the reported psychological alterations of consciousness include feelings of floating, lightness, expansion, euphoria, dreaminess, tranquility, and self-competence. Biofeedback technology may provide an alternative to present drug methods of inducing positive emotional changes. Currently, psychotropic drugs are the primary clinical method of altering mood and emotion, but they are not entirely free of negative side effects, such as dependency. Biofeedback technology offers a second method of altering emotions that is relatively specific, free of serious side effects, and ideal for some patients. For example, biofeedback is effective even with patients who are unresponsive to hypnosis, that is, patients who have only low or moderate trait

(Continued from page 109)

hypnotic ability or who are fearful of hypnosis. Patients who have high hypnotic ability can learn to enter hypnosis easily; "delayed biofeedback" (biological feedback delayed two to five minutes) works better for them than immediate biological feedback. Biofeedback can provide an effective and reliable set of tools to induce positive emotions and to alter biological responses. When biofeedback is associated with psychotherapy, we can not only put out the "fire," or reduce symptoms, but we can also find the "matches" (the causes of the stress).

The body often makes certain physical changes in response to stressful information, and the purpose of biofeedback is to help a person become aware of these biological changes and learn to regulate them. Sophisticated electronic measuring instruments that amplify and give information about such things as blood flow, muscle tension, and skin temperature detect and amplify these small and hard to notice bodily changes. This helps remove a "blindfold" and permits one to regulate bodily reactions that were formerly outside one's awareness and control.

Biofeedback is usually done by licensed psychologists, physicians, or psychiatrists. Some physical therapists, social workers, speech pathologists, dentists, and other professionals do biofeedback therapy as well. However, not all practitioners have had adequate training in this relatively new field, and the client should ask the therapist or doctor about the extent of his or her training and experience. The Biofeedback Certification Institute of America, an interdisciplinary group of health care professionals that includes physicians and psychologists in its membership, has developed certification standards for practitioners interested in assessing their skills and knowledge of this therapy. The potential benefits of biofeedback include reduction of pain and other target symptoms, decreased reliance on medication, and an improved capacity to relax deeply and efficiently.

Length of treatment depends, of course, on many things, such as the severity of symptoms and how long they have been present. Average treatment consists of eight to twelve fifty-minute sessions, administered once or twice a week. Learning to identify the stress response in its early stages and how to respond with relaxation techniques is very much like learning a new language. Once clients have made a good beginning in the therapy sessions, it is important that they continue to learn on their own, without too much dependence on the biofeedback equipment or the therapist. The goal of therapy is for the client to learn to self-manage symptoms whenever possible.

Hypnosis

David Spiegel, M.D.

Hypnosis is a method to highly focus attention. It is a psychophysiological state of attentive, receptive concentration, with a relative suspension of peripheral awareness. Hypnotic phenomena occur spontaneously during periods of intense attention, during trauma, and in certain ceremonies that are designed to elicit trance phenomena. Hypnosis can be understood as involving three main factors: absorption, dissociation, and suggestibility.

Absorption allows one to completely focus attention on one's inner mind, completely ignoring the outside world. As one becomes deeply involved in a central focus of consciousness, one tends to ignore peripheral perceptions, thoughts, memories, or activities. Hypnotized individuals can become so intensely absorbed in their trance experience that often they choose to ignore the environmental context and other peripheral events. There is abundant scientific evidence that demonstrates a correlation between individuals' hypnotizability (capacity to experience hypnosis) and their tendency to undergo absorbing or self-altering experiences. This means that those with hypnotic ability use it spontaneously, not simply when formally instructed to do so.

The process of dissociation is complementary to absorption. The intense absorption characteristic of the hypnotic state permits keeping out of conscious awareness many routine experiences that would ordinarily be conscious. When working properly in our daily lives, it allows us to carry out several complex tasks simultaneously (e.g., knitting while conversing or watching television). Even rather complex emotional states, motor functions, or sensory experiences may be dissociated.

Due to the intense absorption experienced during trance, hypnotized individuals are more responsive than usual to social cues, including suggestions given by the therapist. This enhanced suggestibility allows hypnotized subjects to accept instructions relatively easily. Hypnotized individuals are not deprived of their will, but they do have a tendency to accept instructions in a rather uncritical way. This quality of the hypnotic process allows subjects to suspend the usual conscious curiosity that makes us critically examine reasons for our actions. Because of this, hypnotized individuals are more prone to accept directions, no matter how irrational those directons might be. Nonetheless, no one is deprived of personal will under hypnosis—though they are less likely to exercise it to contradict hypnotic instructions.

The fact that people vary in their ability to experience hypnosis underscores the point that all hypnosis is really self-hypnosis. People learn to enter such states to thc cxtcnt that they have the ability to do so. Hypnosis is not something imposed on them, but rather it is an ability that can be discovered and developed. Being hypnotized is not yielding to an authority but rather mobilizing an inner focus of concentration.

Hypnosis for Pain Control

It has been known since the middle of the 1800s that hypnosis is effective in controlling even severe surgical pain. Hypnosis and similar techniques work through two primary mechanisms: muscle relaxation and a combination of perceptual alteration and cognitive distraction. Pain is not infrequently accompanied by reactive muscle tension. Patients frequently dissociate the parts of their bodies that hurt. Yet, because muscle tension by itself can cause pain in normal tissue and traction on a painful part of the body can produce more pain, techniques that induce greater physical relaxation can reduce pain in the periphery. Therefore, having patients enter a state of hypnosis so they can concentrate on an image that connotes physical relaxation, such as floating or lightness, often produces physical relaxation and reduces pain.

(Continued from page 111)

The second major component of hypnotic analgesia is perceptual alteration. Patients can be taught to imagine that the affected body part is numb. This is especially useful for extremely hypnotizable individuals who can, for example, relive an experience of dental anesthesia and reproduce the drug-induced sensations of numbness in their cheek, which they can then transfer to the painful part of their body. They can also simply "switch off" perception of the pain with surprising effectiveness. Temperature metaphors are often especially useful, which is not surprising given the fact that pain and temperature sensations are part of the same sensory system, as noted above. Thus, imagining that an affected body part is cooler or warmer using an image of dipping it in ice water or heating it in the sun can often help patients transform pain signals.

Some patients prefer to imagine that the pain is a substance with dimensions that can be moved or can flow out of the body as if it were a viscous liquid. Others like to imagine that they can step outside their body to visit another room in the house. Less hypnotizable individuals often do better with distraction techniques that help them focus on competing sensations in another part of their bodies.

Although not all patients are sufficiently hypnotizable to benefit from these techniques, two out of three adults are at least somewhat hypnotizable. Furthermore, clinically effective hypnotic analgesia is not confined to those with high hypnotizability. Hypnosis is especially effective in comforting children who are in pain. Children are more hypnotizable than adults, and they naturally relax when they mobilize their imagination during the sensory alteration component of hypnotic pain relief.

Recent research utilizing measures of electrical activity in the brain (ERP) and blood flow (PET) indicates that when hypnosis helps people alter their perception, their brains actually process these perceptions differently. Thus, hypnotized individuals not only say they feel less pain, they actually feel less pain.

Hypnosis can be helpful as an adjunctive tool for treating stress and anxiety because of its ability to help patients control their somatic or bodily responses to anxiety-provoking thoughts or situations. This enables them to attend to their thoughts long enough to alter their point of view about them and achieve a sense of mastery over them. Most of the strategies used in the treatment of anxiety disorders employing hypnosis combine instructed physical relaxation with a restructuring of cognition, utilizing imagery coupled with physical relaxation. Patients are instructed to maintain a physical sense of relaxation (for example, floating), while picturing the feared situation or stimulus. It is important that the relaxation instruction utilizes an image that connotes reduced body tension, such as "floating" or "lightness," rather than being a direct instruction to "relax." This latter, more thought-provoking term may actually induce more anxiety, while affiliation with a body metaphor usually produces some reduction in tension. When hypnosis is used, a physically relaxed state can be rapidly achieved.

Initially, the use of hypnosis can help in demonstrating to patients that they have a greater degree of control over bodily responsiveness than they had imagined. It is often useful to begin by teaching the patient to create a place in their "mind's eye" where they feel safe and secure. It is also helpful to instruct subjects to learn how to project their concerns onto an imaginary screen. Later, they can learn to manipulate the screen by either making it bigger or smaller, or having the screen being nearer or farther away, as needed.

After they have learned to manipulate the screen and their own physical sensations, patients may, for example, learn to recreate the physical state of relaxation while projecting onto the screen the fearful situation. This, then, becomes a very useful procedure by which to control and obtain mastery over anxiety-producing situations by dissociating the body from the psychological response to the feared thoughts and situations. Initially, the patient is asked to recreate the physical feeling of relaxation. Then, the patient projects

(Continued from page 112)

onto the screen images that remind them of the feared situation, only this time the body reactions associated to anxiety do not develop. On occasion, it helps for patients to foresee likely physical sensations or situations associated with a fearful experience in order to master them.

Patients also may use the trance-state as a means of facing their concerns more directly. For example, they can, in hypnosis, place an image of an upcoming procedure or fearful situation on one side of the screen; then, on the other side, they can test out various strategies for mastering the situation.

Other approaches using hypnosis have included instructing patients in a trance to imagine that they are somewhere else, away from the fearful stimulus, thus separating themselves from the anxiety-producing experience. Positive reinforcement, or "ego-strengthening," techniques have also been used, for example, giving hypnotic instructions to the patient suggesting that their capacity to master the situation and their response to it will improve. Thus, a variety of strategies can be used to mobilize hypnotic concentration on active coping with stress while dissociating the body from psychological distress.

Part II

The Role of the Mind

13

The Will to Live

Ernest H. Rosenbaum, M.D.
Isadora R. Rosenbaum, M.A.
Andrew W. Kneier, Ph.D.
David Spiegel, M.D.

"I, like many others who are ill, went through a period of anguish and decided, yes, life is still beautiful, still precious, and until the last breath, worth fighting for. I have learned to truly value life, to cherish it, to enjoy it, and to appreciate its bittersweet brevity. When you make the momentous decision to live, you suddenly find that you never knew how to live life until you faced the reality of losing it."
—*William Cohen, M.D., a forty-two-year-old patient and physician*

Physicians are always fascinated with the power of the will to live. Like every creature in the animal world, human beings have a fierce instinct for survival. The will to live is the force within each of us to fight for survival when a disease such as cancer threatens our lives. This force is stronger in some than in others, determined by one's innate character and personality, the quality of one's current life, and whether one has a purpose to live.

Often when cancer patients have prolonged or unexpected remissions or cures, we have felt that the added critical factor was the will to live. We have often seen how two patients who are similar in age, diagnosis, degree of illness, and treatment therapy can experience widely different therapeutic results. Each case is different and, of course, the biology of a cancer often dictates the course of events, regardless of the patient's attitude and fighting spirit. Nonetheless, in many cases the strength of a patient's will to live appears to be an important factor in obtaining an unexpected remission.

We are constantly impressed by the spirit and grace with which people cope with chronic disease or disability, even under the threat of death. We have observed how they refuse to let physical debility or discomfort affect their enjoyment of family and friends or prevent them from going to work or pursuing outside interests. Inspired by their fortitude, we asked several of our patients how they were able to transcend their problems and what factors they considered essential to the will to live. Their stories touched on many different elements: hope, faith, perseverance, optimism, courage, goals, love, supportive family and friends, purpose, fear of dying, strong coping skills, and a feeling that it was their destiny to endure and survive. Whatever aspect patients focused on, continuing to live was essential to their inner drive.

It seems that the most critical ingredient of the patients' will to live is having something compelling to live for. They set goals and do whatever they can to get the most out of life. After an initial period of feeling devastated, they decided to make the most of each day.

Maria, who had a mastectomy at age twenty-nine, exemplified this spirit. After nearly eighteen years of chemotherapy, radiotherapy, and hormonal therapy, she died recently—after living with her illness for twenty-six years.

Maria never told her friends that she had cancer. She decided that because she had her husband's support, it was easier not to have to answer questions on how she felt or how her treatment was going. When her friends drove her to Mount Zion for chemotherapy, she told them she was going for a board meeting.

Maria always led an active and productive life as a wife, mother, and real estate agent. Her will to live was one of the strongest we had ever seen. "I got out of bed every morning as if nothing was wrong," she said. "I knew I was going to have to face things and that I might feel sick during the day, but I got out of bed anyway. There was a lot I was fighting for—I had a three-year-old child. I had a wonderful life and a magical love affair with my husband."

Maria's story is similar to the so-called Christmas syndrome, wherein a person summons the will to live until a specific occasion—such as a birthday or Christmas, or to meet a desired goal such as the birth of a grandchild or a graduation. In Marie's case, she lived to raise her child and to be with her husband. After her child was grown and her husband died, she finally let go.

Many of our patients told us that facing the uncertainties of living with cancer makes life more meaningful. The smallest pleasures—eating dinner by the fire, walking the dog, enjoying the smell of fresh-cut grass—are intensified. Much hypocrisy is eliminated. When bitterness and anger begin to dissipate, there is still a capacity for joy.

Some patients have written about what it is that makes them so determined to live. "I love living, I love nature," wrote one, adding that she loved, "being outdoors, feeling the sun on my skin or the wind blowing against my body, hearing birds sing, or breathing in the spray of the ocean."

Another patient also wrote about the newfound meaning: "I don't think I perceive color, sound, all the senses more deeply, but I do relish them more. I really wallow in a good sunset, but I don't think, 'This may be my last sunset.' I try to be honest with my emotional reactions instead of overdramatizing them."

These and many other patients have shown that success and victory have many definitions. For them, victory consists of trying their best to achieve the best quality of life possible under the circumstances, no matter how difficult. As Theodore Roosevelt wrote, "It is hard to fail, but it is worse to never have tried to succeed." Milton, though blind, wrote great poetry. Beethoven, though deaf, wrote beautiful music he would never hear. "Oh how would it be possible to admit the deficiency of a sense that I ought to possess to a more perfect degree than anybody else?" he wrote. "What a dejection when someone next to me heard a flute, and I did not hear anything, or when somebody heard the shepherd sing, and I could not hear even that. Such incidents made me desperate, and I was not far from putting an end to my life. It was only my art, my art that restrained me. Oh, I felt unable to leave this world before I had created what I felt had been assigned to me."

Maintaining a strong will to live when critically ill is easier said than done. Depression, self-pity, and despair are understandable. Experiencing these emotions is part of being human. If you are feeling low enough, your first decision may be whether you want to live. It is natural to have moments of not caring whether you live or die. But in my experience, when the chips are down, most people choose life.

The question that arises, however, is whether to live passively as a person who is resigned to fate, or actively as someone who is ready to make the best of one's fate and surmount bad luck. At some point, you will probably begin to look for ways of regaining control and living as normal a life as possible. Even if the medical crisis passes and you are either cured or reach a long-term compromise with a chronic medical problem, the lesson is not lost.

A threat to our existence typically triggers us to make an objective appraisal of our lives: the kind of people we have become, what is important to us, and how we want to live in the future. And it renews our appreciation of the importance of life, love, and friendship—and of all there is to enjoy and learn in life. We begin taking risks that we haven't had the courage to take in the past.

Sudden ill health or disability is a rude reminder that our time on earth is limited. All of a sudden, your entire life is changed. Everything you took for granted, even the things you complained about, suddenly belong to another life that you'd give anything to reclaim. And yet we are often able to survive a crisis because of the way we have coped with a traumatic situation in the past. At our lowest ebb, there is a small flame, an inner strength that makes us try again to take an active—rather than a passive—role in life.

The Four Horsemen Challenge to the Will to Live

The biblical Four Horsemen of the Apocalypse—conquest, war, famine, and death—were sent to ravage the earth in preparation for its final destruction. The similar imagery can be applied to the threats to one's will to live that come with a life-threatening and debilitating illness. Just as the will to live can be nurtured by a positive attitude, so can it be undermined by fear, anger, loss of self-esteem, and alienation. These feelings are common responses to the diagnosis of cancer. If allowed to go unresolved, they lead to feelings of depression, helplessness, futility, resignation, and loss of the will to live. These feelings can be dangerous if they cause you to give up early rather than fighting for your life.

Fear

Cancer is the most feared of all diseases. In fact, the word "cancer" is one of the most feared words in the English language. After questioning many newly diagnosed cancer patients, we have found that much of the disproportionate fear associated with this disease is due to the anticipation of prolonged periods of suffering and disability. Patients believe that little can be done to control the malignancy or relieve its symptoms. Nothing could be further from the truth.

Some patients react to the diagnosis of cancer in much the same manner that people in primitive societies react to a witch doctor's curse—as a sentence to an inevitable and ghastly death. Being "scared to death" is a well-known consequence of bone pointing, an ancient custom attributed to the Papua New Guinean and Australian Aborigines and other South Pacific cultures. A group of natives sits in a circle and spins a bone on the ground. The person the bone points to receives a tribal curse. Death could take place

in a few weeks. Of course, such a curse is effective only if the person believes in its power.

In modern medical practice, a similar phenomenon may occur when a patient believes the diagnosis of cancer to be a death sentence. For instance, a physician may tell a patient that the surgery or other treatment has been unsuccessful and that nothing more can be done. Such patients may simply accept the idea that they are going to die and extinguish their own will to live. Such patients can die rapidly, long before their disease has progressed enough for it to cause death.

Sometimes a doctor says to the patient, "I'm sorry, Mrs. Jones, but you have advanced cancer and there is no cure." Although the surgeon may feel sympathy and empathy, and may even cry with the patient, all Mrs. Jones hears is, "I can't be cured. I'm dying." How different the outcome might be if the doctor had added, "But we can treat your cancer to help you continue to live—and we can help alleviate your pain. We will soon work out a therapy plan for you."

Cancer is the most curable chronic disease. It is important to know that over 50 percent of persons diagnosed with cancer can be cured. The cure rate climbs to 75 percent when good preventive and diagnostic medicine routines are followed. These include mammograms; yearly physical examinations; colorectal sigmoidoscopy, colonoscopy, and digital (finger) rectal examinations; blood tests; and medical follow-up. As well, people should follow a healthy lifestyle—exercising regularly, quitting smoking, reducing alcohol consumption, and eating less red meat and more grains, vegetables, and fruits.

It is impossible to predict longevity for an individual patient before they begin therapy. Until the response to therapy has been established, no projection is feasible. Furthermore, even if one therapy is unsuccessful, another may work. There is hope that you may outlive any average projection by many months or years.

When a physician makes the effort to carefully explain the nature of cancer, and the anticipated problems and future tests, most patients are surprised to find that their ideas about cancer were considerably more pessimistic than the facts warrant. They find that most of their fears can be resolved by understanding the problems to be faced and the treatments and other supportive measures, and by having a reasonable estimate of the discomfort and inconvenience to be expected. Then they are able to adopt a positive attitude and to accept the compromises that come with the disease and the treatment.

One patient whom we have been treating for advanced cancer for the past six years has taken meticulous precautions to ensure that most of her closest friends do not discover her illness. She does this to protect herself from their possibly negative reactions. Your own fears may be under control, but having to deal with the fears of well-meaning friends can drain emotional energy and cause depression. However, rather than hide your disease, you may feel better including close friends, as well as family, in consultations with your doctor so that they may be able to function as part of your informed support team.

> Every patient runs the risk of encountering fear, pessimism, or other destructive attitudes on the part of doctors, nurses, family, friends, or acquaintances. Patients will also be overwhelmed at times by their own fears, discouragement, or sadness. This is normal. Nevertheless, the patient who is willing to fight and to accept guidance and support in his fight for life will have the basic confidence and equanimity with which to confront the ignorant and the fearful. Although fears and fantasies don't disappear, they are put into a manageable perspective. The individual is free to do more than engage in solitary battle with self-made phantoms.
>
> —Ellen from *Living with Cancer*, 1983

Anger

Much of your reaction to being diagnosed with cancer depends on your personality and on how well you have adapted to life's problems in the past. Some people have difficulty coping with any adversity. Every time they meet a problem they ask, "Why me?" When such people develop cancer, they may spend all their emotional energy being angry that the disease is happening to them. On the other hand, a person with a positive attitude toward adversity sees cancer as a problem that can be attacked in the same way as other problems.

> When people ask me, "How could God let it happen to me? What justice is there from such a God?" I tell them that God is not doing something to hurt them. Illness or death before one's

time is a malfunction of nature just as much as an earthquake or a hurricane.
>
> —Rabbi Joseph Asher, *Living with Cancer*, 1983

Anger is a normal reaction and a way of grieving during the initial period of shock following the diagnosis of cancer. In fact, if anger cannot be felt or expressed, it may turn into depression. If anger remains unresolved, it takes away energy that could be channeled into coping with the disease and living life as fruitfully as possible.

To be able to resolve anger, you must first recognize that you are angry. Often the anger and bitterness about one's disease are displaced; people make major issues out of minor events, like complaining about someone being late or the dinner not being satisfactory, or finding fault with a friend or mate. This displaced anger may be self-defeating: it can alienate people when you need family and friends most.

By recognizing your anger for what it is, you will be setting your mental attitude to cope with it. Letting the anger out by talking about it— even screaming, punching a pillow, or throwing things—can further help to release its hold on you. In the end, you can focus the energy of your anger and apply it in a positive direction by putting it to work to fight against your disease.

Maria also addressed this topic: "Cancer is devastating. At first you can't even think about it. You're smacked hard and all the wind goes out of you. You don't begin to think about yourself and your family and your reasons for living. I have seen people in all kinds of situations destroy themselves with their attitude, and, although I don't believe your attitude can cure your disease, I do believe it can help you. Therefore, I reject my negative thoughts. It sounds insane, but it keeps me healthy. Negative thinking breaks down my energy level. Although my drive and my will and my pace are basically the same as they were before, I have changed in one way. I no longer fly off the handle over unimportant matters. My priorities are being alive and loving my family. I've always loved life, and the biggest pain is that I hadn't had enough of it when this thing happened. So I said, 'Screw you, world! I just ain't leaving.'"

Inner Fire, 1998

Loss of Self-Esteem

The very idea of having cancer may itself threaten your self-esteem. Old superstitions still cling to the word "cancer." Some feel that it is a supernatural punishment or a disgrace. These are only superstitions; having cancer does not mean that you are bad or less worthy, or that you are guilty of some terrible wrongdoing. The disease can happen to anyone; in fact, one out of every two men and one out of every three women in the United States will develop cancer.

Cancer can take away or change the particular things that have given you your sense of self-esteem: body image, independence, and the ability to work and provide for your family. Changes in body image that result from surgery, radiation therapy, or chemotherapy may have a devastating effect on your self-esteem, particularly if the changes are visible to others. You may experience the loss of body parts, voice changes, scars or other skin changes, hair loss, or weight loss. Patients undergoing ostomy surgery (the creation of an artificial opening connecting the bowel to the skin) may feel humiliated because they must wear a bag to collect body wastes. Surgery affecting the genitals or reproductive organs may cause loss of self-esteem if one thinks that one is "not really a man" or "not really a woman" any longer.

Communicating with other cancer patients who have experienced similar body changes will help to remind you that, just as you can relate to them for who they are, so others can relate to you for who you are. Volunteers from various organizations and support groups (see Chapter 24, "Support Groups") can help you to adjust emotionally. In turn, you may be able to reciprocate and be of value to others.

A major problem affecting self-esteem is the loss of independence and control. Until illness deprives us of normal responsibilities, we may not realize how much our sense of self-esteem is related to accomplishment, productivity, and the ability to care for ourselves and others. At the outset, disease and therapy make you dependent on the medical system for your very life. In the hospital, you are dominated by the medical system. Tests are carried out and therapy is given. Others may determine when you eat, bathe, eliminate, walk, or even sleep. You may feel humiliated by having to use a bedpan or by having your body exposed to doctors, nurses, and other hospital personnel. Later, you may not be able to return to work or to carry out former responsibilities at home. You may have to depend on family, friends, or social service agencies for personal care, household help, or financial needs. You may feel guilt at being a burden and feel that you are of no value to others.

Your feelings of independence and self-esteem can be increased by taking responsibility in areas that you can handle. Eating a nutritionally adequate diet, exercising regularly to increase your strength and mobility, and performing as many self-care tasks as possible can help accelerate your recovery. Keeping progress notes on your improvement can help enhance your sense of accomplishment.

Involve yourself in supportive programs, such as patient support groups or special group counseling for cancer patients. Other programs may include meditation, hypnosis, yoga, tai chi, or biofeedback. If there are no support groups in your community, enlist the aid of a social worker, counselor, or clergy, or find other cancer patients and begin a group yourself. At home, choose the tasks you can do yourself. Caring for a pet, growing plants, or giving to family members in thoughtfulness and attention what you may not be able to give in physical effort can be outlets for your ability to nurture and will give you a sense of self-esteem.

If work and former interests must be put aside, find new ways of being productive, such as writing, art, music, sewing, knitting, crocheting, or crafts. You may find talents that you have not had the time to explore before.

Alienation

Nothing is as destructive to the will to live as alienation, the feeling of being cut off from life. Isolation and loneliness cause some patients to lose their will to live. They may "give up" and die very rapidly because they have lost their connection with other human beings. Cancer patients may experience isolation because of physical circumstances, hospitalization, loss of employment, or confinement to the home. You may feel socially isolated because of the attitudes of other people, and you may also experience alienation from within because of your own attitudes.

Hospitalization removes you from the mainstream of life—from family, friends, and all the daily habits and contacts that make you part of society. Although a hospital is full of people, they are busy strangers and you may feel very lonely. When you return home, if you're unable to go back to work or must be confined to home, your isolation there may be greater than in the hospital. In the hospital, you were at least part of a community. Now you may be alone: you may live alone, your family may be gone during the day, or there may be no one to visit you.

Although our society espouses rehabilitation and recovery from disease, in reality we often tend to shut people with chronic diseases out of employment. Some employers resist allowing cancer patients to return to work, out of fear that he or she may not be able to carry responsibilities or that the patient may relapse. If the patient does return to work, fellow workers may avoid him or her because they are afraid cancer may be contagious, or because they do not know how to relate to their coworker. Although laws such as the 1990 Americans with Disabilities Act protect patients' rights, there is still leeway for employers to get around such issues, and unfortunately, some do.

Family and friends sometimes inadvertently isolate the cancer patient. They may at first be sympathetic and attentive, but with time they may drift away; they have their own problems and their own lives to live. They may also find it difficult to carry on a normal conversation with someone who is ill or dying, and they may not know how to relate to you. If these things happen, it can make you feel you're being abandoned by those you care about most.

Even when the patient is not physically or socially isolated, loneliness and alienation may exist for the cancer patient. The uncertain and life-threatening nature of cancer puts us in touch with the essential aloneness with which we all must face death. Even patients who are surrounded by family and friends may feel lonely in this awareness.

In fighting disease, some patients turn much of their energy and attention inward upon themselves. They lose contact with the rest of life and create an isolation and loneliness that they may not recognize as self-inflicted. Other patients withdraw from their connections with the outer world because their focus is on grieving and feeling sorry for themselves. Patients who regard cancer as an automatic death sentence may unconsciously cut their ties with life and live as though they already belong with the dead.

When isolation is thrust upon you from the outside and when old connections to life are broken, you must learn to make new bridges. Loss of independence may encourage you to "wait for things to happen." You may feel frightened or pessimistic about taking any steps toward making a new life; yet we all have the capacity to alter our direction, make changes, and rearrange our strategies.

Getting involved in rehabilitation programs and support groups made up of other cancer patients and their families can be your first step (see Chapter 24, "Support Groups"). You will be aiding your recovery as well as making connections with people who share your experience.

Do not let pride prevent you from asking for help or from admitting your need for other people. And do not be ashamed to express emotions. Sharing with others can deepen and strengthen relationships. The closest bonds are made in times of crisis.

Your nurse, social worker, clergy, counselor, doctor, and patient support groups are there to hear you and to help you. Expressing what you feel and discussing your feelings with others can give you distance and new perspective, as well as heal the alienation that comes from living in a separate emotional world. You will not be abandoned.

Regaining Control

In the face of a disease and treatment effects that are both largely beyond your control, you may feel vulnerable and helpless. Feeling a lack of control, patients often have a sense of, "Why bother?" Although they want to live and they have a desire to fight for their life, they feel that it may be futile to even try. Finding ways of regaining control can offset these feelings. We try to help patients do this by involving them as active participants in combating their disease. In this way, they no longer perceive themselves as helpless victims, but instead become active partners with their medical support team in the fight for improvement, remission, or cure. We have found this is the best action we can take to strengthen a patient's will to live.

Many patients develop their own programs for taking control of their lives. One patient, Joanna, who was diagnosed with breast cancer ten years ago and ovarian cancer five years ago, created her own regimen for handling fatigue and depression that she calls "recharging her batteries." Her program includes "juicing" (drinking a blend of fresh-squeezed apple, cabbage, carrot, and parsley juices every day) and a diet that includes organic produce and hormone-free meat.

She tells us, "I also try to exercise regularly, which really has a good effect. It relaxes not only my body but also my mind, especially when I come back from the office after a stressful day. I love the ocean, and when I feel depressed I walk out to the beach and sit there until I feel better. When I can't get outside, I put on one of my nature tapes with rainfall, the surf, and storms and lie on the floor with my eyes closed listening to them. Classical music has a very calming effect on me, too. If I am really unnerved or depressed, I read one of my favorite spiritual books. Whenever I feel discouraged, I think about one of the survivor stories I've read. I'm not saying it can save you, but it really helps you through the whole mental process."

Each person must find his or her own ways to regain control and thereby strengthen the will to live. Still, there are some essentials, which we have outlined below. Although the purpose of this list is to try to direct the course of your illness toward health by mobilizing your will to live, our experience has been that a significant benefit to the people who use these eleven suggestions is an improvement in the quality of their current lives. This is reason enough to give them serious consideration.

1. Choose a Physician You Can Trust with Your Care.

Find a physician who projects hope, optimism, and confidence—someone you can talk to. Remember, the choice of doctor is yours (if your insurance is through an HMO, your choice may be restricted). You and your physician should have a mutual goal: your getting well, regardless of the diagnosis. As one of our patients said:

> The physician is the most important person in a seriously ill patient's life and has the most telling effect on the kind of life the patient leads. No one—parent, child, husband, lover, or best friend—can take the physician's place. Having had cancer for more than two years, I know what a doctor can mean in liberating one to live actively during the remaining time of one's life.
>
> A doctor should recognize that by his own courage and respect for the patient, he can relieve terror. If he shows confidence that he

can remain in control of the disease and the pain, it removes an enormous burden from the patient's life. This is the approach my doctors have taken with me. It was never spoken, but they communicated it in their actions and manner. It has been a wonderful feeling. Instead of seeing each setback and loss of time as a defeat, we turn it around. Each day, week, and month that we pass—particularly if I am free to enjoy life during that time—is a victory.

If a doctor can add to the quality of a patient's life and can help the patient live more fully, there is no greater gift.

2. Become Partners with Your Physician.

Be an active participant with your physician. Find out everything you can about the nature of your problem and your potential treatment. Try not to see yourself as a victim. The partnership between you and your physician must be based on honesty and open communication about therapy options and rehabilitation.

You and your doctor must also develop a program to help you maintain healthy nutrition, appropriate physical exercise, and proper mental attitude. Becoming well-informed about your medical problem is also an important step. Take advantage of medical libraries and hospital resource centers. Learn as much as possible about your condition. If you have any questions about your cancer or treatment, ask your doctor or seek a second medical opinion.

3. Plan for the Future and Set Goals.

People don't plan for the future if they believe there will be no future. Come up with a list of short-term and long-term goals. Making plans is itself a pleasant and positive experience. Why not enjoy yourself while giving yourself hope for the future? As one of our patients told us, "I'm too busy to die."

4. Seek Psychological Support.

The powerful emotions released by a serious illness—fear, despair, anger, and guilt—fade with recovery, but anxieties can accumulate with an illness that is chronic and possibly fatal. You may worry so much that you lose sight of the possibility of recovery. On the other hand, you also may become so hopeful and confident that you lose sight of reality and fail to follow medical advice. You need to find a balance between undue pessimism and unwarranted optimism.

Choose your support systems carefully. Support groups with skilled leaders can provide a safe atmosphere in which to express your feelings and learn from the experiences of others. The groups not only seem to enhance their members' sense of control over their lives and ability to cope with their illnesses; they also may have positive biological effects.

The best way to judge if a support group is right for you is to attend a meeting. If you feel a group is not helping you, don't go back. You may have to visit several groups before you find one that feels right to you. Many people need one-on-one contact for their support, either by itself or in conjunction with a group.

5. Relaxation and Stress Reduction.

The "relaxation response" is the name used to describe a physical state that can be achieved through acupressure, meditation and directed visualization, yoga, biofeedback, tai chi, and other methods. The relaxation response is important because, when that state is achieved, the immune system may temporarily be enhanced. This may have a beneficial effect on the course of your illness.

Choose a method that works for you and use it regularly. Herbert Benson, M.D., author of *The Relaxation Response*, pioneered studies on the effects of transcendental meditation on health. Dr. Benson found that people who meditate using a simple prayer, word, or phrase show dramatic physiologic changes, including a decrease in oxygen consumption, respiratory rate, heart rate, and blood pressure. Symptoms for a variety of diseases diminish as well.

6. Control Negative Emotions.

Anger, depression, and loss of self-esteem are normal reactions to a cancer diagnosis, as are feelings of isolation and loneliness. You need to use all the means at your disposal to combat them. Allowed to fester, they can destroy hope and lead to a wish to die.

Most important, you should not always believe the statistics concerning your illness. They give you only an average percentage, derived from large population studies on illness and treatment similar to yours. A statistic can give you only a general idea of what the odds are for you to get better or have a recurrence of disease. Even if your odds seem poor, your real chances are anywhere between 100 percent (success) or 0 percent (failure).

7. Find Ways to Enjoy Life.

Positive emotions not only bolster the will to live, they also stimulate the production of natural morphine-like chemicals in the brain called endorphins, which can decrease depression. Activities such as daily walks, enjoying nature, creating art, reading and writing poetry or stories, watching funny movies, getting a massage, and helping others can produce endorphins.

Gardening is also a life-affirming activity. One patient told us, "I had never gardened before, but I was going to be home a lot, so my husband put in a garden and I became a gardener. Nothing makes me happier now than to be out in the backyard when the sun is out and plant my bulbs or prune my flowers or just sit out there and read."

If you're an animal lover, consider adopting a dog or cat. Pets have been scientifically proven to be more than just good company. They have been found to act as a natural sedative, lowering the blood pressure of their owners and promoting wellness.

We frequently encourage our patients to take trips. Most people return rejuvenated because they have had a chance to rest, reflect, reassess, and step out of their daily lives.

8. Avoid Social Isolation.

Spending time alone is important to the healing process. It is normal to want to be alone. However, too much solitude can lead to depression. Nothing can be as destructive to the will to live as the feeling of being cut off from life. Feelings of alienation, isolation, and loneliness are often due to physical circumstances—hospitalization, loss of employment, or confinement to the home—but also may arise because of the attitudes of other people toward you and your illness.

Tell your friends and family what you want and expect of them. Be open and honest about when you need their help and about what you want or don't want to talk about. When you are feeling physically or mentally low, many people will try to raise your spirits by saying, "Don't worry, everything will be fine." This is a common, socially acceptable statement, but the true message seems to be, "Don't tell me that you don't feel good. Tell me you're okay." When you aren't feeling all that great, this isn't what you want to hear. What you want to hear is, "I'm sorry you're feeling down and I'm here for you."

9. Be Open and Honest.

One of the most important realizations is that you have everything to do with how others perceive you and treat you. If you can discuss your disease and medical therapy in a matter-of-fact manner, people will respond without fear or awkwardness. Remember, *you're* in charge.

10. Be Open to Making Compromises.

Compromise involves learning how to adjust to symptoms and treatments while returning to as many of the normal activities of daily living as possible. Maybe you won't be able to take that planned vacation and maybe you won't be exercising as vigorously or as often as you did before. Then again, maybe you will.

You need to continue, adopt, or create a lifestyle and an attitude that will let you function physically and emotionally. You will find that by making compromises, your intellectual and emotional potential have not diminished. On the contrary, they will be enhanced. Illness can be an opportunity to redirect your life in new and productive ways.

In *Creativity and Disease*, Phillip Sandblom, professor of surgery at the University of Lund in Sweden, relates the story of the artist Henri Matisse, who was a lawyer when he suddenly was afflicted by acute appendicitis. This was before the era of successful surgery for this ailment, so Matisse was treated conservatively and spent more than a year recovering from the many complications. During his convalescence, his mother provided him with art materials as a diversion. He became infatuated with colors, and through courage and boldness became a very inventive artist.

"Had Matisse lived in our current era," Sandblom notes, "he would have been hospitalized for a few days and then discharged to continue his career as a lawyer rather than one of the great artists of our time."

11. Seek Inspiration from Others with a Similar Condition.

Physicians and other medical staff will often introduce frightened and apprehensive patients in the early stages of diagnosis or treatment to those who have had a similar experience. Someone who may be starting a course of chemotherapy and is afraid of losing his or her hair, for instance, may benefit from meeting someone who has already gone through that ordeal.

Finally, do not let illness dominate your life.

Hope Helps Patients Live Fuller Lives

Illness generally reduces body function, and forces idleness on the patient. This forced idleness promotes depression and reduces the will to live. Thus, the mind, which can be a powerful ally, is not allowed to fulfill its positive function in the struggle with the illness. Hope promotes recovery.

There is no medicine like hope
No incentive so great
And no tonic so powerful
As the expectation
Of something better tomorrow.
—Orison Swett Marden

Hope is the emotional mental state that motivates you to keep on living, accomplish things, and succeed. It is the expectation when you awaken that today will be a good day. It is what motivates you to get out of bed in the morning. It is a driving force for positive living.

Hope is an essential part of your will to live. Hope can be maintained as long as there is even a remote chance for survival. It is kindled and nurtured by even minor improvements, and when crises or reversals persist, hope is maintained by the positive attitude of family, friends, and your health support team.

But hope will primarily come from yourself, if you are willing to do everything you can to improve your health and if you are willing to fight for your life. Self-motivation and learning what you can do for yourself is critical. By helping yourself, you gain control over your life, thus strengthening your will to live.

Hope can be increased or improved by having good things happen and by enjoying more of life each day through positive activities, such as going to a concert, attending a football game, or enjoying your family and friends. Some of the "good things" come from sheer luck; but you too can help make "good things" happen.

When hope is diminished, a patient can lose the will to live. At these times, "living proof stories"—stories of how others courageously dealt with a similar problem—can be a great help. These stories inspire hope and may be necessary at the time of diagnosis, when everything seems bleak and the future has not yet been imagined.

Hope can last for a long time, or it can be felt during a short burst of activity or thought. You will need to increase your motivation to help maintain a state of hope and not give up. For example, the anticipation of getting well or having a pleasurable event decreases pessimism and anxiety and also gives a sense of control over the future. Sometimes, just supportive care by a physician, family, and friends can help maintain a person during this most difficult time in life.

One of the major themes of this book is that you must become an active partner in the treatment of your illness. You must consider yourself an integral part of the medical team. You should know what is happening in your medical treatment, for with knowledge your role is supported. In this way, your will to live can be channeled into action.

Even when you are very ill, you still have physical and emotional reserves that you can draw on. These reserves will help you to survive yet another day and will become the foundation of your recovery program.

When exhausted soldiers march home after a rigorous day, they sometimes begin to march and sing together. They have a revival of mood and spirit, and find new energies and strength. And you can muster reserve energies too, even when you feel exhausted by disease and illness.

Each of us has the capacity to live each day a little better, but we need to focus on purposes and goals and then set into action a realistic plan that will help us achieve our goals. Only by using the power of the will to live, nourished by hope, can you achieve the sublime pleasures of knowing and experiencing the wonders of life and appreciating its meaning through vital living.

To heal sometimes
To relieve often
To console always

—Sir William Osler, M.D.

Courage and Hope

David Spiegel, M.D.

Plato said that courage is knowing when to be afraid. This chapter is about courageous people, who became very ill or faced some other crisis, yet who counted—and still count—themselves fortunate. In the face of a dismal diagnosis or harsh circumstances, they took stock of their resources and found strength and love.

Many people face sickness, but are not overtaken by it. Just because one part of them becomes ill, they do not give up. Their bodies may suffer, but their spirits remain strong.

Indeed, serious illness is a reminder that we are not immortal. Those who respond creatively to a life-threatening illness hear it as a wake-up call, a reminder of how time is short and life is precious. They do what matters most while they can, experience the joy of living and loving, and let the people around them know how much they are loved and appreciated. They trivialize the trivial, drop useless commitments, eliminate relationships that are taxing and not worth the trouble, and "just say no" to doing things they think they should do rather than what they want to.

A moving section in Chapter 45, "Your Legacy of Love," explores the tradition of writing an "ethical will"—an individual's spiritual legacy, a codification of what that person has learned in life about what has meaning and value. This underscores the importance of feeling embedded in the world of people, using the contemplation of the end of one's life not to deny death but to reaffirm the values of life.

People talk about and illustrate the will to live in a realistic and meaningful way. They do not demonstrate some artificial determination to prolong life no matter what. They assess life's resources, goals, and values. They take stock and see how fortunate they are to have people who care about them and whom they care about. Mind may not triumph over matter, but the mind does matter.

Years ago, a clever graduate student taking a statistics course was wandering through a cemetery and noted that there were two types of data on the headstones: birth dates and death dates. She wondered if they bore any relationship to each other. Theoretically, they shouldn't. When you die, you die—period. That was not what she found. People died more often in the period after their birthday than in the period before. The difference was not large, usually several weeks, but it was statistically significant. People seem to hang on until after their birthdays or some other special event. While this doesn't mean that you can make yourself live indefinitely through mental calisthenics, it does show that meaning makes a difference in the course of disease.

Another crucial theme is the power of social connection: no man or woman is an island. Prisoners of war on Bataan kept themselves alive by giving one another lectures, playing together, and caring for one another. They developed a special relationship with each other and their God.

In my own field of research, we have found that women with breast cancer help one another enormously through support groups in which they can vent their darkest fears and learn how deeply they can still care about each other. To feel part of a network of caring at a time of serious illness is deeply reassuring. The will to live is not the denial of death. Rather, it is the intensification of life experience that comes when you realize how finite life is.

Be willing to make compromises, find the joy in life, find good support groups, and form a partnership with your doctors. Cancer patient stories make it clear that we are not simply happy or sad and that pleasure is not simply the absence of pain. Illness teaches us that we can be both happy and sad and that the threat of progressive disease and death can provide a context in which life can be sweeter. A woman with advanced breast cancer once said to me, "All my life I had wanted to go to

(Continued from page 127)

the summer opera in Santa Fe. This year I went. I brought my cancer with me and it sat in the seat next to me. I loved it."

Adapted from the Introduction to *Inner Fire, Your Will to Live* by Ernest and Isadora Rosenbaum with permission from Plexus, Austin, Texas, 1998.

14

Stress and Cancer: An Overview

Mark J. Doolittle, Ph.D.

The cure of many diseases is unknown to physicians...because they are ignorant of the whole. For the part can never be well unless the whole is well.

—Plato

In recent times, there has been a substantial shift in health care toward recognition of the wisdom of Plato's creed, namely, that the mental and physical are not separate, isolated, and unrelated, but are instead vitally linked elements of a total person. Health is becoming increasingly recognized as a balance of many parts—physical and environmental factors, emotional and psychological states, nutritional habits, and exercise patterns. As part of that balance, the role of stress is well established as the cause of a broad range of disorders.

For example, it is now generally acknowledged that for heart disease—the nation's leading cause of death—emotional stress is a major risk factor, equal in importance to other such recognized risk factors as hypertension, cigarette smoking, elevated serum cholesterol level, obesity, and diabetes. Stress also has been recognized as an important risk factor in high blood pressure, ulcers, colitis, asthma, pain syndromes (e.g., migraine, cluster, and tension headaches; backaches), skin diseases, insomnia, and various psychological disorders. Most standard medical textbooks attribute anywhere from 50 to 80 percent of all disease to stress-related origins.

The role of stress in cancer is unclear. What is important for patients is that the reduction of stress may very well improve chances for recovery, improve quality of life, and provide an opportunity for greater participation in total treatment.

It should also be emphasized that stress is only one element of the mind-body balance that determines your well-being. Like a river with many tributaries flowing into it, health depends on the contribution and equilibrium of many factors. There can be no doubt that exposure to harmful substances (carcinogens) increases the incidence of cancer; but there also is evidence that genetic predisposition, exposure to radiation, and a poor diet also contribute.

The Nature of Stress

We often speak casually of stress as if its meaning was well established, but scientific study has continued to discover new meaning for the concept and attribute new importance to its role in health and disease. While the word may imply a purely mental reaction, research has shown that stress induces virtually every part of the body.

Most research has focused on the "fight-or-flight" response that the body has to threats, and on the long-term effects of chronic stress, in which the body is subjected to repeated arousal.

The fight-or-flight response has been shown to produce a wide variety of mental and physical changes. For instance, when a car swerves toward us on the highway, we may consciously feel afraid, anxious, and angry. Internally, our body is reverberating from head to toe with all the aspects of the stress response: a part of the brain called the hypothalamus stimulates the pituitary gland, which in turn activates the thyroid and adrenal glands, which quickly flood the bloodstream with adrenaline, cortisone, and other stress hormones. The entire body is affected: heart rate increases, blood pressure rises, breathing becomes faster, body muscles tighten, facial muscles constrict, pupils dilate, hearing becomes sharper, sugar is secreted into the bloodstream, blood flows to the brain and muscles and away from the stomach and intestines, the bowels and bladder relax, brain wave activity quickens, palms sweat, and hands and feet become colder as blood flows away from the skin to the brain and muscles.

In addition to its usefulness for physical survival, the fight-or-flight response carries with it an emotional safety valve: by discharging internal tension. Either in physical struggle or escape, the body first releases the built-up pressure, then eventually goes to a post-stress, let-down phase, and finally returns to a neutral, nonstress state. However, what worked in other societies or times often does not work in ours. Recent research has shown that the fight-or-flight response can, ironically, become a threat to our health and survival. The nature of civilization makes this response inappropriate in many situations. For example, being stopped by a police officer may arouse the fight-or-flight response, but to fight or flee would only make matters worse. We therefore stifle those responses for the sake of personal survival and social harmony. But as the number of similarly charged situations increases and tension is not discharged, a state of chronic stress can develop, with the risk of resulting health problems.

It is not difficult to understand how modern life increases the chances for arousal of the stress syndrome: living conditions become more crowded, noisy, and polluted; the pace and intensity of life increases; mass media remind us constantly of the deaths, injuries, and threats all around us; sources of information proliferate and then become increasingly confusing.

When the world around us becomes increasingly stressful, the tendency is for the fight-or-flight response to be chronically activated. If the body is unable to regularly let down, it tends not to swing back to its neutral nonstress point and it becomes pulled more and more toward a chronic stress response. The result is a slowly rising level of internal pressure.

This prolonged buildup of tension and excessive arousal can lead to a host of disorders. Many researchers have found that chronic stress can wear down our body's defenses, lower our immune response, and make us more vulnerable to all sicknesses, including cancer.

Some researchers have attempted to clarify to what degree stressful life events are related to sickness. After long research, Drs. Thomas Holmes and Richard Rahe developed a scale based on forty-three common stressful experiences, in the order they were found to be related to illness. By checking the items that have occurred in the last year, you will arrive at a total score that indicates your supposed level of vulnerability to illness.

This scale reflects that change, *whether positive or negative*, tests our ability to adapt. The higher the score, the higher the probability that a person will become sick. High scores (above 300) do not necessarily mean a person *will* get sick, only that the risk is greater. For instance, in one study using this scale, the 30 percent with the highest scores had 90 percent more illnesses than the 30 percent with the lowest scores. In another study, 49 percent of the people in the high-risk group (scores above 300) became ill; 25 percent of the medium-risk group (200–299) became ill; but only 9 percent of the low-risk group (150–199) became ill.

The life-change scale, though, also shows that there is nothing necessarily health-threatening about life changes. In one of the studies, 51 percent of the high-risk group did not get sick.

Social Readjustment Rating Scale

Rank	Event	Value	Your Score
1	Death of spouse	100	
2	Divorce	73	
3	Marital separation	65	
4	Jail term	63	
5	Death of close family member	63	
6	Personal injury or illness	52	
7	Marriage	50	
8	Fired from work	47	
9	Marital reconciliation	45	
10	Retirement	45	
11	Change in family member's health	44	
12	Pregnancy	40	
13	Sex difficulties	39	
14	Addition to family	39	
15	Business readjustment	39	
16	Change in financial status	38	
17	Death of a close friend	37	
18	Change to different line of work	36	
19	Change in number of marital arguments	35	
20	Mortgage or loan over $10,000	31	
21	Foreclosure of mortgage or loan	30	
22	Change in work responsibilities	29	
23	Son or daughter leaving home	29	
24	Trouble with in-laws	29	
25	Outstanding personal achievement	28	
26	Spouse begins or stops work	26	
27	Starting or finishing school	26	
28	Change in living conditions	25	
29	Revision of personal habits	24	
30	Trouble with boss	23	
31	Change in work hours, conditions	20	
32	Change in residence	20	
33	Change in schools	19	
34	Change in recreational habits	19	
35	Change in church activities	19	
36	Change in social activities	18	
37	Mortgage and loan under $10,000	17	
38	Change in sleeping habits	16	
39	Change in number of family gatherings	15	
40	Change in eating habits	15	
41	Vacation	13	
42	Christmas season	12	
43	Minor violation of the law	11	
		TOTAL SCORE = _____	

Source: Holmes, T.H., and R.H. Rahe, "The Social Readjustment Rating Scale," *Journal of Psychosomatic Research* 11 (1967): 213–18.

When difficult and threatening events occur, it is *how we perceive and respond to them* that determines the intensity of the stress. As any sailor knows, it is not the direction of the wind that determines our course so much as how we set the sails—in sailing parlance, this is known significantly as the "attitude" of the sails. Our attitude about what we feel we should be and our imagined punishment if we fail determine how we see and react to events.

In a classic study of heart-disease patients, Dr. Nanders Dunbar noted the recurring trait of compulsive striving: some patients would rather die than fail. The study showed clearly how attitude could create a chronic life-threatening situation where no real threat exists.

Failure is not death, and it is certainly not worse than death. But as long as we believe that it is, our bodies will respond with the fight-or-flight response; coming events that might be handled with relative ease instead create the constant burden of chronic stress—with the ironic possibility of creating an actual life-threatening illness if the pressure is not removed.

On the positive side, it is equally true that by altering our attitudes and tension-producing habits, we may tip the scales in a more healthful direction. Recent research in areas such as biofeedback and meditation has shown that we can become aware of our stress responses and can influence them.

Stress and Cancer

The possible role of stress-related factors in the onset and course of cancer is certainly not a new or radical notion. As far back as the second century, the Greek physician Galen noted that melancholy women appeared more likely to develop cancer than cheerful ones. Eighteenth- and nineteenth-century physicians frequently noted that severe life disruptions and resulting emotional turmoil, despair, and loss of hope seemed to occur before the onset of cancer. In 1870, Dr. James Paget emphasized that emotional disturbance was related to cancer: "The cases are so frequent in which deep anxiety, deferred hope, and disappointment are quickly followed by the growth and increase of cancer that we can hardly doubt that mental depression is a weighty additive to the other influences favoring the development of the cancerous constitution."

In 1885, Parker made the mind-body connection in a prophetic way by emphasizing the physical results of emotion: "There are the strongest physiological reasons for believing that great mental depression, particularly grief, induces a predisposition to such disease as cancer, or becomes an existing cause under circumstances where the predisposition had already been acquired."

Despite the consistent trend of these observations, the interest in more physical interventions—such as radiation, surgery, and chemotherapy—drew medical attention away from the emotional contribution. Furthermore, the lack of tools for dealing with stress understandably has led to a reliance on these medical interventions.

Emotional Life-History Pattern of Cancer Patients

Recent exploration of the role of stress and emotions in cancer, led by the work of Lawrence LeShan, has aroused new interest. A quarter-century ago, LeShan studied the lives of more than five hundred cancer patients, many of whom he worked with in psychotherapy. He found a distinct emotional life-history pattern in 76 percent of the cancer patients, but the same pattern appeared in only 10 percent of a control group that did not have cancer.

This pattern had four distinctive features:

1. The person's childhood was marked by extreme difficulty in establishing warm, satisfying relationships. Usually, because of the death of a parent, divorce, chronic conflict, or prolonged separation from one or both parents, the child developed a deep sense of isolation and loneliness, with a hopeless view of ever gaining lasting, fulfilling relationships. The child tried to please others in order to win affection.

2. In adulthood, the person found strength and meaning in a relationship or career and poured a great deal of energy into this vital source of support.

3. When this key source was removed—through death, divorce, disillusionment, or retirement—and the childhood wound reopened, the person again experienced that sense of loss, despair, hopelessness, and helplessness.

4. Feelings—especially negative ones like anger, hurt, and disappointment—were constantly bottled up; in fact, others viewed the person as "too

good to be true." But this superficial saint-like quality was a reflection of a deeper inability to express hostility and an overcompensation for feelings of unworthiness.

The pattern described by LeShan in *You Can Fight for Your Life* has been found with remarkable consistency by other researchers. However, it is important to understand that this research identifies emotions as only one possible factor in the development of cancer—not the only one.

Positive Role of the Emotions

Research suggests that there is a positive role for the emotions in cancer. For, just as an attitude of hopelessness and helplessness may hurt a person's chances for health or recovery, so an attitude of determination, hope, and fighting back can help lead to a positive outcome. If bottling up emotional expression and holding a reservoir of tension inside can create a dangerous load of chronic stress, learning to let go can reduce that burden and its risk.

This perspective has led many physicians and patients to recognize that a comprehensive approach to cancer includes dealing with the emotional and stress-related aspects of the disease. Even physicians who are skeptical of the role of stress in the onset of cancer generally speak of the will to live as an important element of treatment. Adding counseling and stress-reduction techniques to traditional medical care is becoming more common.

Cancer treatment is beginning to focus on the "whole" person, as Plato put it, and on how the patient may actively join in the rehabilitation effort.

Coping with Stress

"It is much more important to know what sort of patient has a disease than what sort of disease a patient has."

—Sir William Osler, M.D.

The importance of attitudes, feelings, and beliefs has been revealed by various studies.

The Placebo Effect

First, it is well known, though perhaps not well understood, that if a person has faith in a treatment and believes that it will work, the chances are greatly increased that the treatment will work—even if the treatment has no known therapeutic value. In science this is described as the placebo effect, and it is one of the most powerful tools available to the health practitioner.

The power appears to rest solely on the strength of the patient's positive beliefs and expectations; the placebo effect is stronger if the doctor also believes that the treatment is effective.

The more severe the pain, the more effective the placebo is. The placebo effect goes even beyond pain relief and can change the state of the disease. For example, two groups of patients with bleeding ulcers were given the same medication, but one group was told by a physician that the drug would undoubtedly produce relief, while the second group was told by a nurse that the drug was experimental and its effectiveness was unknown. In the first group, 70 percent showed significant improvements; in the second group, only 25 percent improved. The sole difference was the positive expectation created in the first group.

In another intriguing study, 150 patients were divided into three groups. The first group was the control group and received no medication. The other two groups were told they were going to receive a new drug that would increase health and longevity. One of these groups received a placebo, and the other group received the actual drug. After years of follow-up, the first group showed a normal amount of illness and mortality; the experience of the second (placebo) group was significantly better than the first (control) group, and the third (medicated) group displayed about the same amount of additional improvement over the placebo group as the placebo group had over the control group. Thus, while the drug reduced illness and prolonged life, so did the placebo.

How the power of belief affects the body remains a mystery. Recent research suggests that the placebo may relieve pain by releasing the body's own natural painkilling chemicals. But whatever the mechanism, the fact remains that attitude and belief can play a vital role in the success or failure of any treatment. To ignore or neglect the power of positive expectations and beliefs is to abandon one of the most valuable tools known to medicine.

Biofeedback

Another area that confirms the influence of mind on body is biofeedback—the ability of an individual to have some control over what were previously believed to be involuntary functions. Through the use of sensitive electronic devices, a person can view, for example, his or her own heart rate, brain wave activity, and skin temperature. The startling finding has been that the patient who can "see" internal biological activity can generally learn to exercise some conscious influence over that activity.

Although the study of biofeedback is still in its early stages, it has already proven effective for a broad range of stress-related problems, including heart disorders, high blood pressure, migraine and tension headaches, asthma, ulcers, and chronic pain. The range of applications keeps expanding. Epileptics have been able to reduce seizures by using biofeedback instead of medicine to control their brain wave activity.

Meditation

Recent research into meditation has shown that simple periods of daily deep relaxation may have important and lasting effects on a wide variety of stress disorders, perhaps most notably high blood pressure.

Self-Change

Given the research described earlier and these additional findings, the conclusion seems inescapable: for a person facing cancer, learning to cope with stress in a self-nourishing way can be an important factor in aiding the treatment process, increasing chances for recovery, helping to prevent or minimize flare-up, and maximizing the quality and length of life. Coping with stress is only part of a comprehensive treatment program, but it is the part perhaps most influenced by the patient.

It is often possible, even necessary (although undoubtedly difficult) to see a major illness as an opportunity rather than a tragedy. To become hopeless and feel helpless only makes the situation worse; to go to the other extreme with a denial of feelings and a "business as usual, everything is fine" facade also does nothing about the internal load of stress. Between blindly giving up and blindly charging on is another option—self-examination and change. The two key elements of change are analyzing and restructuring your lifestyle, and practicing and developing enjoyable techniques for reducing stress.

Both of these tasks are easier said than done. The first is no doubt the more difficult and requires real motivation. The key questions you must ask if you are going to alter your stance toward life, are:

- What do I want out of life?
- What is important to me?
- What are my priorities, and where has my own health and happiness been on the list?
- What chronic habits do I have that may have helped lead to the illness? Are they worth dying for?
- What realistic steps can I take to change?

Answering these questions may require the involvement of professionals, family, a number of close friends, and, perhaps, a support group. To establish new priorities and develop realistic ways to reach them takes time, communication, and honest self-analysis. Changing is not easy. But by making a concentrated effort to alter your pattern of stressful life events and the way you respond to stress, you can influence the pace and intensity of your life.

In conjunction with that goal, you may want to seek professional help in developing useful stress-reduction techniques, especially if you feel that tools such as biofeedback may have value for you. In any event, the following relaxation technique will provide a good beginning.

An Easy Introductory Relaxation Method

1. Sit or lie down and get comfortable. Let your arms rest at your sides, and don't cross your legs. (Initially, it's useful to eliminate as many distractions as possible. A quiet, darkened room helps. As you practice, letting go becomes easier and easier, even in less than ideal settings.) Squirm and stretch your muscles a little until you feel more relaxed. Then let your eyes gently close.

2. Take a slow, deep breath in through your nose, feeling your lungs fill up and your stomach expand. When your lungs are full, hold the air in for just a second, then slowly let the air go, feeling yourself letting go all over. When you feel the air exhaled, don't hurry to inhale, just slowly take another smooth, deep breath, feel yourself filling up, hold it for a second, then slowly and completely let it all go and feel yourself relaxing even more. Let the exhale be longer than the inhale, and really let go. Get lost and absorbed in simply listening to your breathing and feeling your body letting go. Do this for a few more

breaths, and then breathe naturally, without trying to take especially deep breaths. Make sure you are breathing deeply and not shallowly (just from the chest).

3. Now let your attention drift down to your toes. Slowly and gently tense the muscles in your toes. Become aware of how the tension feels, then let the toes relax and feel the difference. Notice the sensations you feel in the toes as you let them relax.

4. Repeat this cycle of tensing and relaxing with each major muscle group as you move up your body—your calves, thighs, hips, stomach, back, shoulders, arms, neck, jaws, eyes, forehead, and scalp. Just as you became absorbed in your breathing, get lost in feeling and enjoying the sensations you produce in directly relaxing all your muscles.

5. After going through each muscle group separately, stretch your arms and legs out and tense up all your muscles at once (or as many as you can). Then let your body go limp. Take a few deep, slow breaths. If you notice any residual tension in any part of your body, repeat the tense-and-relax cycle there to see if you can loosen up that area.

6. Finally, before opening your eyes, take a brief journey around your body, sensing how it feels to be more deeply relaxed. Become familiar with the feeling. Then, when you are ready, take another deep breath and slowly open your eyes.

Slow, deep breathing and overall muscular relaxation are perhaps the two easiest and most direct ways to calm down. Most of us breathe sixteen to twenty times a minute; with slow, deep breathing we cut that number in half or more.

Combined with muscular relaxation, the ultimate effect is to slow down heart rate, lower blood pressure, relax muscles, and increase blood flow to the hands and feet—in short, to produce the opposite of the stressful fight-or-flight response.

This relaxation technique can be modified in many ways. One helpful maneuver is to silently repeat a sound, word, or phrase in rhythm with your breathing, such as, "I am…" (as you breathe in) "…relaxed" (as you breathe out).

Buddhists say that the mind is like a drunken monkey. It wanders and rambles all over the place. Thoughts run past in random fashion, like the chatter of several radio programs. Images flash across the internal mental screen like the pictures on a movie screen.

The key to stopping these distracting thoughts and images is to have a simple focus, a home base to return to when you are aware you've been wandering or getting distracted by external stimuli or internal chatter. Then you simply take another deep, slow breath; let the word, phrase, or sound repeat itself in rhythm with your breathing; and let go again. The possibilities for a control focus are endless—music; self-suggestions (such as "My arms and legs are warm and pleasantly heavy"); simple words such as "calm," "peace," "serene," or traditional mantras like Om, Shum, and Mu. One pleasant technique is to imagine yourself in a peaceful, pleasurable setting—a warm beach, a lush green meadow, a refreshing mountain lake, or floating on a soft white cloud.

The key is to keep it simple and enjoyable. If the process isn't enjoyable, chances are good it won't be effective, and eventually it won't be done. Making it into a chore will only tend to maintain your tension. Stress reduction should be viewed along with food, sleep, and exercise as a vital element in maintaining health and resisting disease.

Positive Attitude

Carl and Stephanie Simonton are perhaps the most noted and controversial proponents of the importance of stress in cancer treatment. In addition to providing traditional medical care, they have emphasized a full-scale treatment of the psychological aspects of cancer. Their perspective emphasizes mobilizing the positive attitude of the patient as part of the treatment.

The Simontons reason that if chronic stress increases the probability of cancer, reducing stress and encouraging the will to live should improve the chances of recovery and enhance the quality of life. To that end, they employ relaxation imagery techniques and intensive counseling in addition to the usual medical treatments. They write: "Essentially, the visual imagery process involved a period of relaxation, during which the patient would mentally picture a desired goal or result. With the cancer patient, this would mean his attempting to visualize the cancer, the treatment destroying it, and, most importantly, his body's natural defenses helping him recover."

The Simontons believe that a positive attitude toward treatment is a better predictor of response to treatment than the severity of the disease. Although the extent of "mind over matter" is not known, dealing with stress and encouraging the will to live are undoubtedly important in extending the length of life and enhancing its quality. To what extent we can actually influence our immune system and help it fight cancer remains to be explored.

To have suggested twenty years ago that people with epilepsy would today be stopping their seizures through controlling their own brain waves would have been considered sheer nonsense, yet that, and much more, is now a reality. The importance of mobilizing the mind as a positive ally cannot be questioned. Cancer is a dreaded disease, perhaps the most frightening diagnosis a person can face. Helping the person to cope with that fear is clearly an essential element of any complete treatment.

The perspective emphasizing the relationship between stress and cancer carries with it a new role not only for doctors and other health practitioners, but for patients as well. No longer can patients be seen, or see themselves, as passive recipients of treatment, helpless bystanders awaiting the outcome. In many ways, the patient's motivation, attitude, and behavior can be the key elements that shift the scales from a poor outcome to a good one.

In this light, one anecdote from medical history seems particularly relevant. Louis Pasteur is a well-known name in science: he was the pioneer in exploring the microbe, dispelling the myth of "spontaneous generation," and helping to eradicate such diseases as diphtheria and typhus that ravaged the world in the nineteenth century. Less well known is his colleague, Claude Bernard, who insisted, somewhat in opposition to Pasteur, that it was not so much the presence or absence of microbes, bacteria, or viruses that determined health, but the overall equilibrium of the entire organism. As he put it, "The constancy of the inner terrain is the essential condition of the free life." In other words, microbes hover around and inside us constantly, but it is only when our "inner terrain" is out of balance and vulnerable that they can take root. Pasteur's dying words were reported to have been, "Bernard was right. The microbe is nothing, the terrain, everything."

Both Pasteur and Bernard were right. A total treatment approach encompasses both the physical (the microbe) and the mental and emotional (the inner terrain), and recognizes their interaction. Major illness confronts us with what most of us would rather avoid—the inevitability of death. While death certainly has its tragic aspects, its blunt reality can be a spur to recognizing the importance of really living, here and now, and to reevaluating (as even Pasteur did) our perspective. No matter what quantity of life is left to each of us, we all have a choice about its quality. Nurturing, enjoying, and balancing our "inner terrain" is perhaps the best place to start.

15

Does Stress Cause Cancer?

Andrew W. Kneier, Ph.D.
Ernest H. Rosenbaum, M.D.

There is a widespread belief that emotional stress plays a role in the development of cancer. Many of our patients feel they were somehow "set up" to get cancer, and look back for some specific stressful event or situation (such as financial or marital problems) that may have brought on their disease. Sometimes, patients blame the cancer on long-standing inner stress from some trauma in their life history (such as alcoholism in their family, or being abused when they were children). Patients have also felt that certain aspects of their personality (such as being too submissive or emotionally repressed) made them prone to cancer.

Many claims about stress, personality, and cancer have been made in the popular press and media in recent years. Patients are routinely told to keep a positive attitude, implying that the stress of negative thoughts or emotions is bad for you. We have seen several books and magazine articles on these topics. Woody Allen once quipped that he never got angry, but just grew a tumor instead.

Does scientific evidence support these claims? Certainly the belief that stress can contribute to cancer is not without some basis in scientific literature. However, many studies have also found no such connection.

References for the studies cited in this chapter are available on request from the Cancer Resource Center, UCSF Comprehensive Cancer Center, 2356 Sutter Street, San Francisco, CA 94143-1705.

A Cautionary Note

A recent review of a wide variety of studies over the last twenty-five years on the role of psychological factors in cancer incidence listed more than twenty variables that have been associated with the onset of cancer. This list includes stressful life events, depression, suppression of emotion, social isolation, excessive anxiety, inhibited sexuality, long-standing emotional conflicts, constricted personality type, rigidity, submissiveness, and a facade of pleasantness. It would seem there was a mountain of evidence that such factors (which could all be included under the heading "stress") played a role in the development of cancer.

However, many of the studies that show this connection have a serious flaw—they look at what cancer patients report about past stress, emotional states, or personality traits *after* they have been diagnosed with cancer. The problem is that what patients remember and report may well be distorted by the fact of their cancer.

As an example of this problem, one study asked a group of women who had been diagnosed with lymphoma or leukemia to list the stressful life events that occurred during the four years before their diagnosis. The researchers found that the year just preceding the diagnosis was significantly more stressful for these women than the other three years, and they speculated that this increased stress might have contributed to the development of the cancer. However, we must consider that these women, like everyone, probably had a better recall of stressful events during the more recent year. In addition, the emotional impact of a cancer diagnosis can make a person see past events in a more negative light. These women may have wanted to find an explanation for their cancer that would give them a feeling of control over the outcome; if stress caused the cancer, then reducing stress would help eliminate it. (An additional methodological problem with this study—and one that afflicts most such studies—is that the cancers in question originated, in microscopic form, years before they could be diagnosed. Thus, the stress of the few years before the diagnosis was entirely unrelated to the onset of the disease at the cellular level.)

Some studies have sought to circumvent the retrospective bias problem by interviewing patients who have a suspicious symptom of cancer but have not yet been diagnosed. For example, 160 women who had undiagnosed breast lumps were given psychological tests before biopsies were performed. Those who turned out to have breast cancer showed significantly more emotional suppression (especially of anger) than the women who had benign tumors. But caution is still warranted in interpreting these results. There is evidence that patients are very good at predicting whether biopsies will come back negative or positive for cancer. Furthermore, there is evidence that the diagnosis of cancer, or the suspicion of having it, can cause a greater suppression of emotion, thereby raising questions about cause and effect.

An additional problem concerns the interpretation of "stress." What is stressful to one person may not be stressful to another, and people differ in how they cope with stress. Thus, many studies that look at stressful life events, or at personality traits that are supposed to create stress, have not determined whether the persons involved actually experienced these events or traits as stressful.

Evidence of a Stress-Cancer Link

Even though most studies have these or other flaws, there have been a few well-designed studies that have demonstrated an association between stress and the later development of cancer. These studies have been prospective in nature (unlike the ones described above, which are retrospective); that is, they have obtained psychological information from a large number of people who are then followed over a number of years. Those who developed cancer are then compared with those who did not to determine whether there were any long-standing psychological differences.

For example, in 1957, 2,020 middle-aged men participated in the Western General Electric Health Study. Each was given a standardized personality test and then followed for seventeen years. Those who died of cancer during this period were found to have been significantly more depressed when they were tested at the beginning of the study. This stress-cancer association was unrelated to age, smoking, alcohol use, occupational status, or family history of cancer. The researchers concluded: "The results are consistent with the hypothesis that psychological depression is related to impairment of mechanisms for preventing the establishment and spread of malignant cells." (It is also possible that depression resulted in poor diet, avoidance of regular medical checkups, or ignoring early warning signs of cancer, any one of which could have increased cancer mortality.)

In the 1960s, nearly seven thousand adults were enrolled in the Alameda County Health Study. These participants are being followed for psychosocial and other factors that have a bearing on cancer incidence and mortality. After seventeen years, women who were the most socially isolated and felt lonely had a significantly greater incidence of cancer. Socially isolated men, once they developed cancer, had a significantly shorter survival time. These findings suggest that the stress of loneliness may be a risk factor for cancer.

Numerous studies have firmly established that stress can alter certain measures of immune functioning. For example, depression is associated with a decrease in the number and potency of natural killer cells, which respond to cancer cells. These kinds of changes occur because immune cells, through specific receptors, are sensitive to many of the hormones, neurotransmitters, and neuropeptides that are affected by stress.

These immunosuppressive effects are relevant to the possible role of stress in the development of cancer. It appears that one role of the immune system is to recognize and destroy malignant cells when they develop (which may occur commonly in all of us, although we never know it, thanks to the success of immunological surveillance). It is therefore possible that a weakening of the immune system, caused by stress, could make someone more susceptible to cancer.

Evidence That Stress Does Not Cause Cancer

After seventeen years, the Alameda County Health Study found no association between earlier depression and the later development of cancer. In another study, looking at the association of depression and development of breast cancer, nearly 10,000 women were followed for fourteen years. No association was found between depression and a subsequent diagnosis of breast cancer.

Although bereavement has been found to suppress certain immune functions, this suppression is apparently not related to an increased risk of cancer. For example, 4,032 people who were widowed in Maryland between 1963 and 1974 were not found to have an increased cancer rate during a twelve-year follow-up period. In Finland, nearly 10,000 people who were widowed in 1972 were followed for fourteen years. This group showed no significant increase in cancer mortality.

In 1944, a total of 9,813 soldiers were discharged from the U.S. Army for psychoneurosis. They were matched with 9,942 controls, and the two groups were followed for twenty-four years. The discharged veterans had no greater cancer mortality than the control group during this period. In a similar study by the same author, approximately 10,000 soldiers who had been prisoners of war during World War II or the Korean War were matched with approximately 9,000 controls. The World War II vets were followed for thirty-two years and the Korean War vets for twenty years, during which time the former prisoners of war had no greater

mortality from cancer than the control subjects.

In the Terman Life-Cycle Study, the psychosocial factors and longevity histories of 1,528 participants have been followed since 1921-22 (when they were in elementary school). As of 1991, 663 had died of various causes. These deaths were associated with divorce of parents during childhood, childhood impulsivity and egocentrism, marital instability, and poor psychological adjustment in adulthood. These associations (history of divorced parents, etc., and death) were independent of smoking and alcohol consumption. While these factors were associated with subsequent death from a variety of causes; they did not predict a higher death rate from cancer.

What Conclusions Can Be Drawn?

Obviously, the scientific evidence neither proves nor disproves the role of stress as a cause of cancer. In the majority of cases, the preponderance of evidence suggests that there is no link. It is important to remember, however, that most of these studies involve large groups of patients and are looking at stress-cancer associations in that group as a whole. If there is an association in some individuals within the group, but not in others, then the overall effect will not be significant—although the effect on those individuals is significant. Thus, the evidence is compelling that stress can, and sometimes does, contribute to the development of cancer. That is, in some cases the immune system and/or DNA repair mechanisms are probably impaired enough by long-standing and severe emotional stress that malignant transformation of cells is able to proceed.

Given this, you might ask: "Did stress contribute to my cancer?" Based on the scientific evidence to date, we would answer: "Probably not." We would add that even if stress was a factor, its role was probably very minor compared to the other causative factors that we know exist. But we would also add that stress could have played a role, although it was not the cause itself.

The question is still worth asking, because your cancer diagnosis may help you to identify sources of stress in your life that deserve more attention and that you might be able to change. This process could be helpful to you: it could lead to a better attunement to your own feelings and needs, and help you to make positive changes in your lifestyle, health habits, or priorities. Your emotional well-being would be enhanced, as well as your overall quality of life. This process also might help in a medical sense, by fostering a greater participation in your treatment regimen and by promoting an improved immune response to your cancer.

Reflecting on the role of stress in your own cancer may also be harmful if it causes you to blame yourself. We have heard patients blame themselves for tolerating too much stress in their life, for internalizing their emotions, or for being too submissive—as if this behavior had caused their cancers. Research indicates that such factors probably had nothing to do with the development of cancer.

The belief that stress contributes to cancer—and the self-blame that stems from this—derives in part from how we account for good fortune and misfortune. When things are going well for us—in our lives, our jobs, and in our health—we tend to assume that we are doing something right, living on the right track, and must be deserving of our good fortune. The flip side of this assumption is that misfortune can lead to the thought that we were not so deserving of our good fortune after all, perhaps because of some flaw in our character, having the wrong priorities, or living under too much stress. Therefore, it is not uncommon for people diagnosed with cancer to feel at fault and to search for causes (such as stress) in themselves or in their past. Although cancer is a biological disease, our culture tends to see it as a reflection of the cancer patient's character, personality, or life. Another reason for this view is the influence on our cultural attitudes of the Judeo-Christian view that disease and death are the result of sin.

The themes of domination, mastery, and control also are powerful motifs in our culture, and are quite at odds with our vulnerability to the capriciousness of nature. Rather than accept that we often are victims of natural malfunctions and body processes beyond our control, we tend to think that such imperfections can be fixed with ample understanding and technological intervention. In this context, we look for causes of cancer that we can control. We believe that stress is one of these.

16

Does Your Attitude Make a Difference?
Psychological Factors

Andrew Kneier, Ph.D.
Ernest Rosenbaum, M.D.

The easy answer to the question posed by the title of this chapter is "Yes." Your attitude makes a difference in how you feel about your illness, how you cope with it, and your overall psychological adjustment and quality of life. For example, patients who adopt a fighting spirit feel less vulnerable and depressed than do patients who have a helpless, fatalistic attitude. Your attitude also influences the side effects of your medical treatments and your recovery from surgery. For example, patients who think of chemotherapy as strong and effective medicine are much less distressed over the side effects, and actually experience fewer side effects, than patients who regard chemotherapy as a dreadful poison.

The more complicated question is whether your attitude makes a difference to your medical outcome—that is, does your attitude affect whether a cancer recurs or progresses after treatments, the rate of any progression, and if the cancer is eventually fatal?

The question is not only whether the course and outcome of your illness are influenced by your attitude, but also whether they are influenced by your emotional state, stress level, coping style, personality traits, and degree of personal support you get from others. (In this chapter, we will refer to all of these as psychological factors.)

The question is complicated because some studies indicate that psychological factors do influence medical outcomes in cancer, whereas other studies have found that they do not. Furthermore, we know of cases where certain positive aspects, such as a strong will to live and unshakable hope, appeared to make all the difference in the world; but sadly, we also know of cases where such aspects appeared to make no difference whatsoever.

The issue of how psychological factors might influence medical outcomes also complicates the question. It is often assumed that such factors affect cancer through psychoimmunological processes—that patients' emotional states (which are affected by their attitudes, coping behavior, and social support) cause changes in their immune response, which in turn affects medical outcomes. As we will see, there is evidence to support this possibility. Eastern perspectives on healing, such as the Chinese focus on *chi*, emphasize the balance and flow of energy within the body to explain how psychological factors make a difference.

It is also possible that these factors affect how well a patient adheres to medical treatment, or whether the patient pursues an aggressive treatment approach. Because patients differ on these matters, their medical outcomes could be affected.

Most cancer patients believe that a positive attitude makes a difference to their medical outcome; indeed, patients are often encouraged by family members, friends, and health professionals to maintain a positive attitude and to never give up. This is not surprising. Claims are frequently made in the popular press and media about mind-body connections that affect cancer. If a new study shows some connection along these lines, it usually receives a lot of media coverage, whereas studies showing no such connection are ignored. Proponents of various mind-body approaches to cancer healing often overstate the proven effectiveness of such approaches.

In the discussion that follows, we review the scientific evidence regarding the influence of psychological factors on cancer outcomes. First, we want you to know about some of the positive evidence to encourage you to pursue ways of coping with your illness that might make a difference, and to support you in the constructive efforts you already might be making. Second, we want to offer an objective review of the evidence to correct the claims that are often made in the popular press and media. By exaggerating the medical benefits of a "positive attitude," these claims can make patients feel that their normal "negative" emotions are somehow dangerous, and that it is up to them to deal with their cancer in the "right" ways. Consequently, patients often feel that the progression of their cancer is somehow a personal failure on their part. As we will see, it is actually healthy—psychologically and immunologically—to express an appropriate degree of fear or sadness when dealing with cancer. And there is no justification for burdening patients with the responsibility of their recovery from cancer.

References for the studies cited in this chapter are available on request from the Cancer Resource Center, UCSF Comprehensive Cancer Center, 2356 Sutter Street, San Francisco, CA 94143-1705

Evidence That Psychological Factors Affect Medical Outcome

Most of the studies in this area have a straightforward design: they assess the psychological differences among patients who have a similar cancer diagnosis, and then follow these patients over time to see whether these differences are associated with differences in medical outcomes. It has been impossible for these studies to completely separate out the influence of the psychological factors from all the other factors that affect medical outcomes (such as differences in medical treatments and tumor aggressiveness, and whether the immune system is functioning normally). Nonetheless, some intriguing findings have been reported.

One of the first noteworthy studies was reported in the *Journal of the American Medical Association* in 1979. To their surprise, the researchers found that women with metastatic breast cancer who were visibly angry and upset had significantly longer survival times than those who exhibited less distress. A related study in the same year found that newly diagnosed melanoma patients who acknowledged the adjustment difficulties they were experiencing had a lower incidence of recurrence than those who seemed to minimize their adjustment needs. A similar finding was reported with newly diagnosed breast cancer patients: those who exhibited and acknowledged the severe impact of the diagnosis had a lower incidence of recurrence than patients who appeared to be less distressed.

It is interesting that acknowledging anxiety may be healthy, but that dwelling on it may not be. In one study, leukemia patients who had undergone a bone marrow transplant and who exhibited "anxious preoccupation" with their illness had poorer outcomes than those who were more successful in mastering their anxiety.

A number of studies have found that a patient's degree of interpersonal support, as opposed to social isolation, had an effect on medical outcomes. One such study interviewed two hundred newly diagnosed breast cancer patients about their level of social support and then followed these women for twenty years. Those in the premenopausal group (ages fifteen to forty-five) and the postmenopausal group (ages sixty-one to ninety) who had high social involvement, survived longer than those who had low social involvement. However, those in the perimenopausal group (ages forty to sixty) showed no such differences in survival as related to their social involvement. To complicate matters further, a study involving lung, breast, and colorectal cancer patients found that the benefits associated with social support were different depending on the type of cancer and extent of the disease.

Two widely cited studies found that patients who participated in a group intervention program had improved survival over control patients who did not participate. The best known is a Stanford University study. Women with metastatic breast cancer who participated in a weekly support group for one year (which involved sharing emotions, participating in problem-solving discussions, and undergoing self-hypnosis training for pain control) had significantly longer survival times than the control group. The other study involved newly diagnosed melanoma patients at the UCLA Medical Center. Patients who participated in a weekly support group for six weeks (which involved sharing emotions, teaching about melanoma, and instruction in positive coping skills) exhibited several improvements over the control group. They coped more effectively with their illness, their emotional state was better, their natural killer cell activity and number was higher, and their survival rates were better over the six-year follow-up period.

It is not known why these patients had improved medical outcomes, or whether these findings can be replicated. Perhaps the emotional benefits of a support group are translated into immunological changes that make a difference to the medical outcome. Perhaps patients in support groups take better care of their overall health through diet and exercise, pursue medical treatments more aggressively, cope more effectively with stress, make lifestyle changes to reduce stress, or participate in supplemental approaches such as acupuncture, meditation, and Chinese herbal medicine. Clearly, additional research is needed.

A study in the *British Medical Journal* compared the stressful life events of fifty women who had suffered a breast cancer recurrence with a matched group of fifty patients who remained in remission. Those who had a recurrence reported a significantly greater degree of stress in the years preceding the recurrence then did the patients who remained in remission. A problem with this study is that the emotional effect of a cancer recurrence can distort a patient's memory of past events. Moreover, these patients may have wanted to find a causal explanation of the recurrence (i.e., stress) that would give them a greater feeling of control over the future.

There is a widely held belief among cancer patients, and among proponents of mind-body medicine, that stress contributes to the development of cancer (see Chapter 15, "Does Stress Cause Cancer?"). Insofar as this is the case, it would follow that stress would also influence the medical outcome after cancer was diagnosed.

Psychological Factors and Immune Response

There is considerable evidence to support the possibility that psychological factors affect the immune system, thus influencing medical outcome. For example, depression is associated with a decrease in the number and potency of natural killer (NK) cells, which respond to cancer cells. These kinds of changes occur because immune cells, through specific receptors, respond to many of the hormones, neurotransmitters, and neuropeptides that are affected by stress. Enzyme levels necessary for the repair of mutated DNA have also been found to be lower under stressful conditions.

Although the immunosuppressive effects of stress could theoretically increase a person's susceptibility to cancer, and thereby contribute to the onset of cancer, no studies have demonstrated that this happens.

What about the role of immune suppression, as caused by (or at least associated with) psychological factors on medical outcomes? The evidence here is more intriguing. As we saw above, degree of social support and interaction has been associated with differences in medical outcomes. These connections could result from changes in immune responses that are related to social support. It would follow that separation and loss, such as divorce or the death of a spouse, would be associated with immunosuppression. Several studies have shown that this is the case.

In the UCLA study on melanoma patients, the patients who participated in the group intervention program showed a greater improvement in their emotional state than did the control group, and this improvement was associated with an increase in certain types of NK cells and an increase in the tumor-fighting potential of NK cells. In their follow-up study, the researchers found that these changes were, in turn, associated with improved survival.

With breast cancer patients, certain psychological factors (level of adjustment, degree of social support, energy level, and mood) were associated with variability in NK cell activity three months after mastectomy. It also was found that patients who were most depressed had a greater decrease in NK activity and a higher number of lymph nodes testing positive for cancer involvement. It was not clear whether there was a causal connection between depression, immune suppression, and number of involved nodes, or whether the nodal involvement caused the depression. In a follow-up study, the researchers found that the psychological factors they studied, as well as the variance in NK activity, were associated with the incidence and timing of subsequent recurrences.

Evidence That Psychological Factors Do Not Affect Outcome

The findings summarized above have been contradicted by a number of studies that have found no associations between psychological factors and medical outcomes.

A major study reported in the *New England Journal of Medicine* involved 359 melanoma and breast cancer patients. A number of psychological factors were measured, including social ties, marital history, job satisfaction, use of medication for anxiety or depression, general life satisfaction, hopelessness, and amount of adjustment required to cope with the diagnosis of cancer. These patients were followed three to eight years after their diagnosis. None of the psychological factors were associated with differences in medical outcome—with one exception: patients who reported a moderate degree of hopelessness had longer disease-free intervals than patients who reported either a low or high degree of hopelessness. This is an interesting finding; it may indicate that denying or minimizing hopeless feelings, as well as feeling extremely hopeless, are both associated with poorer outcomes.

Other studies have failed to find a relationship between coping style and medical outcome. A mixed group of patients (ninety-two with hematologic cancers and forty-seven with rectal cancer) were assessed when they were diagnosed and followed for six months. Coping style was not related to length of survival; nor were degree of depression or whether it was felt the disease came from within or without. A similar study with breast cancer patients, who were followed for three years after diagnosis, found no relationship between coping style and outcome.

Researchers have also looked at the associations between marital status and outcome. In a large study in Denmark, 1,782 breast cancer patients were matched with 1,738 controls. No differences were found in the death rates of married patients as opposed to widowed patients. *The New England Journal of Medicine* study described above also found no association between marital history and medical outcome.

One study showed an association between stressful life events and breast cancer outcomes. However, another study of 202 breast cancer patients found no association between stressful events and recurrence during a three-and-a-half-year period. Yet another study found no association between depression and breast cancer outcomes.

Two studies that examined the effectiveness of group therapy found no association with medical outcomes. In one, thirty-four breast cancer patients who participated in Bernie Siegel's intervention program (consisting of weekly peer support, family therapy, individual counseling, and positive mental imagery exercises) were matched with 102 patients who did not participate. The patients were followed for ten years, and no differences in survival time or ultimate survival were found. In the other study, some patients received weekly group psychotherapy and a control group did not. There were no significant differences between the survival times of the two groups. In a third study, 120 end-stage male cancer patients were assigned either to receive weekly individual counseling or to a control group that did not. The patients who received counseling showed an improvement in their quality of life, but did not differ from the controls in survival after one year.

The evidence thus far suggests that psychological factors sometimes make a difference to medical outcomes, but that they do not consistently do so. This conclusion would certainly explain the contradictory findings of these and other studies. The studies in this area have investigated and measured the relationship of psychological factors and medical outcomes in large groups of patients. In order for a relationship to be found, it must be relatively consistent or uniform within the group. If the relationship existed in some patients within the group but not in others, then these would cancel each other out and no consistent relationship would be found. The authors would conclude that there was no relationship between the psychological factors and the medical outcomes; but what they really mean is that no consistent relationship was found in the group being studied. Given the nature of statistical analysis, relationships must be consistent in order to be deemed "statistically significant." The rules for this are very strict. For example, if a relationship was found, but the analysis showed that there was a 10 percent chance that the relationship was due to chance alone, then the relationship would be dismissed as too inconsistent to be "significant."

In an individual case, a psychological factor will, in theory, influence a medical outcome only if a number of conditions are met:

1. The psychological factor in question (e.g., an optimistic outlook) would have to be strong enough to affect the immune response.
2. The right effects on the immune response would have to occur.
3. These effects would have to be strong enough to affect the cancer cells, which in turn would have to be susceptible to the immunological changes that occurred as a consequence of the patient's optimism.
4. The effect on these cancer cells would have to be strong enough, and widespread enough throughout the body, to make a difference to the medical outcome.

These "links in the chain" between a psychological factor and cancer growth sometimes do occur, which is remarkable given the complex and intricate processes involved.

Moving Forward

How should you apply all of this to your own situation? As you go through your cancer experience, it is impossible to predict whether your attitude, emotions, coping style, or degree of support will influence your medical outcome. Because these factors might make a difference, however, we believe you should act as if they will. In other words, try every possible way of responding to your illness in ways that could improve your medical outcome.

But if, despite your best efforts and the best efforts of your doctors, your cancer gets worse, this does not mean that you failed to have the right attitude, that your will to live was not strong enough, that you did not cope as you should have, or that you did something else wrong. It means only that the biological deck was stacked against you from the outset—that is, that the inherent biology of the tumor, the shortcomings of one's bodily defenses against it, and the inadequacies of medical intervention all led to outcomes that were beyond your control. However, no one knows that in advance, just as no one knows in advance whether your attitude will make a positive difference.

We therefore encourage you to respond to your cancer in ways that could make a difference. In every situation, there is a realistic possibility that the patient will achieve medical outcomes that are better than expected; in some cases, there is a realistic possibility that the patient will recovery fully.

You can maximize your own chances of realizing these possibilities by becoming involved in learning about your illness and pursuing the best medical treatments and follow-up evaluation. Make changes in your lifestyle and health habits that are associated with improved outcomes. In other words, become an active participant in the recovery process, as opposed to having a passive, fatalistic attitude.

Medical literature suggests that certain ways of coping with the stress of having cancer can affect the outcome. These include acknowledging stress and expressing the negative emotions that come with it, adopting a fighting spirit, and reaching out for support from others. Participating in a cancer support group could also make a difference.

It is interesting that the belief that attitude makes a difference in medical outcome is so prevalent while the scientific evidence is much more ambiguous. This also is true of popular but unsupported claims about the mind-body connections that affect cancer outcomes. There are two sides to this coin: on the positive side, patients are often encouraged by these ideas to respond to their illness in positive and constructive ways; on the negative side, these ideas often pressure patients to have the right attitude and make patients feel responsible and guilty if their illnesses progresses despite their efforts.

If the scientific evidence is so contradictory, why is the belief that a patient's attitude makes a difference so widespread, and why is the focus in the media and popular press so one-sided? First, there is, as we have shown, good evidence that psychological factors can influence cancer outcomes, and case reports of spontaneous remissions in cancer underscore the remarkable power of these factors—especially the power of emotional catharsis and the patient's total belief that a medical treatment or some other substance (even if it is biologically inert) will be a cure.

Second, most patients want to believe that how they respond to their illness can influence the outcome, as this helps to reduce their feelings of vulnerability and helplessness. Family members and friends also want to believe this and want the patient to act accordingly to reduce their own anxieties.

Third, the nature of cancer lends itself to the notion that the disease implies something about the person who has it. These cells—which have spun out of control and which, if left to their own devices, are ultimately destructive—are part of the person's body, originating from within, and it may seem that they are therefore evidence of some underlying personal pathology or dysfunction. Many patients feel that if they can fix whatever is wrong internally, then the malignancy will go away.

These ideas stem in part from a fourth reason for the emphasis on the patient's role in beating cancer: our culture places a strong emphasis on our controlling our destiny and overcoming obstacles, even natural ones, that stand in our path. The fact that we are susceptible to natural processes beyond our control is not well accepted in our society. The late historian Richard Hofstadter addressed this issue when he wrote: "A great part of both the strength and weakness of our national existence lies in the fact that Americans do not abide very quietly the evils of life. We are forever restlessly pitting ourselves against them, demanding changes, improvements, remedies, but not often with sufficient sense of the limits that the human condition will in the end inevitably impose upon us."

To conclude, we want to return to the defining power of your attitude in shaping how you experience and respond to your illness. We offer the following reflection:

The longer I live, the more I realize the impact of attitude on life. Attitude, to me, is more important than facts. It is more important than the past, than education, than money, than circumstances, than failures, than successes, than what other people think or say or do. It is more important than appearance, giftedness, or skill. It will make or break a company...a church...a home. The remarkable thing is, we have a choice every day regarding the attitude we embrace for that day. We cannot change the past...we cannot change the inevitable. The only thing we can do is to play on the one string we have, and that is our attitude. I am convinced that life is 10 percent what happens to me and 90 percent how I react to it. And so it is with you...we are in charge of our attitudes.

—Charles Swindoll

17

Coping with Cancer
Ten Steps toward Emotional Well-Being

Andrew Kneier, Ph.D.
Ernest Rosenbaum, M.D.
Isadora R. Rosenbaum, M.A.
Diane Behar
Pat Fobair, L.C.S.W., M.Ph.

Coping refers to the attitudes and behaviors that you use to maintain your emotional well-being and to adjust to the stresses caused by cancer. Different people cope in different ways, and some ways of coping are more successful in promoting a person's emotional well-being and psychological adjustment than others. Currently, you might be coping with treatments and their side effects. You may also be coping with a recurrence of your cancer or with pain and disability. Your life has been disrupted and altered by your illness, and you are dealing with the effect on your loved ones of all that is happening to you.

When someone had cancer fifty years ago, there was little discussion of how he or she was "coping." The person just dealt with it. In the last twenty-five years, however, the notion that patients are coping with their illnesses, in better or worse ways, has received an enormous amount of attention by health care professionals. Even the federal government got involved when, in 1980, the National Cancer Institute published *Coping with Cancer.* In the 1990s, more than twenty-five hundred articles on different aspects of coping with cancer have appeared in medical and mental health journals.

In this chapter, we summarize the vast amount of research on coping with cancer by highlighting ten coping strategies that we believe may help you. We also have drawn upon the experiences of the many patients we have cared for over the years.

Ten Coping Strategies

"Coping strategies" reflect the process of coping and the ways of meeting goals and challenges. When you are dealing with cancer, you face many goals and challenges. Some of these are medical and physical, some are emotional, and others are interpersonal and spiritual. In one way or another, they all have to do with the quality of your life, which has been threatened and disrupted by cancer. You have adopted some strategies for pursuing your goals and meeting personal challenges that promote your recovery and enable you to remain emotionally intact. Your ability to carry on is deepened and changed by your cancer experience. This is what coping is all about.

These coping strategies are not applicable to all patients. This is because the method of coping that works best for one person may not work so well for another. What works best for you depends on many factors related to your personality, your current life situation, and how you have coped in the past. Moreover, the goals and challenges you are facing are personal to you, and many of these are dictated by the nature of your illness and medical treatments. Thus, the coping responses that are warranted also depend on these individual matters.

Finally, coping with cancer is a process that goes on over months and years, and patients use different strategies at different times, depending upon the changing situation within themselves and their relationships and with the stage of their illness. It is nonetheless true that research on the coping strategies used by large numbers of patients has found that some strategies, in general, are better than others. More often than not, these strategies are associated with an optimal degree of psychological adjustment.

The positive coping strategies we discuss below may also help to improve your medical condition. They can promote your emotional well-being when dealing with cancer, and thereby enable you to feel more energetic and resilient. These effects may also enhance your immune system's response to cancer cells.

The ten coping strategies suggested here are for all patients, whether you are newly diagnosed, undergoing medical treatment, or dealing with the many stages of cancer, including terminal cancer.

1. Facing the Reality of Your Illness

Patients respond in different ways to their diagnosises, the initial medical work-up, subsequent test results, and the implications of all that is happening to them. Many patients respond by confronting the full realities of their illnesses. They ask pointed and brave questions about the seriousness of their conditions and the pros and cons of the various treatment options. They read up on these matters on their own. They react as if they are strongly motivated to know what they are facing. This way of coping has been found to promote their psychological adjustment.

Other patients react as if the realities confronting them are too much to deal with, and they retreat into states of denial. It sometimes seems that patients in denial are saying, "I can't cope with all this." Yet, denial is just another way of coping. It protects people from being overwhelmed. But it also can prevent patients from coming to terms with their illnesses and getting on with other constructive ways of coping. Denial is therefore associated with a poorer psychological adjustment.

However, denial is often a positive coping strategy because it enables the patient to gradually face the reality of his or her illness, in a piecemeal manner, without feeling overwhelmed. In our experience, patients seldom remain in denial; it fades away over time, as indeed it should, for the good of overall adjustment.

As you read this, you might ask yourself how much you really know about your cancer and your individual case. Are there any relevant questions that you haven't asked? Have you avoided learning more about your illness by not reading about it? You might want to become more proactive in seeking information; the evidence indicates that this will help you.

2. Maintaining Hope and Optimism

After facing the reality of your illness, you should try to maintain as much hope and optimism as possible. Not surprisingly, patients who are hopeful and optimistic about the future course of events show a better adjustment to their illness than patients who are pessimistic. Some studies have also shown that optimism is associated with better medical outcomes. Of course, it would be hard to only feel optimistic (some legitimate fear or is normal); but in most cases, there is a solid and realistic basis for a certain degree of hope and optimism. You should try to focus on that and certainly not lose sight of it when your legitimate fears come to the fore. We'll return to this point when we discuss the importance of balance.

Most patients tell themselves to be positive, but for many, this is easier said than done. There are several reasons for this, some of which may apply to you. Optimism usually involves a feeling of luckiness. However, you were unlucky enough to get cancer and may now feel that you are an unlucky person. You may not expect to enjoy the good fortune of a long remission or cure. You might feel just the opposite: that good luck is unlikely for you.

Optimism can also seem presumptuous: after all, other patients with your diagnosis have not done well. You might think, "What right do I have to expect to recover?" Your optimism can also make you feel that you are not worrying enough about your cancer—that you are not giving cancer its due, that you are acting too boldly or confidently in the face of it, and that you are therefore asking for trouble, as if the cancer might come back to teach you a lesson. Finally, if your prognosis is more favorable than for other patients with your type of cancer, you may feel that it is not right to enjoy this good fortune or to take advantage of it (that is, by being optimistic and going on with your life in a positive and constructive manner).

While these obstacles can be daunting, you should try to feel as hopeful and optimistic as the medical realities of your case allow.

3. Proportion and Balance

Your emotional response should not just be one of optimism and hope. It is also appropriate and helpful for you to be upset and worried, at least to a certain degree.

In most cases, the medical situation provides a basis for hope and a basis for worry. The statistics indicate a certain chance of survival, but also a certain chance of dying of cancer. Of course, the chance of survival and the risk of dying vary greatly from case to case. Ideally, your emotional response would take both aspects into account: you would experience a degree of hope that was proportional to the positive survival chances that applied to you, but you also would experience a degree of worry that was proportional to the mortality rate in similar cases. Your feelings should be in balance. Your feelings of worry or upset should be reduced in intensity, tempered by feelings of hope and optimism.

Alternatively, the nature and intensity of your positive emotions should be tempered by, or take into account, the possibility of death. If you are ignoring this possibility, then your optimism involves a denial or minimization of this threat; in the long run, this will not help you. It is better to acknowledge this threat and to work through the negative emotions that stem from it. In short, it is best if your positive and negative emotions balanced each other out such that you would be neither overreacting nor underreacting to the medical realities facing you.

A number of studies have found that patients who maintain this kind of mixed emotional response—well proportioned to the realities of their illnesses—enjoy a better psychological adjustment than patients who feel too pessimistic or too optimistic. In our experience, patients who have told us of their mixed feelings appear and feel well adjusted. They feel that they are coping well with the uncertainty inherent in their medical condition, neither dwelling on nor denying their legitimate fears, and yet keeping their sights set on getting better. Again, all this is easier said than done.

4. Expressing Your Emotions

People differ in the way they express and communicate how they feel, and in our society women are generally better at this than men. Take stock of how well you express what you are feeling about your illness. Many studies have shown that patients who express their emotions and concerns enjoy a better psychological adjustment than people who tend to suppress their feelings or keep quiet about them.

Emotional expression is usually helpful because it gives you an outlet for your feelings, a means of working through them, and an opportunity to obtain better emotional support. It can be an enormous help just to know that your feelings are understood by others and seen as valid, but this requires open communication on your part.

If you tend to keep your feelings to yourself, it is probably because you have learned to do so. Your earlier experience may have taught you that sharing your feelings led to negative consequences. Perhaps your emotions were not validated by others, or you were criticized for expressing them ("Children are to be seen but not heard," "Big boys don't cry," and so on). You may have felt that your emotional needs were an imposition on others, and that your role was to take care of the feelings and needs of others rather than expressing your own. It is not uncommon for cancer patients to hide their true feelings as a way of protecting their loved ones.

Some people do not express their emotions because they are not very adept at paying attention to what they are feeling. They seldom stop and check in with themselves and try to identify the feelings and concerns that are weighing upon them. Children need permission and encouragement to develop this skill, and then practice and positive reinforcement. In this process, we learn that our emotions are important and valid and thus worthy of attention and expression. Some people just do not have much experience with this essential ability, and even regard it as pointless or self-indulgent. If you find yourself admitting, "Yes, this applies to me," then we encourage you to consider psychological counseling, which could be of great help.

As you probably know, cancer patients are consistently encouraged to "keep a positive attitude." This can make you feel that there is something wrong or dangerous about your "negative" emotions (fear, sorrow, or anger). Research suggests just the opposite: experiencing and expressing such emotions is psychologically and immunologically healthy.

Finally, timing is important. The period after your diagnosis when you are learning about your illness and undergoing the initial work-up and treatments may not be the right time for you to be taking stock of all your emotions. Your plate is already very full. You may need to put your emotions aside for a while as you attend to everything else. Moreover, it will benefit you most to express your emotions with the right people when their support is available to you.

5. Reaching Out for Support

The amount of support available to cancer patients varies across the country, and patients themselves differ in how much they tend to reach out and take advantage of the support. Those patients who have at least a few loved ones available for close emotional support—and who call upon their support or practical help—show a better psychological adjustment to cancer than patients who are largely alone or tend to "go it alone" in coping with their illness.

Reaching out for support often means expressing your feelings and concerns to others—which, as we saw, can be a challenge for many patients. It can also mean that you ask your loved ones for the type of support you need most, and this requires that you first ask yourself what that support might consist of. You will probably identify ways that people can help you that have not occurred to them.

For example, family members and friends often assume that they should provide encouragement and stress the positive (this is sometimes called the "cheerleading" role). Patients generally appreciate the positive intent behind this, yet it can hamper patients from sharing their fears or sorrows. Often, patients would rather hear that others understand how they feel, regard their emotions as valid, and will stick with them regardless of what happens. You might need to tell people that. On a more concrete level, you might ask

others to accompany you during a medical appointment, pick up the kids after school, look up information for you (the Internet is a wonderful resource for up-to-date information, as long as it is from reliable sources), or prepare a nutritious meal for your family.

If you find that you are not reaching out for the support that is available, reflect on the reasons for your stoicism. You may be minimizing your own needs for support because you pride yourself on being independent and self-sufficient. It may seem to you that others would be bothered by your need for support or help and resent your imposing on them. More often than not, this is an assumption based on earlier experience. Perhaps you have found in the past that it is best to rely on yourself. While you should continue to draw upon your own internal resources, you should also realize that other people can and want to assist you in meeting the challenges of your illness, and you allow them to do so.

Obtaining support often means joining a support group, and research has shown that such groups help patients to cope with and adjust to their illness. Support group members find that they have a great deal to offer each other in the way of mutual support and encouragement, discussion of common problems and ways of coping, and sharing of medical information. Groups also offer a safe and supportive haven for confronting one's fears. The American Cancer Society office, or hospitals specializing in cancer treatments in your community, will know of support groups that you could join. See also Part VI, "Resources."

6. Adopting a Participatory Stance

Do you take the initiative and actively participate in your treatment? Some patients tackle their cancer head on. They have a strong fighting spirit, and they find ways of putting it into action. They go out of their way to learn about their illness and the options for treatment. They pursue the best treatments available and also consider alternative or holistic approaches. If you are like this, you will strongly agree with the statement "A lot depends on what I do and how I take part." Research has shown that patients who respond in this manner have less emotional distress than patients who respond in a more passive manner or try to avoid their situation.

Patients who adopt a participatory stance believe they can make a difference, and they put this belief into action. They therefore feel less helpless and vulnerable. This is a main reason why their emotional state is better. The belief in yourself as an active and effective agent is called self-efficacy, and research has consistently documented its positive emotional effects.

Patients who are coping in this way usually ask their doctors about treatment options and alternative therapies that their doctors had not mentioned. Instead of only following what their doctors say, they come up with ideas of their own. Also, they usually embrace some ways of promoting their physical well-being that go beyond the normal recommendations. These include dietary changes, increased exercise, stress reduction, vitamins, herbs, yoga, acupuncture, meditation, prayer, hypnosis, guided imagery, and others (see Chapter 6, "Survivor's Guide to Bone Marrow Transplantation"). These patients often pursue new, experimental therapies that may offer additional hope. In all these ways, the patient is actively participating in an effort to recover fully or, if that is not realistic, to maintain the best physical health possible.

In contrast to those who feel they have an active role to play, some patients adopt a resigned, fatalistic attitude. One reason for this attitude is that it lets the patient off the hook for any extra effort that could make a difference. We have heard patients say, "What will be will be." The research on coping has consistently shown that this attitude is linked to a poorer psychological adjustment to one's illness.

7. Finding a Positive Meaning

While the diagnosis and treatment of cancer is an awful experience in many respects, it also can be a challenge and even an opportunity for positive change. In response to their illnesses, many patients step back and take stock of who they are and how they have been living. They reflect on their values and priorities, and often identify changes that are warranted (and perhaps overdue) in their lifestyles and personal relationships. This is often called the "enlightenment" or "gift" that comes with cancer, or the "wake-up call." Patients who embrace this aspect of their cancer experiences have been found to be especially well adjusted and better able to deal with the many trials and disruptions caused by their illnesses.

It is often noted that growing old forces us to pay attention to what is important in life. The same can be said of a diagnosis of a life-threatening illness. What is important to a person often stems from one's spiritual or religious beliefs. Even if you are not inclined toward spirituality, you probably have a basic philosophy of life that highlights for you the importance of certain goals and values. These are important because of what they mean to your personal integrity and fulfillment.

To what degree does your lifestyle demonstrate these goals and values? This is a question for all of us, but it can become especially compelling if you are dealing with cancer. For many, their illness inspires them to pay more attention to what matters most. This could mean spending more time with family and close friends, making a greater contribution to the causes you believe in, showing more appreciation for all that you have and are, bringing forth aspects of your personality that have been suppressed, taking better care of your physical and emotional needs, and seeking to be more honest and true to yourself. In all these ways and in many more, your illness can become an impetus for positive change.

Sometimes, the idea that there is a message or lesson in one's cancer results in the implication that the person needed to get cancer and perhaps even got it for that reason. This kind of self-blame is completely unwarranted, and it fosters feelings of guilt and depression. A more psychologically healthy response was voiced by one of our patients when she said, "It's too bad that it took cancer to make me see things a bit more clearly, but you know, some positive things have come out of it for me."

8. Spirituality, Faith, and Prayer

Most people in our society have some fundamental spiritual beliefs, and these beliefs can be called upon for help in dealing with cancer. Patients who do so benefit in a variety of ways: they have a greater sense of peace, an inner strength, an ability to cope, and show an improved psychological adjustment and quality of life. These benefits derive especially from the perspective offered by religious faith or spirituality, and from the power of prayer and religious ritual (see Chapter 19, "Religion and Spirituality").

All of us, whether we have cancer or not, are challenged at some point with the question of how to respond to our vulnerability to disease, suffering, and death. For some, these realities lead to a kind of existential despair. Others embrace a perspective that goes beyond these realities, or that penetrates more deeply into them to find meaning and value that transcends their individual existence or plight. This is the perspective offered, in one form or another, by the world's religious and spiritual traditions.

This perspective can help with the "Why me?" question. It is difficult to reconcile how an almighty, loving, and just God could allow cancer to happen to a good person. Patients often believe that the illness is a punishment. In our culture, we often assume that what happens to a person is somehow linked to what the person deserves.

The emotional turmoil and doubt that stem from these issues can be soothed by the themes of consolation and forgiveness that permeate the world's major religions. In the Judeo-Christian tradition, it is emphasized that God is with us in our suffering, providing the grace we need to endure; God is not doling out suffering to those who deserve it.

Through prayer and liturgy, patients are able to connect to the core of their faith and to their religious community and derive the solace and fortitude they need to cope with their illness. Prayer can also have healing effects—most certainly in healing one's soul, but perhaps also in healing the body.

9. Maintaining Self-Esteem

There are many ways that the experience of cancer can harm a person's self-esteem. One of these is the stigma of having cancer—the belief that it can imply something bad about the person who has it. In addition, many of the sources of your self-esteem can be threatened by cancer and the effects of medical treatments: your appearance, your physical abilities and activity level, your personal attributes (such as being healthy and independent), and your role and identity within your family or in your work life. One of our breast cancer patients lamented: "I used to take pride in how I looked, and in being a good mother and working, helping to support the family. Now look at me."

These threats to your self-esteem pose a danger and an opportunity. The danger is depression and, with that, the weakening of the will to live. The opportunity lies in finding additional sources of self-esteem within yourself. For example, you might take pride in the way you are coping with your illness. You might have a new appreciation for how much you are loved—not because of what you do or how you look but because of who you are. Perhaps it has been difficult

for you to depend on others because your independence has been overly important; you might now take pride in your ability to express your needs and ask for help. Perhaps your spirituality has been deepened by your cancer experience, and this can also help to renew your self-esteem. The overall emotional well-being of patients is enhanced when they discover or develop new sources for positive self-regard.

You can also protect your self-esteem by maintaining your normal activities and roles as much as possible. Your illness does not suddenly define you as a cancer patient, as if that is your new identity. Patients who continue to do the things that are important to them, to the extent possible, enjoy a better psychological adjustment than those who too quickly abandon these roles and activities or expect too little of themselves because they have cancer. One study specifically noted that patients need to "deal with the cancer" but also to "keep it in its place."

10. Coming to Terms with Mortality

It may seem that a major challenge when dealing with cancer is to fight against the possibility of death. Certainly, the philosophy and technology of modern medicine are preoccupied with this fight. The practitioners of alternative therapies also stress their healing potential. From all quarters, cancer patients hear that they must maintain hope, keep a positive attitude, and try not to give up. It seems that everything revolves around getting better. And yet many patients die of cancer, and even those who do not are living with the possibility that they might. Very little support is offered to patients coming to terms with this possibility of death, in reaching some sense of peace about it and not feeling that it is a failure and outrage to die.

We are not saying that you should accept the possibility of dying, and therefore not rail against it and do all you can to prevent it. Nor are we suggesting that if your cancer progresses, and death seems inevitable, that you should accept it then. Facing death is profoundly personal and inherently difficult: our survival instinct runs counter to it. The loss of life and everything that entails seems unbearable, and for most of us dying is almost too dreadful to think about. But it is possible to come to terms with death and patients who do enjoy the peace that acceptance brings.

The majority of newly diagnosed patients have a favorable prognosis. You might think that it would be better to confront death when the time comes. But even now, you are facing the possibility of dying of cancer and striving to prevent or delay it. This fight for your life is bound to be filled with fear, desperation, and inner anguish if you are not also striving, in your own way, to come to terms with the possibility of death. This does not mean that you dwell on it; it means that you deal with it and then go on. It is always wise to review your personal and financial affairs (see Chapters 43–46). Having done so, you will be all the better at living in the fullness of life, one day at a time, rather than in the dread of what could possibly happen.

The work of coming to terms with death can draw on our religious, spiritual, and philosophical beliefs about what is important in life, and why. These beliefs can provide meaning and purpose to life, and therefore consolation when facing death. Many people have been able to feel, and to know, that their life has been about something important and of lasting value. This is one of the major ways that our religion or spirituality can help us.

We have found that most of our patients are struggling with these issues and longing for a sense of peace, but they are forced to do so quietly because they have so little support for this important inner work. Many patients abandon this effort, and come to feel hopeless about it. We encourage you to go forward through reflection and reading in the religious or spiritual traditions that appeal to you. One book that many patients have found helpful is *The Tibetan Book of Living and Dying*.

The Benefit for Patients

The coping strategies we have discussed are not right for everyone, but there is good evidence that they generally are helpful to patients who are dealing with cancer. The bottom line is that they help patients feel better and stronger. Patients feel better because they are facing their illness squarely and working through its emotional impacts, and yet also keeping a perspective on it so that cancer does not define them or take over their life. Through all the trials and challenges that cancer can bring, they are keeping their wits about them and are able to carry on. They feel stronger because they have support from other people and from within themselves. They have taken stock of their most cherished reasons for living, which strengthen and sustain them in their fight against cancer. And yet they also feel that their survival is not the only important objective; the quality of their lives and relationships, the values they live by, and their spirituality also deserve attention and effort. They have the peace of knowing that their death from cancer, if it comes to that, will not obliterate the meaning, value, and joy that their life has given to them and their loved ones.

One Patient's Way of Coping

Diane Behar (d.1998)

I have been treated with chemotherapy for more than six years and am now on my fifty-fifth course. My current treatment is an experimental infusion that lasts fifteen days each month. Almost immediately, I experience a nearly imperceptible ebbing away of my physical stamina and soon I prefer to walk rather than run, take an escalator instead of the stairs, and sit down rather than stand. My life moves into slow motion. I gradually witness a change in my personality and the way I react to people and situations. What makes this experience so difficult and frightening is the loss of control that takes place—a transformation from a fully active and vital person into someone who can barely sit up and function effectively, which is overwhelming and disheartening.

Somewhere inside the deepest part of me, my truest self hides out under cover, and tells me that all of this is temporary and that I must just wait out these drug-induced episodes. This kind voice, along with my unwavering faith in God, enables me to conquer and think that somehow I will be able to see my way into the clearing.

(Continued from page 153)

And so I go on. These are the ten coping mechanisms that work for me:

1. I try to live day to day. I focus my thoughts in the present tense and try to deal with matters close at hand.

2. I make myself "stupid," and I try not to think too much about the implications of what it means to have advanced cancer. Instead, I concentrate on concrete and practical things.

3. I try as best I can to compartmentalize the illness and not give it free rein over my existence. I perceive it as unwelcome and boring.

4. I live in a constant state of denial and keep my mind off the disease as much as possible.

5. I surround myself mostly with people and situations that bear no relationship to the illness.

6. I avoid reading or listening to too much about cancer or involving myself with people who are also fighting the disease. Although I am aware they can be beneficial and therapeutic, I avoid support groups in order to prevent myself from allowing any new fears and anxieties about the illness to enter my consciousness.

7. I internalize a belief system that everything I am going through is temporary and will come to an end. I say to myself that in spite of everything, everything will be all right.

8. I stand up to death with a courage I myself do not comprehend, and I do not permit myself to give in to a fear of dying.

9. I acknowledge that it is impossible for anyone to feel like a "normal person" after living with this illness for so many years, and accept the fact that it's okay to feel crazy and alienated some of the time—or even much of the time.

10. I remind myself that no one knows when her last day will be and that, so far, I have lived longer than many people predicted. I then think that maybe I'm doing something right after all and decide to continue to follow my prescription for coping.

Feeling Right when Things Go Wrong: Beliefs I Use to Help Me to Stay Alive

Pat Fobair, L.C.S.W., M.Ph.

In 1955, Albert Ellis, Ph.D., originated a therapy he called Rational Emotive Behavioral Therapy (REBT), an applied philosophy that helps us become aware of our belief system. In his book *Feeling Right when Things Go Wrong* (Professional Resource Press, Sarasota, Florida, 1998), Bill Borcherdt summarized this therapy.

> The only issue more powerful to us than a challenge to our beliefs about life is the possibility of loss of one's survival.

Survival

When it comes to the possibility of loss of one's life, we have a sense of shock, with feelings of isolation and fear. We may notice feelings of being, "out of control." I found that it helped me to notice my feelings of sadness, fear, and anger as soon as possible, and give myself permission to feel disappointment directly. I feel less defensive sooner when I can do this. For example, I have fewer blaming thoughts and use less denial when I can acknowledge my emotional pain. Almost as soon as I get to naming the feeling, I am able to move on to constructive thinking and problem solving. Yet, a source of conflict may emerge within us between our values and beliefs about life and the more immediate reality emerging before us.

Values

When our survival appears to be threatened, some of our basic beliefs in life seem out of line with the new reality. "How could God let this happen to me? I've live a good, clean life. What is true? I feel deceived! The meaning in life seems to have shifted!"

Albert Ellis, Ph.D., addresses this major issue with his Rational Emotive Behavioral Therapy (REBT).

Some ideas are comforting; others challenge us to shift our thoughts to more inclusive humanitarian viewpoints. Here are those that I found comforting:

- Humans are by nature remarkably imperfect and are encouraged not to define themselves by their shortcomings. "If I can be imperfect, I can relax within."
- Humans are not only different from one another, but also differ within themselves by way of thoughts, feelings, and involuntary biochemical sensations. These differences frequently occur spontaneously, often for no special reason, and are best accepted rather than protested against. "You do not have to be like me!"
- Humans do best when they do not try to be islands unto themselves. Nor would it be well to make themselves endlessly dependent on their social group. Rotation and balance between you, me, and us is the socially advisable ideal.
- By putting yourself first and keeping others a close second, you may be able to promote the give and take that is compatible with harmonious social living.
- The essence of good problem solving is to give yourself some emotional slack; to lighten up on yourself rather than tighten up. Permitting yourself an emotional breath of fresh air has value apart from outside changes that you may be able to accomplish.
- Individuals are capable of emotional self-reliance with or without the support of their family or social system. "I can get along alone, should I need to do so!"
- Undamning acceptance of self, others, and life is a fundamental premise of rational living. "You are okay just the way you are, and so am I!"

(Continued from page 155)

- Humans routinely don't practice what they preach. Pledging to more consistently practice affirmed ideals, while not condemning oneself for not hitting the bull's-eye, is suggested. "Thanks for forgiving my discrepancies!"

Here are philosophies that may challenge us to rethink our values and beliefs:

- There is no law of the universe that says others have to do unto us as we do unto them. Although it is nice when others treat us like we kindly treat them, such returns on our emotional investments are not necessities. "I will have to tolerate my disappointments with others who 'let me down.' And, I can allow myself to feel less guilty when I disappoint others."

- The persistence factor is best not underestimated. Getting behind yourself and pushing is habit forming and has a life of its own. Consistently going to bat on behalf of yourself strengthens emotional stamina while increasing the chances of success.

- Everyone is in this life together and no one person is any better than any other. There are no good or bad persons, only individuals who do good and bad things. "This is hard to accept when I feel hurt, angry or disappointed, but blaming others only covers up my feelings and distances me from feeling them fully."

- Happiness is a fleeting thing. It comes and goes in large part by how well you are able to provide for your wants. Vital absorption in a selected project or cause that structures large amounts of your time can improve your sense of meaning in life. "Having projects and completing them gives me satisfaction."

- We all can benefit from a healthy perspective on discomfort in life. Accepting reality rather than intimidating ourselves about discomfort will promote an expanded lifestyle. Worshipping the avoidance of discomfort can lead to an avoidance lifestyle. Humans are in the world to experience the world, which includes a fair amount of discomfort. "It has been hard for me to give up my childhood view of entitlement to unlimited happiness."

- Convincing yourself that you can stand what you don't like allows you to be well grounded in curtailing your frustrations. "The little child in me wants to run away and avoid discomforts and situations that I don't like"

- To damn or condemn a human, including yourself, is immoral and encourages a continuation of problems. "Accepting and forgiving others reduces tension in my life."

- A cornerstone of emotional well-being is not dramatizing the significance of disappointment, by "awfulizing" or "catastrophizing" the consequences. "When I am scared, I immediately think of the worst thing that might happen, then imagine that it has happened. Accepting that I am feeling scared, and that it's just a feeling, helps me let go of the dramatization inside my head."

- Accepting the deficiencies of surety, certainty, and orderliness in this world permits less confusion about and more enjoyment of what it does offer. Uncertainty is part of our daily world. "Accepting this idea encourages me to make the most of each day, and to 'stay in the moment.'"

- Running from pain increases suffering. Taking the long, easy way rather than the short, hard way is central to rational thinking. "Every time I've avoided a problem, it has returned to be struggled with again!"

- Humans are born with the ability to emotionally upset themselves. Rational Emotive Behavioral Therapy takes a dim view of the idea that family of origin or other intrusive background factors are crucial in understanding how humans disturb themselves. "I can choose to upset myself, or to calm down and figure it out!"

- Just because we experience feelings in a situation does not mean that the circumstances caused the feelings. Nor must we presume that if we have a problem we wish to solve, that we must solve it. "Feelings do not equal

(Continued from page 156)

facts! Feelings are just feelings, 'physiological phenomena,' i.e., subjective reactions that may be pleasant or unpleasant, brought about by external circumstances and one's own thoughts and behaviors, and experienced as brief electrical surges in the body."

• People can get by without outside reinforcement by reinforcing themselves with heavy doses of encouraging self-talk. "We can do it, I can do it!"

This philosophy holds us responsible for our emotions. Accepting this higher level of responsibility puts us in the drivers seat to be our own best problem-solving philosophers.

18

Coping with Depression

Andrew W. Kneier, Ph.D.

If you are dealing with cancer, there are many reasons that you may feel depressed from time to time, or at least feel in danger of becoming depressed. Cancer confronts us with our mortality and all of the fears and losses associated with it. It can turn your world upside down, disrupting your life and threatening the roles, purposes, and goals that give you meaning and satisfaction. Cancer therapies may have debilitating side effects and in some cases may cause irreparable damage to your body. Cancer affects not only you but also your loved ones, and this causes you additional emotional distress.

Many cancer patients go through episodes of depression. Depression makes your entire experience with cancer more difficult, weakens your resilience, and may hamper your overall adjustment. It also can undermine your will to live and compromise the courage, fortitude, and determination that you need to face cancer and to endure the necessary medical treatments.

Depression is the exact opposite of what you need: energy and stamina, a vision of a brighter future, hope that inspires and sustains you, and the motivation and commitment to travel through the arduous road of cancer therapy. Depression is therefore a serious threat for anyone dealing with cancer. Fortunately, you can protect yourself from depression, and if it does occur, there are effective remedies for it.

The Nature of Depression

Most of us have been depressed at some time and know what it feels like. The most common complaints are loss of interest in things you used to enjoy (even a simple pleasure, such as listening to your favorite music, could lose its appeal to you); feeling sad, blue, or down in the dumps, and being tearful or crying easily; and feeling depleted of energy and overcome with a paralyzing fatigue.

On some days, a depressed person may feel too drained or apathetic to get out of bed in the morning. You might feel pessimistic and hopeless, begin to welcome death as a relief, and think of suicide. Depression can cause you to feel worthless and guilty, sometimes because of the self-loathing you have developed because of being depressed. Some of the mental problems that accompany depression include difficulty concentrating, difficulty making decisions, and problems with memory. Some of the physical complaints include loss of appetite and libido, sleep disturbances, headaches, and digestive problems.

Causes of Depression

Depression can have psychological or biochemical causes. The psychological causes arise from experiences and events that have a depressing effect; the biochemical (or clinical) causes involve imbalances in the neurochemistry of the brain. Regardless of cause, depression is associated with biochemical change in the brain.

Life experiences may cause depression when they carry certain meanings for the person involved. For example, someone who was abused as a child might conclude that they are undeserving of love or a happy life. Thoughts and feelings of being unworthy, whether conscious or unconscious, can then lead to depression. Other thoughts that commonly underlie depression involve the sense of being helpless, hopeless, and a victim. These thoughts and feelings have their origin in traumatic events in the person's life (although the person may not remember these events). Not only do these events cause depressing thoughts, they can also bring about a biochemical imbalance in the brain, and this imbalance contributes to the depression.

Most of the times that you are depressed you can identify what you are depressed about or are able to identify depressing thoughts (e.g., "Nothing will make a difference"). However, sometimes depression seems to come out of the blue. People have "come down" with depression in ways that feel similar to coming down with the flu, and they may not be aware of why they are depressed. This is because the psychological factors are unconscious or because the depression is caused solely by changes in the neurochemistry of the brain.

Cancer and Depression

Cancer patients often get depressed simply because having cancer can be a depressing experience. However, there is usually more to it than that. Most cancer patients are not clinically depressed. To varying degrees, they are frightened and upset, but this is not depression. When cancer causes depression, there are psychological or biological reasons for it. These causes are understandable, and they are treatable.

The experience of cancer can cause depression because of the various meanings that the illness takes on as a result of the circumstances or psychological background in which it occurred.

Cancer happens to you as a person, not just to your body. You therefore experience it as part of your personal life. The personal issues, themes, perceptions, and feelings that are embedded in your own personal history color your experience of cancer, giving it a certain meaning and feeling or tone.

The clearest example is seen in the reactions to the diagnosis of cancer in people of various ages. In general, cancer patients in their thirties experience a feeling of incompleteness about their life and a strong emotional investment in a long future; to them, the cancer may feel like a threat to that future and to all the goals and purposes that it holds. Patients in their eighties, on the other hand, generally bring some sense of life completion to their experience of cancer, along with an awareness that their future is relatively short; to them, the same cancer may feel more acceptable because of the long life they already have enjoyed.

Of course, chronological age is not the sole influence on how you experience having cancer or whether you become depressed. The following examples illustrate other ways that your psychological context can contribute to depression.

The feeling of sadness (for yourself and loved ones) evoked by a cancer diagnosis is not itself depression, but if it becomes magnified by other sorrows in your life, it can become depression. In this case, a sorrowful life history before your cancer is the context in which the cancer is experienced. The cancer can represent a kind of crowning blow to a long history of abuse, misfortune, or frustration. It can tap into or reactivate many old feelings. The depression that emerges stems partly from having cancer, but it also grows out of one's personal life history and its resulting emotional baggage.

Suppose you had recently achieved an important life goal or were on the verge of doing so. Perhaps you had struggled for years to achieve this goal. Then, on the heels of this important accomplishment, you are diagnosed with cancer. You could therefore feel that you were being thwarted, that the deck was stacked against you, or that you were having to pay a price for your ambition. These are the meanings that cancer could hold for you—derived from the context in which it occurred—and they can cause depression.

The medical treatment for cancer cannot help but cause some degree of physical suffering and damage to your body. The optimal goal of treatment, of course, is to restore your body to health, but this comes at some price. Sometimes the price is severe (such as a mastectomy, head or neck surgery, bone marrow transplant, or skin damage from radiation therapy). Different patients feel differently about the bodily effects of cancer treatments, and one response is sometimes depression. Our feelings about ourselves are to some degree dependent upon our appearance and our physical abilities. When these are compromised by cancer, the loss that we suffer (sometimes to our self-esteem, sometimes to our role and identity) can be deeply depressing.

Our culture often assumes that what happens to a person is somehow linked to what that person deserves. Unfortunately, this assumption, which is often very subtle, can affect a cancer patient. When things are going well for us, we tend to assume that we are doing something right and deserve our good fortune. Misfortune—such as cancer—may make us think that we were not so deserving of our good fortune after all. It is not uncommon, therefore, for cancer patients to wonder where they went wrong. Some patients have felt that things were going too well for them, that their life was too easy, or that they were enjoying more happiness than most people, and that cancer was a way of balancing things out. One woman said of her cancer: "It's all of my repressed resentment and bitterness coming out." Another patient felt that it was an expression of his self-hatred. One referred to it as "a pathetic attempt for the attention I've never had." Such ideas can cause depression.

As already mentioned, there are also biological causes of depression in cancer patients. The emotional consequences of cancer can bring about biochemical changes in the brain. Biochemical changes can also be caused by chemotherapy drugs, hormonal treatments, anti-inflammatory drugs, pain medication, and radiation therapy.

If you are depressed, it does not necessarily mean that you are not coping or adjusting as you should. It often is important and psychologically healthy for underlying feelings to emerge, as this may provide an opportunity for you to confront and work through the emotional traumas from past years.

Whatever the cause, depression is dangerous, especially to your quality of life and your will to live. There are steps you can take to alleviate it.

What You Can Do to Protect Yourself

There are four important ways to protect yourself from depression when you are dealing with cancer:

- Try to become aware of your emotions, and then acknowledge and express these emotions with someone you feel close to. Depression often results from the suppression of painful and upsetting emotions. Research has shown that cancer patients who openly express their feelings and obtain support from others are much less likely to become depressed.

- Maintain close connections and frequent contact with your loved ones and reach out for their support. Studies have demonstrated that interpersonal support is a strong buffer against feelings of isolation and depression.

- Become an active participant in fostering your physical and emotional well-being. Discuss the treatment options with your doctors so that you are informed and can fully embrace the treatment plan, and consider supplemental approaches as well (such as acupuncture, better nutrition, herbal medicine, meditation, and guided imagery). Your active involvement in your recovery will help to counter the feelings of helplessness and passivity that often characterize depression.

- Try to obtain as much exercise as possible. The physiological and mental benefits of exercise help to offset the depressing effect of a serious illness. One reason for this is that exercise increases the brain levels of endorphins, which are natural mood elevators (see Chapters 32 and 33 on exercise and massage).

What to Do about Depression

If you become depressed, try to identify what is bothering you. You might make a list of these problems and ways that you could address them. Discuss these problems and emotions with a relative or close friend.

Depression often results from suppressing our emotions, depriving them of the discharge they need. For example, when depression persists long after the loss of a loved one, it is often because the person's grief has not been adequately expressed. One theory is that unexpressed emotions build up internally and cause depression; another is that the mental energy required to contain such emotions results in the kind of mental fatigue and lethargy characteristic of depression.

It is common to be unaware of what you are depressed about. You might feel that you have no good reason for being depressed, especially because others have far worse problems or because you are grateful for the many blessings you have enjoyed. Try to push yourself beyond that: give yourself the benefit of the doubt—that you have legitimate reasons for your depression—and do some soul-searching to find out what these reasons are. Think about the many ways that cancer can cause depression, as discussed above.

Think especially about your life as a whole, and about the disappointments and sorrows that you have encountered along the way. These may be affecting you now more than you realize. Whatever you come up with in this self-exploration, talk about it with someone you feel especially close to, even if you think you are being foolish, shallow, or self-centered. Permit yourself to feel what you are feeling, honor your reasons for feeling it, and confide in someone about it. Even writing about these matters in a journal can have a relieving effect.

In this process, you might also think about why it is difficult for you to express your feelings. One common reason is not wanting to bother others with your feelings and needs. Some people have difficulty confiding in others because of an underlying belief that they cannot or will not be comforted by doing so. Confiding therefore seems like a setup for more letdown and hurt. Perhaps you let your parents know when something was bothering you, but they did not respond with the comfort or support you needed. Such experiences, over the course of your childhood, could cause you to feel that there was nothing to be gained by voicing your feelings, and that doing so only made you feel worse. While these fears are understandable, it is important to recognize that there is surely someone in your life now (a relative or close friend, a minister or rabbi, a doctor, a nurse, a therapist) who would support you in what you are going through.

Another aspect of depression is that it may cause you to withdraw from others and to turn inward. This can make it all the more difficult to confide in others about your feelings and to obtain the support you need. A vicious circle can set in, wherein a person becomes depressed, withdraws, and therefore has no emotional outlet or personal support and becomes even more depressed. It is essential that you break out of this cycle by finding some way of reaching out for help. If necessary, circle this paragraph, leave it for someone who cares about you to see, and write "Help me" in the margin.

Depression often involves feelings of despair, bitterness, or lack of meaning, resulting in the painful cry of "Why me?" that often arises when someone is subjected to severe suffering. Your religion or spirituality can be a source of meaning and comfort for you, offering a perspective that can soothe the emotional anguish and mental torment that cancer sometimes causes.

Treatment for Depression

Psychotherapy

Often, a mental health professional provides the best help for depression. Research has shown that psychotherapy is an effective treatment for depression in the majority of cases. A therapist will help you to talk about difficult feelings and will create an emotionally safe environment in which to do so. He or she will also help you to explore all the factors that are contributing to your depression, including those that you may not be aware of. You will learn ways of mastering the thoughts that cause depression. In general, your therapy will consist of working through your depression and the life experiences that are related to it. It will not take your cancer away, and you may still feel upset and worried, but you will no longer be stuck in the deep, dark hole of depression.

Antidepressant Medication

Antidepressant medication is warranted in many cases, especially in combination with psychotherapy. The best known of these involve the chemical serotonin, one of the main neurotransmitters. When a neural impulse reaches the end of a nerve cell in the brain, it releases serotonin in the junction (called the synapse) connecting this cell to the next, and this enables the impulse to be transmitted from one cell to the other. Sometimes, the nerve cell sending the signal reabsorbs the serotonin too quickly, and an insufficient amount is left in the junction for the impulse to be transmitted effectively. This phenomenon is apparently associated with the experience of depression.

It is interesting that the mental slowness or lethargy of depression may reflect the state of the brain when serotonin levels are too low. Some antidepressants, called selective serotonin re-uptake inhibitors (SSRIs), block the reabsorption of serotonin, and thereby relieve the symptoms of depression.

There are other types of antidepressant medication besides the SSRIs, and each of these works a little differently. Your physician or psychiatrist will prescribe the best medication for your individual situation. Still, it may take some trial and error to find the medication that works best for you and has the fewest side effects. It may take weeks for some antidepressants to reach their full potential.

The symptomatic relief provided by an antidepressant may be a godsend to a severely depressed person, even though it does not address what the person is depressed about. This relief is often essential in order for the person to even consider ways of addressing the psychological aspects of depression. Research has shown that the best treatment for depression, in many cases, is a combination of emotional support, psychotherapy, and antidepressant medication.

Steps to Overcoming Depression

The depression that stems from cancer and its treatments can make you feel that you can't go on and that it's not worth the effort. However, there are effective ways of combating and overcoming this depression:

- Do not blame yourself for being depressed.
- Identify what you are depressed about.
- Confide in someone you feel close to.
- Express your emotions.
- Engage in problem solving.
- Become an active participant in recovery efforts (do not give in to helplessness).
- Do things that enhance self-esteem.
- Exercise as much as possible.
- Talk with your minister or rabbi.
- Deepen your faith or spirituality (through prayer, reading, and meditation).
- Obtain help from a therapist.
- Explore antidepressant medication.

19

Religion and Spirituality

Andrew W. Kneier, Ph.D.
Rabbi Jeffery Silberman, D.Min.
Reverend Elmer Laursen, D. Min
Reverend John D. Shanahan
Rabbi Joseph Asher
Ernest H. Rosenbaum, M.D.

A life-threatening disease such as cancer makes us confront realities and questions that cause us to step back from our lives and reflect on the meaning and implications of the illness. Our perspective on these realities and questions emerges in large measure from our religious, spiritual, or philosophical orientation, and it influences how we experience the illness—its meaning, how we feel about it, and how well we come to terms with it. A religious perspective can help us as we grapple with these issues and seek to keep our bearing through the mental and emotional turmoil that comes with having cancer.

Cancer and Questions of Meaning

In order to discuss how religion and spirituality can help in dealing with cancer, we must first review some of the religious and spiritual issues, questions, and problems that cancer presents. These are questions of meaning—the meaning of our life and what is important, the meaning behind our personal affliction with cancer, and finding meaning in our suffering.

Mortality

A cancer diagnosis confronts us with the fact that we are vulnerable to disease and suffering, that we are mortal, and that our time is limited. When we are in good health, these realities often reside at the back of our minds; but when a serious illness strikes, they surge forward and challenge us. They challenge us especially with the question of whether we are using our time wisely. This question is linked to what our time is for—to what our life is all about. For many, these questions take on a central and compelling importance, which is why cancer is commonly referred to as a wake-up call.

Usually, the most pressing priority when faced with the diagnosis of cancer is to regain good health; if this is successful, the implications of mortality might once again slip into the background. Sometimes, the illness is regarded as only a temporary bump in the road of life, as opposed to a stark reminder of life's fragility. But more often than not, cancer has a way of capturing our attention, deepening our reflection on what is important, and causing us to live with more awareness of our ultimate priorities.

Patients who are fighting for their lives can be strengthened and sustained by a clear vision of what they want to survive for. Many talk of surviving for the sake of their families, to meet certain life goals, and to fulfill certain inner potentials or strivings. Whatever a person's answer, it reflects deeply held religious, spiritual, or philosophical beliefs about what is important and why.

As cancer patients reflect on their ultimate priorities, they often identify changes that they wish to make in themselves or their lives. This often is referred to as the "enlightenment" of cancer or the "gift" of cancer. Countless patients have commented that they regret that it took a cancer diagnosis to wake them up and capture their attention, but they feel that many positive and overdue changes in themselves and their lives have resulted from it. In making these changes, these patients have found some positive meaning in their illness.

Why Me?

Cancer confronts us with the question of why, as one person among many, we have been afflicted with this disease. Many patients have asked, in open protest or in private anguish, "Why did this have to happen to me?" Of course, the answer is that it did not *have* to happen, it just did. But there often is an emotional poignancy to this issue that cannot easily be dismissed.

One reason for this is religious: those who believe in the God of the Judeo-Christian Bible do not understand how a loving God could allow cancer to happen to a good person. There must be some reason for it. It is not uncommon for patients to wonder whether the illness is a punishment for certain wrongs or failings of character. The Bible teaches that disease and death are the result of sin. Of course, many religiously oriented patients do not feel that they are being punished, but they do feel that their illness is somehow part of God's plan for them, and they struggle and pray to discern the higher purpose for which it is intended.

Even those who are not particularly religious can feel a sense of self-blame about their cancer because of the influence of the Judeo-Christian tradition in our culture. (See Chapter 16, "Does Your Attitude Make a Difference?") Many patients feel that if they can fix whatever is wrong in themselves, or adopt the right attitudes and behaviors, then the malignancy will be stopped. It has been argued, for example, that if

patients heal themselves, or heal their lives, then physical healing will follow.

Why Do We Suffer?

There are many dimensions to the suffering caused by cancer—physical, mental, emotional, and spiritual. The suffering can involve all aspects of the person, including one's relationships, roles, identity, hopes and plans, and the meaning of one's life.

A person with cancer is challenged to respond to suffering in some way. Most patients, of course, strive to gain as much relief from their suffering as possible. Beyond that, some patients feel that their only option is to endure it, either philosophically or stoically. Others seek to deny or downplay it, while some try to rise above it. Some regard it as an opportunity or challenge to demonstrate certain strengths of character or to bear witness to their faith. Some patients rail against it as an outrage, and others are able to find some personal meaning in their suffering, especially in bringing about changes in themselves that they feel are important (such as acceptance or humility).

The religions of the world all contain, in one way or another, a philosophy or perspective on the meaning of suffering. Perhaps the perspective most widely known in our culture is the Judeo-Christian one, according to which suffering serves the positive purpose of deepening one's spirituality. Religious faith can bring a perspective to suffering that offers consolation or strength to those living through cancer.

Religious and Spiritual Perspectives on Meaning

When we talk about the meaning of an experience, we are talking about its relationship or connection to something larger or beyond the experience itself. For example, the meaning of a serious illness can be found in how it is related to the person's life as a whole. The meaning of one's life as a whole can be found in its connection to some larger reality, cause, or purpose. Many people feel that their lives are meaningful because of the contribution they make to the lives of others.

To understand the roles of religion and spirituality in defining meaning for us, we must ask about the larger meaning of the lives of other people. We might argue that the success of a human life contributes to the success of the human experience as a whole. We then might ask, however, whether the success of human evolution (physical, mental, and moral) really matters, because humankind will not survive the eventual demise of our solar system. Suppose there is some realm or cause within or beyond evolution. Fine. But, in order to have any meaning, what is it connected to? Thus, an infinite series of questions is launched here, wherein we can always ask about the larger reality to which something is meaningfully connected. Is there some ultimate reality that finally provides meaning to everything else?

These are the kinds of questions that lie at the heart of religion, faith, and spirituality. All systems of belief acknowledge a transcendent source of meaning and value beyond human beings. At times of serious illness or crisis, it is to one of these systems that we may turn for solace, comfort, and meaning; for the inner strength to endure the physical and emotional challenges of illness; and for guidance in our personal response to it.

Religion describes both the formal area of study of these belief systems and, more specifically, the organized understanding of beliefs shared by groups of people. The Western religious tradition includes—but is not limited to—Judaism, Christianity, and Islam. The Eastern religious tradition includes—but is not limited to—Buddhism, Taoism, and Hinduism. Each religious system is based on a core of beliefs, often articulated through a set of ancient texts that are considered authoritative and sacred. These bodies of literature incorporate that religion's values and teachings, providing the source of answers to many profound human questions.

Faith often refers to the beliefs held by an individual who is an adherent of one of the formal systems of religion. Each of us, whether we know it or not, holds some kind of faith. We may believe in a personal God or in a Divine Clockmaker (that is, a God who created the world, set it in motion, and then left it alone). This faith may be spelled out by a formal systematic theology or comprise pieces of many different religious teachings. This personal faith is frequently deep and forms a foundation of emotional and spiritual strength when we face crisis, cancer, and especially death.

Spirituality is the connection that many people feel to God or to something beyond us, but not in accordance to the formal teachings of traditional religion. Thus, many people speak about being spiritual but not necessarily religious. While some people seek their answers in religious literature and traditional teachings, others search beyond traditional models to find answers that will bring them emotional and existential meaning.

Religion: Coping and Healing

A person's faith or spirituality provides a means for coping with illness and reaching a deeper kind of inner healing. Coping means different things to different people: it can involve finding answers to the questions that illness raises, it can mean seeking comfort for the fears and pain that illness brings, and it can mean learning how to find a sense of direction at a time of illness. Religious teachings can help a person cope in all of these dimensions.

Religious teachings can also point the way toward healing, which can be something very different from curing. Modern medicine has been able to recognize that a medical cure is not always possible; nor is it the only appropriate goal for treatment. Sometimes, when treatment is futile, the healing of soul or spirit can provide a deep and sustaining comfort. Religion has long focused upon this as its central purpose. Healing of the soul or spirit means recognizing the values in one's life and striving to bring these in line with the teachings of one's religion or the fundamentals of one's faith.

The Quest for Meaning

The meaning of life and death, humanity's purpose or direction, and the struggle with suffering and pain have long been central themes in religious literature.

Within the context of many traditional belief systems, the ultimate answer to meaning, suffering, and death resides with God alone. One conservative religious answer is that God's ways are beyond human understanding, but we must trust in God's goodness and purpose. Many people feel a great sense of confidence and assurance in the belief that an all-powerful, all-knowing deity controls the world. The idea that the reward for a life well lived is eternal life in heaven is usually associated with this conservative belief.

Liberal theologies offer other explanations about God's place in human experience. Some hold that God has created an imperfect world and that it is our task and responsibility as humans to work toward the world's repair or perfection. This means that we share an obligation to help one another face the struggles of human existence, including illness and death.

Some humanistic religious traditions assert that God has no direct influence on contemporary human events. They assert that when we suffer, all that God can do is to be present with us. The comfort in this belief system comes from the conviction that God feels our pain and knows what we are going through when we suffer.

Religion and "Why Me?"

For many patients, the "Why me?" issues are essentially religious in nature. Religious people are sometimes concerned that illness relates to sin that they have committed. Most religions today reject the idea that God punishes us through illness. Many people hold to an alternative view—that illnesses such as cancer demonstrate the presence of evil in the world. Religion gives us the opportunity to help others and thereby overcome evil or imperfection by creating good.

Most theologians and religious leaders today acknowledge that there are no simple answers to these questions. They also recognize that the question "Why me?" is really not so much a question requiring an answer as a cry of emotional and spiritual pain. Rather than try to address this question with theological formulas that bring little consolation, they strive instead to honor the emotional anguish behind these questions and to point to the comfort, reassurance, and broader perspective offered in religious teachings.

Emotional Comfort

In the face of a serious illness, we are often challenged by a range of emotional reactions that can be unfamiliar and more intense than anything we have ever encountered. We feel ourselves vulnerable and in need of a stable and solid support. Religion steps in with comfort and reassurance.

One of the great sources of emotional support in times of illness is the Book of Psalms. For those familiar with the Western religious canon, the Psalmist speaks compassionately and with great understanding of the emotional upheaval of crisis. The 23rd Psalm (King James Version) reads: "Yea, though I walk through the valley of the shadow of death, I will fear no evil: for Thou art with me; Thy rod and Thy staff they comfort me."

When we are confronted by cancer or other serious illness, our sensory experience is often heightened, both in regard to the beauty of life and its more frightening, ugly, and painful side. Our emotional connection to the world can become more intense. Religious tradition places this experience in an ancient perspective. We recall the stories of great sages and saints who also faced hardship and death. They instruct and show us about the intensity and how our path has been traveled before by so many others. Our feelings direct us to a new connection to the world and God's presence in it.

Religious Guidance

Another dilemma confronting cancer patients relates to what can be done. They wonder how to act and how to function at this time. It seems that the ordinary ways of living and functioning are inappropriate or trite. Religion again assists us with models of behavior to demonstrate the values we hold as important. Spiritual disciplines and teachings of various kinds can instruct us in structured exercises.

Asceticism—simplifying our life and living for others—is an example well known through religious history. Religion teaches us that we can find order and direction by doing things that foster our spiritual well-being and energy. These can include some of the following practices.

Religious Resources and Practices

Many conventional religious resources and practices help us cope with cancer by offering comfort, support, and direction.

Rituals and prayer are the central and best-known religious techniques. Prayer extends comfort in many ways. It offers us consolation, encouragement, connection, and solace. We experience a sense of divine presence and divine love as we pray. Prayer and ritual touch deep feelings within us. They allow us to give voice to our pain, joy, grief, loss, isolation, alienation, and loneliness. Prayer evokes memories of our youth and of our family and long-standing relationships. It also brings a sense of power and awesome mystery. Prayer reveals a side of ourselves that may be needy, that we may not want to reveal, and that struggles with uncertainty.

Prayer techniques, such as centering, traditional prayer, meditation, guided meditation, and anointing, have long been recognized as effective tools in dealing with illness. Recent scientific studies reported in books such as Dr. Larry Dossey's *Healing Words* prove beyond doubt that prayer makes a difference. Four nondenominational prayers for healing, selected by the pastoral care staff at the UCSF/Mount Zion Medical Center, are found at the end of this chapter.

The *religious community* is a powerful ally in dealing with crises in our lives. People who know us and care about us from within a community of faith are important partners in the healing process. Apart from the effectiveness of their love and prayers, the religious communicants can often provide practical support for the necessary tasks of daily living.

We should not underestimate the value of clergy visits for helping us to cope with cancer. In many ways, the presence of clergy powerfully conveys the message of God's care to those who are ill. Clergy tangibly represent God's caring presence, both through their being there and through the words they speak.

Healing practices associated with religion and focused upon cancer and other illnesses have become much more common today than ever before. Some of these practices come from fringe groups and charlatans seeking to prey upon frightened people. Yet mainstream religion also has recognized the value of healing prayer services and rituals as an addition to more typical prayers and rituals. Some rituals of this kind are ancient. Some are contemporary. Many people have sought and found spiritual healing and comfort through religious tradition and practice.

Nondenominational Prayers for Healing

These four nondenominational prayers for healing have been selected by the pastoral care staff at the UCSF/Mount Zion Medical Center.

My God and God of all generations, in my great need I pour out my heart to you. Long days and weeks of suffering are hard to endure. In my struggle, I reach out for the help that only you can give. Let me feel that you are near, and that your care enfolds me. Rouse me with the strength to overcome my weakness, and brighten my spirit with the assurance of your love. Help me to sustain the hopes of my loved ones as they strive to strengthen and encourage me. May the healing power you have placed within me give me the strength to recover so I may fulfill my journey in the Divine Plan.

In sickness I turn to you, O God, as a child turns to a parent for comfort and help. Strengthen within me the wondrous power of healing that you have implanted in your children. Guide my doctors and nurses, that they may speed my recovery. Let the knowledge of your love comfort my loved ones, lighten their burdens, and renew their faith. May my sickness not weaken my faith in you, nor diminish my love for other human beings. From my illness may I gain a truer appreciation of life's gifts, a deeper awareness of life's blessings, and a fuller sympathy for all who are in pain.

Send me, O God, your healing, so that I may quickly recover from the illness that has come upon me. Sustain my spirit, relieve my pain, and restore me to perfect health, happiness, and strength. Grant unto my body your healing power so I may continue to be able to bear testimony to your everlasting mercy and love, for you, O Lord, art a faithful and merciful healer.

Be at Peace
Do not fear the changes of life—
Rather look to them with full hope as they arise.
God, whose very own you are,
Will deliver you from out of them.
He has kept you hitherto,
And He will lead you safely through all things;
And when you cannot stand it,
God will bury you in His arms.
Do not be afraid of what may happen tomorrow;
The same everlasting Father who cares for you today
Will take care of you then and every day.
He will either shield you from suffering,
Or He will give you unfailing strength to bear it.
Be at Peace—
And put aside all anxious thoughts and imaginations.

—St. Francis de Sales

The Role of the Clergy

Reverend Elmer Laursen, D.Min.
Reverend John D. Shanahan
Rabbi Joseph Asher
Ernest H. Rosenbaum, M.D

Men and women of the clergy occupy a unique position. Whether ministers, priests, or rabbis, they have authority and respect in the community. One of their many functions is to comfort the sick, at home or in the hospital. The patients they visit in a hospital are not necessarily limited to members of one congregation, or even one religion. Some patients may no longer have any religious affiliation. Yet the clergy still can be welcome figures, sympathetic listeners, and sources of emotional and spiritual sustenance.

Many people under the stress of illness or dying call upon God to help them. Severe stress and fear may also cause them to revert to previously held religious views. For these people, as well as for regular members of religious groups, the clergy represent faith, salvation, and the authority of God. They are expected to have special insight into the mysteries of life and death.

Ernest H. Rosenbaum interviewed representatives of three faiths—Chaplain Laursen, Father Shanahan, and Rabbi Asher—to ask them how they approached individual patients and how those patients reacted. What follows is not a comprehensive discussion of religion; it is an attempt to understand the role of the clergy with regard to the patient who has cancer. In spite of the many differences among the three faiths, in both concept and practice, it was found that in dealing with the cancer patient the three clergy differed only in style. Their objectives were similar: to help people to live, and also to die. In this respect, their roles do not differ from those of doctors, nurses, social workers, or volunteers.

Interview

Father John Shanahan: There are, of course, certain expectations, somewhat vaguely conceived, of what a clergyman should do. He is expected to minister to the patient, to provide the opportunity for sacraments and prayer, to bring comfort and solace in some way, to deal with spiritual problems, to lift the patient's morale, and to spread comfort and cheer. In the popular dichotomy, the doctor cares for the body, and the chaplain cares for the soul. The clergyman has the opportunity to make a unique and valuable contribution to the spiritual, mental, and emotional well-being of the sick, the seriously ill, and the dying.

As a priest in a hospital setting, I am, among other things, acting as a representative of our religious community. The patients don't know me personally. They come from various parts of the San Francisco Bay Area. They are separated from their families. My being there says, "We care about you. We want you to get well. How can we help?" Maybe these people haven't seen a priest in a long time. But my presence might remind them of a time when they attended church and thereby give them strength for the present. On the other hand, some people with tenuous ties to our religious community don't care about seeing a priest, so my visit to them will not be supportive. Each patient reacts differently. Therefore, I don't have a planned approach.

Slowly and painfully I have learned one general approach. I think this approach helps me, as a priest caring for the seriously ill, to listen, and I hope it has helped the patients I visit. Unaware of the dynamics behind the emotional stresses or moral disorders in a man or woman about to die, with not the faintest idea of what to say, I listen. I have learned to hold my tongue, learned what not to say. I try to show sincere interest, to reflect understanding of the person's feelings. I try to accept the person as a fellow human being. As a

(Continued from page 168)

listener, I have learned that I can create an atmosphere of solicitous permissiveness in which the troubled patient feels free to share the burden he or she is unable to carry alone. I try to be compassionate, to touch the emotional pulse of the patient by identifying in some personal way with his anguish, his bewilderment, his interior conflict. I try to understand. I need hardly say a word. Someone is interested; someone understands; someone is in no hurry to run, to belittle, to disparage, to explain away the worry, or to trot out pious clichés. I am, primarily, a listener whose contribution is a wholehearted acceptance of the patient. I try to create a climate in which the sick person feels he or she may speak without fear.

Rabbi Joseph Asher: I feel that my function is to try to be an empathic person who relates to people not as a rabbi but as a friend. The only rabbinic component of this kind of relationship is that perhaps the person has more respect and regard for me because he recognizes that I have seen other people in his same situation and may even have some direct communication with the divine. But I don't. I really don't think I have ever contributed to a person to the extent that I have evoked resources of strength he did not have before I came. The best I have been able to do is maybe awaken resources that this person was planning to set aside or was unaware he possessed.

I may say to a patient, "Now look, every day that you live is one more opportunity for an improvement in your condition, because with medical science the way it is today, what is impossible today may be possible tomorrow." I also explain to him or her that much of survival—and this may be impression rather than fact—depends on a person's will and a person's desire to survive.

Recently, a member of my congregation had a stroke and simply did not want to live. He would not participate in such therapy as was available to him and after a period of months he just died. The physician who took care of him told me that this man could have lived longer and could have lived an active life. He simply did not want to live. So what I can do, as a rabbi, is constantly reassure a

patient that a great deal of his recovery depends on that person's will to live. If I can help strengthen that will to live, I have made a contribution.

Nevertheless, I'm terribly aware of my impotence in these things. It's very difficult for an outside force to have any effect in a situation like this. People's lives cannot be influenced to such an extent that a person can say, "The rabbi was here and he told me I'm going to live. Therefore I'm going to live. I'm going to try harder than I did before he came in." The person may do this for five minutes, in my presence, but if his nature is inclined toward giving up, that's what he's going to do.

However, I think we often underestimate both the patients' abilities to cope and their need for comfort arising from an apprehension of the truth. We always think they need to be babied when they are in such situations. It is really more the function of the rabbi to relate to the family, to help them accept the inevitable with grace and with a certain amount of consolation. They, in turn, convey this composure to the sick person. The entire Jewish tradition teaches us to confront reality. If a person is about to die, then we have to recognize the fact that this is about to happen. We do not, under any circumstances, encourage a kind of covering up of what is about to occur, nor do we hold out a description of life beyond. That is why it's sometimes much more difficult for a rabbi to comfort a family, particularly when a death occurs that is out of the ordinary.

In such instances, the family's first response is often, "How could God let this happen to us? What justice is there from such a God?" I tell them that God is not doing something to hurt them. The untimely death of the person they love is simply one of the malfunctions of nature just as much as is an earthquake or a hurricane.

Reverend Elmer Laursen: Patients have fear of cancer as a disease, and they need to share their fear and anxiety with someone who will listen. Many physicians and nurses listen to patients, but a clergyman may do it in a different way. He comes to listen to their questions, which often include

(Continued from page 169)

"Why did this happen? What did I do?"

Our objective is to support patients in the most appropriate way. We try to keep hope alive, but not to foster false hope. We share the bad times that depress patients. We try to help them accept illness as a part of their lives instead of just to fight it. We try to emphasize the positives in their lives, but when there are few or none of these it is harder to help them.

I attempt to console, share and be alongside people during their suffering. I listen to their questions in a supportive way, helping them tap and enlarge upon their religious resources. I listen, and sometimes in silence I give aid and comfort. Frequently my main function is just to be there. I try to hear patients' verbal and nonverbal cries and concerns and, if possible, to help them achieve a new perspective. It seems to me that by sharing I contribute the important element, which is to help them feel less alone and less deserted.

When there are family members, relatives, and friends who are a part of the supportive system for a patient, I can at times also help them with their feelings and enable them to be supportive rather than hindering to the patient.

I have become increasingly aware that in our work with people and their problems, we need not pretend to have any great answers for them. They sometimes find answers for themselves, or at the least they find someone with whom they can share their questions.

While as a chaplain my desire is to work closely with the physician, he is not always ready to involve me in patient care. Often, I am able to minister effectively in spite of his reluctance to include me. However, we both do a better job when we can work together.

The acceptance of the problem of illness and the incorporation of that acceptance into one's life and trying to deal with it is an upward process. People who learn to accept and reconcile themselves to dying often seem to live more effectively. Given the opportunity to vent their anger at God in the presence of an understanding clergyman, they may be relieved of their guilt feelings. It is normal to be angry, curse, or swear at God and ask, "Why?" Eventually they learn that they can be as angry as they wish at God because He is big enough to handle it. Then they can begin a more dynamic process of living for their remaining time. Somehow, it is helpful to most of us to be able to accept that death is a part of life.

The process of learning how best to support a patient is long and arduous. It involves going into a patient's room, letting him say whatever he wishes, and then helping him to look at what is going on, to reflect on it. I feel it is unnecessary to confront a person too heavily or bluntly. I have better ways of being with a patient than saying, "You know, you have to take a look at this for your wife and family. You can't just give up." Rather, I try to help him take hold of the problem and deal openly with it.

Finally, the time arrives when all I can do is to help a patient to die graciously. In doing that, I believe I am helping people to live right up to the last moment.

Ernest Rosenbaum: The three of you have a similar concept of the role of the clergy in supporting a cancer patient. You help by supporting, encouraging, listening, empathizing, and giving both faith and hope to a patient, his family, and his friends. You absorb the anger of a patient. You can be trusted with confidences and yet you are accepting and not shocked.

Ritual is often followed in ministering to patients. Father Shanahan, do you still administer the last rites to a patient who is coming to the end of his life? If so, what effect does this have on him?

Father John Shanahan: There has been a change in the administration of the sacraments that makes them more meaningful. The Sacrament of Extreme Unction is now called the Sacrament of the Sick. It is administered frequently and quite normally when a person is ill but not about to die. Last rites is a term reserved for the use of the funeral liturgy.

Ernest Rosenbaum: Rabbi Asher, how does

(Continued from page 170)

the Jewish ritual help people to come to terms with grief?

Rabbi Joseph Asher: As with every aspect of life, Judaism's rituals seek to provide outlets for emotions rather than submerge them. Our tradition understands the immediate response to the crises we experience and seeks to vest them with meaning in the context of our relationship with the divine. Thus, when death comes the family's anger and their total withdrawal is acknowledged. Certain normal religious functions are suspended. In our anger, we can hardly be expected to praise God. After the funeral, the family remains at home for seven days, desisting from its regular habits and inviting friends to come to the house for communal prayer rather than going to the synagogue. After that week, and until thirty days after the death, normal activities are resumed, while some personal habits—for which one would have no inclination anyway—are still restricted. For the ten months following, one does not engage in any activities that might be interpreted as unduly entertaining or engaging in levity. Eleven months after the death, family and friends gather to consecrate a memorial at gravesite. This ritual demonstrates the "closing of the grave," a symbol that grief must now be set aside and we must come to terms again with life.

The most modern understanding of the grief syndrome acknowledges stages of emergence from it. Jewish ritual is designed to guide us from the most abject sorrow to renewed composure, allowing for time to bring its healing to the bereaved.

Ernest Rosenbaum: Chaplain Laursen, what extra help can a person find in dealing with death and grief?

Elmer Laursen: Workshops, seminars, and retreats for clergy and laypersons are effective in helping them express their feelings and thoughts about death and grief. People of all ages have participated in these groups. Most of them have felt threatened at first, but after permitting themselves to become involved in the dialogue and in the process of reflection, they have found that some of their fears were lessened. These are subjects that we all prefer to avoid, but by bringing them into the open and confronting them we may be able to deal with death, and life, in a more realistic and wholesome manner. Members of communities in which such experiences take place have developed rich resources for ministering to one another when confronted by death and grief. They can be open with one another to a far greater degree than exists in the usual "denial" of real feelings.

I am convinced that this entire process of opening up to each other makes it possible for persons suffering all kinds of diseases of body, mind, and spirit to live more fully and to limit to some degree the destructive element that threaten us.

Ernest Rosenbaum: Unlike most of the people who support the patient and his family, the clergy continues to serve the family after the patient's death by helping them through the process of grieving. The ritual of a funeral service and a post-funeral meal for family and friends is as much a supportive gesture toward the bereaved as an opportunity to say farewell to the deceased. Following these brief distractions, the survivors may experience a deeper state of shock than they did at the time of death. The period of mourning begins. There is no way to shorten or lessen the grieving process, although it can be shared and the pain, in part, alleviated through the compassion of others.

Many thanks to Tina Anderson for her assistance with this section. Reprinted from *Living with Cancer*, 1982.

20

Visualization
The Power of Imagery and Mental Participation

Andrew W. Kneier, Ph.D.
Janet Amber Damon, M.S.W.

If you have ever made up a story, painted a picture, or created a sculpture, you know about the creative power of your imagination. Images or scenes just pop into your mind, seemingly from nowhere. Sometimes the image is so right for the story that you are both delighted and taken aback, wondering, "Where did that come from?" It often seems that the image was given to you, not created by you, or that you somehow found the image in your mind. Writers of fiction and artists of all types owe their craft and livelihood to the resourcefulness of their imagination as they draw upon this wondrous source of creativity that resides within all of us.

Cancer patients also have discovered the power of their imagination in dealing with the many challenges posed by their illness. In the most general sense, they do this by mentally visualizing what they hope to achieve, whether it be the destruction of their tumor, relief from pain, or overall inner peace. In their mind's eye, they visualize an image of what they are striving for and how they might achieve it. They have found that imagination is not only a wellspring of ideas and images but also a powerful tool for promoting emotional, spiritual, and physical well-being.

In *Healing Yourself*, which has helped countless patients to employ this versatile inner resource, Martin Rossman, M.D., described imagery this way:

> An image is an inner representation of your experience or your fantasies—a way your mind codes, stores, and expresses information. Imagery is the currency of dreams and daydreams; memories and reminiscences; plans, projections, and possibilities. It is the language of the arts, the emotions, and most important, the deep inner self.
>
> Imagery is a window on your inner world—a way of viewing your own ideas, feelings, and interpretations. But, it is more than a mere window—it is a means of transformation and liberation from distortions in this realm that may unconsciously direct your life and shape your health.

This chapter discusses the many uses of imagery by cancer patients and offers a firsthand account by a psychotherapist who used imagery in coping with her own cancer.

The Simonton Approach to Fighting Cancer

In 1978, O. Carl Simonton, M.D., and Stephanie Matthews Simonton presented a method of using imagery to combat cancer in *Getting Well Again*. Their approach was to visualize the process of medical treatments and the immune system successfully destroying cancer cells. After guiding patients into a state of deep relaxation, they offer the following instructions:

Mentally picture the cancer in either realistic or symbolic terms. Think of the cancer as consisting of very weak, confused cells. Remember that our bodies destroy cancerous cells thousands of times during a normal lifetime. As you picture your cancer, realize that your recovery requires that your body's own defenses return to a natural, healthy state.

If you are now receiving treatment, picture your treatment coming into your body in a way that you understand. If you are receiving radiation therapy, picture it as a beam of millions of bullets of energy hitting any cell in its path. The normal cells are able to repair the damage that is done, but the cancer cells cannot because they are weak. (This is one of the basic facts upon which radiation therapy is built.) If you are receiving chemotherapy, picture that drug acting like a poison. The normal cells are intelligent and strong and don't take up the poison so readily. But the cancer cell is a weak cell so it takes very little time to kill it. It absorbs the poison, dies, and is flushed out of your body.

Picture your body's own white cells coming into the area where the cancer is, recognizing the abnormal cells, and destroying them. There is a vast army of white blood cells. They are very strong and aggressive. They are also very smart. There is no contest between them and the cancer cells; they will win the battle.

Picture the cancer shrinking. See the dead cells being carried away by the white blood cells and being flushed from your body through the liver and kidneys and being eliminated in the urine and stool. Continue to see the cancer shrinking, until it is all gone.

According to the Simontons, a key aspect of successful visualization is the *type* of imagery used, not just the process of using it. They believe the cancer cells should be visualized as weak, confused, and extremely vulnerable; the medical treatments and immune response should be visualized as powerful, aggressive, and invincible. This makes good intuitive sense in that the response of immune cells against the cancer can certainly be characterized as an attack. Images of combat and victory can also help a patient feel less vulnerable and helpless against the cancer.

However, some clinicians in this field argue that aggressive imagery is not the best for everyone. Depending on a person's temperament, a more gentle imagery may feel more comfortable and appropriate— for example, the imagery of the cancer melting away or being quietly put to sleep. Some patients feel more protected and healed by soothing images or memories of being held or rocked than they do by images of a relentless military-like attack.

The Simontons' work also raises the question of whether imagery that is anatomical in nature is any more or less powerful than symbolic representations. (They acknowledge that the answer to this question is unknown.) Is it better to picture in your mind what the cancer and immune cells actually look like (photographs of a cancer cell surrounded by immune cells can be found in medical books), or is it better to imagine a shark devouring terrified little sand crabs as a symbol of this process? Again, it is important for each person to find the imagery that works them.

In their book, the Simontons touched on an important issue that has been further developed by other clinicians who use imagery in working with cancer patients. We can learn from the images that come to us. Just as we can interpret the meaning behind images in our dreams, we can also find meaning in the images that present themselves when we visualize cancer and the healing process. As Dr. Rossman noted, often the images that arise spontaneously come from our unconscious. If we picture the cancer as dark and foreboding, it suggests the ominous nature of cancer that we hold in our minds. If we imagine chemotherapy as a corrosive acid, it could indicate our fear of the treatment rather than our perception of its healing power. Picturing cancer cells as cockroaches and the treatment as total house fumigation may betray the person's pessimism about ever completely eradicating the cancer. The image of cancer being stoned to death by an angry mob of immune cells—which implies that the cancer is being punished—may be a reaction to a person's feeling punished or victimized by cancer.

When the images that spontaneously come to us have negative connotations—about ourselves, the future, the nature of cancer, the effects of treatment, and so forth—the opportunity arises to grapple with these underlying assumptions and to develop imagery that is more positive and optimistic.

You can choose to do this on your own or to be guided in your imagery by a therapist or guided-imagery tapes. For more information about negative versus positive imagery, consult *Imagery in Healing*, by Jeanne Achterberg and Frank Lawlis.

Does Visualization Work, and If So, How?

Whether or not visualization can impede or reverse the course of cancer has not been proven definitively one way or the other. The scientific evidence on this issue is reviewed in Chapter 12, "Alternative and Complementary Therapies"; the conclusion there was that a patient's active participation in combating cancer—and the feelings of hope, optimism, and a strong will to live that underlie this effort—appear to make a positive difference to the medical outcome in some cases. Many studies have documented this effect. However, there are also many studies that have failed to find evidence of this effect. However, the evidence to date makes a solid case that visualization could have beneficial medical effects and should at least be tried.

There is no controversy, however, about whether visualization is emotionally and psychologically beneficial. The scientific studies on this issue have consistently documented a positive effect on a patient's emotional state and psychological adjustment. The main reason is that visualization offers an active and potentially effective means for self-help in the healing process and thereby diminishes the feelings of vulnerability, helplessness, and lack of control that so often accompany the experience of cancer.

How visualization works in assisting recovery from cancer is one of the many mysteries having to do with mind-body communication. Some people can lower their heart rate by imagining themselves in a peaceful, natural setting. Others have lowered their body temperature by imagining that they are in a tub of ice water. Under hypnosis, people have caused warts to go away by directing and imagining their dissolution. Countless studies on the placebo effect have demonstrated the physical changes caused by a person's *belief* in the healing effects of what they *thought* was a real medicine. In classical conditioning studies, a stimulus (such as sugar water) is given along with an immuno-suppressive drug; later, the stimulus alone leads to a decrease in certain immune measures. People afflicted with multiple personalities sometimes exhibit certain physical conditions in one personality state that are not present in another state. There have been cases where cancer has regressed spontaneously, sometimes in association with a strong emotional catharsis. We do not know the mind-body mechanisms by which these wonders occur.

It is also unknown why these mechanisms sometimes appear to result in marvelous outcomes while in other cases they seem to have no effect. Often, for example, a person's belief in a placebo counts for nothing; only the real medicine works independent of expectation. Some highly suggestible subjects, under hypnosis, will develop a blister when they are told (and imagine) that the ice cube they are touching is really a hot coal; others will just feel the ice.

Although we do not understand the why and how of the mechanisms involved, the powerful effect of mental images on bodily processes has become an added source of hope for cancer patients and provides an additional means for their active participation in the recovery effort. To many, it makes good sense that mentally participating in the healing processes at work within their bodies (such as the immune response to a tumor, or the poisoning of cancer cells by chemotherapy) will assist these processes. This is the major application to cancer treatment that has grown out of the mind-body interactions that have been documented in recent years.

The improved emotional state of patients who practice visualization also may help explain why these patients sometimes enjoy better-than-expected medical outcomes. Research in the growing field of psycho-neuroimmunology has consistently demonstrated the connections between emotions and the immune response.

Applications of Imagery

Cancer patients have used their own visualization and the guided imagery offered by others in a variety of ways and for a variety of purposes. Here are some of the many ways in which imagery may help you in your own struggle with cancer:

- **To Maintain Hope.** Several times a day, imagine yourself completely healthy, and hold this image in your mind. Let this be the image that inspires and sustains you. In their tapes and their book, the Simontons advise: "Imagine yourself well, free of disease, full of energy. Picture yourself reaching your goals in life. See your purpose in life being fulfilled [and]…your relationships with people becoming more meaningful. Remember that having strong reasons for getting well will help you get well, so use this time to focus clearly on your priorities in life."

- **To Promote an Effective Immune Response.** Try to find images that feel right for you, whether they are biological pictures in your mind or powerful symbols of the body's defense processes at work. Add to those images scenes of your body's own defenses working to destroy the cancer. In this way, you may be able to assist this process by mentally participating in and supporting it through imagery.

- **To Prepare For and Heal From Surgery.** Surgery for cancer can create intense anxiety because of the vulnerability involved and the uncertainty about the outcome. Before surgery, you might imagine the operation and the active presence of your will or soul in preventing the cancer cells from evading the scalpel. You might imagine yourself at peace in the caring and competent hands of your surgeon. To promote your healing from surgery, you can visualize the opening of blood vessels and the increased flow of blood (and infection-fighting white blood cells) to the surgical site.

- **To Participate Mentally in Chemotherapy.** It is not uncommon for patients to dread chemotherapy and to feel that something awful is being done to them. Through imagery, you can embrace the process and participate in it. Try to welcome these medicines into your body and visualize how they expel the cancer and restore you to health. You can use the images suggested by the Simontons or develop your own. Invite your imagination to help you: it is often best to let the images come to you, as a gift from an inner source of wisdom, rather than to force an image that you intellectually think is right.

- **To Reduce Side Effects.** The nausea and vomiting caused by chemotherapy are partly due to the anticipation and dread of these side effects. Patients have successfully reduced these effects by visualizing, during chemotherapy, that the healthy cells in their gastrointestinal tract are being protected from the drugs or bouncing back rapidly from the toxic effects. Sometimes, the smell of the rubbing alcohol used to cleanse the skin before infusion causes nausea; patients who attach a more positive image to this smell have been able to offset this effect. Positive imagery can reduce the nausea and stress that often comes in anticipation of receiving chemotherapy by substituting it with happier images.

- **To Cope with Pain.** You can use imagery to reduce pain by distracting yourself from it and by altering the meaning behind the pain. Pain often creates anxiety, which can make the pain worse. Try to find an image for your pain that has a blunting effect on it, or an image that soothes and heals the source of the pain. To quote the Simontons again: "If you are experiencing pain anywhere in your body, picture the army of white blood cells flowing into that area and soothing the pain. Whatever the problem, give your body the command to heal itself. Visualize your body becoming well."

- **To Offset Stress and Anxiety.** Learn to take a deep breath, close your eyes, and imagine yourself in a special place that makes you feel peaceful and strong. Symptoms of anxiety can be banished when your mind substitutes a tranquil image for a stressful one. You can even infuse yourself with energy to banish the weariness of fear and foreboding. Dr. Rossman's book contains a lovely exercise that escorts you to a serene imaginary location of your own creation.

A Firsthand Account

Janet Amber Damon, M.S.W.

My cancer diagnosis came totally out of the blue. I was forty-eight years old, had been working as a psychotherapist for more than fifteen years, and was about to leave for Paris to study art. Two weeks before leaving, I had my annual gynecological exam. I learned I had ovarian cancer, Stage Four. It already had metastasized to other organs.

Before this moment, I had always been a fighter. I always found a way to cope with the tragedies, stresses, and struggles of life. Now—unexpectedly—attack came from within my own body. I had no knowledge of cancer or what I was facing. It all felt overwhelming!

I had a hysterectomy and four tumors removed, and then began chemotherapy. I was a basket case. I withdrew; I isolated myself; I was immobilized, fragile; I had no energy for anything. I was undone. I had used up my bag of hope; the blackboard was erased and I had run out of chalk.

My journey through cancer then turned toward greater hope and strength. I met a doctor, Bernard Towers, who was doing research on the body-mind connection. I began weekly visits to learn visualization techniques. It was a process that helped me connect with my internal world. My strength began to return despite the massive doses of chemotherapy.

I experienced the healthful effects of the visualization on my healing and recovery. Later, from reading and hearing about others who had similar experiences, and through teaching visualization to other patients and seeing their benefits, I am convinced that it is a valid, effective path for releasing tensions and stresses and for increasing the body's ability to fight disease.

For me, visualization became a means of focusing my mind in order to release the healing forces of my body and to encourage the healthy parts of my body to maintain and protect themselves while chemotherapy worked at killing the cancer. It also was a way to take control. I felt empowered. At the very least, it improved the quality of my life. I also believe that visualization can release enough of the healing forces in the body to effect a cure.

When I first learned of visualization techniques, I was surprised to realize that I had been visualizing all the time. It's something we all do without being aware of it. We think in images, but we usually don't focus and concentrate on these images or change them in order to reach certain goals.

Something that I learned from the research on imagery was the idea that images in the mind are perceived as real events to the body. For example, athletes who practice their toning and muscle-strengthening exercises in their imagination often receive similar benefits to those received by athletes who physically do the exercises.

In a state of deep relaxation, with images coursing through the mind, the body moves into a state of heightened alertness and heightened ability to achieve whatever it is you are attempting to achieve. There are phrases that describe this phenomenon: athletes refer to it as being "in the zone," and religious people refer to it as ecstasy.

How I Got Started

I was introduced to visualization by listening to guided-imagery cassette tapes. I found this to be a simple and effective way of getting started. These tapes are available in bookstores, some health food stores, and catalogs.

I also used guided-imagery scripts from books such as those suggested by the Simontons and Martin Rossman. I later developed my own visualization script, which I offer for your consideration. I created my own tape of this script to help me through the process.

I also took advantage of biofeedback in order to reduce stress and obtain inner calm. I found that biofeedback can be easily learned from written or spoken instructions. The process employs an

(Continued from page 176)

electronic device to measure your body's reaction to stress. There are small, inexpensive models available. A light or a tone emanates from these devices, and the intensity of the signal reflects many of the body's reactions to stress, such as increased brain wave activity and skin temperature. I found it invaluable to learn from the device I used when a state of total relaxation was attained, how to create that state mentally, and what factors would raise or lower the relaxation response in my body.

I also sought professional help from a therapist who helped people learn visualization techniques. For a referral to someone in your community who specializes in this work, call your local American Cancer Society office. I found it essential to work with a therapist who helped me develop the type of imagery that was right for me—one that fit my temperament and interests.

You might want to keep this in mind in creating your own imagery. Think of your hobbies and of activities that interest you and that you know something about; try to develop a visualization exercise that builds on these. For example, if you are a gardener, you might want to visualize weeds growing, the bugs and poisons that destroy them, and the fertilizers and sunlight enriching healthy plant life.

A Sample Visualization

This is a visualization exercise that I developed and found to be a powerful tool in dealing with my cancer. I recorded it onto a tape and listened to it every day. You could also have someone quietly read the steps to you. It is good to follow the steps carefully the first couple of times.

Before you start, think of something that you consider a healing liquid. This could be a particular medicine, a tonic your parent used to fix you when you were sick, the honey from flowers, a magician's potion, a particular hue of spray paint that stops rust, or whatever has a certain poignancy for you.

1. Find a comfortable, quiet, darkened place to sit or lie down and relax completely. If this is difficult, get earplugs and a dark material to put over your eyes. Do whatever is necessary to get about twenty minutes of uninterrupted time. Turn off the phone, and put a sign on the front door. Ask your family to help.

2. Breathe gently and slowly five times, drawing your breath down into your lungs and stomach, feeling your ribs moving and expanding with each breath, and then fully exhale your breath.

3. Keep breathing gently and regularly. Focus all your attention and imagine that you are bringing that warm breath into any place of tightness or tension in your body.

4. Release the tension with each exhalation as though the warm air was gradually being released from a balloon. Let it drain away.

5. Imagine the healing liquid in a container. This is your healing force.

6. Imagine the container is at the location where cancer cells exist.

7. Pour or spray the liquid over the cancer so it covers or coats it.

8. Picture the cells beginning to melt away as the healing force coats and covers them.

9. Allow that coating to remain in place as you slowly open your eyes and become aware once again of the room around you.

10. During the coming hours, take a moment to close your eyes and imagine the coating on the cells as you left it. The cells are being smothered and are dying.

11. Repeat the visualization at least three times a day. Return to the site of the cancer, using the same method, and add more of the healing force to the now dissipating and dissolving cancer cells.

12. Do this visualization at bedtime, but when you are done do not open your eyes. Let yourself drift off to sleep with the image of the dying cancer cells in your mind.

I believe not only that visualization helped me to recover from my cancer, but that it also provided a direct means of encouraging the healthy parts of my body to maintain and protect themselves while

(Continued from page 177)

drugs and radiation did their job. Our medical doctors work at destroying the cancer, and each day they are discovering better techniques and drugs to carry out their work. We have tools to help them. Visualization gave me a way of participating in what my doctors were doing, a way of using the power of imagery to fight cancer. Although I placed myself in the hands of the medical team, I also found a way of doing my part to see to it that the best results were achieved.

Our body wants to be well. There is great wisdom in the way the systems of the body work each day for our benefit. Our job is to encourage and help those systems to become strong. If you take charge of your body and become part of the team of medical people who are working to return you to health, then I believe your chances for survival are heightened. In my case, there is no doubt in my mind that the combination of the medical care I received and the visualization skills I learned (and have continued to practice for ten years) are the two major reasons for my regaining and maintaining my health.

21

The Art of Forgiveness

Frederic Luskin, Ph.D.

One of the most challenging tasks we face in life is how to remain peaceful when something frustrates us. Not getting what we want is one of the main challenges to dealing with illness, abandonment, dishonesty, or any other difficulties that humans experience. Most of us never fully accept that life often does not give us what we want. We often react with outrage or offense when a normal, but difficult, life experience emerges. Most of us will make the situation worse by insisting and complaining that the specific difficulty is wrong instead of focusing our energy on how to best deal with the situation.

We have the choice to either forgive the parts of life we do not like or to continue suffering by insisting that life be run on our terms. Many of us have trouble with forgiveness because there are so many different views about it. To some it means that their religion compels them to get over something that hurts them. To others it means that they have to become friends again with people who mistreated them. Finally, some people think that forgiveness is the same as saying what happened was okay.

Actually, no one has to forgive—forgiveness is a *choice*. Forgiveness means that we release our suffering over difficult situations; it does not mean we have to put ourselves back into hurtful situations. Forgiveness means that even though what happened is not OK, you can move on and make peace for yourself.

There are three different kinds of offenses that can be forgiven. It is common for people to think that different processes of both creating a grievance and learning to forgive are involved. However, in each situation the problem is essentially the same: something we really wanted to happen in a certain way did not.

The first kind is the most common: where another person has committed the offense against you. This kind of forgiveness is called interpersonal forgiveness. The second kind of forgiveness, where you are upset with something that you did, is called intrapersonal forgiveness. In this case, you are forgiving yourself. The third kind of forgiveness is existential, where you forgive God or nature for what they have done to you. Existential forgiveness often is a critical component of either interpersonal or intrapersonal forgiveness and is seen when we ask the question "How could this happen?"

It is my belief that making the choice to forgive can be a liberating practice. Forgiveness is only possible because we have the ability to make choices. We have the choice to forgive or not to forgive and no one can force us to do either. Forgiveness is choosing to take the offense less personally, blaming the offending situation less for how we feel, and changing how we describe the situation to reflect our choice to forgive.

In this model, the development of forgiveness moves along four steps or stages.

Four Stages of Forgiveness

Step One
You are filled with self-justified anger. At some point in your life, you have been wounded and you are mad or hurt by an experience you feel wronged you. You blame the person who committed the wrong for how you are feeling. It is their action and not your choice of response that you believe to be the cause of your distress. You have forgotten that you have choices about how you can react. Perhaps you are so wounded that you are convinced it would not be right to forgive the offense. At this stage, there usually is both active and submerged anger, as well as a great deal of pain.

Step Two
After feeling upset with something for a while, you realize that your hurt and anger do not feel good. It may be affecting your emotional balance or physical health. You may wish to repair the damage to the relationship and take steps toward forgiveness. You may begin to gain perspective on how common the problem is or you may simply decide to let go of your pain. In either case, after an extended period of time, you are no longer aggrieved and have forgiven the situation/person causing you distress. This process of forgiveness can be applied to anger at oneself, at another person, or at life in general.

Step Three
The third stage of forgiveness comes after you have seen the results of forgiveness in action and choose to let go of a new grievance fairly quickly. In this stage, you choose to feel the hurt for a shorter period of time and then work to either repair the relationship or let go of seeing the situation as a problem. In either case, you

decide to forgive because you have had more practice with it and see the clear benefit in your life. This could happen when something simple occurs, such as being cut off by another car on the expressway or in a complex situation like an affair in a marriage. At this stage of forgiveness, you are aware that the length of time you experience a situation as a grievance is primarily up to you.

Step Four
The fourth stage of forgiveness involves the choice to rarely take offense in the first place. This means you are prepared to forgive in advance of a specific trigger. This stage often emerges simultaneously with all or some of the following thoughts:

- I don't want to waste my precious life in the discomfort caused by anger or hurt, so I will decide to feel differently. I am able to forgive myself, forgive others, forgive life, and forgive God.
- I know how it hurts when people don't forgive me. I do not want to hurt other people by my actions, so I will perceive the problem in such a way that I can either deal with it or let it go.
- Life is filled with incredible beauty and wonder and I am missing these experiences if I am stuck in the remembrance of old hurts or disappointments. I forgive myself for getting sidetracked.
- Everyone, including myself, operates primarily out of self-interest. I must expect that sometimes I, in my self-interest, will be annoyed by someone else's expression of self-interest. If I can understand that this is an ordinary part of life, what is there to be upset about?

Often, people with cancer have grievances or hurts that fall into each of the three kinds of forgivable offenses. Generally speaking, the way one forgives a specific grievance is the same, no matter whether the grievance is with yourself, another person, or God.

Nine Steps toward Forgiveness

1. Know exactly how you feel about what happened and be able to articulate precisely what is not acceptable to you. Then tell a couple of trusted people about the hurtful situation and how you feel about it. After taking these preliminary steps, you are ready to start working toward forgiveness.

2. Make a commitment to yourself to do what you must do in order to feel better. You need not

continue to suffer because of some difficult situation. Remind yourself that you deserve to feel better and at peace. Forgiveness is for you and not for anyone else. No one even needs to know about your decision.

3. Understand your goal. Forgiveness is not simply reconciliation with the experience that upset you, though you may achieve that. What you are seeking is to feel better. Forgiveness can be defined as the "peace and understanding that comes from lessening the blame of that which has hurt you, taking your life experience less personally, and seeing the cost of holding a grudge." Your forgiveness goal is to find peace in your life now.

4. Get the right perspective on what's going on. Recognize that your primary distress is coming from your hurt feelings now, not what happened in the past.

5. When feeling upset, practice a simple stress management technique to counter your body's fight-or-flight response. When you remember an unresolved problem, your heart speeds up, your blood pressure rises, your hands get cold, and you can't think straight. To counter these symptoms and regain calm, at the very moment you start to get upset or recall what happened, bring your attention fully to your stomach as you breathe in and out for two slow and deep breaths. Then picture something in your life that is beautiful or reminds you of something you love. Hold the feelings that emerge from this visualization in the area around your heart and relax. This simple two-step technique cuts your experience of distress and lets you think more clearly about how to deal with the problem that you are struggling to forgive. Practice doing this whenever you feel upset.

6. Give up expectations of other people or your life that they do not choose to give you. Recognize the "unenforceable rules" that you have established for your health or how you or other people must behave. For example, if you have been seeking emotional support from someone who does not provide it, ask yourself, "How many times will I hit my head against the wall of that person's coldness hoping that that person will be different?" The forgiving response is to stop making demands of whatever it is that has hurt you. Remind yourself that you can actively strive for health, love, friendship, and prosperity and work hard to get them. However, you will suffer needlessly if you demand that these things occur when you do not have the power to make them happen.

7. Put your energy into looking for another way to fulfill your goals rather than investing in an experience that has hurt you. If you've been waiting for a loving relationship with an indifferent parent, for instance, look for a mentor who can provide the love, guidance, and approval that you crave. I call this step finding your positive intention. Instead of mentally replaying your hurt and distress, seek out new ways to have your needs met as you move on from a situation that is unsatisfying.

8. Remember that a life well lived is your best revenge. A person who lives such a life often finds things to appreciate in each moment. Instead of focusing on your wounded feelings, and thereby giving the person who has wounded you power over you, look for the beauty and kindness around you. Spend time appreciating the good things in your life and remind yourself of pleasant and loving experiences. One important tool in this process is to list the things for which you are grateful. The moment you shift your thoughts in this fashion, the less you will feel hurt by life's unfairness. You will start to see that the sun still shines, people still fall in love, and beauty still exists everywhere.

9. Amend the grievance story you are telling and focus on your choice to forgive. By doing so, you reclaim the power you gave to this offending situation to hurt you. When you are able to change the story you tell yourself and others, then you will not give the difficulty so much space in your mind and peace will be the result. That feeling of peace is the experience of forgiveness.

22

Mindfulness-Based Stress Reduction

Mark Abramson, D.D.S.

Stress is a major factor in life-threatening illness. With a diagnosis of cancer, there is an immediate change in your life that profoundly affects your ability to cope. There is enormous fear and anxiety related to the challenges of the ensuing treatment—the fear of the unknown.

Mindfulness-Based Stress Reduction is a meditation technique based on a stress reduction program created by Jon Kabat-Zinn twenty years ago at the University of Massachusetts. He started teaching patients mindfulness meditation, which comes from Buddhist meditation practice, as an adjunct to traditional medical treatment.

The working definition for mindfulness is nonjudgmental awareness. It is being present in this moment and being "open" to this moment as it presents itself. The word "open" for me is a key word. Once when I was waiting to teach a class at Stanford, I picked up David Lerhner's book on choices in breast cancer and read the chapter on what he terms "healing." He uses the word "openness"—openness of mind, openness of spirit, openness to life. Openness is a necessary component to healing.

When I first started learning meditation, one of my teachers was Steven Levine, who works with conscious living and conscious dying. I remember one time when we were in a group with a young woman aged thirty-five who had brain cancer. She had just a couple weeks of life left. She had done so much healing work with her life that her relationships were clear and whole. All there was left was a state of love. She literally radiated it! I was jealous because I saw so many places where I was stuck. I was not free as she was. It really helped me to look at the values that I wanted to cultivate more deeply in my life. She was a shining example of a healed human being.

I haven't had the diagnosis of cancer and the stress that it brings. I did have an experience in my life that was a great challenge, one that was educating and has motivated me more than anything else. When I was fourteen years old, I was walking on the sidewalk on my way home. My mother had asked me to buy a loaf of bread on the way home. It was raining and I should have taken the bus. She would have understood why I had not bought the bread and walked home, but I wanted to buy her the bread so I stopped, bought it, and went on my way.

As I was walking along, I heard a loud crash and I went flying through the air. I was hit by a car that had come up on the sidewalk, struck me, and crashed into two houses.

Immediately my life had changed. Somehow, I had this inspiration about the relationship between my experience of trauma/pain and the medical treatment. I had a sense that I should pay careful attention to the experience. I observed my physical sensations, my emotions, and my reactions to these experiences. I did not know it then, but it started my practice of mindfulness meditation. The experience was actually a blessing because I developed a commitment to trust the course of my life and made a commitment to actually try to feel and deeply experience my physical and emotional sensations. When I first started to read about meditation, I realized that I already was practicing mindfulness. I had a wealth of direct experience in the benefits of living in the present moment with openness to the sensations of the body and mind. The pain was more tolerable and the emotions were less discomforting.

The practice of mindfulness is like reading a book. You're going along and really into the story and, all of a sudden, your mind goes off somewhere. Your eyes keep moving along totally unaware that the mind is disconnected from the experience of seeing. They're going through paragraph after paragraph and at some point you "wake up" and realize that there was no connection to the words. There was no meaning. Your eyes somehow are still reading and seeing, but there has been no connection with that.

Mindfulness is like reading the book and staying connected to the words and their meaning. Mindfulness can be practiced at the beach by staying with the experience of the beach, just the waves and the experience of the colors and the sounds. It could be a time when you were really connected to somebody, a grandchild perhaps, and you were really present. In some ways, unfortunately, that's the exception because the tendency of the mind is to be in the imaginary future or a rehashing of the past. It's exceptional when we're really in the present moment.

How do we have the courage to really be present when we are faced with cancer? It's terrifying. Cancer evokes unfamiliar and uneasy emotions. How do you stay open? How do you stay connected? That's really what meditation is.

I'm going to tell you what it is not. A lot of people report to me that they tried meditation and couldn't do it because they couldn't control their thoughts. They had a belief that if they were correctly practicing meditation, all thoughts would stop and they would experience eternal bliss. In every class I hear the same thing, "I tried to meditate, but I couldn't because my mind wouldn't stop. I couldn't get to that state other people can." That interference discourages many people from getting the benefits of meditation practice. Meditation is simply being present to life as it is right now. Whatever you're feeling right now in your body—your mind states, your emotions, and physical sensations in your body—that's where you pay attention.

That's the wonderful thing about mindfulness. You don't have to be in any certain way. You don't have to handle your emotions at all. The goal is not eliminating stress in your life—it's having a relationship with yourself that's whole and open in the middle of stress. Something may come up, and you might have a reaction that causes you to experience certain feelings and physical sensations. Your muscles may contract. That is the physiological response. You have emotional and mental responses as well. Mindfulness is paying attention to all of this, becoming the observer as it is happening.

As you bring yourself to your life experience, you begin to cultivate a direct relationship with your life. You begin to realize that you have the ability to choose how you respond to life. You can be nurturing to yourself when these difficult times arise. Healing is about the ability to be kind and loving to yourself in the middle of whatever is arising.

Many times, life takes us to the edge before we're really willing to look deep into our lives, values, and what's really important to us. The times that I've been at the edge, where a major crisis has occurred, are also the occasions that I've learned the most. I had to pay close attention to myself and my life and make clear choices. Meditation helps me to pay better attention.

Mindfulness helps deal with stress by focusing on the finite experience of what is actually present at this moment in time. We can begin to observe the continually changing sensations of our experience. We can choose how we "respond' to ourselves and to our environment appropriately for a more beneficial outcome. We usually have an unconscious, habitual way of "reacting" to the infinite possibilities of past and future. Long-term habits can be very destructive both physically and emotionally.

Beginning the Practice of Mindfulness Meditation

Mindfulness meditation uses the observation of breathing as a focus of awareness to anchor our attention to the present moment. Breathing is a constant companion, always available as part of our experience.

Begin by setting aside twenty to forty-five minutes to sit in a comfortable chair or on a cushion on the floor. Bring your attention to your breathing. Notice the awareness of your body as you draw in air. As you begin to breath out, be aware of the body releasing the air. Be aware of the body's natural rhythmic pattern of breathing; do not try to control or force the flow of air, just be mindful of it as an experience. You can use what is referred to as "noting": as you breathe in quietly, repeat inwardly in your mind "breathing in"; as you experience the awareness of exhaling breath, say to yourself "breathing out." Noting is a useful tool to focus your attention.

Continue to note your breathing as it flows in and out. The natural habit of the mind is to drift away into thoughts, bringing up memories of the past or imaginations of the future. When this happens, simply bring your attention back to your breathing. Be careful not to be harsh or unkind to yourself if you should drift away, choose to be kind and gentle with the habits of the mind. Each time one drifts away and returns can be seen as an opportunity to practice self-kindness.

Meditation is like sitting by a stream and watching the water flow by. We stay concentrated on the water. We may notice leaves and twigs in the water and bugs flying around but we choose to stay focused on the water itself.

With practice and formal meditation sessions, the focus of conscious breathing will spread gradually to other areas in our lives. We begin to take showers, eat, walk, read, write, and talk with more awareness. Our breathing is an anchor to being in the present moment, to feeling fully alive.

23

The Waiting Process
Hurry Up and Wait!

Ernest H. Rosenbaum, M.D.
Isadora H. Rosenbaum, M.A.
Susan Diamond, L.C.S.W.
David Spiegel, M.D.
Andrew W. Kneier, Ph.D.

The doomsday scenarios you conjure up during stressful waiting periods are usually far worse than reality.

Waiting for appointments and test results can turn living with cancer into a full-time occupation and preoccupation. You count the weeks and days until your next appointment and make note of every ache and pain, thinking it might be a signal that your disease is worsening. On the day of your appointment, you are so anxious that you arrive early at your physician's office, only to discover that he is behind schedule, increasing your waiting time as well as your apprehension. During your visit, your physician orders the required tests and tells you to go home and wait for a phone call—or suggests that you call back in a few days or a week to get your test results.

You are always waiting for something: the initial diagnosis following surgery; a biopsy, mammogram, or fine needle aspiration; the results of treatment; and when in remission, your next checkup. The most difficult aspect of waiting is the open-ended uncertainty of not knowing what is happening inside your body. Conversely, "knowing" can be a relief—even when the news is not good—because you and your physician then can take action and discuss therapeutic alternatives.

You should also be aware that the time you spend waiting for appointments and for information on your medical status is often determined by circumstances beyond your control or that of your physician. For example, because of economic pressures, most physicians see more people per hour today than they saw in the past, resulting in shorter office visits. This can make you feel that you have received insufficient consideration of your psychosocial needs. Physicians' increasingly heavy workloads also lead to longer waiting periods for an appointment, whether for an initial consultation or for subsequent therapy.

The operating procedures of insurance companies and Health Maintenance Organizations (HMOs) can also lead to delays that, in turn, increase your apprehension. These organizations generally require that physicians obtain an authorization from them before ordering certain types of tests, therapies, and surgical procedures. You or your primary physician must also request permission from the insurance company or HMO to consult with a specialist and you must, of course, choose one who belongs to your plan. If you choose a specialist who is not on your plan, you may find

Reprinted by permission from *Coping* magazine.

that the plan will not pay (or will pay less) for the services. Any or all of these negotiations can mean added hours or days of fretfulness for you.

In short, facing delays is a part of the treatment of cancer, but with a little mutual understanding and effort, you and your physician can attempt to lessen those that are occasioned by heavy patient loads, complex diagnostic tests, and insurance company and HMO requirements. Hopefully, in the last instance, future legislative action will streamline some of the medical management procedures that currently prolong certain waiting periods and exacerbate what is already a highly stressful time in anyone's life

---

Reducing Stress in the Stressed-Out World of Cancer

Susan Diamond, L.C.S.W.
Ernest Rosenbaum, M.D.
David Spiegel, M.D.

Coping with cancer entails navigating effectively between being so overwhelmed by threat that you feel helpless and denial that the threat exists. Getting that balance is a constantly shifting and demanding process. It involves accepting temporary crisis situations and utilizing the disruption to formulate new plans of action.

The pattern of response you establish during an acute crisis is likely to become cemented in place, regardless of its relative effectiveness. *Effective* coping involves taking in and processing the emotional reaction to the danger and seeking the opportunity for a response that at least mitigates the danger.

Acknowledge the problem. It is better to face head-on whatever is threatening you than to try to deny or avoid it.

Be specific. See the problem as being on a continuum, more or less difficult, rather than as an all-or-nothing catastrophe.

Seek information. The more you know about a problem, the more likely you are to figure out a better way of dealing with it.

Feel what you feel. Difficult situations bring strong emotions with them. Let them come and learn from them. Emotions can point out to us what is important, and, when shared appropriately, can build intimacy and support.

Seek social support. Don't do it alone. Family and friends often feel more helpless than you do. They welcome any opportunity to help. Give them many.

Find an Active Response

You will feel better about any problem when you can find a way to be active about it. Even if you can't solve the problem or make it go away, you will feel better if you can do something about some aspect of it.

False Positives

Don't force yourself to be more upbeat than you feel. Indeed, defining what constitutes a truly positive attitude is a complex problem. Being too positive all the time can verge on denial. This can inhibit obtaining necessary medical information and treatment. It also can lead family and friends to actively discourage the expression of appropriate sadness and fear.

One of our patients related to her support group that when she started to cry in front of her husband about the progression of her inflammatory breast cancer, he said: "Don't cry, you'll make the cancer spread." Another member of the support group referred to this as the *prison of positive thinking.* We see many people with cancer whose family members are afraid that giving vent to these negative feelings will somehow unleash the cancer itself, as though the feeling uncontrolled is the same as the disease uncontrolled. Many people are desperate to do anything they can to control the illness, and are willing to exist in an emotional straightjacket if it will somehow improve their odds of survival. Yet another downside of the positive attitude often recommended to someone with

(Continued from page 186)

cancer is that progress of the cancer provides fertile ground for inappropriate guilt : "If I can control the spread of disease through my attitude, and the disease has progressed, then there must be something wrong with my attitude." There is simply no medical evidence that a positive attitude *per se* has any effect on the course of cancer.

Group Support

Harboring fears and anxiety about cancer can be absolutely paralytic. The opportunity to share thoughts and concerns and express even the most frightening feelings, such as "I'm terrified I'm going to die," offers enormous comfort, allows you to realize you are reacting normally to an abnormal situation, and helps you regain your emotional balance while significantly reducing your stress (Spiegel, 1993).

Sharing experiences with other people who have cancer is a potent experience. Many people find that being a member of a cancer support group offers multiple benefits. The very thing that has made you feel separated from the rest of the world is your admission ticket into the group. Thoughts and feelings that previously seemed bizarre are normalized. It is the rule rather than the exception to feel terrified, enraged, grief-stricken, immobilized, and wondering if you're going to die. You can experience tremendous relief in finding out that you are not alone and that others sharing your dilemma accept you and understand.

Just as the group helps you integrate a new sense of self, it simultaneously helps you define and revise what is important to you. The issue of how to make the best use of time becomes paramount in the face of an uncertain future. This usually involves seizing the moment and taking full advantage of the present instead of becoming exclusively focused on the future. You may begin rearranging your priorities as you develop new interests, or expand on or drop old ones. Cultivating experiences that are enriching and pleasurable should become a key goal; eliminating those that no longer interest you is another.

For example, a woman with progressive, metastatic breast cancer decided to undergo a bone-marrow transplant as a "last ditch" treatment. Not knowing what the outcome of this procedure would be, she determined that there were certain things she wanted to accomplish in the event she died. She and her partner took a long-delayed vacation to Hawaii where they agreed to make a more formal commitment to their relationship prior to her hospitalization.

Another woman, a prolific poet with incurable brain cancer, was encouraged by her partner to take up painting. She did and, to her delight, found herself immersed with an almost child-like fascination in a new world of shapes and colors (some of her paintings were exhibited at the hospital where she was treated). Rather than giving in to her cancer, she viewed it as an opportunity for creative growth and unanticipated pleasure.

Some people with cancer continually reorder their priorities. A lovely woman of forty-one with advanced ovarian cancer chose to forgo a level of pain medication that, essentially, would have left her pain-free but unconscious. She wanted to stay alert, aware, and connected to the people she loved. For her, the importance of this far outweighed being physically comfortable.

Clearly, openness and expressiveness—emotionally and in other areas—is critical to your overall recovery and goes a long way toward helping you manage the inevitable stresses of the disease. Using family and friends as a resource is a crucial part of this process. Early involvement of your family in both decision making and treatment helps you integrate your experiences with cancer into the rest of your life. Family and friends can encourage you to talk about how you feel and about what is happening to you. A simple statement from someone close, such as "I'm scared too, but we'll fight this together" is both encouraging and comforting. The relief in knowing that you can give voice to what is frightening and painful can remind you that you're not fighting this battle alone.

As barriers to communication are overcome, you can benefit from and help your natural support

(*Continued from page 187*)

system while feeling sustained through the cancer experience. In sharing all emotions, both the positive and the negative, you don't hide or deny any aspect of your experience. It also offers those who care about you a way of better understanding your experience, as well as the means to feel closer to one another and to you.

Some people diagnosed with cancer find that they need the privacy of individual counseling or therapy to work through some of their feelings about their cancer. A therapy session with a specially trained and caring professional at the time of diagnosis or recurrence, with the potential for continued visits, provides a safe place for you to discuss your feelings about and experience with the cancer. This can help lessen fear and offers a setting for the diagnosis and treatment of more serious forms of anxiety and depression.

Serious sleep and appetite disturbance or persistent suicidal thoughts call for professional evaluation. Although the thought of living with cancer will never be free of anxiety, you may need help in recognizing that while cancer is now an undeniable part of your life, it is not the only part.

Your renewed ability to see yourself as an active participant in your life will help you maintain your emotional perspective, which will help keep the stresses of living with cancer from constantly intruding into your life.

Reprinted by permission from Coping magazine.

When Your Spouse Has Cancer

Andrew W. Kneier, Ph.D.

What you can and should do when your partner contracts cancer depends on your partner's personal needs. Each situation is different. Your partner may be newly diagnosed, dealing with metastatic cancer, or living in a kind of limbo, not knowing whether the cancer has regressed. Here are some general guidelines that could help you provide the kind of support your partner needs.

Face Cancer Together

Although your spouse has cancer, the illness is really happening to both of you. Your life is being disrupted in many of the same ways. You are sharing many of the same emotions and concerns. You are both challenged to find constructive ways of dealing with the disruptions and threats posed by cancer and with the side effects of medical treatments. It can be tremendously reassuring and comforting to your loved one to know that the two of you are facing the illness together and that your support and involvement will be steadfast and unwavering regardless of what happens.

Here are some of the specific issues that you should try to face together:

- How serious is the cancer?
- What is the best treatment, and what are the pros and cons of different options?
- Are there clinical trials to consider, or perhaps complementary or holistic approaches?
- What roles or division of labor should we take in learning about these matters?
- What should we tell our children, and how can we best help them in dealing with this frightening situation?
- What changes do we need to make in our daily routine to accommodate the need for treatments and to deal with side effects?
- What does our family need in the way of support and practical help from relatives, friends, and our religious community?

- How can we best reach out for the support we need?

Discussion Is Better than Assumption

Do not assume that you know what your spouse is thinking or feeling about the cancer, or that you know what he or she needs from you. You might think your spouse is mostly scared, when actually he or she feels more sad or perhaps guilty about the consequences of the cancer for you. You might think that your spouse is strong and resilient, when actually he or she feels vulnerable and dependent on you, but may not want to let you know that. You might think that your loved one wants you to offer encouragement and hope, when actually he or she just wants you to say "I'm with you in what you are feeling, and we'll face this together no matter what happens."

The point is to talk with your spouse about his or her emotional reactions and concerns and to ask what your spouse needs from you. Some of these needs may be concrete or practical: going together to doctor's appointments, becoming educated about his or her cancer and the treatment options, handling all the phone calls from friends and relatives, and taking over more household chores. Other needs may be more emotional: being attuned and responsive to what your spouse is feeling, encouraging your spouse to confide in you, and offering empathy and support during difficult times.

Support Your Partner's True Feelings

Most cancer patients feel pressure to maintain a positive mental attitude, and too often this pressure prevents them from expressing their true feelings. Your partner might hold back in sharing legitimate fears because he or she does not want to disappoint or burden you, or because he or she thinks that negative emotions might jeopardize healing. Actually, it is the suppression of fears,

(Continued from page 189)

sorrow, or anger that could jeopardize your partner's psychological adjustment and immune response. Your loved one probably has good reasons to be worried and upset, as well to feel hopeful and optimistic. You should try to support and validate both sets of emotions (not only the positive ones).

Confront Sexual Issues

Your spouse's cancer and the treatments have probably affected his or her sexual interest, sexual functioning, or feelings of attractiveness. Some common examples are the loss of libido caused by chemotherapy and hormonal therapy, the impotence caused by prostate cancer treatments, and the body image effects of mastectomy and reconstructive surgery. Even without such specific problems, the depression that cancer can cause can reduce libido and sexual functioning. The bodily or mood changes in your spouse can also cause you to lose interest.

The key to dealing with these issues is open communication. Because your partner might be reluctant to broach these topics, you could take the lead by acknowledging these issues and conveying your desire to face them together. You might also go out of your way to reassure your spouse of your love and devotion and that your feelings are not motivated just by physical attractiveness or sexual performance, that your main priority is his or her survival, and that you continue to desire an intimate physical relationship.

I know of hundreds of couples who have followed these principles. They have told me that the bond between them has actually been deepened and strengthened. "It's ironic," one husband told me, "but somehow having to face death, and having to say good-bye to each other if that happens, has made us hold on tighter and cherish what we have."

Reprinted by permission from *Coping* magazine.

David Spiegel, M.D.
Pat Fobair, L.C.S.W., M.P.H

24

Support Groups
The Benefits of Talking with Others

Rationale

Why join a support group? Do they exemplify the adage that "misery loves company?" Do cancer patients became more miserable by being exposed to the fears of others with the same illness?

Robert Watts, a football player with Hodgkin's lymphoma, explained how joining a group of fellow cancer sufferers helped him. "When I was diagnosed, I was a professional athlete," he recalled. "I was used to putting problems aside. I could not think about injuries when I was playing or I would get injured and instead I would picture myself doing what needed to be done, picture myself winning. That didn't work when I found I had cancer, although I used it as my model for getting through treatment."

"It was after treatment that problems began. I would find myself getting overwhelmingly anxious, feeling tight in the chest. I remember working out in my gym at home and after fifteen seconds of skipping rope my chest tightened up; my muscles were tight from the radiation and I didn't know how to deal with that. I was scared I was going to die. But I wasn't allowed to be scared. It got to where I found myself driving in my car on the Golden Gate Bridge thinking, well if death is going to get me, let's just get it over with. I can't live with this. I needed a checkup from the neck up. I called up my doctor and he said, 'Get down here.' Sometime during treatment, someone needs to lead you by the hand and take you to the group. I felt overwhelmed at the thought that I wasn't the same man I was when started treatment, that I couldn't solve things by just working out more. I couldn't accept being someone who was sick, who faced the risk of dying. Since I have been to the group, I have cried. I feel better because I can accept better who I am now."

For Robert, his physical strength represented his sense of well-being. It took the experience of feeling the emotional pain caused by the disease in his body before he could reach out to others for help.

Methods

Groups provide an opportunity for people to see their own problems as others see them, through the eyes and ears of other group members. This helps them gain a new perspective on their illness and reduces the inappropriate guilt that often besets cancer patients. They learn that many of their problems are due to cancer, rather than personal failings. At other times, group members develop and consolidate their own sense of personal competence in dealing with cancer by helping others who have less experience with it. Groups can also assist in developing a more active coping stance and in finding something to do about even the worst aspects of the illness, such as fears of dying and death. Group discussions of these issues help members to experience shared anxiety and sadness. This can be invaluable to an individual who is about to sink into the despair that loneliness causes. Our recent book, *Group Therapy for Cancer Patients*, provides a detailed description of the methods of leading such groups.

Gaining Perspective

Many patients report a psychic numbing that characterizes their initial response to learning they have cancer. Before patients can speak fully about their grief, they need to talk together, a process characterized by Freud as "remembering, repeating, and working through." Something therapeutic occurs when you hear your own voice while talking with others about your problems. The experience of a life threat and the need to grieve the loss of one's health is better handled when shared with others in the same predicament. For example, perhaps you've always believed that life should be fair, or that "bad things do not happen to good people." The discrepancy between this view and your present life situation conjures up many feelings, many of them negative.

When you ask yourself the question, "Why has this happened?" you're really asking, "How could this have happened to me?" There is a human need to find a positive purpose for a negative event. Examining old beliefs can lead to finding meaning in the new situation. Illness threatens our dreams and diminishes our illusion of autonomy and control over life. Cancer threatens the illusion that life is predictable and controllable. Group discussions can lead to the discovery of smaller but potentially controllable new domains. Taking charge of treatment decisions, family relationships, priorities in life, and managing relationships in the group can be a powerful antidote to the helplessness engendered by illness.

Some topics that frequently emerge in support groups are the impact of the cancer diagnosis, the sense of loss and grief, the overwhelming emotional reactions that overcome us from time to time, physical losses, communication problems with family and friends, the reactions of others to us, the changes in our values and goals, and a view of the meaning of life.

Expressing Emotions

The ability to be in touch with one's feelings is a very important part of dealing effectively with the disease. Robert Watts recalls, "The greatest thing that turned me back towards my feelings is what I learned with the Survivors' Group. One night when I was feeling bad, a young Latin woman entered the group. She had recently completed her therapy for lymphoma. She cried every time she attempted to talk about her pain. Finally, she spoke about not being able to feel good about anything, about not feeling lovable. For the first time, I heard someone talking about experiencing what I had experienced, and suddenly I realized that I was not the problem, but instead that I had a problem."

The moments of clarity, identification, and connection that come with discussing deep concerns are part of the emotional healing process that group therapies offer cancer patients, a process that helps patients return to a sense of inner control. Just as illness has biochemical and emotional components, healing requires emotional as well as physical assistance.

Benefits of Group Support

There is growing evidence that educational, supportive, and psychotherapeutic interventions for the medically ill can have a variety of positive effects, including distress reduction, improved coping, enhanced interaction with family and friends, improved interactions with health care professionals, and adherence to treatment. Social support also can be an important factor in mediating individuals' ability to cope with stress.

Support Group Are Safe and Inexpensive

Support groups have proved helpful to cancer patients. For example, support groups have been shown to reduce traumatic stress symptoms, reduce other psychological symptoms and distress, improve coping, enhance disease knowledge, improve quality of life, and reduce pain. Such programs have been developed in oncology centers, private practices, and in supportive care programs. Recently, efforts have been made to establish and evaluate chat room programs on the Internet for cancer patients and those with other medical illnesses. While maintaining quality control is a difficulty, electronic support has already opened new worlds of information for patients, and also may provide increasing amounts of emotional, as well as intellectual, support at little or no cost.

Group members often remain in touch with one another for years after their formal participation ends. Typical comments are:

"When I joined the support group, I realized I was not alone."

"I needed time to talk with others about what I had just been through."

"I thought I was healthy and then this thing came along! I felt wounded, and nobody else seemed to get it!"

"Sometimes I found that what I said seemed to register with others in the group."

"It felt so good just to get my feelings out in the open."

Cancer patients benefit from sharing their feelings with others and from finding understanding in their responses and stories about themselves. Having cancer presents an immediate life threat. Treatment offers hope as well as new problems. The life threat may subside with treatment, but many need to talk about it with others in order to reclaim a sense of inner control.

25

Creative Expression
Improving the Quality of Your Life with Art, Music, Poetry, and Humor

Ernest H, Rosenbaum, M.D.
Isadora R. Rosenbaum, M.A.
Cynthia D. Perlis, B.A.
John Fox, C.P.T.
Malin Dollinger, M.D.
Stu Silverstein, M.D.
Jim Murdoch

A merry heart doeth good like a medicine.

—*Proverbs 17:22*

Courage, hope, faith, sympathy, and love promote health and prolong life. A contented mind and a cheerful spirit is health to the body and strength to the soul. How you live has a major effect on your health and your life—not only your attitude but also your activities can promote better health. Enhancing and enriching your quality of life heightens your emotional experiences and reduces depression. Your attitude depends in part on what you expect from life and how good you think your life has been. Health depends on the interaction between mind and body and between joys and sadness, as well having a sense of security and of being loved and appreciated.

To achieve a better quality of life, you need to involve yourself in a positive living program for the promotion of a healthy mind. The quality of life can be enhanced by the spiritual uplift and relaxation provided by interests and hobbies such as art, music, writing, and humor. These can enrich your life through positive experiences. We achieve a special satisfaction through things that we create ourselves. Becoming involved in creative activities improves feelings of self-worth, decreases depression, and promotes a sense of well-being.

The Role of the Mind in Health

Good health is one of the greatest assets we have in life, for without it our future is uncertain. The mind plays a key role in promoting good health. If your health is impaired, through an accident or illness, your life may become limited. Some of the new problems you may face will be physical, economic, social, emotional, or psychological.

Recently, there has been a shift in the philosophy of health care to a more "holistic" way of medical care, as suggested by Plato a few thousand years ago. We can't separate the mental from the physical because they are related as part of the whole person. Being a health care provider is like being a juggler trying to balance many balls—the medical, physical, environmental, psychological, and nutritional—in an attempt to keep the heart, brain, and body healthy. Many authorities feel that 50–80 percent of illnesses are stress related, including high blood pressure, colds, depression, and certain skin diseases. Certainly, facing continued ill health can be stressful.

Research at the University of Utah evaluated the role of stress during a recent economic depression. The rate of fatal strokes and heart attacks was higher than predicted. Continuing studies are looking at how stress relates to a decrease in the function of the immune system. If a direct link is found, an immune defect could precede many diseases. There is a relationship between anger, stress, and disease. One of the secrets of good health and longevity is knowing how to control stress. (See Chapters 14, 15, 17, 20, and 22.)

We have known for more than two thousand years that there is a relationship between the mind, the body, and one's health. It is an accepted fact that attitude and the will to live can, in part, determine one's future. How one accepts and deals with adversity or controls stress and anger reflects one's coping skills.

Norman Cousins found a way to use humor to cope with his incapacitating arthritis, fight his way back to good health, and increase his longevity. When told by doctors that his health would never improve—that he would be bedridden and either in pain or so drugged that he wouldn't know what was going on around him—Cousins rebelled. He obtained every Marx brothers, Three Stooges, and other comedy tape that he could lay his hands on, and watched them continuously. He found that laughing made his pain go away without the debilitating drugs. After some weeks of taking his own "cure," he could move without pain. Then he could walk. His self-treatment is living proof that "laughter is the best medicine."

Attitude

Attitude has a major influence on our lives and has become identified as one of the important ingredients in living well and longer. Attitude is in part shaped by our experiences and education, by our failures and successes. A positive attitude can help to increase our ability to cope with life's problems or with a disease. We have a chance each day when we get up to make this a great day for us and to achieve what we wish, or to merely accept events that occur and not try to improve our situation or to set new goals. Some things in life are more difficult to change than others. Thus, how we live is in part controlled by our attitude toward life. Because we can change our attitude, we can change our outlook, and thus our life.

The Will to Live

The will to live is nurtured by a positive attitude. A negative attitude can diminish or undermine the mind through fear, anger, or loss of self-esteem. These emotions, when unresolved, can lead to hopelessness, futility, resignation, and the loss of the will to live. (See also Chapter 13, "The Will to Live.") Here are a few examples:

- The phrase "frightened to death" is more than a figure of speech. An early reference to stress and fear is recorded in the Bible, in Acts 5, when Ananias and his wife Sapphira suddenly die after being castigated by Peter for withholding from the disciples some of the money paid for the sale of land. This has been attributed to a sudden coronary death from stress.

- In primitive societies, people have been literally frightened to death by the imposition of a curse or spell, known as bone pointing. When a person who believed in the phenomenon was "boned," he or she withdrew from the world, stopped eating, and waited to die. Death could take place in a few weeks. Such deaths have not been explained medically, even with an autopsy, but it seems apparent that the paralyzing effect of fear played an important role. The victim's fear stems from ignorance and superstition. He has been encouraged to believe in the power of the curse. Thus, ignorance and superstition play a role in how the mind functions to help or hinder a person in living.

People with a positive attitude are able to be open—to talk about their problems with their family, friends, and physicians. They feel good about themselves and generally have been that way all their lives. It often is very hard to change lifelong patterns such as your psychological reaction to daily living.

The will to live is therefore a spiritual, emotional, and ethical commodity. It needs nurturing and developing; if controlled, it can strengthen a person's resolve to survive. There is a direct correlation between a person's mental and emotional states.

We measure successes and failures in life by our standards and ideals as we strive for goals in work, relationships, and health. To live just for survival makes for a shallow life. Victory is for those who have the courage and stamina to fight and endure each of life's many struggles and who always have goals and the satisfaction of aspiring to reach them—whether they succeed or fail. This is the "challenge of life."

We can help ourselves and others live better if we:

- Live in the present *and* in the future, not in the past.
- Set reasonable goals as to what can be accomplished.
- Accept new problems and attempt to solve them through understanding and increased awareness.
- Try to resolve depression and negative emotions.
- Actively do things to help ourselves and others.
- Learn techniques to relax and practice mind control by using simple methods to calm down, such as yoga or tai chi, or practice biofeedback or visualization.

The Role of Creating Art in Health

Cynthia D. Perlis, B.A.
Ernest H. Rosenbaum, M.D.
Isadora R. Rosenbaum, M.A.

A hundred years ago, it was commonly believed that people could not be creative past middle age. Now, reports Lydia Bronte in *The Longevity Factor*, most Americans can expect a "second middle age"—a stage of adulthood between fifty and seventy-five created by our increased longevity and good health. Today, people in middle age and beyond sometimes feel that life is just beginning. A new sense of identity is discovered and defined along with an enhanced sense of self. During these years, art can be a healing force.

Artistic expression is an important psychosocial activity. We can create art by ourselves or we can attend classes ranging from beginning drawing to advanced printmaking. Sometimes we can express ourselves visually when we are unable to express ourselves verbally. Art can help us express what we are feeling in the present, yet it also can help us to express a memory, a moment that has happened that we do not want to forget. Music, drawing, painting, and creating sculpture provide a means of communication and self-expression—and a way to alleviate stress. Art also helps us to change our moods, come out of depression, or simply relax.

Art can be richly therapeutic for people, including the elderly, with a serious illness such as cancer. Suzanne, a woman approaching eighty who is living a full and energetic life in spite of her advanced cancer, has continued to teach art classes, take printmaking classes, and work in her home studio. Her recent works have included drawings and watercolors that express what it feels like to cope with life-threatening illness. She has created drawings that tell the story of her disease. One watercolor, *The Cell of Positive Thinking*, was created when she began a course of chemotherapy.

Creating art, says Suzanne, improves her self-worth and leaves a permanent gift to be enjoyed by all. She has received constant encouragement and support from her friends and family. They drive her to art classes and create along with her. Together they are participating in a shared experience, a shared community of meaning; the essence of what it means to be human.

You do not have to have artistic ability to be creative. Sometimes, just doodling or experimenting with art materials can open up a wide range of ideas. People often become too critical of their work—or are afraid others will judge their ability. It is important to express yourself for yourself and not for other people's approval. There really is no right or wrong in expressing who you are. For instance, if you feel you cannot draw, try making collages from pictures cut from magazines.

Creating art at any age gives people an opportunity to express what they are feeling. Creating art provides the ability to make decisions for oneself. With the opportunity to make

(Continued from page 196)

decisions and to exercise control over choice, people enhance their quality of life, improve self-esteem, and create ways to relate to others in a meaningful way.

A whole life or one experience can be shared in a work of art. One artist writes, "No, I will never say my work is finished. I must live forever—on and on. The reason we artists enjoy such longevity is that we are always looking ahead to the 'masterpiece' to come."

Here are some recommended creative art activities:

- Draw a self-portrait. Include words to describe who you are.
- Create a family tree—ask family members to draw their own portraits on the tree.
- Take painting, drawing, or sculpture classes at your local community college. If you feel you're not good enough, take a beginners' class—everyone will be in the same boat.
- Draw your dreams.
- Make a collage with pictures cut out of magazines. Decide on a theme before you start or let the theme evolve.
- Do a drawing with a friend, child, grandchild, or spouse.
- Take photographs.
- Learn needlepoint, quilting, crocheting, tatting (lace making), or knitting.
- Buy fabric paint and paint on T-shirts.

Don't be judgmental—there is no right or wrong, no rules, no grades. Smile as you create. Share with others. Be encouraging—to yourself and others. Enjoy!

Breast Cancer Quilts

Cynthia D. Perlis, B.A.
Ernest H. Rosenbaum, M.D.
Isadora R. Rosenbaum, M.A.

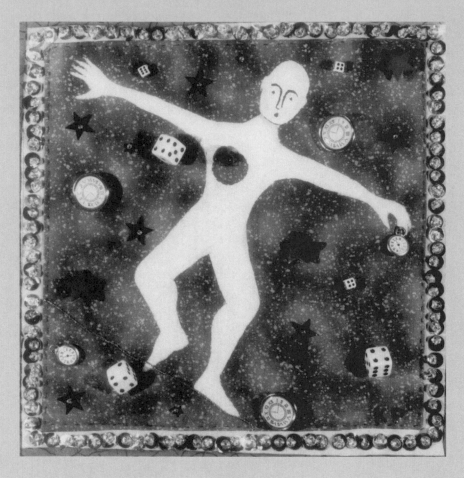

Inspired by the AIDS quilt, in 1996 a project was suggested to the Susan G. Komen Foundation that was designed to give women with breast cancer a creative voice. Because the tradition of quilt making has been nurturing and creative for countless women throughout history and, as it had for people with AIDS, could serve to bring the terrible epidemic of breast cancer before the public in a moving and beautiful way, Dr. Rosenbaum suggested that women who had had breast cancer touch their lives create their own quilt.

Cynthia Perlis, director of Art for Recovery, remembered the touching stories and drawings that women with breast cancer had shared with her. It was time to give these women a voice in the larger community, to let them speak through their creative spirits and to share their pain, their hopes, and their dreams along with their families' and friends' visions and wishes. Women recovering from and coping with breast cancer would be able to express visually their feelings about this illness. The Breast Cancer Quilts Project became a project of Art for Recovery through quilt workshops and meetings with women at their bedsides.

These squares began to represent the entire scope of this devastating illness. One square read: "I WON THE LOTTERY NO ONE CARED TO ENTER." On another piece of fabric, written in ballpoint pen, was the entire story of one woman's breast cancer experience. Another woman

(Continued from page 198)

embroidered "THE GIFT OF A LIFETIME" and dedicated the square to her doctor. The quilt makers then sewed the squares into a beautiful quilt.

One year later, there were five quilts, each measuring eight feet by eight feet, and each including images by twenty-five women with breast cancer or in memory of a loved one. Now, in the year 2001, there are thirty-six quilts, and the number is growing by five quilts a year. The quilts have been on display across the country. One of the most poignant parts of this project are the stories that women have written about their own squares that tell the painful reality of breast cancer. Here is one example:

> I wanted to make this square as a thank you to my three daughters who have been so loving and supportive these past ten months. The design idea came from a beautiful Christmas tree ornament given to me by my second daughter. I was extremely touched by this gift and displayed it prominently on our tree.
>
> I didn't really understand why it made such an impact on me and I'm not sure I know the answer yet. However, I suspect one of the reasons was that it was possible to have something beautiful represent a difficult and challenging time in my life. It also served as a daily reminder to be ever vigilant and to never forget. I wear a pink ribbon of some kind every day now to continue to remind myself, my daughters, and the world that the ENEMY is still out there ready to strike 180,000 more women this year alone.

—Elisa Bambi Schwartz

The Breast Cancer Quilts Project continues to invite women from around the country to create images for the quilts. In May 1998, eleven quilts were exhibited at the National Institute of Health as part of the National Cancer Institute's Breast Cancer Think Tank to support women battling cancer and increase public awareness of the disease. As a result of this prestigious exhibition, calls continue coming to Art for Recovery from all over the United States wanting information about participating in this significant project.

The Role of Poetry and Prose in Health

Ernest H. Rosenbaum, M.D.
Isadora R. Rosenbaum, M.A.

Poster Girl

I want to be the poster girl
For this cancer that has invaded me
I want the doctors, (after treatments)
To say, "There's no cancer I can see"
How did this cancer get inside of me?
I did not invite it here
And since it is not welcome
Why should I fear it?
It's true that it is awesome
But my God is awesomer.
So, cancer, you got to go
As I'm sure you must know
Do you think that I saved this body
For a poison such as you?
Do you think that I will lay down
And accept you as my due?
Not 'til I've declared war
And fought my very best
I won't let up until I've destroyed you
You most unwelcome pest
—Josie Teal, July 2000

Since the development of written language, humans have tried to capture their lives and history through writing. The ancients used pictures and signs to record their lives and thoughts. Over the centuries, this has evolved into written history as well as literature. Like art and music, literature—whether prose or poetry—is another way to support and enhance patient care and well-being. Like art and music, literature can be "the best medicine" and, through the benefits of self-expression, can have healing powers.

Reading or writing poetry or prose can reduce boredom and help relieve depression. It can divert your mind from your medical situation, provide creative stimulation, and help you to communicate your feelings with your family, friends, and medical team. Enjoying the use of your creative spirit and intelligence can provide a vital force to improve your state of wellness, daily living, and quality of life.

You may feel unsure about your ability to create literature, but do not be too critical of your early efforts because it takes time to learn techniques and to discover your unique "voice." Your talent will develop if you give yourself a chance. Many people find that taking a creative writing class or joining a poetry or fiction writers' group provides guidance and reduces their initial frustrations.

When people are seriously ill or depressed, they often feel hopeless. Receiving bad news about their disease or treatment can heighten such feelings. Even during the recovery process, people may feel sadness and a heaviness of heart. Reading great literature, whether prose or poetry, as well as attempting to express your own feelings of sorrow and loss through writing can raise your spirits, provide relaxation, and give creative satisfaction. Working with others in a class or group also can help to prevent isolation.

A patient who is a poet described the deep effect that reading Pushkin, Lermontov, and Pasternak has on her heart and spirit. She also said, "Sometimes when I have had a sad or hard day, I create poetry myself. Poetry makes my heart 'burn bright' through its magical strength. It also pleases me with an unusual inner feeling when people read my poetry, which for me is a 'lyric confession.' They appreciate my lyric confession when they understand my point of view and this creates an impulse to create more and more poetry."

This poet is also a journalist and writes articles and reviews on art, dance, and music. She says, "I have also enjoyed the recognition I have received. It has led to important moments in my life during the past two-and-a-half years, such as when a small, four-page newspaper, *Odessky Listok*, reprinted

(Continued from page 200)

stories [I had written] of people from other cities and countries. Readers appreciated the stories about people's adventures and lives, which is not only a personal declaration of their importance on earth but for mankind as well."

> "I want to live—to think and suffer"
> The poet said, and I agree.
> I want to live to sing in poems
> The taste of life, its smell, its joy, its dreams.
> I want to share my deepest feelings
> How free and happy—I am blessed to live
> In Golden State—unique and gorgeous
> In the mysterious Bay waves.
> I want to suffer, but not from pain
> Not from the evil—my inevitable fate
> I want to cry from love, to love again,
> Be loved, forget my age, be able to create.
> —Tamara Belorusets, translation by
> Yelena Nechay

Alexander Morrison, also a poet, said, "I also have written poetry for many years. I find it interesting to observe how, in different ways, I expressed the same philosophy at eighteen as I do now. I was amazed then, as I am now, at how the human being, screwed by circumstances beyond all belief, can manage to stand up despite the unmitigating bullshit that presses down on him. I'm talking about mankind and people like myself—the survivors and the contributors, the people I think have become successful human beings."

> Trace the affinity
> Of the will to be
> with the ability
> To Be no longer.
> Ah...such a narrow way divides.
> And yet, in the precarious clime
> Of this most eccentric inch
> A world of men lived
> Triumphant!
> —Alexander Morrison

"I'm looking for the same answers I looked for at eighteen. I haven't changed, but I do know that even with the odds tremendously against you, most of us manage somehow to make it."

> The vulgar splendor of a noise
> Contents the appetite of ears
> Insensitive to subtleties
> The really loud occurrence falls
> without the benefit of sound
> How silently are these:
> The awakening to love,
> The audacity to dream,
> The will to live.
> —Alexander Morrison

The Recovery
No longer can I bear
To dwell in this misbegotten state
Of involuntary confinement
The sorrow is too deep
The truth of it too great
For human comprehension
And so, with anxious hands I break away
The larval crust and shake myself free!
Outside carillon bells
Sing of my resurrection and celebrate
My reawakening with soft murmurs
Bird songs and forgotten lullabies
They call to me, beckon me
Into the blazing light of day
And direct me toward the path
Of undisturbed freedom!
With grateful tears
I squint into the blinding sun
And with an innocence of childhood born
I join the living once again
All is forgotten
> —Diane Behar

(Continued from page 201)

My breast, my womanhood, my life.
These things I took for granted.
But that all changed just
as the New Year began.
No, it couldn't be happening—not to me.
It just doesn't happen so fast.
I was just checked.
It doesn't run in my family.
It's just my imagination.
It's probably nothing.
Or is it?
It's a Saturday night.
How long should I wait?
Then Monday came.
My doctor's on vacation.
Find someone else, I can't wait.
"Just a cyst," they said,
"This doesn't look good."
"What does that mean?" I said.
"Don't worry, it's probably nothing,
but get it checked IMMEDIATELY."
"Don't panic," they said, as if I could stop.
It's all so unreal,
like I'm in a padded tunnel.
More tests, more worried looks, no answers.
"See a surgeon," they said, "ASAP"
I felt so alone, so small, so scared.
Why me? Will I die? Will I be mutilated?
Will Chris still want me?
"We'll call you tomorrow, just relax."

As if I could!
Who are they kidding?
Somehow I slept that night.
I can't remember what I dreamed.
It's probably better that way.
We met the surgeon the next morning;
I vaguely remember.
"I'll have to operate," he said,
"Go home, wait for the results."
The hours seemed endless.
Then the call came.
Oh, God! It can't be true!!
Not cancer! Not me!
I nearly collapsed.
Chris looked so helpless.
My life flashed before me.
Not so much the past,
but the future I was so scared of losing.
I'm too young to die.
I'm not finished living.
So back to the surgeon we went.
"It's a nasty one," he said.
"We'll operate tomorrow,
no time to wait."
What will I look like?
How much will they take?
Has it spread?
Will it come back?
Will my life ever be the same?

—Holly Kurzman, 1999

Poetic Medicine: Using Poetry to Deepen Your Connection to Self and Others

John Fox, C.P.T.

We human beings are at our best when we enjoy poetry. Sometimes all you need is to reflect in your mind one poem that says, "I can make it through."

—*Maya Angelou*

Support is a major issue when coping with cancer or any illness that requires intense medical intervention and time. The sheer logistical requirements of doctor visits and hospital treatments can be exhausting! Indeed, it can be difficult when you are ill to make it through a day without the help of a friend or family member acting as advocate and companion, the support of a medical professional offering treatment, or the help of a counselor or minister. Support may come in the form of stress-relieving practical information, advocacy, friendship, and counsel: but there is a particular kind of support that offers nourishment to your creative spark. This creative spark is accessible to us even when we are ill. We may experience a pull towards imaginative expression as a form of healing, but when dealing with the necessities of illness, your creative voice may be given short shrift.

The previous chapter spoke of the role of poetry and prose in health. The encouragement to write down your feelings will nourish your creativity. How can you get even more out of your creative expression and the healing art of poem-making?

Giving attention to this creative spark may support your desire to live life as fully as possible. People find that the expression of feelings, images, and metaphor meets some of their deepest needs in being human while coping with cancer and, at the same time, taps into their spiritual strength, playfulness, and search for meaning. Creative expression helps you hold on to your core self while facing the demands of a disease like cancer. Poetry reminds you that you are more than a disease.

How can you get started? You can start by putting your pen to the page! You don't have to share your writing with anyone; however, you might find it a surprising source of inspiration and support when you do so.

Ask a receptive friend (perhaps a few friends) or a family member with whom you are comfortable to share in the writing and reading of poems. Ask someone to share their favorite poem with you. Robert Pinsky, former Poet Laureate of the United States, appears regularly on the News Hour to share Americans' favorite poems.

You could ask a nurse, caregiver, or doctor if they are open to listening to your poems, and perhaps to share their own. There is a growing interest among nurses and doctors in poetry. Medical humanities courses are increasingly popular at medical schools. Poems regularly appear in the *Journal of the American Medical Association*. You can encourage this healthy trend!

The opportunity to share poems, to speak poems you've written, and to listen to others read their poems can deepen your connection with what matters to you. There is a spiritual dimension to this creative bond that allows for a deep and vulnerable place in a person to be received and honored. This is sharing at a level that fosters honesty and compassion.

Your poetry can explore joy and grief, insight and confusion, pain and pleasure, fear and love, what you do and do not know, your enjoyment of the natural world, and your intuitive awareness. Spirit poems that speak to these things feed the bonds of relationship and the soul of each person. Laura is a close friend of Kathy, a woman with ovarian cancer. Laura accompanied Kathy through many aspects of her illness and treatment. They formed a special bond by sharing poems together.

When, because of her illness, Kathy had to leave a writing group she had joined with Laura,

(Continued from page 203)

she continued to meet with Laura to share the writing and reading of poems. Laura says of their experience, "Having the chance to work on poetry together brings Kathy back from getting lost in the medical reality. I know it is a return to wholeness for her and it helps me to see her wholeness too. To be with someone coping with serious illness can at times be heavy and stressful, but because we are sharing with one another in this creative way, there is a deepening of our friendship that is nourished by poetry. Poetry keeps us receptive to moments of joy, connection, and compassion. Writing makes us aware of a place that holds a deeper meaning than the medical reality. It carves out a time and a space where the illness is not totally in control. Listening to the voice of poetry is liberating. It's a chance for both of us to be ourselves"

It is important to establish a safe environment when exploring healing issues through writing. Trust and empathy, openness and honesty, playfulness and respect—these are threads that weave the fabric of relationship. These qualities become more crucial in a relationship when we are ill. Nurturing these qualities will be helpful in drawing out creative expression when, under the pressure of illness, our safety is threatened. Illness forces us to enter the unknown, a loss of identity for instance, that can be frightening. Poetry can be a companion for this difficult journey and offer a way to navigate in the darkness.

Kathy comments about her writing and sharing poems, "Writing poems helps me to remember who I am. What I love. The writing brings me to life again. It brings back my love of creating things I enjoyed before I got sick. I feel so much more of my value and worth—both in writing and sharing. There is something about writing that sometimes has nothing to do with illness. The following poem came to me after waking from a dream.

The Spring of Inner Joy
Around the spring of inner joy
We gathered, just we three
Father, Son & Holy Ghost
and their invisible me.
Out amongst the pines at night
We heard the owl call
"Strengthen, Deepen, Darken, Flyers.
I will fly for all."
And but for their abundant joy,
A gift beyond us all
We fed together in the night
All those who heard the call.

"This is a mysterious poem for me. It is a celebration. I think the 'invisible me' is a part of myself that came back to me in the writing the poem. This poem is very promising. Like an underground seed, this poem is a truth I am not quite aware of.

"My sister begged me for a copy of this poem, as did my friend Jan who said it spoke to her about her own spirituality. I was so pleased that my poem was deeply meaningful to them! That meant a lot to me.

"Laura just bought me a new blank journal and I love it. The cover is wine-colored—magenta and a couple of shades of blue. It is very personal, especially when you can also include drawings. I love the colors; I want to hug it. It's perfect for me."

The benefit of people supporting one another's creative voice is profound, especially when we are exploring the unknown that we all face.

Art for Recovery/Brandeis Pen Pal Project

Cynthia D. Perlis, B.S.

In 1992, I developed the Art for Recovery/ Brandeis Pen Pal Project for patients to enjoy the art of writing letters to teenage pen pals. The idea developed from my Art for Recovery program hospital visits, where I noted that although these people in many cases were quite frail, weak, and in pain, their spirits were very much alive. I felt that they had much to offer in the way of personal experiences, insight, and wisdom.

Seriously ill patients could become, in effect, teachers. During the first year of this program, I matched twelve patients, half with cancer and half with AIDS, with twenty-four seventh- and eighth-grade students (aged twelve, thirteen, and fourteen). The teens wrote letters to the patients, including drawings if they chose to do so. They could ask absolutely any question, such as, "Are you afraid to die?" "How did you ever tell your parents that you had cancer?" One twelve-year-old girl wrote to a thirty-two-year-old woman with leukemia, "How did you ever tell your parents you had cancer? I could never tell that to my parents." The patients would respond by writing about their jobs, their families, and their illnesses. They would answer the teens' questions about their conditions and difficulties and tell them about all their experiences.

The students and the patients exchanged letters for nine months. To date, more than one hundred students and as many patients have built bridges and have created their own community. Thirty patients have died, some during the school year. At the end of each school year, there is a healing service, where the students and the patients meet face-to-face for the first time. The students read aloud blessings that they have written and the patients bring the students symbols of healing. This experience defines the true meaning of the word *mitzvah* (a Jewish word for a good deed). Further plans for this project include a book and a performance piece.

The following letters are excerpted from the correspondence between a woman with leukemia and her twelve-year-old pen pal.

Dear Katharine,

How did you know you had cancer? My sister has a muscular disease, so I know about muscular problems, but I don't really know anyone with a serious disease. Was it really scary when you found out you were ill? How long have you had cancer?

I'm really looking forward to writing you.

Love,

Lily,

P.S. Please send a picture.

Dear Lily,

It was really nice to get your letter.

I have breast cancer and I found a lump in my breast that felt big and hard. I could also feel swollen lymph nodes under my arm. It was very scary when I first found out.

I had to go through a lot of treatment and make decisions about the treatment. That was hard. I seem to be doing well so far and hope it continues this way.

Because I am a physician, I see a lot of children with serious diseases and also a lot of children who are healthy. I'm sorry to hear that your sister has a muscular disease. How has it been for you to deal with this and help her?

Thank you for your very nice picture—Write soon.

Katherine

Dear Emily:

I got some bad news recently. My leukemia is back. The doctors are very surprised; it is unusual for someone who has done well for two years to get their cancer back now. I always knew there would be a chance for it to come

(Continued from page 205)

back, but I was hoping it would be longer (or not at all).

I had thought there was nothing more the doctors could do. But they want to try a procedure on me where they get some cells from the man who donated some of his bone marrow to me before. These cells are white blood cells and they fight off infections. The doctors hope by giving me these cells, it will help boost my immune system to fight off and maybe destroy the leukemia.

It is a hard decision for me to make. It might be hard to understand why I might decide to just let the leukemia kill me. The procedure will make me pretty sick again. And the doctors are not too sure it will work anyway. I was not very happy last time I was in the hospital and I am not looking forward to being sick again. But my friends and family seem to really want me to try this procedure because it is my only chance to live.

It is hard to realize that I have to make these kinds of decisions. I am just a regular, normal person. These kinds of things happen in the movies or on TV.

Whatever happens, I would like to keep writing you. We can write about all sorts of things still. And you can ask me questions about what is happening to me if you want. The leukemia is part of my life, but not all of it.

My knees are better; I almost walk normal. But I am still pretty weak. Only my left leg can go up the stairs. It is like someone is holding me back if I try with my right leg.

Jana

Dear Jana,

I am very sad right now because you have got leukemia again. I had no idea this could happen again and I am very sorry. But I have a lot of hope that you will get better and I know you will too.

When did the leukemia come back? Is it as bad as it was before? How does your family feel about this? Are you afraid? How do you feel about coming back to the hospital after you've been out of it for so long? I have so many questions about this.

I heard from Cindy that you feel okay right now and I'm really glad about that. I hope that the new procedure the doctors are going to try will work.

It really is going to be a hard decision for you to make, but I think that if I were in this same situation, I would just try whatever the doctors think might work. I don't know why, but I hope whatever they do works and I hope you'll feel better soon.

I would like to keep writing to you too. Thanks for saying I can ask questions about what is happening....I'm glad your knees are better.

Bye,
Emily

The Role of Humor in Health

Ernest H. Rosenbaum, M.D.
Malin Dollinger, M.D.
Stu Silverstein, M.D.

Humor and laughter have been found to have a positive effect on the body's physiology and to induce relaxation. They help people cope and produce improved relations among family members and friends. A light-hearted attitude can reduce the chance of illness, reduce depression, and thereby promote longevity.

Humor reduces stress almost immediately. It also helps alleviate pain. Laughter has even been used as an aide in treating disease. As Norman Cousins stated, "I made the joyous discovery that ten minutes of genuine belly laughter had an anesthetic effect and would give me at least two hours of pain-free sleep." He discovered that watching funny movies with the Marx Brothers or the Three Stooges was therapeutic. Cousins wrote in *Anatomy of an Illness* that he deliberately tried to increase his laughter to help improve his health.

There is an old joke that a man was wondering what the meaning of life was, and he became morbidly depressed over this question. He even tried to shoot himself in the head, but missed. Finally, in desperation, he wandered randomly into a movie theater, where a Marx Brothers movie was showing. There he realized that as long as there is laughter, there is meaning to life.

Thus, humor can do wonders to help lift the spirits. Some studies have shown that if you just smile, the body has a positive response. Try it and see what happens.

The Physiology of Humor and Laughter

Humor usually results in laughter, which arouses the emotions, resulting in physical changes. These include short-term increases in blood pressure, heart rate, and respiratory rate, and reduction of stress.

Laughter stimulates the brain to produce endorphins (morphine-like relaxants that have a euphoric or analgesic effect). The result is muscle relaxation, an improvement in mental and spiritual well-being, and often a decrease in hostility and anger. Laughter also confers several long-lasting benefits on your body; it lowers blood pressure and it also serves as a mini-aerobic workout. Scientific studies are looking at exactly how laughter, joy, and a humorous perspective can have a positive effect on health and improve quality of life.

Laughter from jokes, speeches, comedies, plays, movies, operas, or other humorous events is a socially accepted way of getting a message across. It is sometimes a means of getting through personal tragedy or crisis (for those creating the humor as well as for those responding to it). Some people find that telling jokes about themselves removes some of the heaviness they may feel about their lives.

Humor can be spontaneous or specifically created, but no matter how it comes about, it can make a difference to your life. It has healing power for both body and soul as well as helping to sustain oneself through some of the depressing episodes of life.

Benefits of Humor

There are many benefits of humor. Here are some of them:

1. Humor can help us expand our perspective on life and enhance creativity.
2. The more we laugh, the better our chance of decreasing depression and promoting the healing process. Promoting the laughter factor injects more happiness into daily life.
3. Humor can improve family relations and smooth communications.
4. Humor provides physical and mental energy and rejuvenation through emotional relaxation.

(Continued from page 207)

5. Humor helps people cooperate and communicate, and decreases anger and fear.

6. Humor can promote a will to live, manufacture energy, improve self-esteem, and increase one's sense of self-worth.

7. Humor is considered by many to be one of the great medicines of all time.

8. Humor can reduce anxiety and thereby improve the enjoyment of social experiences such as dining.

There is an old Dutch saying that humor often comes from telling a tragic story after enough time has passed. In this way you can laugh at many hard times in your life. It wasn't funny at the time, but after you triumph over the tribulations of life, the stories can later be uproariously funny.

How to make humor work for you:

1. Collect or write down humorous anecdotes, memories, cartoons, and jokes. Refer to them often to improve your emotional energy and revive sagging spirits.

2. Create humorous cards and cartoons to make you laugh every day. Often, telling personal or family stories about life is a way of sharing humor and funny events.

3. Take a class on writing or telling jokes.

4. Keep humorous books, articles, or cartoons nearby. Refer to them frequently to make yourself smile and laugh.

5. Try to avoid frequent contact with depressing people who drain your emotional energy. Associate with positive people who use humor.

6. Promote parties and fun social events, such as birthdays. You need to make them happen.

7. Arrange a get-together with friends or relatives to tell jokes, recall happy and funny events, or share a funny video or movie.

8. Regularly visit a local comedy club.

9. Maintain a compendium of humor and philosophy to help you reduce isolation, anger, despair, or loneliness.

By using vignettes, jokes, or philosophical or practical sayings or words, you can improve your coping skills and reduce despair. A bit of humor, when appropriate, can make a sad event a little lighter and more positive. For grave or serious situations, a little humor can decrease your level of unhappiness. Apply the techniques of Norman Cousins.

Don't leave it to chance. Actively seek humor in your life. Those who laugh last laugh best!

The Role of Music in Health

Ernest H. Rosenbaum, M.D.

Jim Murdoch

Isadora R. Rosenbaum, M.A.

Malin Dollinger, M.D.

Music has healing powers. It has been said that "music soothes the savage beast." Plato believed that health in body and mind is obtained through music. Florence Nightingale used the healing powers of music as part of nursing the ill. Music affects the physiological and psychological aspects of an illness or disability. In the Bible, David, the shepherd boy, played his harp to help the psychologically anxious, insomniac King Saul relax and sleep. And music was used to calm shell-shocked soldiers in World War II.

Music has a personal meaning to each of us, often recalling or eliciting a positive emotional response. It has a universal appeal, it is inexpensive, and it crosses cultural barriers. It is available by Internet, radio, TV, tape player, CD player, vinyl records, and live. It can be listened to quietly, through earphones, or out loud for all to enjoy.

There always is a place for music in our daily lives. It gives a special pleasure and enjoyment and improves our mood. It affords us a way of expressing ourselves in a nonverbal way that can give us joy, calm us down, or lead to great excitement. It can provide us an escape or reach down into our deeper soul and elicit emotions that are pent up. For some people and their relatives and friends, music offers a special way to pass time that may sometimes seem endless.

Music can provide a way to decrease stress, promote emotional recovery, and provide relaxation. It also can afford a means of communication without the need to use a common spoken language.

Physiological and Psychological Effects

Music can increase or decrease heart rate and blood pressure, depending on the tempo and type of music. It can relax and reduce anxiety, or it can stimulate and heighten awareness. The intense emotions evoked by music can affect the nervous system and induce production of endorphins (natural painkillers). Music can help relax muscles to decrease nervous tension. It also can reduce alienation and feelings of isolation, and improve self-control and confidence.

Both age and illness and its therapies can affect a person's psychological equilibrium, causing depression as well as negatively affecting spiritual and emotional feelings and social interactions. Music offers a bridge in helping to support a person through many of the crises in life. It reduces stress and thus reduces stress-related illnesses.

Emotional Enhancement

There is a type of music to fit any emotion or mood. John Philip Sousa playing the "Stars and Stripes Forever" brings cheers and elicits patriotism. Verdi's *Requiem* or Rossini's *William Tell* may elevate the mood and give waves of relaxation to reduce stress or help alleviate grief. Listening to Mendelssohn's *A Midsummer Night's Dream*, or a Count Basie or Turk Murphy jazz program, can provide an emotional lift. Listening to the soft sentimental music of Nat King Cole, Glenn Miller, or Tommy Dorsey is relaxing; it also can provide fun and exercise if you get up and dance.

Music offers immediate gratification. You can sit and tap your feet to the rhythm, play simple instruments, or stand up and march. You can hum a tune to yourself or sing it out, but you also can sing songs, clap your hands, or even sing in the shower. Pretend for a moment that no one else is around. Think of your favorite song, the one that brings back pleasant memories—especially of someone close to you. How do you feel now? Do

(Continued from page 209)

you understand how powerful music can be in helping us gain emotional peace and happiness? Music is a form of communication that can be enjoyed with others. It requires no active participation, unless you wish it to.

A music program:

- reduces boredom and disillusionment;
- creates and enhances a happy mood;
- recalls pleasant experiences, bringing pleasure;
- offers immediate gratification;
- creates distraction from problems of daily living;
- may improve bonding among family and friends; and
- leads to an opening up of communication as people reminisce after enjoying music together.

In the hospital or treatment setting, music:

- helps improve coordination when used with physical therapy rehabilitation;
- gives psychological, social, physical, emotional, and supportive benefits;
- enhances—through rhythm—the effectiveness of speech training in persons who have had brain damage; and
- helps reduce anxiety commonly seen during medical therapy, thereby making therapy more acceptable.

Music is truly a vital part of our lives—when we are well and especially when we are ill. We can see the positive benefits live music can have for hospital patients and their friends and families from their reactions to a musician playing for them in their rooms.

Part III

The Care of the Body

26

Nutrition for the Cancer Patient

Bernadette Festa, M.S., R.D.
Ernest H Rosenbuam, M.D.
Isadora R. Rosenbaum, M.A.
Julie Matel, M.S., R.D.
Robert Ignoffo, Pharm.D.

Good nutrition is needed for general good health and is particularly crucial when you are ill. During this time, it is important to give yourself the calories, protein, fat, carbohydrates, vitamins, and minerals that are necessary for energy and the repair of normal tissue, and which will keep your immune system strong. Food is not only something to delight the taste buds, it is an essential ingredient in the fight against disease. It is as important as your medicine or medical therapy. Because of your illness or treatments, you may not be able to eat in the same way, and you might find that your eating experiences are affected.

When you are ill, you will be more attuned to the smells, tastes, and textures of foods. As your senses will be acute, it is important to savor and enjoy foods now more than ever. However, you may find that your tastes have changed and that you are turned off by foods that you once enjoyed. This is called food aversion. Allow your memory of the enjoyment to encourage you to eat these foods, as well as to develop a taste for new foods.

Think of yourself as an explorer. Sample small portions of the foods you used to eat, try new foods, and note the reaction your body and spirit have to them. Even an explorer needs a map to chart unknown territory. With the help of a registered dietitian, you can learn to explore alternative tastes and foods.

In the following chapters, we will:
- discuss the basics of good nutrition—what foods you need to eat, and how much you need to eat;
- describe the various side effects of therapy that may interfere with adequate nutrition;
- recommend ways for you to deal with these problems through diet and medication; and
- provide a variety of special diets that will make it easier for you to eat if you are unable to eat a regular diet.

You will not be asked to follow any difficult and unpleasant diets. Rather, it is our intent that you can use the information here, along with the guidelines your health care experts have given you, to plan a nutritious diet around your own food preferences. In Chapter 29, "Recipes for the

Chemotherapy Patient," you will find a large selection of recipes. Always consult your health care team experts if you are having problems or plan to change your diet.

NOTE: The dietary principles discussed in this chapter apply to most cancer patients, but if you have special dietary needs because of other problems, such as diabetes, heart disease, liver disease, kidney disease, etc., it is especially important for you to consult your medical team experts before changing your diet in any way.

Nutritional Needs of Cancer Patients

To help your body function at its best, it is vital to choose a variety of nutritious foods each day. Good nutrition is very important for people with cancer for the following reasons:

- Well-nourished patients are better able to cope with the side effects of treatment and may even be able to handle higher doses of certain treatments.
- A healthy diet can combat fatigue, give you more energy, and improve your quality of life so that you have more stamina to do the things you desire.
- A well-balanced diet can prevent the breakdown of body tissue and help rebuild tissues that cancer treatment may harm.
- A healthy diet can maintain the body's immune system, which will help prevent and treat infections.

The following elements are essential to your diet when you are starting cancer treatment.

Calories

A calorie is a unit of energy derived from food. Calories are required to keep our bodies functioning. The body has the ability to store excess calories as fat, and, when needed, convert this fat to energy. The body may require more calories during an illness, for healing after surgery, or for recovering from the side effects of radiation or chemotherapy treatment.

It is important to maximize caloric intake by selecting calorie-dense foods. You may find that you are uncomfortable with eating more fat, since diets to prevent cancer often emphasize lower amounts of fat. However, during this period, eating foods higher in fat than you might typically eat will make it a lot easier to obtain the calories you need to deal with problems such as nausea, loss of appetite, and unwanted weight loss. Sometimes, certain medications can increase your appetite, and thus result in undesirable weight gain. In these situations, it is important to choose vitamin- and mineral-rich foods that are lower in calories.

Protein

Protein is made up of individual units called amino acids. The body uses amino acids to build and repair tissues, to manufacture antibodies that fight infection, and to assist in many other body functions. Your body requires more protein for healing if you have lost weight, had surgery, or been through radiation or chemotherapy. Keep in mind that in order for your body to use protein efficiently, you must obtain adequate calories.

Good sources of protein include meat, fish, poultry, eggs, milk and milk products, soy and soy products, beans, nuts, and dried peas. Nutritional supplements, such as Ensure Plus, Boost Plus, Carnation Instant Breakfast, Scandishake, or homemade shakes can supply extra protein when you are unable to eat enough high-protein foods. According to the food guide pyramid, the suggested number of servings from the food groups high in protein are two servings of lean meat, fish, chicken, and meat substitutes (two to three ounces each) and two or three servings of milk or milk products. However, your protein needs may be increased at this time. Consult with a registered dietitian about recommendations for your age, sex, weight, and medical condition.

Good examples of low-cost, high-calorie/high-protein nutritional supplements are Carnation Instant Breakfast, fortified milk, high-protein smoothies, and milkshakes.

Fat Requirements

A higher-fat diet may be necessary for those who have lost weight or who are underweight. A lower-fat diet is suggested for those gaining nonfluid weight.

Vitamins and Minerals

Vitamins and minerals are essential nutrients that help to activate, regulate, and control many of the body's metabolic processes. The National Academy of Sciences has established recommended dietary allowances (RDA) for thirteen essential nutrients.

Most people can get all of these vitamins and minerals from eating a balanced diet. A multivitamin may be required, however, if you are unable to eat properly. Make sure that the vitamin and mineral supplement that you choose supplies all of the needed nutrients at about 100 percent of the RDA. (See Chapter 30, "Choosing a Multivitamin").

Although megavitamin therapy (vitamin dosages far in excess of recommended levels) has been suggested as a treatment for cancer and other diseases, no reliable scientific evidence proves that it is effective. In fact, some vitamins taken in excess can be harmful. For example, while the body has the ability to excrete excess amounts of the water-soluble vitamins (vitamins B and C, for example) in the urine, the fat-soluble vitamins (A, D, E, and K) are stored in the tissues and can accumulate to toxic levels if consumed in excess. Do not take any vitamins in high doses unless prescribed by a physician.

Antioxidants

Human studies show that antioxidants, including beta-carotene, selenium, and vitamins A, C, and E, may reduce the risk of cancer. Antioxidants act by destroying harmful molecules—called free radicals—that form in the body naturally. Free radicals can damage DNA, RNA, and fat and protein molecules, and they may be involved in the development of cancerous cells. Antioxidants decrease DNA damage, and it is possibly through this route that they help prevent the transformation of normal cells into malignant cells, thus acting as protective substances. However, there is no conclusive evidence that a diet rich in these antioxidants is able to reduce the incidence of cancer, or to produce a cure. Taking high-dose antioxidants during radiation and chemotherapy may reduce the effectiveness of these treatments in destroying cells. Consider waiting until after radiation and chemotherapy is completed to start taking these.

Fluids and Hydration

It is important to maintain adequate hydration by drinking enough fluids daily. Drink at least eight glasses of water a day unless your physician has told you to restrict your fluid intake. Avoid too many caffeinated drinks, as these act as diuretics and can increase water loss. Some chemotherapeutic agents increase your need for water. Therefore, be sure to follow your health care provider's instructions concerning your fluid intake.

Complementary Diets

Vegetarian Diet

Many Americans have elected to follow a vegetarian diet, which, when planned well, can be a healthy alternative to the conventional diet. Several terms are used to describe vegetarian diets. Lacto-vegetarians include milk and seafood, and lacto-ovo-vegetarians include eggs as well. Those who consume vegetables only—excluding all animal flesh, dairy products, and eggs—are referred to as vegans. There are more details about following a balanced vegetarian diet in Chapter 28, "Modified Diets."

Vegan Diet

If you are undergoing radiation or chemotherapy, it is often difficult to prevent weight loss on this eating plan due to its inherently high bulk and low calories. More careful planning is required if you are following a vegan diet. It is limited in calcium, iron, riboflavin, and vitamin B_{12} and lacks concentrated protein sources. In order to provide an adequate supply of essential amino acids, include whole grains and cereals with each meal. In addition, a complementary protein, which can be provided by legumes, vegetables, or a combination of nuts and seeds, should be included each day. Furthermore, the iron from grains, beans, and leafy green vegetables is not absorbed by the body as well as the iron from meat. Therefore, to increase iron absorption include a source of vitamin C (e.g., orange juice, citrus fruits, kiwifruit, or strawberries). Be sure to include dark green vegetables and nuts for calcium, and cereal for riboflavin. Vitamin B_{12} is found almost exclusively in animal products; vegans may need to use vitamin B_{12}-fortified products or supplements.

Maintaining an adequate vitamin intake is a concern for people with cancer and can be a challenge when following a strict vegan diet. Therefore, include plenty of nuts and seeds, one to four servings of additional fruits and vegetables, and three to five extra servings of grains and cereals.

Macrobiotic Diets

Another vegetarian diet is the Zen macrobiotic diet. Macrobiotic diets are not recommended for people with cancer.

This diet is based on the Zen Buddhist belief that one's health and happiness depend upon a proper balance between the "yin" and the "yang" foods. This balance is achieved by progressing through ten steps, which range from the lowest-level diet—made up of 30 percent vegetables, 30 percent animal products, 15 percent salad and fruit, 10 percent soups, 10 percent cereals, and 5 percent desserts, to the highest-level which contains 100 percent cereals. Avoid the higher and more extreme level, as it will be difficult to obtain all the nutrients you need and it may result in dietary deficiencies.

What Foods Should You Eat?
Basic Nutrition—The Food Guide Pyramid
One of the most important ways you can help yourself to get well is to eat the right amount of the essential nutrients needed by your body to repair tissue and maintain your weight. These essential nutrients—proteins, fats, carbohydrates, vitamins, and minerals—are also vital for normal body functioning and for maintaining good health.

The food guide pyramid has been developed as an outline to assist you with daily meal plans. Foods are divided into groups according to the nutrients they contain. Each group provides some, but not all, of the nutrients you need each day. Be sure to choose a variety of foods from each group daily.

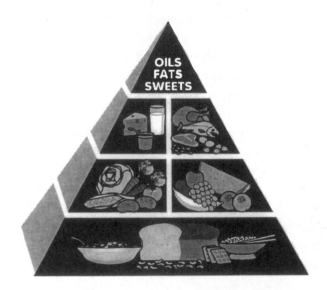

Bread, Cereals, Rice, and Pasta Group
The recommended emphasis in the diet is reflected in the base of the pyramid. This group provides primarily the B vitamins and carbohydrates for energy. Include six to eleven servings from this group on a daily basis.

Examples of one serving are: 1 slice bread, ½ cup (125 ml) cooked rice or pasta, ½ cup (125 ml) cooked cereal, 1 oz. (25 g) ready-to-eat cereal. Ideally, choose higher fiber whole wheat and grain products

Vegetable Group
Include three to five servings from this group daily. Choose at least one serving of a dark green or a deep yellow vegetable for beta-carotene (the plant form of vitamin A).

Examples of one serving include: ½ cup (125 ml) chopped, cooked vegetables, 1 cup (250 ml) of raw vegetable.

Fruit Group
The recommended amount of fruits is two to four servings daily. Include at least one serving of a fruit rich in vitamin C, such as orange, kiwi fruit, strawberry, or grapefruit.

Examples of one serving size include: 1 piece fresh fruit or 1 melon wedge, ¾ cup (175 ml) fruit juice, ½ cup (125 ml) canned fruit, ¼ cup (50 ml) dried fruit.

Milk, Yogurt, and Cheese Group
The two to three recommended daily servings of this group are a good source of calcium, phosphorus, vitamin A and D, protein, and riboflavin.

Examples of one serving size are: 1 cup (250 ml) milk or yogurt, 1½–2 oz. (40–50 g) cheese. Choose low or nonfat products unless trying to gain weight.

Meat, Poultry, Fish, Dried Beans, Eggs, and Nuts Group (includes peanut butter and tofu)
Protein, B vitamins, and iron are the important nutrients found in this group. Include two to three servings per day.

Examples of one serving size are: 2–3 oz. (50–75 g) cooked lean meat, poultry, or fish; ½ cup (125 ml) cooked beans; 2 eggs; 2 tbsp. (25 ml) peanut butter (equivalent to 1 oz./25 g of meat); 4 oz. tofu (125 g).

Fats, Oils, and Sweets Group
This group includes butter, cream, margarine, and vegetable oil, along with candies and sweet desserts.

NUMBER OF SERVINGS RECOMMENDED FOR CALORIC REQUIREMENT

Calories	Milk	Meat	Vegetable	Fruit	Bread	Fats
1,600–1,800	2	2	3	2–4	6	3–5
2,000–2,400	3	2	4	4–5	9	6–7
2,600+	3	3	5	5–6	11	8–9

Foods from this group contain calories, vitamin E, and negligible amounts of other nutrients. Therefore, most people should limit their intake of foods from this group.

Examples of one serving include: 1 tsp. (5 ml) margarine, oil, or mayonnaise; 1 tsp. (5 ml) salad dressing.

A range of servings is shown for each group of the food guide pyramid. The number of servings that is right for you depends on the number of calories you require each day. You will learn how to calculate your estimated calorie needs in the next section. If your calorie needs are low (1,600–1,800 calories or fewer), select from the lower number of servings from each food group. If your calorie needs are in the average range (2,000–2,400 calories), select from the middle number of servings from each food group. If you have high calorie needs (2,600 calories or more), select from the higher number of servings from each group.

Use the table below to determine the number of servings you should eat from each of the food groups.

Monitor your weight weekly to determine whether you are getting enough calories. If you find that you are losing weight, start including more calorie-dense foods from the fats, oils, and sweets group. However, if you cannot tolerate fat, consider increasing your consumption of calorie-dense, low-fat foods such as dried fruit and fruit juices. Note the range of the fruit and fat serv-

DESIRABLE WEIGHT

Height*	Weight for Age 19–34†‡	Weight for 35 and Older†‡
5'0" (152 cm)	97–128 (44-58 kg)	108–138 (49-63 kg)
5'1" (155 cm)	101–132 (46-60 kg)	111–143 (50-65 kg)
5'2" (157 cm)	104–137 (47-62 kg)	115–148 (52-67 kg)
5'3" (160 cm)	107–141 (49-64 kg)	119–152 (54-69 kg)
5'4" (163 cm)	111–146 (50-66 kg)	122–157 (55-71 kg)
5'5" (165 cm)	114–150 (52-68 kg)	126–162 (57-74 kg)
5'6" (168 cm)	118–155 (54-70 kg)	130–167 (59-76 kg)
5'7" (170 cm)	121–160 (55-73 kg)	134–172 (61-78 kg)
5'8" (173 cm)	125–164 (57-74 kg)	138–178 (63-81 kg)
5'9" (175 cm)	129–169 (59-77 kg)	142–183 (64-83 kg)
5'10" (178 cm)	132–174 (60-79 kg)	146–188 (66-85 kg)
5'11" (180 cm)	136–179 (62-81 kg)	151–194 (69-88 kg)
6'0" (183 cm)	140–184 (64-84 kg)	155–199 (70-90 kg)
6'1" (185 cm)	144–189 (65-86 kg)	159–205 (72-93 kg)
6'2" (188 cm)	148–195 (67-89 kg)	164–210 (74-95 kg)
6'3" (191 cm)	152–200 (69-91 kg)	168–216 (76-98 kg)
6'4" (193 cm)	156–205 (71-93 kg)	173–222 (79-101 kg)
6'5" (196 cm)	160–211 (73-96 kg)	177–228 (80-104 kg)
6'6" (198 cm)	164–216 (74-98 kg)	182–234 (83-106 kg)

*Without shoes
†Without clothes
‡ The higher weights in the ranges generally apply to men, who tend to have more muscle and bone; the lower weights more often apply to women, who have less muscle and bone.

Source: Adapted from *Nutrition and Your Health: Dietary Guidelines for Americans*, Third Edition. Washington, D.C.: U.S. Government Printing Office, 1990.

ings listed. These ranges are to allow flexibility in your food choices, depending on your ability to tolerate fat. More ideas on how to increase calories will be discussed later in this chapter.

How Much Should You Eat?

Protein and Calorie Requirements

This section shows you how to determine your desirable weight and the amounts of protein and calories you require in order to maintain that weight.

The table on page 217 shows average desirable weights for healthy adults. You may want to make allowances for the effects of your illness. If you are overweight, maintain your weight, as this is not a good time to lose weight. Try to maintain your weight within your range. Ask your dietitian for advice and determine a realistic desirable weight to maintain during your therapy. You may wish to keep track of your weight by using a Personal Daily Requirements table.

Minimum Daily Protein Requirement

A healthy adult has a daily nutritional requirement of approximately 0.5 grams of protein per pound of desirable body weight. Cancer patients may have *increased* protein and calorie needs. In addition, if you are already malnourished because of your illness or treatment, you will need to consume an even greater amount of protein (0.7–0.9 grams per pound of desirable body weight).

To find your minimum daily requirement of protein in grams, multiply your desirable body weight (in pounds) by 0.5 (or by 0.7–0.9 if you have already lost weight). Enter this figure in a food journal. When planning your daily menu, try to get at least this amount of protein from the foods you choose.

Minimum Daily Calorie Requirement

Your sex, age, and activity level affect the amount of calories you need. Men need more calories than women. Children need extra calories for growth, while the elderly need fewer calories. The more active you are, the more calories you need.

To estimate your daily calorie needs, multiply your desirable weight by eighteen if you are a man (by twenty if you have already lost weight) or by sixteen if you are a woman (by eighteen if you have already lost weight). Enter this amount in a food journal. Plan your daily menu to get at least this estimated amount of calories.

Meeting Your Daily Requirements

You can determine whether you are meeting your daily protein and calorie requirements by keeping a list of everything you eat, and then adding up your total protein and calorie intake each day and keeping track of it in a food journal. The protein and calorie content of most foods can be found in *Bowes & Church's Food Values of Portions Commonly Used*, which you can find in the resource center at your hospital, a bookstore, or a library. There are also computer programs, such as Nutritionist IV and Foodworks, that can help you to keep track of protein and calories.

Weigh yourself weekly rather than daily, because daily weights reflect your body's fluid content rather than overall changes in body weight. Track your weight in your food journal. If you are losing weight, increase your daily calorie intake by using high-calorie/high-protein recipes.

Reading Food Labels

Nutrition information on food packages can also help you make informed food choices to suit your specific needs. Food labels will assist you with maximizing your calorie and protein intake and developing an awareness of the fat content of various foods. When reading food labels, keep in mind that the amounts of calories, protein, fat, and so forth are stated per serving. Almost all bagged, wrapped, and canned items contain more than one serving. The same food item made by different manufacturers may have different per-serving sizes.

If you are usually careful about the amount of fat you eat, you can afford to relax a bit while you are undergoing cancer treatment and possibly losing weight as a result of it. At this time, the calories in fat may be beneficial (unless you are significantly overweight).

Sample Menu for Good Nutrition for Cancer Patients

The following menu is an example of a well-balanced meal plan that includes the recommended number of servings from each food group. If you have lost weight and need to include extra calories in your diet, add more servings of snacks, appetizers, desserts, and drinks.

Breakfast (265 calories, 5 g protein)
½ cup (125 ml) cooked cereal

$\frac{1}{2}$ cup (125 ml) fruit or juice

1 slice toast with 2 tsp. (10 ml) margarine or butter

Midmorning Snack (440 calories, 21 g protein)

1 cup (250 ml) milk

3 crackers

2 tbsp. (25 ml) peanut butter or $1\frac{1}{2}$ oz. (40 g) cheese

3 crackers

Lunch (365 calories, 20 g protein)

Sandwich:

2 slices bread

2 oz. (50 g) meat/fish/poultry or 2 tbsp. (25 ml) peanut butter or $1\frac{1}{2}$ oz. (40 g) cheese slices

1 tsp. (5 ml) mayonnaise

1 slice each lettuce, tomato

1 piece fruit

Mid-afternoon Snack (160 calories, 12 g protein)

$\frac{1}{2}$ sandwich:

1 slice bread

1 oz. (25 g) meat/fish/poultry

$\frac{1}{2}$ cup (125 ml) raw vegetables

Dinner (510 calories, 30 g protein)

2 oz. (50 g) meat/fish/poultry

$\frac{1}{2}$ cup (125 ml) vegetables

$\frac{1}{2}$ cup (125 ml) grain product (rice, pasta, etc.)

1 slice bread

1 tsp. (5 ml) margarine, butter, or oil

1 cup (250 ml) milk

This menu is a guideline. You may find that your day-to-day intake varies. For example, some days nausea and taste changes may prevent you from eating adequate amounts of food in all food groups. On these days, high-calorie/high-protein shakes or supplements that contain added vitamins and minerals may be helpful.

Helpful Hints for Better Nutrition

Whether you are at home or in the hospital, you can make good use of a planned approach to your eating. You may have to work hard to overcome the obstacle of a poor appetite, but there are techniques to help you.

Nutrition in the Hospital

1. **Consult with the hospital dietitian.** When you are in the hospital, you have the advantage of being able to consult with the hospital dietitian. Have him or her help you plan a balanced daily menu that includes the proper amounts of protein and calories. Ask for advice if you are having any eating problems. The hospital dietitian can also help you plan an at-home nutrition program.

2. **Consider adding a high-protein or high-calorie diet supplement to your menu.** Ask the dietitian to discuss various diet supplements with you. He or she may let you taste-test brands of supplements and can advise you about the pros and cons of the various brands.

3. **Snack between meals**. The dietitian will arrange for you to have snacks such as high-protein diet supplements, milkshakes, eggnogs, puddings, or sandwiches. If you must interrupt or miss a meal for a test, therapy, or examination, ask that your food be saved or order another meal when you return to your room.

4. **Fill out your daily menu when you are feeling well enough to plan your meals imaginatively**. Have someone help you if necessary. Order food that you like. Find out if the hospital has any menu choices not listed on the printed menu. Consider the protein and calorie values of the foods you order, but also give thought to its eye appeal and aroma so that it will be as appetizing as possible. Giving variety to your menus will improve your appetite. You may want to save some of your menus to use as examples when you are planning your meals at home.

5. **Have your family and friends bring your favorite foods.** Favorite foods from home will often help your appetite. In some hospitals, families are allowed to use the ward kitchen to prepare special food or to warm up food brought from home.

6. **Make your mealtimes pleasant.** Your mealtime atmosphere is important to make you feel like eating. Your family and friends can bring flowers and pictures to your hospital room. Ask for candles or wine, if permitted. Whenever possible, eat with family, friends, or other patients. If you are alone, turn on the radio, television, or music for company. Try to make mealtime a social time.

HIGH-CALORIE/HIGH-PROTEIN SMALL MEAL AND SNACK IDEAS

Food item	Calories	Grams Protein
Apple slices and cheese	175	7
Apple slices and peanut butter	250	8
Bagel with cream cheese	350	10
Baked potato and cheese	340	10
Buttered popcorn with Parmesan cheese	60	3
Carnation Instant Breakfast Drink	130	7
Cheese nachos	345	10
Cinnamon toast and milk	270	10
Cold or hot cereal and milk	240	11
Commercial supplements: Ensure, Boost, Resource	250	8
Cornbread and buttermilk	200	10
Cottage cheese (½ cup) with fruit	245	28
Crackers or pretzels and dip	175	10
Crackers with peanut butter or cheese	370	10
Dried fruit, nuts, granola	245	5
Egg custard and graham crackers	250	7
Eggnog and cookies	480	12
English muffins with butter and preserves	220	3
Fruited yogurt (1 cup)	225	9
Granola bar	100	2
Hard-boiled or deviled egg	75	6
Hot chocolate (cocoa) and cookies	350	10
Milkshakes and graham crackers	450	14
Muffins with cream cheese	350	10
Popsicles (pudding or regular)	80	2
Sandwich with protein	400	2
Sherbet or ice cream and topping	300	6
Soups, cream	200	6
Soups, with meat and vegetables	150	14
Tomato or V-8 juice and crackers	130	3
Tomato stuffed with egg or tuna salad	200	16
Waffles with syrup and butter	350	6

7. **Avoid stress at mealtimes.** Relaxation exercises before meals may help reduce tension and may improve your appetite. If your doctor gives you permission, you may find a glass of beer or wine before meals relaxes you as well as stimulates your appetite.

8. **Exercise before meals.** Light exercise for five to ten minutes approximately one-half hour before meals may stimulate your appetite. The nurse or physical therapist can show you simple range-of-motion exercises you can do in bed; or if you can get out of bed, take a walk up and down the hospital corridors.

Nutrition at Home

In addition to many of the above suggestions (frequent

HIGH-CALORIE FOODS

Food	Calories	Protein
Butter (1 tbsp./15 ml)	100	0
Cheese (1 oz./25 g)	112	7
Cottage cheese (½ cup/125 ml)	120	16
Cream, heavy (¼ cup/50 ml)	202	1
Gravy (¼ cup/50 ml)	50	2
Hard-boiled eggs (2)	150	12
Peanut butter (1 tbsp./15 ml)	115	5
Sour cream (2 tbsp./25 ml)	50	1

small meals, snacks, high-protein supplements, attractive surroundings, exercise, etc.), there are some additional techniques to use at home, when you no longer have the hospital facilities and staff available.

1. **Plan your daily menu in advance.** Include the proper number of servings from the food guide pyramid and your required amounts of protcin and calories. In addition to planning your menu, plan the time you will eat. If you have no appetite, you will need to rely on specified times to eat, rather than on your hunger mechanism.

2. **Get help preparing your meals.** If you are not feeling well, you may not feel like making the effort to prepare a nutritious meal. A friend or relative may be able to help you by preparing foods for several days in advance. Home aid in preparing meals or delivered meals are available in many communities. Some grocery stores have shopping services that you can access online—or order take-out from your favorite restaurant.

3. **Fix small portions of favorite foods and store them.** Prepare several portions at the same time and freeze them. Then you won't have to think about what to fix. It lessens the problem of figuring out what to eat when your appetite may be poor or you do not feel like cooking. Remember to protect against bacterial contamination that can cause food poisoning: do not leave food at room temperature for long periods, and refrigerate or freeze foods immediately.

4. **Add extra protein to your diet.** Drink fortified milk and use it for cooking. Use peanut butter, cheese, cottage cheese, and hard-boiled eggs as snacks, and devise ways to add them to recipes.

5. **Add extra calories to your diet.** Add cream or butter to soups, cooked cereals, and vegetables. Use gravies, sauces, and sour cream with vegetables, meat, poultry, and fish. Add a high-calorie dietary supplement to your normal recipes. The table below provides some suggestions for ways to add calories to your diet.

6. **Make food visually appealing.** The eye appeal of food can stimulate your appetite. Choose foods with attractive colors. Garnish your meal with parsley, lemon wedges, olives, cherry tomatoes, shredded raw vegetables, and so on. Use a small plate if you cannot eat normal portions of food, so that your meal will not look too small.

7. **Appeal to your sense of smell.** Cook dishes with tantalizing aromas and special sauces. Gravies and sauces are aromatic and enhance the taste of food; they also add calories and make swallowing easier. The smell of bread baking can stimulate hunger and contribute to a sense of well-being. Avoid foods with odors that trigger queasiness.

8. **Be creative with dessert.** Desserts are an appealing part of the meal. Take advantage of this for a caloric boost.

9. **Follow your own preferences in eating.** Even if you have dietary restrictions, there still is room to improvise, choose foods that you like, and mealtimes that work for you.

Myths of Nutrition Therapy for Cancer

Many people have their own ideas about treating cancer with special vitamins, particular foods, or avoidance of chemicals. It is important to discuss these ideas with your health care team to partner your personal needs with the best scientific evidence available.

Natural and Organic Foods

Patients are often curious about the superiority of "natural" or "organic" foods over regularly grown and processed foods in the dietary management of cancer. "Natural" is a general term covering all foods that are processed without artificial coloring, preservatives, or any kind of synthetic additives. "Organic" is a more specific term that refers to foods grown without chemical fertilizers, pesticides, or herbicides. There is no scientific evidence that either natural or organic foods offer any nutritional advantage over regular foods, but often patients find organic foods, while more costly, to be more tasty.

Concerns about the relationship between additives and cancer are based, for the most part, on speculation, and there is no good evidence that a person eating regular foods from the supermarket is at any greater risk than a person who eats natural foods. Cancer existed long before food additives were invented.

Starving the Tumor

Probably the most commonly held myth is that you can starve the tumor by starving yourself. Many patients have expressed the fear that by eating proper diets they will be feeding the tumor more than they will be feeding their normal body tissues. There is no scientific evidence to support this theory. Some experimental studies on animals with cancerous tumors found that those animals put on a starvation diet did not show any improvement over those on a regular diet. On the other hand, we know for certain that patients who are malnourished have more toxic side effects from therapy, do poorer medically, lose their strength earlier, heal more slowly, have reduced immunity, and become invalids or bedridden more quickly.

Megavitamin Therapy

Much attention has recently been focused on megavitamin therapy for certain diseases, including cancer. In some animal studies, certain vitamin A or E compounds have been shown to be related mainly to the *prevention* of tumors, rather than to the *treatment* of them. These results have yet to be confirmed in humans. Experts generally agree that there is no benefit to any form of megavitamin therapy for cancer.

Ideally, vitamins and minerals should come from the foods you eat. A properly planned diet makes vitamin and mineral supplements unnecessary, although, at times vitamin and mineral preparations may be prescribed for patients unable to eat a balanced diet. A trained professional should prescribe such supplements and should do so only on the basis of a dietary analysis and assessment of individual needs.

Recently, much has been written about the role of minerals, such as zinc, copper, selenium, and magnesium, in human nutrition. These metals are present in the human body (and in our foods) in minute amounts and are, therefore, termed "trace minerals." They are important for nutritional health, but their precise functions in the body are just beginning to be understood. The effects on cancer of ingesting increased amounts of minerals have not been well studied. Animal experiments have shown that some metals can actually *cause* cancer, but we do not know the implications for human cancer treatment.

It has been shown that zinc deficiency in humans may result in a loss of appetite, slower wound healing, and sometimes a loss of sense of taste and smell. However, it is not clear whether some of the loss of appetite and taste distortion experienced by cancer patients is due to zinc deficiency or to the cancer itself.

One fact is clear: a well-balanced diet supplies adequate amounts of the trace minerals for known human requirements. The first and best nutritional goal is to prioritize eating the recommended servings from the food guide pyramid. Eating whole foods first will ensure that you are receiving the nutrients that you need, even ones that haven't been discovered yet.

Nutrition-Related Internet Resources

If you need additional information regarding nutrition, the following websites may be helpful:

- www.aicr.org
- www.eatright.com
- www.mayohealth.org
- www.navigator.tufts.edu
- www.oncolink.com
- www.cancersupportivecare.com
- www.cancernet.nci.nih.gov
- http://dietary-supplements.info.nih.gov

27

Nutrition Problems: Causes and Solutions

Bernadette Festa, M.S., R.D.
Ernest H Rosenbuam, M.D.
Isadora R. Rosenbaum, M.A.
Julie Matel, M.S., R.D.
Sol Silverman, M.A., D.D.S.
Robert Ignoffo, Pharm.D.
Jillian Chelson, M.S.C.C.C., S.L.P.

Maintaining adequate nutrition can be challenging for patients with cancer. Many problems—most commonly loss of appetite—occur as side effects of cancer therapy. The foods you eat can affect these problems—they can make them worse or they can relieve them.

Physical problems may interfere with food intake and proper nutrition. Patients with head and neck tumors may have mouth or throat pain or difficulty swallowing. People who have had a part of their stomachs or gastrointestinal tracts surgically removed may be presented with problems, such as early filling, diarrhea, cramps, and decreased absorption. Removal of parts of the intestine or blockage of the intestine can also inhibit absorption. Patients with ileostomies or colostomies may have difficulties with salt and water balance because of diarrhea. Diarrhea also causes poor absorption of calories and nutrients, because food moves through the gastrointestinal tract so rapidly.

Radiation therapy to the head and neck frequently results in a loss of taste perception and decreased production of saliva, along with inflammation of the mouth lining (mucositis), pain, and difficulty swallowing. This suppresses the appetite and adds further to the problems of inadequate nutrition and insufficient caloric intake. Radiation to the abdomen may cause some damage to the bowels, resulting in cramps, diarrhea, poor calorie and nutrient absorption, or obstructions.

Chemotherapy can inhibit appetite by the same mechanisms as radiation. This is often worsened because of nausea. Decreased food intake is common for a short period around the time of treatment. It is important to try to compensate for weight loss during this time by making a conscious effort to eat more.

When you experience any of these problems, first consult your physician, nurse, or the dietitian on your health care team. With their help and with the suggestions in these chapters, you should be able to plan a diet designed to minimize these problems. Prescription medications may be required. Your dentist and pharmacist may also be of assistance.

In this chapter, we discuss the problems you may encounter and offer suggestions—what foods to eat, what foods to avoid, medication that can help, and other tips.

Surgery to the Head and Neck Area

Surgery to the head and neck area often affects the ability to eat. Proper planning before surgery should include a visit to a dentist to ensure optimal oral/dental health, whether that involves tooth decay, gum disease, or dentures. If necessary, a special dental appliance can be made to replace any teeth or tissues to be removed for cancer control. These dental applications will help your drinking, speech, chewing, and swallowing.

Your diet may have to be modified because of a change in your ability to chew some foods. Adapting to surgery involving the tongue or other oral structures often takes time, and it may require swallowing rehabilitation with a speech pathologist or occupational therapist specifically trained in head and neck swallowing disorders.

Colostomy and Ileostomy Dietary Guidelines

A colostomy is formed when part of the colon is surgically moved so that it opens on the surface of the abdomen, usually just below the waist. This forms a stoma, or artificial anus, through which stools are excreted. An ileostomy is an opening leading to the small bowel. The person with an ostomy wears a bag attached to the stoma to catch the excretions. He or she can lead a normal life in most respects, including choosing what to eat.

The following foods can cause problems for those with colostomies and ileostomies. You may wish to experiment with these foods to find out if they are problematic for you.

Foods That May Irritate
- Foods with seeds, such as strawberries, raspberries, tomatoes
- Nuts, popcorn, coconut, skin on fruits and vegetables such as apples and corn
- Some fresh vegetables such as coleslaw and salads

Foods That May Produce Gas
- Carbonated drinks and beer
- Dried beans or peas, broccoli, brussels sprouts, cabbage, cauliflower, corn, cucumbers, green peppers, onions, sauerkraut, turnips, winter squash

Foods That May Produce Odor
- Onions, eggs, fish

What You Can Do

Keep a record of what and when you eat so that you can identify (and avoid) any food that causes symptoms. The general guidelines for avoiding digestive problems can be helpful, such as eating in a pleasant, relaxed atmosphere and chewing your food slowly and thoroughly. Avoid swallowing air, which can lead to gas formation. Yogurt, buttermilk, and cranberry juice have proven effective in helping to control odor. Using Beano and/or soaking beans and discarding the soaking water before cooking can help reduce both gas and odor.

Be sure to drink plenty of fluids to prevent dehydration. Contact your physician if you are experiencing severe diarrhea or severe constipation.

Radiation Therapy to the Head and Neck Area

Radiation to the head and neck area frequently results in a loss of taste perception, decreased production of saliva, along with inflammation of the mouth lining (mucositis), pain, and difficulty swallowing. This suppresses the appetite and adds further to diminishing adequate nutrition and caloric intake.

Radiation Effects

Ionizing radiation delivered in doses large enough to kill cancer cells induces unavoidable changes in the surrounding normal tissues, causing compromises in function and host defenses, along with severe complications.

Mucocutaneous Changes

Unless intraoral or interstitial treatment is used, most patients will develop some redness (erythema) and moderate tanning of the skin in the treatment portal. Hair follicles are quite radiosensitive, therefore if hair is in the radiation treatment beam field, it will cease to grow and will fall out. This is often transient.

The acute oral mucosal reaction (mucositis) is secondary to radiation-induced cell division (mitotic) death of the basal cells in the oral mucosa. If the radiation is delivered at a rate equivalent to the ability of the oral mucosa to regenerate, then only mild mucositis will be seen. Oral microorganisms probably play a role in aggravating the impaired epithelium. Smoking is also a factor. Clinically observed late or post-radiation-induced atrophy (tissue damage) and telangiectasis (blood vessel red spots) of the mucosa often increase the risk for pain and/or necrosis.

Management of acute mucositis may sometimes require a one-week interruption of therapy. Topical anesthetics (Viscous Xylocaine) may be of some value, but the pain usually requires systemic analgesic drugs. Since infections may be associated, appropriate diagnosis and antimicrobial agents must be considered for either fungal or bacterial organisms. Viral infections are rarely a complication of radiation-induced mucositis. A short course of systemic prednisone (40–80 mg daily for not more than one week) has been helpful in reducing inflammation and discomfort.

Loss of Taste

Taste buds, which occur primarily in the tongue (circumvallate and fungiform) papillae, are very sensitive to radiation. Because of their location in the tongue, they are included in the beam of radiation for most oral cancers. Therefore, patients will develop a partial decreased taste (hypogeusia) or, most usually, complete (ageusia) loss of taste during treatment. The cells comprising taste buds usually will regenerate within four months after treatment. However, the degree of the resulting long-term impairment of taste is quite variable from patient to patient.

Dietary consultations regarding recipes with pleasing texture and perceptible and pleasing tastes are essential to improve intake of food. However, there are tremendous patient to patient differences, which preclude standard recommendations. Failure in taste perception, in addition to pain, dysphagia, hyposalivation, and depression, is associated with the loss of pleasure in eating, thus, a loss of appetite. Weight loss, weakness, malaise, and dehydration often follow. This is further complicated when prior surgery has caused problems in mastication and swallowing. Trials with zinc supplements such as zinc sulfate (ZnSO4) exceeding the usual recommended daily doses (RDA) appear to be helpful. We have prescribed 50–100 mg elemental zinc daily with success in some patients (220–440 mg ZnSO4). While zinc serves as a critical enzyme in many biochemical reactions, its role in taste and saliva remains unknown. Saliva probably has a modulating effect on the acuity of some tastes (sour, bitter, salt, sweet) through biochemical interactions, as well as providing an ionic environment in signal transduction for taste cells.

Salivary Function

Exposure of the major salivary glands to the field of ionizing radiation induces fibrosis, fatty degeneration, glands (acinar) atrophy, and cellular necrosis within glands. A critical dose level has not been identified. The serous glands (acini) appear to be more sensitive than the mucinous. During irradiation, the glandular secretions are usually diminished, thick, sticky, and very bothersome to the patient. Some patients are unable to produce more than 1 ml of pooled saliva in ten minutes. The duration of this depressed salivary function varies from patient to patient. Some regeneration can occur several months after treatment, and the undesirable signs and symptoms of xerostomia (dry mouth, discomfort, difficulty in speech, and swallowing) may be modified. However, recovery of adequate saliva for oral comfort and function may take up to twelve months; in others, the saliva remains inadequate indefinitely and is the source of major post-treatment complaints. When both of the parotid glands are exposed to the treatment beam, saliva diminution is most marked, and the prognosis for recovery is the worst. Obviously, the higher the dosage of irradiation, the worse the prognosis for xerostomia.

Frequent sips of water and water rinses are essential for partial control of radiation-induced xeroxtomia. Sugarless chewing gum and tart candy may be helpful. In some patients, pilocarpine hydrochloride as a solution or tablets (Salagen) has been effective in stimulating saliva production (5 mg three or four times daily). Side effects can include sweating and stomach discomfort. Another salivary gland stimulant, cevimeline (Evoxac), administered as 30 mg capsules three times daily, has been helpful in many xerostomic patients.

Synthetic saliva solutions and saliva substitute lubricants have been of limited help in the majority of patients with dry mouth, although some favorable reports have been published. Oral Balance, an over-the-counter gel, is a good example. In some patients, in whom the salivary complaint is related to the "thickness" (excess mucous-type secretions), guaifenesin (Organidin NR) as a liquid or tablet may help as a mucolytic agent (200–400 mg, three to four times daily).

Because of the painful mucositis, loss of taste, and xerostomia, the lack of desire or frank inability to eat is a common and almost universal complaint from patients receiving external irradiation to the oral cavity.

A resultant weight loss tends to weakness, inactivity, discouragement, further anorexia, and susceptibility to infection. Therefore, close attention is given to food intake and weight maintenance during treatment and follow-up. Anemia, bleeding, or immune deficiencies have not been complications of head and neck radiation.

Dental Caries

Patients who have not shown any degree of caries activity for years may develop dental decay and varying degrees of disintegration after irradiation. This condition appears to be due to the lack of saliva as well as to changes in its chemical composition.

To prevent or at least minimize radiation caries, oral hygiene must be maximal, including intensive home care and frequent office visits for examination and prophylaxis. Mouth rinsing is essential. Antiseptic mouth rinses, for example, chlorhexidine (Peridex, Periogard), if tolerated, are helpful in eliminating debris and controlling microbial flora. Daily topical fluoride applications, either as a solution for mouth rinsing, a gel delivered by means of a tray, or brushed on as a paste or gel, are all effective (as examples, Prevident and Gel Kam). Prevident is a sodium fluoride paste, and Gel Kam is a stannous fluoride gel. Attempts should be made to increase salivary flow either by local or systemic means. Foods and beverages containing sucrose should be avoided. If carious lesions develop, removal and restoration should take place immediately. Appropriate use of dental X-ray imaging is in order when indicated to monitor caries activity.

Candidiasis (Thrush)

Infections of the mouth by *Candida albicans* are commonly seen in irradiated patients, and are related to the alterations in the saliva. Clinically, the signs may be confused with radiation mucositis or other sources of infection. Candidiasis is usually painful. Management is primarily with the use of antifungal drugs. Systemic administration (200 mg ketoconazole daily with food, or fluconazole 100 mg daily) is usually more effective for both response and compliance. Duration of treatment depends upon control of signs and recurrences, since complete elimination of Candida from the oral flora usually does not occur. Topical administration entails the use of nystatin or clotrimazole tablets dissolved orally. Because of pain from mucositis and dry-

ness, patients may experience difficulty in dissolving tablets topically. Suspensions are another alternative form of treatment, but often this is not as effective because of limited contact time between drug and fungus. Antiseptic mouth rinses similar to those used for caries control may be helpful, if tolerated. In addition, topical (Viscous Xylocaine) or systemic analgesics may be required. Keeping the mouth moist is essential. There is always the possibility of developing fungal resistance, or the need of higher dosages, when these agents are used for prolonged periods of time.

Osteoradionecrosis

Osteoradionecrosis is one of the more serious complications of head and neck irradiation for cancer. Bone cells and vascularity may be irreversibly injured. Fortunately, in many cases devitalized bone fragments will sequestrate and lesions will spontaneously heal. However, when radiation osteonecrosis is progressive, it can lead to intolerable pain or fracture and may necessitate jaw resection.

The risk for developing spontaneous osteoradionecrosis is somewhat unpredictable, but it is related to the dose of radiation delivered and bone volume (usually more than 6000 cGy). The mandible is at higher risk than the maxilla. The risk is increased in patients without dentures and even more if teeth within the treatment field are removed after therapy. Spontaneous bone exposure usually occurs more than one year after radiation is completed. The risk for osteonecrosis continues indefinitely following radiation therapy.

If osteonecrosis does not progress clinically or radiographically, the usual management involves periodic observation. If flares (swelling, suppuration, pain) only occur occasionally, antibiotics are usually effective. If pain and/or flares occur too frequently or present other difficulties for the patient, surgery must be considered. Hyperbaric oxygen treatments along with surgery and antibiotics may be helpful in healing, promoting the formation of new blood vessels induced by increased oxygen.

Soft Tissue Necrosis

Soft tissue necrosis may be defined as the occurrence of a mucosal ulcer in irradiated tissue that has no residual cancer. The incidence of soft tissue necrosis is related to dose, time, and volume irradiated. The risk is far greater with interstitial implantation and intraoral techniques because of the higher irradiation doses.

Soft tissue necrosis is usually quite painful. Optimal hygiene is required and analgesics are usually helpful, but antibiotics are generally of little help in relieving pain and promoting healing. Since these ulcerations are often at the site of the primary tumor, periodic assessment for recurrence is essential until the necrosis heals.

Dental Treatment Planning

In view of the risk that accompanies high-dose irradiation, special attention to preradiation dental planning is critical. Factors important in the dental management of these patients include the following: (1) anticipated bone dose; (2) pretreatment dental status, dental hygiene, and retention of teeth that will be exposed to high-dose irradiation; (3) extraction techniques; (4) allowance of adequate healing time for teeth extracted before radiotherapy; and (5) patient motivation and capability of compliance to preventive measures.

Since many infections occur months or years after treatment, it is evident that the tissue changes induced by radiation persist for long periods of time and may be irreversible. Therefore, extreme care must be taken in evaluating the status of the teeth, and periodontal hygiene must be maintained because of the lowered biologic potential for healing in response to physical irritation, chemical agents, and microbial organisms. Such attention is critical because of the potentially progressive nature of radiation osteonecrosis, which may involve large segments of bone and present a major therapeutic problem, possibly requiring extensive resection.

It is impossible to establish precise formulas for managing preradiation and postradiation dental problems. Extractions are considered primarily for teeth with a poor prognosis due to such conditions as advanced periodontal disease, extensive caries activity, and periapical lesions. Other considerations are sources of chronic soft-tissue irritation (trauma), and the degree of patient cooperation and compliance in preventive home care and dental office programs. The decision is modified further for each patient on the basis of the prognosis, age, desires, economic aspects, and radiation delivery.

Reported studies and personal experience don't substantiate the advisability of extracting all teeth

before treatment as a good preventive measure. When teeth are extracted before or after radiation, the alveolar bone must be evenly trimmed and carefully smoothed so that a primary tissue closure is possible. This is necessary because suppression of bone cell viability diminishes remodeling, and if a suitable alveolectomy is not performed, the resulting alveolar ridge will be irregular and may increase the risk of subsequent bone exposure and discomfort. It may also compromise effective wearing of dentures. A minimum of one week to ten days is arbitrarily allowed for initial healing before radiation is instituted. However, if the situation permits, more time is preferable, up to fourteen or even twenty-one days. Since dosages are fractionated, healing can usually continue before damaging levels of radiation are delivered to a surgical area. Obviously, teeth completely out of the treatment field are not affected similarly.

The use of antibiotics during the healing period is important to minimize infection. Whenever possible, an attempt is made to retain teeth to support tooth-borne appliances for the tentatively planned rehabilitation of these patients.

The periodontium is maintained in optimal condition by periodic routine periodontal procedures. When areas exposed to radiation are treated, extreme care is exercised and antibiotics may be selectively administered. Fluoride applications (daily, in the form of mouth rinses or gels) appear to aid in minimizing tooth decalcification and caries in these patients. There are no unusual contraindications for endodontic procedures.

Radiation Therapy to the Chest and Esophagus

Radiation is frequently delivered to the chest and esophagus to treat lung cancer, esophageal cancer, and lymphoma. Doses in excess of 3,000 cGy may, within three weeks, result in esophagitis (inflammation of the esophagus), with symptoms of painful swallowing. Reducing the daily dose or a short interruption in the treatment will usually allow rapid healing.

Radiation Therapy to the Abdomen and Pelvis

Radiation to the upper abdomen or pelvis may cause radiation enteritis (inflammation of the bowel). However, only a very small percentage of patients treated with radiation to the abdomen will develop chronic problems. Because of their rapidly dividing cells, the mucosa (soft lining) of both the large and small bowel, including the rectum, are sensitive to even modest doses of radiation. The severity of symptoms depends on the extent of the irradiated area, the daily dose, the total dose required, and if chemotherapy is used simultaneously. In addition, patients with a history of abdominal surgery, pelvic inflammatory disease, atherosclerosis (inflammation of the lining of the arteries), diabetes, or hypertension are predisposed to radiation-induced nausea and vomiting.

Treatment to the upper abdomen is more likely to lead to nausea and vomiting, while pelvic irradiation is more likely to result in rectal irritation or in frequent bowel movements or diarrhea because of faulty absorption of fat, bile salts, and the B vitamins.

Your physician will evaluate the extent of the intestinal inflammation by assessing the frequency of diarrhea, the character of the stools, and the presence of rectal bleeding or abdominal distension, as well as dehydration or electrolyte imbalance resulting from diarrhea or faulty absorption.

What You Can Do

Treatment of inflammation caused by radiation includes adjusting the diet, medication, and, in severe cases, interrupting radiation treatment. Patients receiving abdominal or pelvic radiation should follow a low-fiber/low-residue diet, beginning with the first radiation treatments or first symptoms of intolerance such as loose bowels or diarrhea. ("Residue" refers to indigestible material in food, sometimes called fiber.) Patients should limit their intake of milk products, except for buttermilk, yogurt, and acidophilus, or lactose-free milk. Milk or milk products may be hard to digest. The milk sugar lactose may cause bloating, gas, or diarrhea. However, yogurt may be beneficial to your gastrointestinal tract. Other food guidelines to follow include:

- avoid greasy, fried, or fatty foods, as they tend to be difficult to digest;
- vegetables should be cooked;
- whole-grain and high-fiber products—such as whole wheat bread, brown rice, nuts, popcorn, and beans—should be avoided and replaced with food such as white bread, potatoes, and white rice;

- patients can drink fruit juices (except prune juice), but they should avoid raw fruits, as these may be irritating to the digestive tract;
- some fruits and vegetables contain pectin and gums that may help symptoms; especially with diarrhea choose bananas, applesauce, and vegetables such as carrots, white and sweet potatoes, butternut and acorn squash;
- remember the "BRAT" diet, Bananas, Rice, Apple juice or Applesauce, and Toast or weak tea in addition to the other food groups needed daily; and
- reduce alcohol consumption.

Medication

If bowel inflammation (radiation enteritis) persists despite diet changes, medications will be needed. A 250 mg 5-ASA suppository every night can help reduce or control symptoms during and after radiation therapy. For small bowel inflammation, oral 5-ASA may be helpful.

Relief from abdominal pain may be obtained with narcotics. If proctitis is present, a steroid foam given rectally may offer relief. If you have pancreatic cancer and are experiencing diarrhea during radiation therapy, your doctor may recommend oral pancreatic enzymes (pancreatin) or Ultrase to be taken with meals to assist with digestion and absorption of food.

Chemotherapy

Detailed information on nutrition and chemotherapy is often not easily available. The specific dietary recommendations in this book show that many drug side effects can be reduced or controlled. Ideally, a registered dietitian should be included on your health care team to work with the oncologist and you.

Loss of Appetite (Anorexia)

Cancer therapy or the cancer itself may cause changes in your body chemistry that result in a loss of appetite. Pain, nausea, vomiting, diarrhea, or a sore or dry mouth may make eating difficult and cause you to lose interest in food. It is common to lose your appetite because of anxiety or depression about your disease. Often, patients who have been informed of the possible diagnosis of cancer lose five to ten pounds while waiting for their test results.

The brain produces chemicals (cytokines and serotonin) that can cause loss of appetite. The reduction of calorie intake can lead to a loss of muscle mass and strength and other complications by causing:

1. interruptions of medical therapy, impeding effective cancer therapy;
2. poor tolerance of surgery;
3. impaired efficacy of chemotherapy and radiotherapy;
4. decrease in quality of life; and
5. decrease in immunity.

A totally different approach to eating is required when you no longer have an appetite to nourish you. You will need to learn to eat even when you do not feel like eating and to approach eating as an important part of your therapy. Talk to a dietitian, nurse, or your doctor about ways to improve your appetite. It is important both for your general well-being and your ability to fight disease that you eat a nutritious diet and try to maintain your weight.

As appetite may no longer motivate you to eat well, now you will need a planned approach. You may improve your appetite by experimenting with different ways of preparing and serving food. Choose foods high in calories and proteins, so you can get the maximum energy possible and avoid losing weight, which will cause weakness. If you don't seem to be making progress, you might ask your doctor about medications that can stimulate your appetite such as Megace, Decadron, or Marinol—a legally available, synthetic form of THC (the active ingredient in marijuana) in capsule form. It is usually used as an antinausea drug, but it also stimulates the appetite. Some states allow marijuana to be used to reduce nausea symptoms for patients receiving chemotherapy under the supervision of their physicians.

More tips for reducing loss of appetite are found under "Nutrition" in Chapter 26. Also choose from the high-calorie/high-protein small meal or snack ideas in that chapter.

Abnormalities in Smell and Taste Perception

Abnormalities in smell and taste perception are common, especially for those who are receiving radiation therapy to the neck and mouth area. "Taste blindness," or an altered sense of taste and smell, is a temporary condition that occurs when the tongue's lining and taste buds are altered by surgery, radiation therapy (especially of the head and neck), chemotherapy, or because of the cancer itself. The most common complaints are of food tasting too sweet or too bitter, or of a continuous metallic taste or smell.

A loss of taste perception makes it more difficult to eat, which leads to weight loss. Taste loss tends to increase in proportion to the aggressiveness of treatment. With time and healing, the sense of taste returns. Often, a strong aversion to certain tastes or foods follows an illness. Taste aversions may also be associated with chemotherapy, so avoid eating your favorite foods on the day you receive chemotherapy.

What You Can Do If Foods Taste Too Bitter

1. Add sweet fruits to meals.
2. Add honey or sweetener to foods and drinks.
3. Eat meat cold or at room temperature.
4. In place of meat, eat blandly prepared chicken and fish, mild cheeses, eggs, dairy products, or tofu. All of these foods may taste better when prepared in casseroles or stews.
5. Marinate meats or fish in pineapple juice, wine, Italian dressing, lemon juice, soy sauce, or sweet-and-sour sauces.
6. Good mouth care can help. Brush your teeth several times a day, and use mouth rinses (water mixed with salt, hydrogen peroxide, or baking soda, or diluted Cepacol or Chloraseptic).

What You Can Do If Foods Taste Too Sweet

1. Gymnema Sylvestra, an herbal tea that often is used by professional wine tasters, will deaden the taste buds to sweet tastes for about twenty minutes if it is held in the mouth for about five minutes before eating.
2. Dilute fruit juice or other sweet drinks with half water or ice.
3. Avoid sweet fruits; vegetables may be more appealing.

What You Can Do If Foods Taste "Off"

1. Drink water, tea, ginger ale, or fruit juices mixed with club soda to remove some of the strange tastes in your mouth.
2. Use sugar-free gum or hard candies to reduce aftertastes.
3. Add wine, beer, mayonnaise, sour cream, or yogurt to soups and sauces to disguise the off tastes of other foods.
4. Eat starchy foods such as bread, potatoes, rice,

and plain pasta. Do not add butter, margarine, or other fatty substances to these foods.

5. Choose bland foods. Eggs, cheeses (including cottage cheese), hot cereals, puddings, custards, tapioca, cream soups, toast, potatoes, rice, and peanut butter are less likely to taste strange than foods with more distinctive flavors.

6. Remember that what tastes "off" today may taste normal next week.

What You Can Do in General

1. Eating in relaxed and pleasant surroundings can help reduce problems of taste blindness.

2. You may have cravings for spicy and salty foods. Spicy, highly seasoned foods are irritating to many people. However, if your doctor does not advise against such foods, and if you can tolerate them, by all means satisfy such urges.

3. Often, flavorings such as herbs, spices, or other food seasonings may help your food taste better to you. Acidic foods, such as grapefruit, may stimulate taste buds, but avoid them if they irritate your mouth.

4. Experiment with different food textures, such as crunchy, creamy, and crispy foods.

5. High-protein foods and supplements are particularly important when taste-blindness prevents you from eating properly.

Nausea and Vomiting

Nausea and vomiting are a frequent side effect of cancer therapy. They can also be brought on by an obstruction in the intestine, irritation of the gastrointestinal tract (gastritis), or a brain tumor.

Constant vomiting makes it impossible for you to eat or take fluids, so whatever can be done to reduce nausea should be done before vomiting starts. Paying attention to psychological causes and using antinausea drugs, as well as antianxiety and relaxing medications, will help control symptoms.

Nausea and vomiting may begin one to three hours after treatment or even as long as two to four days later. You may start to fear therapy, a fear that can gnaw at you and make you want to avoid treatment. Nausea and vomiting may also make pain control and maintaining an overall good quality of life much harder. A wide variety of antinausea drugs are available to minimize or prevent the problem.

Medications for Nausea and Vomiting

Medications are available to combat nausea and vomiting. These include Compazine (prochlorperazine), Ativan, Benadryl (diphenhydramine), Decadron, Dramamine, Inapsine (droperidol), Reglan (metoclopramide), Zofran (ondansetron) and Kytril (granisetron). Marinol is also effective. The FDA has also approved Marinol, the active ingredient in marijuana, in capsule form. Many patients obtain marijuana from private sources and add it to brownies, cookies, or other food; brew it as tea; or take it in gelatin capsules by mouth or in rectal suppositories.

Medications

Two areas in the brain have been identified as being responsible for nausea and vomiting, and certain drugs and other methods can selectively block these areas. Your doctor can work out a program to combat your nausea, although if one drug or a combination of drugs doesn't work as well as you both would like, you may have to experiment with various programs.

Generally, antivomiting drugs (antiemetics) should be taken thirty minutes before chemotherapy so that they have time to take effect. If vomiting has already started and you cannot keep a pill down, antinausea suppositories such as Compazine or Tigan may help. Long-acting capsules such as Compazine Spansules can be very helpful, since they work for six to twelve hours.

Ativan (lorazepam) and Decadron (dexamethasone), both sedatives, may help block the brain's vomiting center. This is also a powerful combination for blocking anticipatory nausea and vomiting. During severe nausea, Ativan can be taken under the tongue for rapid absorption. Xanax (alprazolam), another sedative, or other antidepressants, may also help to reduce anxiety. Ativan is an antidepressant, antianxiety, and sleeping tablet that can cause amnesia, which might take the edge off any memory of vomiting once the episode is over.

Some forms of marijuana—the natural tetrahydrocannabinol (THC) and the synthetic Marinol—may control nausea and vomiting. However, they can also cause drowsiness, dry mouth, dizziness, a rapid heartbeat, and sweating. The use of marijuana to alleviate cancer therapy's side effects is legal in some states.

Granisetron (Kytril), ondansetron (Zofran), and dolasetron mesylate (Anzemet) are the most significant new drugs used to control nausea and vomiting caused by intensive chemotherapy and radiotherapy; they may be needed when you cannot get relief with other antinausea agents. They are often given with Decadron IV. They suppress vomiting in 60–80 percent of patients and are even more effective in combination with other antinausea drugs. Anzemet and Kytril last longer, often for one day.

Delayed nausea and vomiting can occur after cis-platin, carboplatin, and cyclophosphamide chemotherapy. The most effective antinausea medications for delayed nausea and vomiting are Reglan and dexamethasone. However, these drugs have more side effects than the "setrons" (ondansetron, granisetron, and dolasetron). A setron should be used after Reglan and dexamethasone has been tried. If effective, a setron may be used as a preventative therapy during the next cycle of chemotherapy.

Anticipatory Nausea and Vomiting

It is estimated that up to half of all people receiving chemotherapy experience some nausea or vomiting before, not after, they receive the drugs. This is known as anticipatory nausea and vomiting (ANV), and it usually makes the nausea and vomiting even more severe when the chemotherapy is actually given. ANV can become such an established psychological pattern that the amount of chemotherapy given must be reduced. And once the psychological pattern of ANV is established, it is much harder to control nausea and vomiting before and after treatment. (This behavior pattern was described ninety years ago by the Russian physiologist Pavlov and is referred to today as Pavlov's syndrome.)

The aim in chemotherapy is to deliver a therapeutic amount of drugs with the fewest side effects. But each chemotherapy agent and each drug combination has a potential for causing nausea and vomiting. Receiving three or four drugs at a time, which is typical, can make the reaction even more severe. The dosage and the number of cycles to be given also contribute to the reaction.

You, your family, and even your friends should talk with your doctor about the type of chemotherapy you will be getting. For each drug or drug combination, a program should be established that allows you some control over the situation. With psychological factors playing such a big part, it is very important that you be a participant in preventing nausea and vomiting.

Your level of anxiety, how you feel about yourself and your cancer, and how you respond to stress and disease are all important factors in setting up this psychological pattern. And once the pattern is established, all kinds of stimuli can trigger feelings of nausea: the colors or smells in the room where the chemotherapy is given, the smell of rubbing alcohol used to prepare you for the IV needle, the sight of the nurse entering the room, or even the sight of the hospital.

What You Can Do

To deal with anticipatory and general nausea and vomiting, you will have to take steps both to relax before your chemotherapy and to not inadvertently set up situations that become associated with nausea. Some patients benefit from meditation, self-hypnosis, psychological support, and nonaversion training (through media such as audiotapes to help prevent fear and nausea). Our patients have found the following suggestions helpful:

- Try to relax in a quiet, darkened room before your treatment sessions.
- To help yourself relax and control any triggering stimuli, use behavioral techniques such as hypnosis, relaxation therapy, imagery, or listening to a tape of your favorite music.
- Try acupuncture or acupressure, which have been effective in controlling nausea and vomiting in some cases.
- Try seasickness wristbands available at any drugstore.
- The time of day when you get treatment can sometimes make a difference. If you usually

(Continued from page 231)

get nauseated in either the morning or the afternoon, try to change your appointment schedule.

- Avoid eating spicy foods if they upset your stomach or gastrointestinal tract.
- Replace fluids and electrolytes. Drink extra fluids before a chemotherapy treatment to help your body get rid of chemotherapy byproducts.
- Avoid eating for at least two hours before your treatment. Eat foods that are easily digested (high-carbohydrate, low-fat). Take a snack with you to treatment. If you experience "dry heaves," you may be able to get relief by eating something light, such as crackers or dry toast, before your therapy. Pregnancy antinausea programs can provide helpful suggestions.
- Eat and drink slowly. Do not force foods past the point of tolerance. Eat smaller, more frequent meals. Take clear, cool foods and chilled drinks at first, especially apple and cranberry juices, fruit drinks, Gatorade, ginger ale, 7-Up, and tea or iced tea. Try peppermint or ginger teas. Try one-half to one cup of cooked white rice with pearl barley.
- Popsicles, salty foods, soda crackers, and toast are often well tolerated. Avoid overly sweet, greasy, hot or spicy foods, and foods with strong aromas if they aggravate your nausea. Food served chilled or at room temperature may be more appealing.
- Avoid cooking odors that may bring on nausea by having friends or family prepare your meals at their own homes and bring them to you, or order in from a restaurant. To reduce the smell of beverages, drink them through a straw.
- *Always* avoid your favorite foods when you are receiving chemotherapy. You might start to associate these foods with treatment, nausea, and vomiting and develop a strong aversion to them. You need your favorites to entice you to eat when you don't feel hungry.

HOW TO TALK WITH YOURSELF ABOUT FOOD

Negative talk	Positive and Supportive Talk
I'm too tired or weak to eat	I'll feel stronger after my frozen dinner. It will take only three minutes to microwave.
I'm already nauseated, I don't want to eat.	Having light foods in my stomach (crackers, Jello, apple juice) may help me to feel better.
I'm eating as much as I can and haven't gained a pound	Have patience, it takes time to gain weight. Just keep on eating high-calorie foods every few hours.
I'm sick. I can always eat more tomorrow.	I need to do the best I can do today. I'm in control of this aspect of my life.
My medication has caused me to gain weight.	Eating low-fat food will prevent weight gain.
I'm not going to eat today.	Eating the right foods will help me to fight my illness.

Sore Mouth and Throat

A sore or ulcerated mouth or throat is a frequent side effect of chemotherapy or radiation therapy to the head and neck area. This condition will clear up in a few days, unless your recovery is slowed by malnutrition. If symptoms persist, consult your physician; you may have a viral or fungal infection, such as monilia (also known as thrush).

The mouth and digestive tract are composed of cells (mucosa) that are more sensitive to chemotherapy. The lining, or mucosa, of the gastrointestinal tract, which includes the inside of the mouth and throat, is one of the most sensitive areas of the body. Thus, during or after chemotherapy or radiation therapy, a cancer patient may develop some sort of mouth problem, ranging from dryness to ulcers. Many chemotherapy drugs can inflame the lining, a condition called mucositis. Many drugs can also cause small ulcerations or sores to develop.

These mouth problems are more often due to chemotherapy or other medication. From three to ten days following chemotherapy, patients may experience a burning sensation, followed by ulcers. When ulceration develops, treatment is mostly supportive until the cells regenerate themselves, which takes about seven to fourteen days. This can impact oral comfort and nutrition, but adequate care can minimize these effects.

Oral Hygiene

Basic mouth hygiene is of primary importance, and should be initiated before chemotherapy starts. When using cytotoxic chemotherapeutic drugs, it is extremely important to keep patients free from the oral foci of infection and pain to minimize local infection and bacteremia, and to enable them to maintain a nutritious diet. The chemotherapeutic agents utilized to eradicate tumor production also adversely affect normal cells, particularly those that have relatively high turnover rates, such as oral epithelial tissues. The depressant effect of therapy on oral epithelial mitoses can result in thinning and ulceration of the tissues as well as salivary glands and taste dysfunctions. The oral ulcerations may be due to direct cellular cytotoxicity from the cheomtherapeutic agents, increased susceptibility to microorganisms owing to neutropenia (bone marrow suppression), a trauma, or a combination of these factors. A good oral hygiene program includes dental cleaning and scaling, followed by daily brushing and flossing to reduce plaque. Make sure your mouth stays clean and moist and that you eat the proper foods and get the proper medication for any infection that develops.

Any scaling, cleaning, tooth extractions, or repair of cavities should be done before your cancer therapy begins. Extractions, especially, should be completed at least two weeks before therapy to give your mouth a chance to heal. Ill-fitting dentures should be fixed or replaced. Any peridontal or dental work has to be coordinated with your oncologist.

Before any dental work is to be performed, your blood counts should be checked to be sure that your body can take care of any infection or bleeding (low white blood cell counts can lead to infections, and a low platelet count may lead to excessive bleeding). If you sustain any mouth injury because of a dental procedure, antibiotics are recommended if your white blood cell count is low or there is an infection. Unless there is an emergency, dental procedures should be delayed until the blood counts return to a normal range.

Patients should brush their teeth three to four times a day with a *soft* toothbrush or sponge and use floss. Patients at high risk (those receiving 5-FU or methotrexate) should rinse their mouths frequently with salt water, baking soda, or chlorhexidine (Peridex) following chemotherapy. The use of floss, electric toothbrushes, and Water-Pik appliances should be curtailed if gums are swollen, sore, or tend to bleed.

Xylocaine is a local, short-term anesthetic available as a 2 percent orabaseB gel or spray (Hurricane) and used to decrease pain. It should not be used prior to meals, as it can cause choking. Protective agents (sucralfate, kaopectate) can be used to cover ulcers and decrease irritation. It is important to stay away from irritant substances like peroxide, as they may worsen the ulcers. Topical steroids should be used with caution, as they may facilitate infections. In addition, patients should not eat spicy, hot, acidic, or coarse foods or beverages. Soft, moist foods are best.

The following daily steps will help your mouth stay in good shape:

- Use a soft-bristle toothbrush and soften it more by soaking it in warm water.
- Brush with Biotene toothpaste or a paste of baking soda and water; it is less irritating than commercial toothpaste.
- If brushing your teeth is painful, use a cotton swab or Toothetes, a sponge-tip stick impregnated with a dental cleaner.
- Avoid commercial mouthwashes—some have ingredients, especially alcohol, that can irritate your mouth.
- Avoid lemon glycerin swabs because glycerin can dehydrate and will make your mouth drier.
- Using a Water-Pik to cleanse your mouth is helpful.
- An oral rinse, such as Peridex, will help soothe gum inflammation and prevent bleeding, but it contains alcohol which may sting your mouth.

ANTI-NAUSEA DRUGS

Drug Name	Usual Dose	Side Effects	Cost
Compazine (Prochloperazine)	10 mg every 8 hours as needed	Sleepiness, dystonic reactions, lockjaw	$0.20/ tablet
Lorazepam (Ativan)	Orally every 4 to 6 hours as needed 0.5 to 1 mg	Sleepiness, confusion	$0.50/ 1 mg
Ondansetron (Zofran)	Orally every 2 to 3 times daily 4 to 8 mg	Constipation	$15.00 8 mg tablet
Granisetron (Kytril)	Twice a day or 2 mg once daily 1 mg orally	Headache	$35.00/ 1 mg
Dolasetron (Anzemet)	Orally once daily 100 mg	Headache, constipation, sleepiness	$20.00/ 100 mg tablet
Dronabinol (Marinol)	Orally four times daily 2.5 to 5 mg	Appetite stimulation, confusion	$1.00/ tablet
Dexamethasone	Orally twice daily with meals 4 to 8 mg	Insomnia, stomach upset	$.50/ tablet
Metoclopramide (Reglan)	10 to 20 mg orally four times daily	Diarrhea, anxiety, sleepiness	$0.60/ tablet

If You Have Mucositis

In chemotherapy, the mucositis is usually due to the low white blood cell count; in radiation to the head and neck, it is usually due to the necrotic and inflammatory effect of radiation energy on oral mucosa.

If the soreness in your mouth becomes severe, there are quite a few anesthetic agents that you can use on a short-term basis. If your symptoms persist, you should have a complete dental hygienic evaluation. There is an increased risk of mucositis for those who wear dentures or tooth devices, who have a history of oral lesions (herpes, canker sores, monilia, or gum infections), or who smoke.

The following treatments may be helpful to you:
- Benadryl elixir, lozenges, and analgesics to help reduce mouth pain.
- Swishing and swallowing the anesthetic jelly Xylocaine or Hurricane (benzocaine) can help to reduce pain in your mouth, pharynx, or esophagus so that you can eat.
- Cepacal or Chloraseptic spray and lozenges.
- Swishing or gargling with a tea or 1 tsp. baking soda and salt dissolved in warm water (less harsh than a commercial mouth wash).
- Swishing diluted milk of magnesia, Carafate slurry, or Mylanta around your mouth.
- Orabase, with or without Kenalog, will cover mouth sores while they are healing.
- A GI (gastrointestinal) cocktail of 1 tbsp. (15ml) Cherry Maalox (analgesia) 1 tsp. (5ml) Nystatin (antifungal), and 1/2 tsp. (2ml) Hurricane Liquid (analgesia) immediately before each meal, swish and gargle for one minute, then swallow.

Infections

Mouth infections can be dangerous. Examine your mouth every day for any irritation or early fungus growth (white spots inside your mouth that don't wash off). Look under your tongue and at the sides of your mouth and report any changes to your doctor. If you do get an infection, it should be treated promptly.

If you have a herpes virus—acute or recurrent—your doctor may prescribe oral acyclovir tablets or cream. Monilia requires antifungal agents, such as Mycostatin (nystatin) oral suspension, Mycelex Troches, Mycostat Pastilles, Nizoral (ketoconazole)

TREATMENTS AND DRUGS COMMONLY USED TO TREAT MUCOSITIS

Drug Name	Usual Dose	Side Effects	Cost
saline mouthwash	10—30 ml; swish and swallow every 2 to 6 hours	Few	None
baking soda mouthwash	dissolve 1/2 tsp. salt and 1/2 tsp. baking soda in 1 cup warm water; rinse every 3 or 4 hours	Few	None
chlorhexidine (Peridex, Periogard)	dilute 1:1 with water; rinse every 4 hours	taste, teeth staining	$
betadine mouthwash	as needed	teeth staining, iodine allergy	$
xylocaine, 2 percent viscous	gel: 5 to 15 ml every 4 hours; spray: 1 spray every 4 hours	possible systemic effect; choking if taken before meals	$$
sucralfate or kaopectate	10 to 30 ml every 2 to 6 hours; swish and spit	taste	$$

ANTIFUNGAL DRUGS COMMONLY USED TO TREAT INFECTIONS OF THE MOUTH

Drug Name	Usual Dose	Side Effects	Cost
clotrimazole troches (Mycelex)	place 10 mg troche in mouth 4 to 5 times a day, for 7 to 14 days	well tolerated, taste	$$
nystatin suspension	1 tsp. every 4 to 6 hours; swish and swallow	well tolerated, irritation	$$
fluconazole (Diflucan)	100 mg oral capsule every day	nausea, vomiting, itching	$$$
amphotericin B	intravenous; dose varies	headache, fever, chills	$$
amphotericin B suspension mouthwash	10 mg once daily; swish and swallow every day	taste	$$$

tablets, Diflucan (fluconazole) capsules, fluconazole oral solution, Fungizone (amphotericin), or Sporanox (itraconazole) oral solution. You can freeze the liquid form of nystatin in medicine cups or ice cube trays and let it melt in your mouth. Use mycolog cream for sores at the corner of the mouth.

Damage to the mucosa can make it easier to get some infections, such as candida or herpes simplex virus infections. Appropriate treatment should be started. Thrush (monilia) can be treated with topical antifungals, such as clotrimazole or nystatin. When infection is more severe, oral ketoconazole, fluconazole, or intravenous amphotericin may be used.

Nutrition

A normal high-protein, high-calorie diet with supplements as needed will help your sore mouth or tongue heal faster. Drinking lots of fluids will also help with healing, as well as make your mouth sores more comfortable.

A high-calorie, high-protein diet includes scrambled eggs, custards, milkshakes, malts, gelatins, creamy hot cereals, macaroni and cheese, and blenderized and pureed foods. Commercial supplements, such as Ensure, Boost, and Carnation Instant Breakfast Drink can be helpful.

Until your mouth sores heal, you should avoid:

- very hot or very cold foods;
- tomatoes and citrus fruits, such as grapefruit, lemons, and oranges, which can cause a burning sensation;
- salty foods, which can cause a burning sensation;
- hot, spicy, coarse, or rough foods—including toast, dry crackers, potato chips, pretzels, nuts, etc.
- alcoholic beverages and tobacco, which irritate the lining of the mouth; and
- any medications that contain alcohol, such as mouthwashes or cough syrups.

Your diet should consist of soft, bland foods. Solid foods should be soft or cooked until tender. A liquid diet or a pureed diet may be necessary if you find solid food too irritating. Frequent small meals served warm or at room temperature will be more tolerable than large meals or foods that are very hot. Foods that are especially well tolerated are applesauce, cool or room temperature drinks, cooked cereal, strained cream soups, custards and puddings, eggs, plain ice cream (no nuts, chips, chunks of fruit, etc.), sherbet, Jell-O, milkshakes, mashed potatoes, and popsicles.

Dry Mouth (Xerostomia)

Saliva serves many functions. It initiates the digestion of starch. It mixes with food to form a soft mass that can be swallowed. It is the first line of defense to protect the teeth from oral bacteria and fungus. Radiation therapy to the head and neck area affects the salivary glands. Saliva production is decreased and becomes thicker, resulting in a dry mouth, a condition called xerostomia. This can interfere with chewing and swallowing, speech, and hygiene. It is an uncomfortable sensation. This may be temporary, but if radiation therapy doses exceed 4,000 cGy, you may be left with some degree of permanent dryness.

What You Can Do If You Have Dry Mouth

Dry mouth (xerostomia) can occur in certain patients and can be easily treated by drinking fluids, sucking ice chips, eating fresh fruits, or chewing gum. Preparations containing alcohol or glycerin should not be used because they may irritate the lining of the mouth or aggravate dryness. Artificial saliva (MoiStir, Artisial) is commercially available and can be useful for some patients. Dryness should not be overlooked, as it may predispose the patient to ulcers or infections.

Choose foods with a high liquid content, such as applesauce, custard, puddings, hard candies (especially sugar-free lemon drops), ice cream, sorbet, most fruits, yogurt and cottage cheese

Tips for Moistening Foods

- Add gravies, sauces, melted butter or margarine, broth, or salad dressing.
- Dunk breads or other baked goods in beverages.
- Drink generous amounts of nutritious liquids with meals, but be aware that you may eat less because you fill up on the liquid. Try eggnog (pasturized) yogurt and milkshakes.
- Add lemon juice to water.
- Suck on sugar-free hard candy or chew sugar-free gum. This may help to stimulate saliva production. Avoid sweet products because your teeth have lost the natural protection that saliva provides. You also can suck on sugar-free popsicles or flavored or plain ice cubes.

Other Tips

- Artificial saliva products may be helpful. Ask your physician, dentist, or speech therapist about these.
- Salagan (pilocarpine) is a medication in pill form that increases saliva production.
- Commercial preparations such as MoiStir and MouthKot, oral saliva substitutes, or Oral Balance, a moisturizing gel, may help.
- Use a special dry-mouth toothpaste, such as Biotene.
- Make your own mouthwash with liquid lidocaine (Xylocaine), baking soda, and salt dissolved in 1 quart (1L) of water; or mix 1 quart water, 1 tsp. (5ml) salt, and 1 tbsp. (15ml) baking soda.
- Use lip balms or chapstick if your lips are dry.

Heartburn, Reflux, and Indigestion

More than one million people experience heartburn (also called GERD or gastroesophogeal reflux disease), which commonly is caused by acid reflux (the movement of acid from the stomach into the esophagus). Heartburn is a sensation of burning or pressure in the upper stomach and the esophagus. It can cause an inflammation of the esophagus called esophagitis.

Indigestion, an uncomfortable feeling in the abdomen after eating, is usually caused by eating too

Swallowing Difficulties

Bernadette Festa, M.S., R.D.,
Jillian Chelson, M.S.C.C.C., S.L.P.

Difficulty swallowing may be a result of surgery to the mouth and throat, radiation therapy, or generalized weakness. The severity of your swallowing problem will vary depending on the type of surgery you have had and whether you have undergone radiation therapy. You may experience only temporary discomfort due to pain and swelling, or you may have more severe problems requiring supplementation by tube feeding until your ability to swallow is restored. If your swallowing difficulties are minor, and you feel you can manage them without a swallowing therapist, the following suggestions might help.

What You Can Do

If swallowing difficulties prevent you from eating your normal meals, eat frequent small meals and snacks to ensure that you get enough calories. Choose soft foods or foods that can be cooked until tender. This will make chewing and swallowing easier. Many people find liquid nutritional supplements, in addition to their meals, an easy way to get all the protein and calories they need.

Cut your food into bite-sized pieces or grind them so that less chewing is required. If you are having trouble using your tongue to move the food from the front to the back of your mouth or around your mouth, moisten foods with gravies, sauces, or yogurt.

If you continue to have trouble swallowing (coughing, choking, changes in breathing, frustration with eating) or experience weight loss, ask your doctor for a referral to a swallowing therapist.

A Swallowing Training Program

If your swallowing difficulties are more severe, you may need a swallowing training program to relearn how to swallow safely and comfortably. The basic components of this program are (1) proper food consistency, (2) proper positioning of body and head, (3) specific, prescribed swallowing techniques, and (4) appropriate feeding methods.

Food Consistency

The consistency of your food will be critical to your success. Ideally, a team that includes a dietitian, a swallowing therapist, and your physician will choose the type of food and consistency most appropriate for you. Their evaluation will take into account your ability to move and feel the structures of your mouth, to cough, to clear your throat, and to handle secretions.

While relearning how to swallow, you will need to progress from those foods that are easier to swallow to those that are the most difficult. For many people, thin liquids are the most difficult because of the highly complex coordinated movements and sensory perception required to swallow them. The following paragraphs give some examples of food consistencies that may be prescribed for you.

Foods That Tend Not to Fall Apart in the Mouth. These include applesauce, avocados, bananas, custard, egg dishes, ground foods with sauces or gravies, hot cereal, mashed potatoes, puddings, most pureed foods, quiches, soft vegetables with sauces, soufflés, and tapioca.

Foods That Fall Apart in the Mouth. These include crackers, dry breads, dry cereals, meats, nuts, seeds, rice, and raw vegetables.

Thin Liquids. These include alcohol, broth, coffee or tea, Ensure or Sustacal, hot chocolate, ice cream, juices, Jell-O, milk, Popsicles, sherbet, soda, and water.

Semithick Liquids. These include pureed or cream soups, buttermilk, Ensure or Sustacal (or equivalent supplement with 2 tbsp./25 ml thickening agent such as Thicken-up), milkshakes, nectars, and tomato or V-8 juice.

Thick Liquids. These include pureed fruits, thickened shakes, and Ensure or Sustacal (or

(Continued from page 237)

equivalent supplement with 3 tbsp./50 ml thickening agent, such as Thicken-up).

Solid Diets for Swallowing Difficulties

Solid food diets vary in consistency; there are four levels. Your swallowing therapist or dietitian will help you choose the right level for your needs. In most cases, you will want to eat foods that do not fall apart on your tongue. Some people may need to eat food that is smooth and nonfibrous. Still others may only be able to drink their nutrition. Your choices will depend on your specific type of swallowing problem.

Level 1—Pureed. These include baby foods; pureed cottage cheese; cream of wheat or rice; custard; mashed potatoes; puddings; pureed fruits and vegetables; pureed meats, fish, and beans; pureed soft-cooked egg; and thinned plain yogurt.

Level 2—Ground. These include custards, finely chopped pasta, ground meats, junior baby foods, macaroni and cheese, moist cakes, pancakes in bite-sized pieces, soft canned fruits in bite-sized pieces, moist scrambled eggs, soups without chunks, and cooked vegetables in bite-sized pieces. Avoid nuts, seeds, skins, and connective tissue on fruits and in meats.

Level 3—Chopped. These include beans, boiled eggs, breads without crusts, seeds or nuts, casseroles, chopped tender cuts of meat, poultry and fish, cooked cereals, corn flakes and puffed rice, French toast, fresh peeled fruits in bite-sized pieces, omelets, pasta dishes, peanut butter, potatoes without skin, puddings, soft-cooked vegetables in bite-sized pieces, and waffles.

Level 4—Soft-textured. These include breads without seeds, nuts, or dried fruit; all cheeses; all cooked cereals; dry cereal without nuts or dried fruit; cooked fruits and vegetables; cream soups; eggs; raw fruits and vegetables without skins or seeds; and whole moist tender meats, fish, and poultry.

Amount and Pacing

In most cases, foods should be eaten in small bites ($^1/_2$ tsp.). Sometimes a larger amount (1–2 tsp.) will provide the sensation required to swallow. Be careful when you experiment with sizes. Until you are once again proficient at swallowing, eat with someone nearby.

Completely swallow each bite before taking another bite. Run your tongue around your mouth or look in a mirror to see if the food has cleared the mouth. "Sense" whether food has cleared the throat. Do you feel or see any food in the mouth? Do you feel food stuck in your throat? If you answer yes to either of these questions, attempt dry swallows until you can no longer see or feel any food pieces.

Hydrating the Mouth

A dry mouth can make it difficult, or even impossible, to swallow. There are a few tricks to hydrate (moisten) the mouth and increase saliva. Use popsicles, hard sugarless candy, or crushed ice, or take frequent sips of water throughout the day. You can buy artificial saliva products such as Salivart at a drugstore. When saliva production is a problem, choose sour foods, which increase saliva production, and avoid sweet foods, which decrease saliva production. Always be sure that you are capable of swallowing your own saliva and thin liquids.

Positioning of Body and Head

The proper position can often markedly reduce swallowing difficulties. In the beginning, eat without the distraction of conversation or noise so that you can concentrate on the swallowing process. The standard position for swallowing is sitting as upright as possible with your hips at a right angle to your body. Sit in a firm chair, preferably one with a high back, so you can place a pillow behind your head. Place your feet on the floor or another firm surface. After you swallow, tilt your chin down toward your chest to close off the trachea (windpipe) and help prevent food moving into the lungs, which can cause pneumonia.

If you have to eat in bed, sit up and use a wedge-shaped cushion behind your back to achieve as upright a position as possible. If you are in a hospital bed, put the head of the bed in a full

(Continued from page 238)

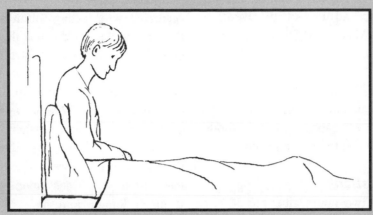

upright position. Never eat lying down or in a reclining position, unless your swallowing therapist has suggested these positions.

The position of your head is also important to effective and safe swallowing. Your swallowing therapist will prescribe the best head position for your particular swallowing needs.

Feeding Methods

The following tips may be helpful while you are learning to swallow and to manipulate foods of different consistencies. Be patient with yourself during all stages of your swallowing rehabilitation.

- Never rush feeding. Time and patience are needed on your part and the part of your caregiver.

- Always make sure your mouth, tongue, and teeth are brushed and clean before you start to eat.
- After eating, sit upright for at least twenty minutes.
- Do whatever exercises for lips, tongue, jaw, and swallow response your swallowing therapist prescribes. Do these four to eight times a day. The more frequently you do them, the faster you will recover.

You may wish to keep a record of your progress. The goal of your training program is to be able to swallow safely and enjoy your normal diet. By achieving this goal, you will help achieve another vital goal, a highly nutritious diet, which is crucial to your healing and well-being.

much or by eating foods that are too spicy or too fatty. Indigestion may also accompany stress, constipation, bloating, or eating when you have no appetite.

Tips to Avoid Heartburn

- Avoid spicy, acidic, tomato-based, or fatty foods such as citrus fruits, fruit juices, onions, garlic, and chocolate.
- Limit your intake of tea, alcohol, colas, coffee, and chocolate (including decaffeinated versions of these). Herbal teas are acceptable.
- Stop, or at least reduce, smoking.
- Watch your weight. Obesity causes an increases in intra-abdominal pressure, which can aggravate reflux.
- Eat small, frequent meals.

- Avoid exercising too soon after eating.
- Walk around after meals rather than sitting or lying down.
- Avoid bedtime snacks. Eat meals at least three or four hours before lying down.
- Elevate the head of your bed with 4- to 6-inch blocks to use gravity to drain stomach and gastric acids. Or, you can use several pillows to elevate your head when you are lying down or sleeping.
- Increase proteins.
- Use stress-reduction techniques.

Medications for Heartburn

An antacid taken one or two hours after meals and at bedtime may provide relief. If heartburn is excessive or recurrent, consult your doctor about stomach-acid blocking medicines such as Tagamet, Zantac, Pepcid, Axid, Prilosec, Prevacid, and Propulsid. Over-the-counter antacids include Maalox, Mylanta, Gaviscon, Tums, and Gelucil.

What You Can Do about Indigestion

Again, frequent small meals and a bland diet can be helpful. In general, avoid overeating and avoid foods that you have found cause you to get indigestion.

Medications for Indigestion

An antacid taken one or two hours after meals may help relieve indigestion discomfort. Antispasmodic drugs such as Donnatal help block acid production in the stomach.

Esophagitis

Esophagitus, or inflammation of the lining of the esophagus (the tube leading from the throat to the stomach), may be a side effect of chemotherapy or radiation therapy to the head and neck area. It may also occur because of infection.

The recommended dietary approach is similar to that used with a sore or ulcerated mouth or throat. In general, eat slowly and eat only small amounts at a time

Medication

Any medications should be prescribed by your physician. You might ask your doctor about gargling with and swallowing an analgesic solution such as liquid or Viscous Xylocaine gel before meals to lessen irritation. A similar solution may be made by dissolving 1 tbsp. (15ml) baking soda and 1 tsp. (5ml) salt in 1 quart (1L) warm water. Use 2–4 tbsp. (25ml–50ml) before each meal. Systemic analgesics such as Tylenol or codeine may be needed to relieve pain. Carafate (sucralfate) suspension may reduce symptoms and discomfort and help healing by coating the esophagus.

If symptoms persist, a candida (monilial fungal) infection may be present, which can be effectively treated with ketoconazole (Nizoral), nystatin (Mycostatin), fluconazole (Diflucan), amphotericin (Fungizone), itraconazole (Sporanox), or Mycelex.

Early Filling and Bloating (Satiety)

A common problem during radiation therapy or chemotherapy is early filling—a feeling of being full after having taken only few bites of food.

Bloating may be defined as an over-full feeling occurring after eating, often after just a few bites. Bloating is due to the inability of the stomach and intestines to properly digest the food you eat. It may also occur because of a slowdown of the passage of food from one part of the intestines to another, which may be caused by nervousness and tension; anticancer drugs, narcotics, strong pain-relieving and other medications; lack of adequate exercise; or constipation. Bloating may also be related to the type of food you eat. Fatty, fried, and greasy foods tend to remain in the stomach longer and may cause you to feel full. Carbonated drinks, gas-producing foods, and milk may also cause bloating.

What You Can Do

Eat frequent small meals instead of three large meals a day and emphasize starchy foods and low-fat protein foods. Sit up or walk around after meals.

Avoid fatty, fried, and greasy foods, gas-producing vegetables (such as dried beans and peas, broccoli, brussels sprouts, cabbage, cauliflower, corn, cucumber, green peppers, sauerkraut, turnips, and winter squash), carbonated drinks, chewing gum, and milk. Use Lactaid milk and yogurt, which are usually well tolerated. Stir carbonated drinks to remove gas bubbles.

Medications

Mylanta gas tablets or Tums Gas (simethicone) help relieve and reduce symptoms of excess gas.

Diarrhea

Several anticancer drugs can damage the digestive tract, at times leading to diarrhea. Specific drugs particularly associated with diarrhea are 5-FU, high dose methotrexate, cytarabine, capecitabine (Xeloda), and irinotecan (Camptosar). Because it is difficult to predict which patients will develop diarrhea, prevention is not an effective management strategy and antidiarrheal therapy is the mainstay of treatment. Diarrhea is a condition marked by abnormally frequent bowel movements that are more fluid than usual. It is sometimes accompanied by cramps. You may get diarrhea because of chemotherapy, radiation therapy to the lower abdomen, malabsorption because of surgery to the bowel, or sometimes a bowel inflammation (ileitis or colitis) or infection. Some antibiotics, especially broad-spectrum antibiotics, can cause diarrhea. Diarrhea may also develop because of an intolerance to milk (see "Milk (Lactose) Intolerance" on page 242), difficulty in absorbing fats, sensitivity to a specific food or group of foods, food allergy, or emotional or psychological problems.

Treatment

Adequate fluid intake is critical in preventing dehydration. Drinking water, soup, or noncaffeinated beverages are adequate in mild diarrhea, while an oral fluid replacement preparation (such as Gatorade) is often necessary for moderate cases. Intravenous fluid support might be required in a severe case of dehydration. Diarrhea can be controlled with Lomotil or Imodium, unless the diarrhea is caused by an infection.

Effective treatment depends on finding the cause. Patients who have had radiation therapy should avoid caffeine and drink 8–10 glasses a day of water or weak herbal teas. Rehydration formulas may be necessary. Loperamide or Lomotil are both effective antidiarrheal drugs.

Diarrhea caused by irinotecan (Camptosar) (CPT-II) is treated in a different manner. If diarrhea occurs less than twenty-four hours after the infusion, often before administering chemotherapy IV, atropine is given to control the symptoms. For late-onset diarrhea (more than twenty-four hours after infusion), the patient should take two caplets (4 mg) of Imodium (loperamide) after the first episode of loose stools, followed by one or two caplets (2–4 mg) every two hours until the patient is diarrhea-free for twelve hours. During the night, the patient should take two caplets (4 mg) every four hours. This regimen is tailored for irinotecan-treated patients and should not be used for others, unless indicated otherwise.

- Kaopectate (30 cc to 60 cc after each loose bowel movement).
- Lomotil (One or two tablets every two to six hours as needed to a maximum of eight tablets a day. Most patients require only two or three tablets per day after the diarrhea has been controlled).
- Imodium (loperomide) (two tablets initially followed by one tablet after each loose stool, not to exceed sixteen tablets per day); Imodium is also available in liquid or tablet form without a prescription.
- Donnatal (one or two tablets every four hours for abdominal cramping).

- Paregoric (1 tsp./5 ml every four hours) (requires a physician's triplicate prescription).
- Tincture of opium is very successful for severe uncontrollable diarrhea (requires a physician's narcotic triplicate prescription).
- For severe diarrhea from drugs, infections, or post-surgery, octreotide (Sandostatin) injections can be helpful.

A general approach is to limit your diet solely to fluids to allow the bowel to rest. Drink plenty of mild liquids, such as low-acid fruit juices and Gatorade, ginger ale (regular, not diet), peach or apricot nectar, water, and weak tea. Hot and cold liquids and foods tend to increase intestinal muscle contractions and make the diarrhea worse, so they should be warm or at room temperature. *Allow carbonated beverages to lose their fizz or stir them before you drink them.* Inform your physician, nutritionist, or health care team if you are on this diet longer than one day.

When you are feeling better, gradually add foods low in roughage and bulk. Examples include steamed rice, cream of rice, bananas, applesauce, mashed potatoes, and dry toast and crackers. These foods should be eaten warm or at room temperature.

As your diarrhea decreases, you may move on to a low-residue diet (see Chapter 28, "Modified Diets"). Frequent small meals will be easier on your digestive tract.

Foods to Avoid

Many types of foods are likely to aggravate your diarrhea and should be avoided. These include:

- fatty, greasy, and spicy foods
- coffee, regular (not herbal) teas, and carbonated drinks containing caffeine and/or artificial sweetener
- citrus fruits, such as oranges and grapefruits
- popcorn, nuts, and raw vegetables and fruits (except apples)
- drinks and foods that are served too hot or too cold
- milk not containing Lactaid

What You Can Do

- Talk to your physician and other health team members to determine the cause of the problem. It may be due to a variety of causes as mentioned earlier, including an intestinal blockage (adhesions), antibiotics, or the cancer.

- Diarrhea can cause dehydration, so you will have to drink plenty of fluids (see "Clear Liquid Diet" in Chapter 28.) When you have diarrhea, food passes through the gut more quickly, so many nutrients are not absorbed. You also lose electrolytes (sodium, potassium, chloride, and bicarbonate), which are vital to the fluid balance of your body. To replace the fluid, sugar, and salt you will lose, a general formula is: 1 quart (1 l) boiled water, 1 tsp. (5 ml) salt, 1 tsp. (5 ml) baking soda, 4 tsp. (20 ml) sugar, and flavor to your taste. As with any specially prepared concoction, however, check with your dietitian or doctor to make sure you can tolerate the ingredients.
- Potassium is lost when you suffer from diarrhea. It is a necessary mineral and must be replaced. Foods high in potassium include bananas, apricot and peach nectars, tomatoes, potatoes, broccoli, asparagus, and citrus juices. A potassium supplement may be needed if diarrhea persists.
- Gatorade may be useful for replacing fluid, potassium, and electrolytes.
- Try the BRAT diet: bananas, rice, applesauce, tea, and toast.
- Eat foods that are high in protein and calories.
- Reduce your intake of foods that are high in roughage and residue.
- Talk with your dietitian about ways to improve your diet.
- Ileostomy and colostomy diarrhea may be severe enough to require specific medical and dietary treatment and foods.
- An antidiarrhea medication, such as Kaopectate, may be prescribed.

Milk (Lactose) Intolerance

Lactose intolerance sometimes can develop after intestinal surgery, radiation therapy to the lower abdomen, or chemotherapy. Some people are also born with lactose intolerance or develop it later. The intolerance results from a deficiency of lactase, an enzyme that digests milk sugar (lactose) in the intestine; the intolerance is marked by bloating, cramping, and diarrhea.

- If your diarrhea is caused by lactose intolerance, avoid milk and milk products such as ice cream, cottage cheese, and cheese. Depending on how sensitive you are to milk, you may also have to avoid butter, cream, and sour cream.
- If you are very sensitive, use lactose-free, nonfat milk solids or soy milk.
- You can make your own lactose-free milk by adding Lactaid—a tablet containing lactase—to your milk and then keeping it in the refrigerator for twenty-four hours before drinking it.
- You can use buttermilk and yogurt because the lactose in them has already been processed and is easily digested.
- Try some processed cheeses to see if your body can tolerate them.
- Try Mocha-mix, Dairy Rich, and other soy products, or lactose-free substitutes, such as Imo (an imitation sour cream), and Cool Whip.
- See the "Lactose-Free/Lactose-Restricted Diet" in Chapter 28.

Constipation

Constipation may be due to a number of drugs used in the management of patients with cancer, including narcotic analgesics (painkillers); "vinca" chemotherapy drugs, including vincristine (Oncovin), vinblastine (Velban), and vinorelbine (Navelbine); and calcium-containing antacids (Tums). Patients administered any of the above drugs should be given a bowel regimen in order to maintain normal bowel functioning.

Narcotic analgesics administered by any route (oral, topical, or injection) may cause substantial decrease in bowel movements by inhibiting the nerves in the gastrointestinal tract. Drugs such as oral morphine (MS Contin), oral oxycodone (Oxycontin), fentanyl (Duragesic) topical patch, injectable morphine, and hydrocodone (Dilaudid) have been implicated. The vinca chemotherapy drugs frequently cause constipation beginning within seven days of therapy. Elderly patients are particularly susceptible to constipation from both narcotics and vincas.

Any patients started on these drugs should also be taking adequate fluids and fruits (prunes or raisins) to stimulate bowel functioning. In addition, a stimulant laxative such as Senokot or Dulcolax, along with a stool softener such as Ducosate (Colace), should be taken concurrently with narcotics. If Senokot is ineffective, a prescription medication may be required such as lactulose or Miralax or an over-the-counter solution of citrate of magnesia may be required. The usual doses of medications to prevent and treat constipation are shown in the table below.

Constipation is defined as infrequent bowel movements, compared with your normal pattern. It is often accompanied by decreased appetite and a bloated feeling. It commonly results from inadequate fiber or bulk-forming foods in the diet, not drinking enough fluid, emotional stress, or lack of exercise.

Constipation may be caused by some chemotherapy drugs such as vincristine, vinblastine, and vinorelbine. Other drugs that are constipating include pain-relieving narcotics such as morphine and codeine, gastrointestinal antispasmodics, antidepressants, diuretics, tranquilizers, sleeping pills, calcium- and aluminum-based antacids, and iron. When prescribing these drugs, your doctor should anticipate the need for a stool softener or a laxative. Enemas or suppositories might also be needed.

What You Can Do

Add foods to your diet that are high in fiber and bulk, such as fresh fruits and vegetables, dried fruits, dried beans, whole-grain breads, cereals, and bran. If you are not used to eating these foods, proceed slowly. A product such as Beano may help eliminate the bloating sometimes associated with eating these foods.

- Drink plenty of liquids.
- A glass of prune juice or hot lemon water taken in the morning may help.
- Eat fresh fruits and vegetables, including their skins. (Check with your medical team first if your white blood cell count is lower than 1,500 and absolute neutrophil count is less than 500.)
- Eat cooked dried beans and peas such as lentils, split peas, and kidney, garbanzo, and lima beans.
- Eat whole-grain products—cereals such as bran cereals or shredded wheat, foods made with whole-grain flours, and other whole grains, such as bulgur and wheat berries.
- Add unprocessed wheat bran to homemade breads, cereals, pancakes, casseroles, and baked goods.
- Add bran to your diet. Start with 2 tsp. (10 ml) per day. Increase your fluid intake when you eat bran, as bran works by absorbing fluid, increasing stools, and promoting a bowel movement.
- Exercise routinely. Your doctor or physical therapist can help design a program for you (see Chapter 32, "Rehabilitation Exercises").
- Check with your doctor before taking any medications.

Medication

Laxatives and enemas are sometimes needed in addition to these other measures, but they should be used only under the direction of your physician. Many types of laxatives are available; your physician and other health care team members will help you find the best one to fit your specific situation.

Patients requiring narcotics should not take bulk-forming laxatives because the combination causes constipation; stool softeners may be used instead. Certain other laxatives, when used continually, irritate the digestive tract and often make it difficult to regain normal bowel habits once they are discontinued. Increasing doses may also make your colon and rectum insensitive to the normal reflexes that stimulate a bowel movement.

Don't try to diagnose and treat yourself, as there may be more to the situation than you realize. For example, diarrhea can occasionally develop at the same time as a stool impaction (one that is not moving through the system), with the liquid stools moving around the impaction. If you take antidiarrheal drugs, you can make the situation much worse.

- Stool softeners help the stool retain water and so keep it soft. Stool softeners such as Colace (docusate) should be used early, before the stools become hard, especially as it can be days before any effect is noticeable.
- Mild laxatives help promote bowel activity. Examples are milk of magnesia, Doxidan, cascara sagrada, and mineral oil (a lubricant).
- Stronger laxatives include Phospho-soda (Fleet's), magnesium citrate, and sennoside (Senokot).
- Contact laxatives, such as castor oil, glycerin suppositories, and Dulcolax suppositories or tablets, cause increased bowel activity. (Dulcolax may cause cramping.)
- Bulk laxatives include dietary fiber, bran, methyl cellulose (Cellothyl), and psyllium (Metamucil).
- Laxatives with magnesium should be avoided if you have kidney disease. (Laxatives that contain magnesium can also cause diarrhea.) Laxatives with sodium should be avoided if you have a heart problem.
- If you are taking narcotics, use stool softeners and mild or strong laxatives rather than bulk-forming laxatives (Metamucil), because the

CONSTIPATION MEDICATIONS			
Drug Name	**Usual Dose**	**Side Effects**	**Cost**
Senokot	tablets twice daily until regular bowel functioning, then 1 tablet/day	Stomach upset	$
Colace (Ducosate)	capsules (100mg each) twice daily	None	$
Dulcolax	1 or 2 tablets daily until regular bowel functioning, then 1 tablet/day	Stomach upset irritation	$
Lactulose (Chronulac)	15–30 ml two to three times daily to induce bowel functioning	Diarrhea (excessive dose); flatulence	$ $$$
Miralax	17 grams (1 teaspoon)	Nausea, bloating, cramping	$

combinaton can cause high colon constipation. A good prescription is Colace and Senokot.

- Nonstimulating bulk softeners such as Colace (ducosate) help to soften the stool, and mineral oil or olive oil can be used to loosen the stool.
- Bowel stimulants such as Reglan may be useful.
- Lactulose (Chronulac) has an osmotic effect, drawing water into the gut to soften the stools and stimulate an increase in the number of bowel movements. This is usually effective and well tolerated.

Treating Stool Impaction

A stool impaction develops when all of a stool doesn't pass through the colon or rectum. The stool gradually gets harder as the bowel absorbs water from it, and then it gets larger. If you cannot pass it, it may partly obstruct the bowel or irritate the rectum or anus. If you do pass it, it may cause small tears or fissures in the anus. You may need to see a proctologist (rectal specialist) to treat the problem.

The primary treatment is to get fluids into the bowel to soften the stool so it can be passed or removed. Using enemas—oil-based, tap or saline water, or phosphate (Fleet's)—may help accomplish this goal. Sometimes it might be necessary for a health professional to use a gloved finger in the rectum to break up and extract a large stool or to give you a high warm saline colonic enema.

Malabsorption

Cancer sometimes results in calories and nutrients from food not being absorbed normally from the intestines into the bloodstream. For example, a decrease in the digestive juices that regulate absorption may be caused by cancer of the pancreas, the organ that produces many of these juices.

If you decrease your normal food intake, the intestines become unable to absorb nutrients as well as they did before. A healthy gastrointestinal tract requires food to stimulate it and maintain it in a healthy state. When you resume eating after decreased food intake, bloating or diarrhea occur, and your ability to correct this cycle by eating lessens as your nutrition becomes poorer. So to keep your gastrointestinal tract healthy, you must continue to eat, even though you may not necessarily feel like it.

Dehydration

Dehydration is a lack of fluid in the body. It may occur after surgery, radiation, or chemotherapy, or as a result of diarrhea, sweating, fever, nausea, or an inability to drink fluids.

What You Can Do

Increase your sources of fluid; try fruit and vegetable juices, fruit drinks, Gatorade sports drink, punch, soft drinks, decaffeinated and herbal teas, milk, milkshakes, eggnogs, soup, low-salt broth, fruits with a high fluid content such as grapes or watermelon, Jell-O, ice cream, sherbet or sorbets, fruit ices, and Popsicles (see Chapter 28 for high-protein, high-calorie beverages). If you cannot drink liquids or if you eat and become dehydrated, you may need to go to your doctor's office, infusion center, or emergency room for IV (intravenous) fluids.

Water Retention

The body may retain excess salt and water in the arms or legs because of removal of or radiation of the lymph glands, which filter excess fluid from body tissues. Water retention may also occur in the abdomen, chest, head, or neck because of cancer therapy or the cancer itself. Hormonal drugs, such as cortisone, Prednisone, testosterone, and estrogens, also may cause the body to retain excess salt and water.

What You Can Do

Decrease your intake of salt, because salt causes you to retain fluids. There are two levels of salt-restricted diets: one allowing a small amount of salt, the other restricting salt severely.

Low-Salt Diet

This diet restricts sodium to about 2–3 grams a day, the equivalent of 1–1½ tsp. (5–7 ml) salt. Do not add any salt to food while it is being cooked, and (depending on your diet) add only a very small amount to food at the table. Foods vary in their natural salt content. Ask your dietitian for guidance.

Salt substitutes such as Morton's Salt Substitute and Adolph's Salt Substitute may help satisfy your need for a salty taste without adding to fluid-retention problems. Salt substitutes may add potassium instead of sodium. Check with your doctor to be sure that this is appropriate for you. Some salt substitutes taste better than others, and you may need to try several before finding the one that suits you best. Also, some, even though they are salt substitutes, still contain sodium (which you are trying to avoid), so read the label carefully before you buy.

You must also read the labels on all foods you eat to avoid foods with naturally high salt content, such as:

- bouillon and canned soups
- canned, cured, and dry meat and fish, such as bacon, cold cuts, corned beef, canned herring, and sardines
- salted crackers, nuts, potato chips, corn chips, and other snack foods
- packaged foods, such as rice mixes and macaroni and cheese
- soy sauce, catsup, and barbecue sauce
- cheeses (you may need to limit total dairy consumption)

Restricted-Salt Diet

This diet restricts salt to about ½ gram a day, equivalent to ¼ tsp. (1 ml) salt. It requires the use of special milk, bread, and other food products low in salt. If you need to restrict salt, your physician will prescribe a special diet for you.

Medications

Your physician may prescribe a diuretic, a drug that will cause you to lose excess fluid and salt through the urine.

Diuretics may cause you to lose too much potassium, a mineral that is important to body functioning. If you are taking diuretics, you may need to eat foods that are high in potassium, such as apricots, bananas, cantaloupe, dates, dried figs, milk, orange juice, potatoes, prunes, raisins, tangerine juice, and tomato juice. Your physician may also suggest a potassium supplement.

Kidney Stones

Some drugs can cause patients to form kidney stones. There may be no symptoms, or patients may have an ashen pallor combined with very severe back pain. The degree of pain depends on the amount of urine that is backed up behind the obstruction caused by the kidney stone.

If a stone is small enough to pass through the urinary tract, collect it and give it to your doctor. It is important that your doctor determine the type of kidney stone you have (uric acid or calcium oxalate) before prescribing a special diet.

If You Have Calcium Oxalate Kidney Stones

Take these steps to acidify the urine:

- Reduce intake of foods high in phosphate, such as dairy products, eggs, organ meats, and whole grains.
- Reduce intake of foods high in oxalic acid, such as asparagus, spinach, cranberries, plums, tea, cocoa, and coffee.
- Drink at least ten to twelve glasses of water a day, (if local water is "hard," substitute distilled water).
- Consider taking vitamin B_6 and magnesium supplements.
- See your dietitian to determine other diet changes.

If You Have Uric Acid Kidney Stones

These are the most common type of kidney stone among those caused by chemotherapy. Take these steps to alkalinize the urine:

- Increase intake of alkaline-forming foods such as dairy products, fruits (especially dried fruts), vegetables (especially green beans and peas) and breads prepared with baking soda or baking powder.
- Reduce intake of meat, eggs, fish, poultry, cereals, breads, pasta, rice, cranberry juice, prune juice, and plums.
- Your physician may prescribe allopurinol (Zyloprim) to prevent uric acid crystals.

What You Can Do for All Types of Stones

- Drink large amounts of water—except "hard" (high-mineral-content) water—and fluids throughout the day and night. Aim for twelve glasses every twenty-four hours.
- Drink plenty of fluids with meals and snacks.
- Choose foods with a high water content.

Weight Loss

When you are being treated for cancer, it is important to try to maintain your desirable weight as closely as possible. The key is to maintain adequate calorie and protein intake.

Cancer patients (like patients being treated for burns, stress, or infections) may need up to 25 percent more calories than their bodies normally require. Keep a daily record of your calorie and protein intake. If you are losing weight, increase your calorie intake until you are no longer losing weight. It can be particularly helpful to develop a regular pattern of nibbling on high-calorie snacks.

Here are some ideas you can use at home to add extra calories and proteins to your everyday cooking:

- Add cream, evaporated milk, or fortified milk to cooked cereals, cream sauces, puddings, and soups.
- Use sour cream on baked potatoes and in cream soups.
- Use gravies and sauces on meats and vegetables.
- Add extra butter or margarine to cooked cereals, noodles, rice, sauces, soups, and vegetables.
- Add cheese or hard-cooked eggs to casseroles, noodles, rice, or sauces.

- Spread peanut butter or other nut butters on apple wedges or celery, and in cookies, frostings, and sandwich fillings.
- Use avacados freely.

Weight Gain

Weight gain can result from chemotherapy, hormonal therapy (Tamoxifen), prescribed steroids, abnormal fluid retention, and eating because of anxiety or frustration about your cancer.

Steroids (e.g., prednisone, dexamethasone, Decadron) may change your metabolism or the way your body uses calories when taken over an extended period of time. Steroids may also increase your appetite and cause fluid retention.

Keep track of how much weight you have gained and where you have gained it. If you are being treated for cancer, do not go on a strict weight-loss program, as your body requires nourishing food. However, there are things you can do to reduce weight gain. If you are gaining weight because of chemotherapy, hormonal therapy, or steroids, switch to a low-fat diet. If you are retaining fluid, a low-sodium diet or diuretics may be needed. Your dietitian can suggest appropriate food choices.

Pain

Pain is a problem for many cancer patients. Its effects can be mild or totally disabling. Pain can result in nutritional problems because pain can cause loss of appetite and seriously limit your ability to eat.

What You Can Do

Your physician's guidance in taking pain medications is important for effective pain control. Your physician can also help you learn special pain-control techniques. Mental relaxation and reduction of stress and anxiety will also work to reduce pain.

One point of great importance should be stressed: be sure your doctor is aware of all the medications you are taking. You may be treated by more than one doctor or dentist, and anyone prescribing medication must know of all medications you are receiving.

Depression, Anxiety, and Fear

Most people eat less when they are depressed. Seeing their bodies waste away may further convince depressed patients of the hopelessness of their situation—an often unfounded fear. Anxiety and fear can also take away appetite. The best treatment here is a positive approach toward your cancer therapy at all stages. (See Chapters 16, 17 and 18.)

28

Modified Diets

Bernadette Festa, M.S., R.D.
Ernest H Rosenbuam, M.D.
Isadora R. Rosenbaum, M.A.
Julie Matel, M.S., R.D.

The liquid and special diets described in this chapter are designed for various special needs. Your physician will recommend a diet appropriate for your medical condition and your dietitian will plan an individualized program based on your personal preferences and your cancer treatment.

Liquid and Soft Diets for Illness

On days when you are not feeling well because of illness or therapy, you may not feel like or may not be able to eat your normal diet. You will find you have to eat lighter foods or even liquid foods. As you start to feel better, you can add more solid foods and gradually progress back to your normal diet.

The following diets progress from simple, clear liquids that require little digestion, through liquids of thicker consistency, to a diet of soft-consistency solid foods. These dietary progressions are: clear liquid diet, full liquid diet, and soft diet.

Clear Liquid Diet

The clear liquid diet is your first step to returning to a regular diet when you are unable to eat solid foods because of surgery, a partial gastrointestinal obstruction, diarrhea, or your therapy. The diet consists of clear fluids or foods that will become liquid at body temperature. There is no fiber or residue in the diet.

The clear liquid diet alone—without supplements—does not provide adequate protein, calories, vitamins, and minerals and is not intended to be used for more than forty-eight hours.

Full Liquid Diet

The full liquid diet contains foods that are easy to eat. You may also progress directly to a clear liquid or a soft diet. A full liquid diet is good if you are experiencing a sore or dry mouth because of your therapy or if you have had oral surgery, but it may not provide adequate vitamins and minerals. Your health care provider will recommend high-calorie/high-protein

FOODS ALLOWED ON CLEAR LIQUID DIET

Food	Calories	Protein (grams)
clear broth	5–25	0
clear juices (apple, cranberry)	80–120	0
coffee or decaffeinated coffee	0	0
tea (regular or herbal)	0	0
fruit-ades (Kool-Aid, Gatorade, etc.)	60	0
mild carbonated beverages (ginger ale, 7-Up)	113	0
plain jelly dessert	65	1

supplements if you need to be on the diet for longer than two days.

In addition to the foods in the clear liquid diet, milk and milk proteins are allowed. Where no specific serving sizes are given, refer to *Bowes & Church's Food Values of Portions Commonly Used.*

Modified Consistency Diet

When a patient has problems chewing or swallowing, a soft, pureed, and blenderized diet is usually recommended. A soft or pureed diet contains whole foods that are tender and easy to chew. Foods containing coarse, whole grains or tough connective tissue, as well as raw fruits and vegetables and seeds and nuts, are omitted. A blenderized diet is similar to a full liquid diet except that it allows any foods that can be passed through a straw. It, too, is used by patients with mouth, jaw, and esophageal problems after surgery or during therapy. A pureed diet provides foods that are soft, smooth, and semi-liquid.

Soft Diet

The soft diet is used when your digestive ability has improved and you are able to advance from liquids to whole cooked foods. You may find, however, that you are still unable to tolerate some foods you normally eat, such as fried or spicy foods, raw or gas-forming vegetables, or hard foods such as nuts, popcorn, and pretzels. You may, therefore, need to eat a soft diet before resuming a normal diet. Frequent small meals may be better tolerated than three large meals a day if you are experiencing a lack of appetite or if you fill up after eating just a few bites of food. Between-meal snacks of eggnogs, milkshakes, and liquid high-protein diet supplements are recommended for extra calories and protein. Use lactaid milk or lactose-free supplements if you have trouble digesting milk products.

In addition to the foods in the full liquid diet, the following foods are allowed. Where no specific serving sizes are given, refer to *Bowes & Church's Food Values of Portions Commonly Used.*

FOODS ALLOWED ON FULL LIQUID DIET

Food	Calories	Protein (grams)
cooked cereal made with fortified milk	215	9
custard	205	9
eggnog	342	10
fortified milk	161	8
fruit juice (1 cup/250 ml)	120	0
high-protein supplements (e.g., Ensure Plus)	355	14
ice cream (¾ cup/175 ml)	174	4
milkshake	500	16
plain yogurt (low fat, 8 oz.)	122	8
popsicle	40	1
pudding	219	4
sherbet	130	1
strained cream soup	145	6
vegetable juice	17	1

FOODS ALLOWED ON MODIFIED CONSISTENCY DIET

Food	Calories	Protein (grams)
avocado, 1	167	2
banana, 1	125	1
butter and margarine, 1 tsp. (5 ml)	45	0
canned fruit, ½ cup (125 ml)	60	0
cooked mild vegetables (125 ml)	25	2
cottage cheese, 1 cup (250 ml)	240	31
cream cheese, 1 oz. (25 g)	105	2
cold or hot cereal, ¾ cup (175 ml), with milk ½ cup (125 ml)	235	10
egg, boiled or poached	75	6
eggs, scrambled	125	6
*fish, 3 oz. (75 g)	164	24
macaroni, 1 cup (250 ml)	151	5
mayonnaise, 1 tbsp. (15 ml)	101	0
*meat, 3 oz. (75 g)	225	21
mild processed cheese, 1 oz. (25 g)	112	7
omelet, 3 eggs, with 1 oz. (25 g) cheese	355	25
papaya, 1	115	2
pasta noodles, 1 cup (250 ml)	200	7
plain soft cakes and cookies, 1 oz. (25 g)	140	3
potato, 1 med.	80	2
*poultry, 3 oz. (75 g)	225	21
rice, cooked, 1 cup (250 ml)	164	3
salad dressing	75	0
smooth peanut butter, 1 tbsp. (15 ml)	115	5
soufflé cheese, ½ cup (125 ml)	10	9
tofu (soybean curd), 4 oz. (125 g)	75	8
white bread/toast, 1 slice	80	3

*baked, broiled, roasted or stewed until tender

The following foods are difficult to digest and should be avoided:

- bread with hard crusts, nuts, or seeds
- dried fruit
- fried foods
- horseradish, olives, pickles, and relish
- nuts, seeds, and coconut
- popcorn, potato chips, and pretzels
- raw fruit
- rich pastries

Special Diets

Sometimes your cancer or cancer therapy will cause problems that require a special diet. Your physician or dietitian may recommend one of the following diets to help you with these problems.

1. Pureed diet
2. Lactose-free/Lactose-restricted diet
3. Bland diet
4. Fat-restricted diet
5. Low-residue diet
6. Neutropenia diet
7. Vegetarian diets
8. Alternative nutrition
9. Nutritional supplements

Suggested recipes for foods recommended in these diets are given in Chapter 29, "Recipes for the Chemotherapy Patient."

Pureed Diet

A pureed diet provides foods that are soft, smooth, and free from whole, minced, or ground chunks of food. It

SAMPLE MENU FOR SOFT DIET

Breakfast (445 calories, 15 g protein)

Food	Calories	Protein
fruit juice, ½ cup (125 ml)	60	0
cooked cereal, ½ cup (125 ml)	65	3
fortified milk* or cream for cereal, ½ cup (125 ml)	80	4
soft-cooked egg, 1	81	6
toast, 1 slice, with butter, 1 tsp. (15 ml) and jelly, 1 tsp. (15 ml)	157	2
coffee/tea, 1 cup (250 ml)	2	0

Midmorning Snack (405 calories, 13 g protein)

Food	Calories	Protein
milkshake or liquid high-protein supplement, 1½ cups (375 ml)	405	13

Lunch (745 calories, 30 g protein)

Food	Calories	Protein
meat, poultry, or fish (roasted, baked, broiled, or stewed), 3 oz. (75 g)	225	21
gravy, ¼ cup (50 ml)	20	1
potato, boiled, baked, or mashed, ½ cup (125 ml)	70	2
green beans, ½ cup (125 ml)	16	1
bread, 1 slice	62	2
butter, 1 tsp. (5 ml)	45	0
canned fruit, ½ cup (125 ml) or banana	100	0
whole milk, 1 cup (250 ml)	160	2
coffee/tea, 1 cup (250 ml), with cream, 1 tbsp. (15 ml), sugar, 1 tsp. (15 ml)	50	0
herbal tea, such as peppermint	0	0

Midafternoon Snack (405 calories, 13 g protein)

Food	Calories	Protein
custard or pudding, ½ cup (125 ml)	200	6

Dinner (630 calories, 27 g protein)

Food	Calories	Protein
meat, poultry, or fish (roasted, baked, broiled or stewed), 3 oz. (75 g)	225	21
rice, ½ cup (125 ml)	82	2
gravy, ¼ cup (50 ml)	20	1
carrot, ¼ cup (50 ml)	15	1
bread, 1 slice	62	2
butter, 1 tsp. (5 ml)	45	0
sherbet, ½ cup (125 ml)	130	1
fruit juice, ½ cup (125 ml)	60	0

Evening Snack (405 calories, 13 g protein)

Food	Calories	Protein
milkshake or liquid high-protein supplement, 1½ cups (375 ml)	405	13

eliminates the need for chewing. It is used for people with chewing and swallowing difficulties.

Pureed foods can be purchased in the form of baby food or you can prepare them at home in a blender or food processor. If you are experiencing a loss of appetite or tend to fill up easily, you may find it better to eat frequent small meals instead of three large meals a day. Adding eggnogs, milkshakes, and liquid

FOOD ALLOWED ON PUREED DIET

Food	Calories	Protein (grams)
avocado, 1	167	2
banana, 1	185	1
canned, pureed, stewed fruits, ½ cup (125 ml)	100	1
cooked/dry cereals, ¾ cup (175 ml), with milk	235	10
cooked pureed vegetables, ½ cup (125 ml)	25	2
cottage cheese, 1 cup (250 ml)	240	31
cream cheese, 1 oz. (25 g)	105	2
cream soup, ¾ cup (175 ml)	145	6
custard, ½ cup (125 ml)	205	9
eggnog, 1 cup (250 ml)	42	10
egg, boiled or poached	81	6
egg, scrambled	125	6
fish, meat, poultry (finely ground/pureed), 3 oz. (75 g)		
served in broth	250	25
served in cream sauce	285	22
high-protein diet supplements, 1 cup (250 ml)	250	14
malted milk drinks, milkshakes, 1 cup (250 ml)	200	12
mashed potatoes, ½ cup (125 ml)	70	2
papaya, 1	115	2
popsicles	60	1
pudding, ½ cup (125 ml)	175	6
regular ice cream, 1 cup (250 ml)	250	4
sherbet, 1 cup (250 ml)	250	1
soufflés	210	9
tofu (soybean curd), 4 oz. (125 g)	75	8
vegetable juices, ½ cup (125 ml)	20	1
yogurt, low fat with fruit, 1 cup (250 ml)	200	8
If you are able to chew, you may add:		
graham crackers, 4	120	2
macaroni with cheese, 1 cup (250 ml)	151	5
plain soft cakes (1) and cookies (3)	140	3
rice, 1 cup (250 ml)	164	3
saltines, 6	80	2
white bread toast, 1 slice	80	2

high-protein supplements as between-meal snacks will increase your protein and calorie intake.

The foods above are tolerated well. Unless otherwise indicated, the amounts are for one serving.

Foods Not Well-Tolerated
- bread with hard crusts
- coconut, nuts, and raisins
- fish, meat, and poultry pieces
- jams and preserves containing seeds or tough skins
- olives, peppers, raw vegetables
- raw fruit that is not pureed, except bananas and papayas
- smoked, spiced, or processed meats
- tart juices if they irritate the mouth

SAMPLE MENU FOR PUREED DIET

Breakfast (495 calories, 15 g protein)

Food	Calories	Protein
fruit juice, ½ cup (125 ml)	60	0
cooked cereal, ½ cup (125 ml)	67	3
soft-cooked egg, 1	75	6
bread, 1 slice, with butter, 1 tsp., and jelly, 1 tsp.	157	2
fortified milk or cream (for cereal), ½ cup (125 ml)	80	4
coffee/tea, 1 cup (250 ml), with cream, 1 tbsp. (15 ml), sugar, 1 tsp. (15 ml)	50	0

Midmorning Snack (405 calories, 13 g protein)

Food	Calories	Protein
milkshake/liquid high-protein supplement, 1½ cups (375 ml)	405	13

Lunch (715 calories, 36 g protein)

Food	Calories	Protein
finely ground or pureed meat, poultry, or fish, 3 oz. (75 g)	225	21
potato, mashed, boiled, or baked, ½ cup (125 ml)	70	2
gravy, ¼ cup (50 ml)	20	1
pureed cooked vegetables, ½ cup (125 ml)	25	2
bread, 1 slice, with butter, 1 tsp. (15 ml)	107	2
pureed fruit, ½ cup (125 ml)	60	1
whole milk, 1 cup (250 ml)	160	8
coffee/tea, 1 cup (250 ml), with cream, 1 tbsp. (15 ml), sugar, 1 tsp. (15 ml)	50	0

Midafternoon Snack (200 calories, 6 g protein)

Food	Calories	Protein
custard or pudding, ½ cup (125 ml)	200	6

Dinner (530 calories, 27 g protein)

Food	Calories	Protein
finely ground or pureed meat, poultry or fish, 3 oz. (75 g)	225	21
boiled rice, ½ cup (125 ml)	82	2
gravy, ¼ cup (50 ml)	20	1
pureed cooked vegetables, ½ cup (125 ml)	25	2
sherbet, ½ cup (125 ml)	130	1
coffee/tea, 1 cup (250 ml), with cream, 1 tbsp. (15 ml), sugar, 1 tsp. (15 ml)	50	0

Evening Snack (405 calories, 13 g protein)

Food	Calories	Protein
milkshake or liquid high-protein supplement, 1½ cups (375 ml)	405	13

Lactose-Free/Lactose-Restricted Diet

Milk (lactose) intolerance results from a deficiency of lactase, an enzyme that breaks down milk sugar (lactose) in the intestine. It is marked by bloating, cramping, and diarrhea. Sometimes it is caused by chemotherapy, intestinal surgery, or radiation herapy to the lower abdomen. If you were not previously lactose-intolerant, you should be able to return to your normal diet once your treatment has ended.

What You Can Do

- Read food labels and avoid foods containing lactose. Lactic acid or lactate will probably not be a problem.
- Buy Lactaid, a lactase enzyme, at your drugstore

or supermarket. This breaks down the milk sugar for proper digestion and absorption in the body.

There are different degrees of lactose intolerance. To determine the degree of your sensitivity, first eliminate all sources of lactose (see the Foods Prohibited list). Three days later, add back milk treated with Lactaid. Every two or three days, add Lactaid to a previously excluded food and try it again in your diet. If you tolerate that food, keep using it; if you don't, exclude it for now and try it again later. Follow this regimen as long as symptoms are a problem.

Foods Allowed

Beverages: Mocha-Mix; Poly Rich; carbonated drinks; coffee (read the labels); Lidalac and other lactose-free milks or milks treated with lactase enzyme (Lactaid); yogurt; and lactose-free products such as Ensure, Ensure Plus, Resource soy milk, and Vitasoy.

Breads and Cereals: breads and rolls made without milk; bagels; Italian bread; some cooked cereals; prepared cereals (read the labels); macaroni; spaghetti; rice, and soda crackers.

Meat, Fish, Poultry, Tofu: beef, chicken, turkey, lamb, veal, pork, and ham; strained or junior meats; meat combinations that do not contain milk or milk products; kosher frankfurters; eggs prepared without milk or prepared with Lactaid-treated milk; and tofu.

Vegetables: fresh, canned, and frozen artichokes, asparagus, beets, broccoli, cabbage, carrots, cauliflower, celery, corn, cucumbers, eggplant, green beans, kale, lettuce, lima beans, mustard greens, okra, onions, parsley, parsnips, pumpkin, rutabagas, spinach, squash, tomatoes, white and sweet potatoes, and yams. Beware of cream-based sauces.

Fruits: all fresh, canned, and frozen fruits that are not processed with lactose (read the labels).

Fats: margarine and dressings that do not contain milk or milk products; oils; bacon; some whipped toppings; some nondairy creamers (read the labels); and nut butters and nuts.

Soups: clear soups; vegetable soups; consommés; and cream soups made with Mocha-Mix, Lactaid, or nondairy creamer.

Desserts: water and fruit ices; frozen fruit bars (read label); gelatin; angel food cake; homemade cakes; pies and cookies made from allowed ingredients; and puddings made with water or milk treated with lactase enzymes.

Miscellaneous: carbonated drinks; carob powder; cocoa powder; corn syrup; gravy made with water; instant coffees that do not contain lactose (read the labels); jelly, jam, or marmalade; molasses (made from beet sugar); olives; pickles; popcorn; pure seasonings and spices; soy sauce; sugar; pure sugar candy; and wine.

Foods Prohibited

Beverages: untreated milks of animal origin and all milk-containing products (except lactose-free milk), such as skim, dry, evaporated, and condensed milk, yogurt, ice cream, sherbet, malted milk, Ovaltine, hot chocolate, cocoas, and instant coffees that contain lactose (read the label); powdered soft drinks; and milk that has been treated with *Lactobacillus acidophilus* culture rather than lactase.

Bread and Cereals: prepared mixes that contain lactose (read the label) for making muffins, biscuits, waffles, or pancakes; and Bisquick or similar mixes. Prepared foods include cornbread; some dry cereals, such as Total, Special K, and Cocoa Krispies (read the label); Instant Cream of Wheat; commercial breads and rolls to which milk solids have been added; Zwieback; and french toast made with milk.

Dairy, Meat, Fish, Poultry: creamed or breaded meat, fish, or fowl; sausage products, such as frankfurters; liver sausage; cold cuts containing nonfat milk solids or cheese; egg dishes, omelets, and soufflés containing milk or cheese; and cheese, cottage cheese, and yogurt.

Vegetables: any vegetables to which lactose is added during processing, such as creamed vegetables, breaded or buttered vegetables, instant potatoes, corn curls, or frozen french fries processed with lactose.

Fruits: any canned or frozen fruits processed with lactose (read the labels).

Fats: margarine and dressings containing milk or milk products; butter, cream, cream cheese, and sour cream; peanut butter with milk-solid fillers; salad dressings containing lactose (read the label).

Desserts: commercial cakes, cookies, and baking mixes; custards and puddings; sherbet and ice cream made with milk; ice milk and frozen yogurt; anything containing chocolate; pie crust made with butter; gelatin made with carrageenan; and whipping cream.

Miscellaneous: chewing gum, peppermints, butterscotch, caramels, and chocolate; cocoas, coffee, and

SAMPLE MENU FOR BLAND DIET

Breakfast (525 calories, 19 g protein)

Food	Calories	Protein
fruit juice, ½ cup (125 ml)	60	0
cooked cereal, ½ cup (125 ml)	67	3
boiled or poached egg, 1	75	6
white toast, 1 slice, with butter, 1 tsp. (15 ml) and jelly 1 tsp. (15 ml)	157	2
fortified milk or cream (for cereal), 1 cup (250 ml)	160	8
herbal tea, 1 cup (250 ml)	0	0

Midmorning Snack (405 calories, 13 g protein)

Food	Calories	Protein
milkshake or liquid diet supplement, 1½ cups (375 ml)	405	13

Lunch (525 calories, 26 g protein)

Food	Calories	Protein
meat, poultry, or fish, 3 oz. (75 g)	225	21
potato (boiled, baked or mashed), ½ cup (125 ml)	70	2
green beans, ½ cup (125 ml)	16	1
white bread and butter, 1 slice	107	2
canned peaches, ½ cup (125 ml)	96	0

Midafternoon Snack (575 calories, 19 g protein)

Food	Calories	Protein
custard or pudding, ½ cup (125 ml)	575	19

Dinner (550 calories, 27 g protein)

Food	Calories	Protein
meat, poultry or fish, 3 oz. (75 g)	225	21
boiled rice, ½ cup (125 ml)	82	2
cooked carrots, ½ cup (125 ml)	15	1
white bread, 1 slice, with butter, 1 tsp. (15 ml)	107	2
sherbet, ½ cup (125 ml)	130	1

Evening Snack (405 calories, 13 g protein)

Food	Calories	Protein
milkshake or liquid diet supplement, 1½ cups (375 ml)	405	13

spice blends that contain milk products; MSG extender; artificial sweeteners containing lactose, such as Equal and Sweet 'n Low; some nondairy creamers containing lactose (read the label); dips made with milk products; some antibiotics; and vitamin and mineral preparations.

Bland Diet

The bland diet consists of foods that are soft and do not irritate the stomach. It eliminates fried, highly seasoned, and raw foods. The bland diet is recommended if you are experiencing heartburn or indigestion. All foods recommended on the soft diet are included. You may find it easier to tolerate frequent, small meals rather than three large meals a day. Between-meal snacks of eggnog, milkshakes, and liquid diet supplements are recommended for extra protein and calories.

The following foods are highest in protein and calories: cottage cheese; custard; eggnog; eggs; fish, meat, and poultry (baked, broiled, steamed, roasted, or stewed); liquid diet supplements; milk and fortified milk; milkshakes; puddings; smooth peanut butter; tofu (soybean curd); and yogurt made with whole milk.

LOW-FAT/HIGH-PROTEIN FOODS

Food	Calories	Protein
buttermilk, 1 cup	100	8
custards/puddings made with nonfat milk, ½ cup	205	9
egg (2 per week)	81	6
eggnogs made with nonfat milk	250	10
fish, lean meat, poultry (without skin)	165	21
high-protein diet supplements made with nonfat milk, juice, or water	400	13
nonfat milk or fortified milk	103	10
nonfat yogurt	122	8
tofu (soybean curd)	75	8

The following foods are potentially irritating and should be avoided: coffee and tea; fried foods; raw and dried fruits (except avocados, bananas, and papayas); garlic; highly seasoned foods; horseradish; fresh and dried legumes; smoked, spiced, or processed meat, such as bacon, luncheon meats, and sausage; nuts, seeds, and coconut; olives; pepper; potato chips; relishes; gas-forming vegetables, such as broccoli, brussels sprouts, cabbage, cauliflower, corn, cucumber, green peppers, onions, rutabaga, sauerkraut, and turnips; and raw vegetables.

Fat-Restricted Diet

The fat-restricted diet is helpful if you are experiencing a full feeling or bloating after eating only a few bites of food. This diet eliminates rich, greasy, and fatty foods, which tend to "sit" in the stomach. You may tolerate frequent small meals better than three large meals a day. Between-meal snacks low in fat will help add calories without ruining your appetite. Nonfat milk or buttermilk should be substituted for whole milk. Plain cakes and cookies, fruit ices, Jell-O, puddings made with nonfat milk, and sherbet make good low-fat desserts. All nonfatty foods are included in the fat-restricted diet.

Foods Prohibited

Prohibited foods in the fat-restricted diet include avocados; bacon; more than 1–2 tsp. (5–10 ml) butter, margarine, or mayonnaise per day; chocolate; cream and whipping cream; duck and goose; fish packed in oil; french fries and other fried foods; greasy gravies; ice cream; luncheon meats; nuts; peanut butter; potato chips; rich desserts; sausage; rich or highly seasoned sauces; and whole milk.

Low-Residue Diet

The low-residue diet consists of soft, easily digestible foods. "Residue" refers to indigestible material in food, sometimes called fiber. When the intestines are irritated, as in diarrhea, fiber may add to the irritation. The purpose of the low-fiber, low-residue diet is to minimize stool output.

Foods Allowed

These include white breads, rolls, and biscuits; refined grain products; plain bagels; plain cake and donuts; cookies without nuts; cold cereals such as corn flakes, Rice Krispies, and Cheerios; cream of wheat; instant oatmeal; cooked, peeled, seedless fruits; ripe bananas; applesauce; canned fruit; fruit juices without pulp; jellies without seeds; meats and other ground or well-cooked protein foods including tender beef, lamb, ham, pork, poultry, organ meats, fish, eggs, and cheese; pasta, white rice, and tortillas; sherbet; cooked peeled seedless vegetables; and vegetable juice without pulp.

Foods Prohibited

These include whole-grain products and baked goods; raw fruits and vegetables; seeds, nuts, and legumes. Milk is restricted to 2 cups (500 ml) per day, including that used in cooking, and is prohibited entirely if you have diarrhea.

Neutropenia Diet

During chemotherapy or radiation therapy, there may be a decrease in blood counts—white blood cells, red blood cells, and platelets. Neutropenia is a lack of special white blood cells called neutrophils or polymorphonuclear cells (PMNs or polys), which fight

SAMPLE MENU FOR FAT-RESTRICTED DIET

Breakfast (330 calories, 19 g protein)

Food	Calories	Protein
fruit juice, ½ cup (125 ml)	60	0
egg, boiled or poached	81	6
cooked cereal, ½ cup (125 ml)	67	3
toast, 1 slice	15	2
nonfat milk, 1 cup (250 ml)	88	8
coffee/tea, 1 cup (250 ml)	19	0

Midmorning Snack (400 calories, 13 g protein)

Food	Calories	Protein
high-protein supplement made with water, nonfat milk, or juice, 1½ cups (375 ml)	400	13

Lunch (675 calories, 35 g protein)

Food	Calories	Protein
broth, 1 cup (250 ml)	23	2
meat, poultry or fish, 3 oz. (75 g)	225	21
potato (mashed, boiled, or baked), ½ cup (125 ml)	70	2
cooked vegetables, ½ cup (125 ml)	25	0
bread with 1 tsp. (5 ml) butter, 1 slice	107	2
applesauce, 1 cup (250 ml)	119	0
nonfat milk, 1 cup (250 ml)	88	8
coffee/tea, 1 cup (250 ml)	0	0

Midafternoon Snack (350 calories, 10 g protein)

Food	Calories	Protein
sherbet shake, 1½ cups (375 ml)	350	10

Dinner (525 calories, 28 g protein)

Food	Calories	Protein
meat, poultry or fish, 3 oz. (75 g)	225	21
boiled rice, ½ cup (125 ml)	82	2
cooked vegetables, ½ cup (125 ml)	25	2
bread with 1 tsp. (5 ml) butter, 1 slice	107	2
nonfat pudding with peaches	100	4
coffee or tea with sugar, 1 cup (250 ml)	19	0

infections caused by bacteria, fungi, or viruses. Neutropenic patients are more susceptible to serious infections.

Some basic guidelines:

- Washing hands before eating reduces the risk of infection.
- Refrigerate leftovers immediately.
- Sanitize chopping boards.
- If purchasing deli foods, avoid the first slice of cold cuts.

Vegetarian Diets

A vegetarian diet generally refers to a diet that omits meat, fish, and poultry. However, a number of variations exist.

- A vegan or total vegetarian diet includes only plant foods.
- An ovo-vegetarian diet includes eggs.
- A lacto-vegetarian diet includes dairy products.
- A lacto-ovo-vegetarian diet includes dairy products and eggs.

SAMPLE MENU FOR LOW-RESIDUE (HIGH-CALORIE, HIGH-PROTEIN) DIET

Breakfast (450 calories, 16 g protein)

Food	Calories	Protein
orange juice without pulp, ½ cup (125 ml)	60	1
boiled or poached egg, 1	81	6
cooked cereal, ½ cup (125 ml)	65	3
toast, 1 slice, with butter, 1 tsp. (15 ml) and jelly, (15 ml)	157	2
milk (if tolerated), ½ cup (125 ml)	80	4
coffee/tea, 1 cup (250 ml)	50	0

Midmorning Snack (595 calories, 21 g protein)

Food	Calories	Protein
lactose-free, liquid, high-protein supplement, 1½ cups (375 ml)	535	21
canned mandarin orange, ½ cup (125 ml)	60	0

Lunch (565 calories, 31 g protein)

Food	Calories	Protein
broth, 1 cup (250 ml)	23	4
potato (mashed, baked or boiled), ½ cup (125 ml)	76	2
meat, poultry, or fish, 3 oz. (75 g)	225	21
green beans, ½ cup (125 ml)	16	1
bread and butter, 1 slice	107	3
applesauce, ½ cup (125 ml)	119	0
coffee/tea, 1 cup (250 ml)	0	0

Midafternoon Snack (200 calories, 6 g protein)

Food	Calories	Protein
custard or pudding, ½ cup (125 ml)	200	6

Dinner (700 calories, 34 g protein)

Food	Calories	Protein
meat, poultry, or fish, 3 oz. (75 g)	225	21
boiled rice, ½ cup (125 ml)	82	2
cooked carrots, ½ cup (125 ml)	15	1
bread and butter, 1 slice	107	3
plain cake, 1 slice	140	3
milk (if tolerated), ½ cup (125 ml)	80	4
coffee/tea, 1 cup (250 ml)	0	0

Evening Snack (185 calories, 3 g protein)

Food	Calories	Protein
Jell-O or fortified Jell-O, ½ cup (125 ml)	65	1
plain cookies, 2	120	2

- A semivegetarian diet may include fish and poultry, as well as dairy products and eggs.

A well-planned vegetarian diet has been associated with lower blood pressure, less obesity, and less constipation than the norm. It has also been shown to reduce the risk of several diseases, among them colon cancer, coronary artery disease, and adult-onset diabetes.

A poorly planned vegetarian diet can result in many nutrient deficiencies. The more restrictive the diet is, the more danger for deficiency diseases. The are many "self-proclaimed" nutritionists who, although they are

VEGETARIAN DAILY FOOD GUIDES

(number of servings)	Lacto Vegetarian	Lacto-Ovo Vegetarian	Vegan
breads and cereals	4–6	6–7	7–10
fats/oils	0	1 tbsp. (15 ml)	1 tbsp. (15 ml)
legumes (dried beans and peas, lentils)	1+	1+	2+
milk and milk products	2–4	0	0
nuts	1+	1+	1+
other fruits and vegetables	2+	2+	2+
vegetables and fruits rich in vitamin A†	1–2	1–2	1–2
vegetables and fruits rich in vitamin C‡	1–2	1–2	1–2

Note: One egg can be substituted for one serving of milk/milk product for the lacto-ovo vegetarian.
Milk: 1 serving=1 cup (250 ml) milk or yogurt; 1 oz. (25 g) cheese
Breads/cereals: 1 serving=1 slice bread; 1 cup (250 ml) cooked grain/pasta; 3/4 cup (175 ml) cold cereal
Legumes: 1 serving=1 cup (250 ml)
Nuts: 1 serving=1/4 cup (50 ml) nuts or 1/3 to 1/2 cup (75–125 ml) seeds
Vegetables/fruits: 1 serving=1/2 cup (125 ml) cooked or 1 cup (250 ml) raw vegetable or 1/2 to 1 whole fruit
† Vegetables and fruits rich in Vitamin A include beet greens, broccoli, brussels sprouts, carrots, escarole, pumpkin, spinach, and sweet potatoes; V-8 juice; apricots, cantaloupe, mango, nectarines, papaya, and peaches.
‡ Vegetables and fruits rich in vitamin C include bell peppers, broccoli, cauliflower, kale, spinach, and tomatoes; V-8 juice; cantaloupe, grapefruit, mango, orange, and citrus juices.

not qualified to do so, may make claims and recommendations that can be dangerous. A registered dietitian is an expert on nutrition and can assist you in planning a safe and well-balanced vegetarian diet. It is especially important to plan vegetarian diets for children and adolescents carefully, to ensure meeting their nutritional needs for growth and development.

If you opt for a vegetarian diet of any type, choose a wide variety of nutrient-dense foods, which may include fruits, vegetables, whole grains, nuts, seeds, legumes, low-fat dairy products or fortified soy substitutes, and a limited number of eggs. To improve the value of the vegetable protein sources, your dietitian can show you how to combine complementary proteins (see below). Special attention should be given to assuring adequate intake of protein; calcium; riboflavin; iron; zinc; and vitamins A, D, and B$_{12}$.

Complementary Proteins

Proteins are made up of amino acids. There are eight essential amino acids, which must be obtained from the diet. Each serving of foods derived from animals, such as meat, fish, poultry, dairy products, and eggs, contain all eight essential amino acids. This makes them a "complete protein." Foods derived from plants do not contain all eight essential amino acids in one food, but with complementary combining, a complete protein can be formed. Complementary foods can be eaten over the course of the day; it is not required that they be eaten at the same meal.

Complementary Foods

Grains and Legumes:

- barley-bean soup
- bread and baked beans
- brown rice and tempeh (a soybean food product)
- corn and beans
- corn tortillas and black beans
- cornbread and black-eyed peas
- crackers and split-pea soup
- flour tortillas and pinto beans
- millet and tofu
- pasta and kidney beans
- rice and beans
- rice and bran casserole
- rice and lentil curry

Nuts, Seeds, and Legumes:

- chopped nuts/tofu vegetarian burgers
- dry roasted soybean and seed snack mix
- hummus (blended seasoned tahini—a paste of sesame seeds—and garbanzo beans)
- nuts with any bean dish
- seed/nut tempeh
- sesame seeds on a bean dish
- sunflower seeds in bean chili

Grains and Dairy Foods

Dairy foods are complete proteins by themselves. In addition, they contain extra lysine, an amino acid that is in low quantity in grains. When grains and dairy products are eaten together, there is enough lysine from the dairy

High-Calorie Foods and Supplements

	Calories (per cup/250 ml)	Protein (grams)	Lactose
Ensure, Boost	250	9	No
Fortified milk	220	14	Yes
Häagen-Dazs honey vanilla ice cream	426	8	Yes
Homemade milkshake	405	13	Yes
Raspberry and cream sorbet	300	0	No
Instant Breakfast (made with whole milk)	280	14	Yes
Resource Plus, Ensure Plus, Boost Plus	360	13	No
Whole Milk	160	8	Yes

product to complement the grain.

- cereal and milk
- cheese and crackers
- cottage cheese and wheat germ
- flour tortillas with cheese
- macaroni and cheese
- milk and toast
- ravioli, manicotti, tortellini
- rice and cheese casserole
- rice pudding
- yogurt and oats

Alternative Nutrition

Nutritional support can help reduce the risk of malnutrition as well as help improve the quality of life. Sometimes you may not be able to eat, which means you can't maintain your weight or take in an adequate amount of calories, protein, and fluids. Feeding by tube on a short-term basis will provide your body with enough nutrition to enable you to fight your illness and keep your immune system strong until you can eat normally again. Tube feeding also frees you from pressure or anxiety around eating. The tube is passed through the nose, down the throat and esophagus, and into the stomach. The procedure may be unpleasant but it is painless. In some cases, depending on your health or the location of your cancer, tube feeding may be more permanent. Parenteral nutrition may be needed when your digestive system is not functioning or does not absorb nutrients properly.

Nutritional Supplements

Recipes for cooking with nutritional supplements are in Chapter 29, "Recipes for Chemotherapy Patients."

To obtain more detailed nutritional information about dietary supplements contact the manufacturer or ask your doctor. See Chapter 29 for nutritional supplement resources.

29

Recipes for the Chemotherapy Patient

Bernadette Festa, M.S., R.D.
Ernest Rosenbaum, M.D.
Isadora Rosenbaum. M.A.

When you're sick and not feeling well, it is difficult to focus on eating. It is, of course, very important to get the calories and protein to rejuvenate yourself. These recipes are a sampling of ideas that have helped other patients during cancer treatment. Let this be a guide for you or your family and friends who are helping with your recovery.

On high-energy days, or when someone else is doing the cooking, make your favorite recipes in larger quantities and freeze them for days you really don't feel like cooking.

Sweet Potato Custard

1 cup mashed, cooked sweet potato
½ cup mashed banana (about 2 small)
1 cup evaporated skim milk
2 tbsp. packed brown sugar
3 egg whites, beaten
¼ cup raisins
1 tbsp. sugar
1 tsp. ground cinnamon

In a medium bowl, stir together sweet potato and banana. Add milk, blending well. Add brown sugar and egg whites and mix thoroughly.

Spray one-quart casserole dish with nonstick spray coating. Transfer sweet potato mixture to casserole dish. Bake in a preheated 300° oven 45–50 minutes or until a knife inserted near the center comes out clean. Serves 6.

* Note: If you need to add more calories, try evaporated (not skim) milk and whole eggs. Adapted from: *Down Home Healthy*, by the National Cancer Institute and the Henry J. Kaiser Family Foundation.

Calories 142, Fat 0.33 g, Cholesterol 1.5 mg, Sodium 85 mg

Chicken Soup with Matzo Balls

1 large chicken fryer (almost 4 lbs.)
3 quarts water
1 large onion, cut in half
3 to 4 carrots cut up
4 to 5 celery stalks with tops
1 parsnip
1 to 2 chicken bouillon cubes
Salt and pepper to taste
Matzo balls (recipe follows)

Cut up chicken into quarters; place in large pot and add 3 quarts water. Add vegetables, bouillon cubes, salt, and pepper. Bring to a boil, cut to medium heat, then to low heat, and simmer about 2 hours. Strain (reserving 2 tablespoons broth to make matzo balls) and add matzo balls.

Serves 4.
188 calories, 12 g protein per serving (3 matzo balls)
10 grams fat per serving, 48 percent fat

Matzo Balls

2 eggs
2 tbsp. melted fat
1 tsp. salt
½ cup matzo meal
2 tbsp. chicken broth

Beat eggs and add melted fat. Mix salt with matzo meal and pour into egg mixture. Mix thoroughly. Add broth and mix once more. Refrigerate at least 1 hour. Form into 12 balls the size of walnuts and place in 4 quarts salted, boiling water. Cover and cook 1 hour over medium heat. Drain and use in soup or stew.

48 calories, 2 g protein per ball
2.8 g fat per ball, 53 percent fat

Hummus

1 can garbanzo beans
1 clove of garlic or to taste
2 tbsp. tahini (optional)
Lemon to taste
1–2 tbsp. olive oil
Water to desired consistency

For additional spiciness, add cumin.

Serve with crackers, bagels, or pita bread

High-Protein Munch Mix

Keep on hand a mixture of any of the following:
- dry-roasted soybeans
- sunflower seeds
- walnuts
- peanuts
- cashews
- raisins

You can coarsely chop this mixture to make it easier to chew.

160 calories, 6 g of protein per ounce

High-Protein, High-Vitamin Crunchy Granola

5 cups (1250 ml) old-fashioned (not instant) oatmeal
1 cup (250 ml) soy flour
1 cup (250 ml) wheat germ
1 cup (250 ml) nonfat milk powder
1 cup (250 ml) slivered almonds*
1 cup (250 ml) unsweetened shredded coconut
1 cup (250 ml) unrefined sesame seeds*
1 cup (250 ml) hulled sunflower seeds*
1 cup (250 ml) safflower or soy oil
1 cup (250 ml) honey

*May be irritating.

Combine dry ingredients in a large bowl. In a separate bowl, stir together oil and honey. Stir into dry ingredients. Spread on cookie sheets and bake at 250°, stirring occasionally, until lightly browned. Mixture burns very easily, so watch it closely.

Makes 15 cups (3.75 l).
270 calories, 8 g protein per ½ cup

Sesame Rolls

¼ cup sesame paste (tahini)
3 tbsp. honey
½ cup wheat germ
¼ cup sunflower seeds, ground in blender or food processor

Combine all ingredients, and when thoroughly blended, form into a roll one inch in diameter and twelve inches long. Wrap in foil or waxed paper and store in refrigerator.

78 calories, 3 g of protein per 1-inch slice

Deviled Egg

Because it is moist, a deviled egg is much easier to eat than a plain, hard-boiled egg for anyone with a dry mouth or some swallowing difficulties. These don't freeze well.

6 hard-boiled eggs, peeled
½ tsp. dry mustard or curry powder
3 tbsp. mayonnaise
Salt and pepper to taste

Cut eggs in half lengthwise, slip out yolks, and mash them with a fork. Mix in rest of ingredients. Fill whites with egg yolk mixture.

142 calories, 6 g protein per 2 filled halves

Bran Muffins

These hearty bran muffins add bulk and fiber to your diet.

2 cups (500 ml) whole-wheat flour
1½ cups (750 ml) bran*
2 tbsp. (30 ml) sugar
¼ tsp. (1 ml) salt
¼ tsp. (1 ml) baking soda
2 cups (500 ml) buttermilk
1 egg, beaten
½ cup (125 ml) molasses
¼ cup (50 ml) margarine, melted
1 cup (250 ml) raisins (optional)

*May be irritating to the bowels.

In a large bowl, mix together the flour, bran, sugar, salt, and baking soda. In a separate bowl, beat together the buttermilk, egg, molasses, and melted margarine. Add the wet ingredients to dry ingredients, stirring just until mixed. Stir in raisins. Fill well-greased muffin cups ⅔ full and bake 25 minutes at 350° until a tester comes out clean.

Makes 20 muffins.
100 calories, 3 g protein per muffin

When You Don't Feel Like Cooking
Quick Snacks or Small Meals:

- Canned tuna (drained): add olive oil, lemon, salt, and pepper as desired, eat with saltine-type crackers.
- Sardines topped with sour cream and chives and eaten on crackers or dark bread.
- Melt cheese over broccoli or asparagus, or mix cheese into a white sauce and add broccoli. Serve on toast or crackers.
- Try canned chicken soup, lentil or split pea soup, or vegetarian chili.

Avocado and Cheese Omelet

1½ tsp. melted butter
2 eggs
¼ cup (50 ml) sour cream
½ cup (125 ml) grated cheese
½ avocado, sliced

In frying pan over medium heat, melt butter. Beat together eggs and sour cream. Pour into frying pan. When eggs are half set, sprinkle with cheese and layer avocado slices on top. Cover and cook a few more minutes until the eggs are set and cheese is melted. Fold omelet in half and slide onto warm plate.

This is a great recipe if you are loosing weight or having any swallowing difficulties.

Serves 1.
790 calories, 31 g protein per serving

Green Delight

½ pound of Swiss chard

2 small potatoes, peeled and cut into 1-inch pieces, cooked until tender

Preferably cook the chard in a nonstick fry pan, covered in a small amount of water and cooked until tender. Add the cooked potatoes, then add olive oil to taste, salt and pepper, and sprinkle with parmesan or grated cheese. For additional protein, add ¼ cup canned white beans, and heat.

Pasta with Egg and Cheese

This dish is really easy to eat and glides down without much effort.

Pastina or any other small macaroni, cooked.

Take cooked pasta off the burner and drain, reserving a small amount of liquid. Add a beaten egg to it. Add olive oil and canned chicken or vegetable broth. Return the pot to the burner and cook until the egg is well cooked. Add grated Parmesan or Romano cheese.

Cream Cheese and Nut Bread

Banana nut bread

Cream cheese

Honey

Spread banana nut bread with cream cheese and drizzle with honey

125 calories, 2 g of protein

Soothing Soup

"When I was going through chemotherapy, I didn't want or feel like I could tolerate solid foods. I found it very nourishing to create the following soup"—Pat

¼ package Lipton Onion soup mix

2 potatoes, Yukon gold preferred

3 carrots

1 large or 2 small zucchini

½ onion

1 clove garlic

You can improvise with additional vegetables like spinach, string beans, seasonal green vegetables, and tofu.

Cook all the vegetables in 1–2 cups of water with the soup mix, covered. When the vegetables are soft, puree them in a food processor or blender. Enjoy!

Egg Salad Sandwich

hard-boiled eggs

mayonnaise to taste

Sweet Potato

2 sweet potatoes (preferably garnet sweet potatoes), microwaved until soft

2 tbsp. of brown sugar

2 tsp. of butter

While potatoes are still hot, slice lengthwise, add brown sugar and butter.

Carrots Elegance

½ pound baby carrots

1–2 tbsp. brown sugar

1–2 tbsp. butter

2 tsp. orange juice

Combine all ingredients and microwave until desired consistency.

South of the Border

1 corn tortilla

2 slices of cheese such as Monterey Jack, mozzarella, or cheddar

1 tomato, chopped

In a nonstick fry pan, add olive oil, then lightly brown the tortilla. Take the pan off the burner. Add the cheese and chopped tomatoes to the top of the tortilla. Return to the heat, cover, and cook for a few minutes.

Fresh Green Soybeans

These are a good protein source. They are known as Edamame and can be found in the frozen section of your supermarket. You can also buy them fresh, especially in Japanese markets.

Bring water to a boil, add the beans, and cook uncovered 5–10 minutes or per the package directions. Use your hands to split open the pod and enjoy the nutty tasting bean. You can also dip these in your favorite dip.

When You Really Don't Feel Like Cooking

Be prepared for those times when you don't feel well enough to grocery shop and cook. Keep a list of grocery delivery services and restaurants that will deliver. Stock up on canned soups, peanut butter crackers, packaged macaroni and cheese, and healthier TV dinner brands such as Amy's.

Breakfast can be your best meal of the day. Most breakfast foods are easy to eat because they are soft, moist, bland, and light. These foods are good at any time of the day. Remember them when you are not feeling up to heavier food.

You can increase the protein and calorie content of recipes calling for milk by using fortified milk or cream in place of regular milk. If you must restrict the fat content of your diet, use skim milk or fortified skim milk instead of regular milk. If you are lactose-intolerant, use a milk substitute such as Mocha-Mix or Dairy Rich, or you can make milk lactose-free by adding Lactaid.

Easy Cream of Vegetable Soup

1 jar pureed baby vegetables, such as creamed spinach, creamed corn, or peas
1 cup milk.

Mix and heat.

Serves 1.
250 calories, 11 g protein
11 g fat, 40 percent fat (using milk)

Beverages and Special Shakes

These beverages and shakes are high in calories and protein and make nutritious additions to your diet as between-meal snacks or drinks that can be sipped throughout the day. These beverages can be adjusted to meet your tolerances and tastes, by making the following additions and changes:

- To boost protein, add cottage cheese, tofu, creamy peanut butter, frozen pasteurized egg product, or fortified milk.
- Wheat germ adds B vitamins.
- Bran adds fiber to aid with constipation.
- If swallowing is a problem, you can change the thickness by adjusting the fruit and liquid.
- Substitute soymilk if you are lactose-intolerant.

Fortified Soy Milk

1 quart of soy milk
Soy powder, without added isoflavones

Combine and stir until smooth.

Fortified Milk

Use this extra-high-protein milk for drinking and in all recipes calling for milk.

1 cup (250 ml) nonfat milk powder
1 quart (1 l) whole milk

Combine ingredients and stir until smooth.

220 calories, 14 g protein per cup

Fortified Skim Milk

If you must restrict the fat content of your diet, you can make fortified milk with skim milk.

1 cup (250 ml) nonfat milk powder
1 quart (1 l) skim milk

Combine ingredients and stir until smooth.

149 calories, 14 g protein per cup

Berry Milk

1 cup (250 ml) milk
½ cup (125 ml) fresh or thawed frozen
  strawberries
¼ cup (50 ml) blackberry nectar
1 tbsp. (15 ml) sugar

Put all ingredients in a blender and blend until smooth.

Serves 1.
200 calories, 9 g protein per serving

Berry Power

½ cup strawberries, fresh or thawed frozen
¼ cup cherry juice
1 tbsp. honey
1 cup milk

Combine all ingredients in a blender and blend until smooth.

Serves 1.
180 calories, 9 g protein per serving
8 g fat, 36 percent fat

Tofu Madness

¼ lb. Tofu
½ banana
½ cup orange juice
2 tsp. honey to taste

Serves 1.
235 calories, 11 g protein per serving
5.9 g fat, 23 percent fat

Peanuts and Bananas

1 tbsp. peanut butter
½ banana
½ cup vanilla ice cream
½ cup milk

Serves 1.
354 calories, 12 g protein per serving
24.2 g fat, 61 percent fat

Melon Shake

½ cup chopped cantaloupe, honeydew, or watermelon
½ cup half-and-half
½ cup vanilla ice cream
1 tbsp. honey (if desired)

Serves 1.
402 calories, 8 g protein per serving
25.6 g fat, 57 percent fat

Almond-Peach Milkshake

1 cup milk
1 cup sliced peaches
1 to 3 drops almond extract
1 cup vanilla ice cream

Combine all ingredients in a blender and blend to desired thickness. Garnish with shaved almond and fresh mint on top.

Serves 1.
650 calories, 15 g protein per serving
32.3 g, 44 percent fat

Sherbet Shake

This is a lighter shake than the milkshake and is a good snack for a fat-restricted diet.

¾ cup nonfat milk
1 cup sherbet, any flavor

Combine ingredients in a blender and blend to desired thickness.

Serves 1.
325 calories, 8 g protein per serving
4.3 g, 12 percent fat

Orange Juice Shake

1 cup orange juice
½ cup vanilla ice cream

Combine ingredients in a blender and blend to desired thickness.

Serves 1.
260 calories, 5 g protein per serving
12 g fat, 41 percent fat

Orange Freeze

¾ cup orange juice
1 tbsp. lemon juice
1 cup orange sherbet

Combine ingredients in a blender and blend to desired thickness.

Serves 1.
340 calories, 3 g protein per serving
3.8 g fat, 10 percent fat

Orange Buttermilk Shake

1 cup buttermilk
½ cup orange juice
2 tbsp. brown sugar
1 cup vanilla ice cream

Combine ingredients in a blender and blend to desired thickness.

Serves 1.
530 calories, 15 g protein per serving
26.2 g fat, 44 percent fat

Orange Juice Float

¾ cup orange juice
½ cup orange sherbet

Pour orange juice into a tall glass and top with a scoop of orange sherbet. Serve with a straw.

Serves 1.
215 calories, 2 g protein per serving
1.9 g fat, 8 percent fat

Peach Yogurt Shake

1 cup sliced peaches
1 cup plain yogurt
1 cup skim milk

2 tbsp. honey

Combine ingredients in a blender and blend until smooth. Variations: instead of peaches, use 1 cup of sliced bananas, fruit cocktail, strawberries, raspberries, or blackberries. If you use raspberries or blackberries, strain after blending to remove seeds.

Apricot Yogurt Smoothie

1 cup chilled apricot nectar
1 cup plain yogurt

Combine ingredients in a blender and blend until smooth.

Variations: instead of apricot nectar, use peach or pear nectar or your favorite fruit juice. Add honey to taste.

Mooless Smoothie

½ cup tofu, silken if available
1 cup vanilla soymilk
½ cup fresh or frozen berries
1 tbsp. honey

Puree in a blender or food processor to desired consistency.

Strawberry/Banana Protein Smoothie

1 cup soy milk, vanilla flavor
½ cup frozen strawberries
½ ripe banana
1 scoop soy frozen dessert
1 scoop protein powder, soy, or whey

Whirl together in a blender until frothy. You may use different berries if you like. I found this to be one of the only drinks I could have on mornings when I was nauseous. It packs about 25 grams of protein and will help to build your blood volume if you are anemic.

Banana/Peanut Butter Smoothie

1 cup soy milk, vanilla flavor
1 ripe banana
1 scoop soy frozen dessert

1 tbsp. crunchy or smooth peanut butter
1 scoop protein powder, soy or whey

Whirl together in a blender until frothy. Whey protein powder is easier to blend and less chalky tasting than soy protein. It is, however, much more expensive.

Carrot Shake

1 cup of carrot juice
1 ripe banana
1 cup vanilla yogurt
milk or soymilk to thin

Blenderize to desired consistency.

Ginger Drink

1 cup ginger ale
½ cup unsweetened applesauce
½ cup orange juice
optional: ¼ tsp. finely chopped ginger

Put all of the ingredients in a blender and blend on high for five or ten seconds.

Refreshing drink: good for nausea, dry mouth, loss of appetite

How To Select a Liquid Nutritional Supplement

Liquid nutritional supplements, when taken in addition to your meals, are a nutritious adjunct to your diet, and the extra calories can help you return to your usual weight. You will also find them soothing when you have a sore or dry mouth.

- Most commercially available supplements are lactose or milk free.
- Choose a drink with at least 250–500 calories and at least 8 grams of protein per 8-ounce can.
- If the supplement tastes too sweet, ask your dietitian about unflavored products.
- Generic products are often cheaper and quite similar. You can find these at pharmacies and large grocery chains.
- If you have diarrhea or loose bowel from the product, a supplement with soluble fiber may help.

Foods for When You're Having Swallowing Difficulties
Riced Fruit

Pears: using a spoon, mash pears through a coarse sieve or ricer.

Bananas: using a fork, mash a banana very finely. May be served covered with a small amount of orange juice.

Applesauce: canned applesauce may be served with no special preparation

These are fruits that will produce the desired consistency. Check with a swallow therapist for additional suggestions.

Blended Cottage Cheese and Fruit

½ cup (125 ml) cottage cheese
1 jar baby fruit

Blend cottage cheese and fruit together until mixture has applesauce consistency. Mixture should not be smooth.

Serves 1.
222 calories, 15 g protein per serving

Thick Soup-Like Pureed Meat

½ cup (50 ml) baby pureed meat or blended cooked meat
¼ cup (50 ml) well-mashed potatoes
2 tbsp. (25 ml) broth.

Combine baby pureed meat or blended cooked meat and the well-mashed potatoes. Add the broth. Mix well. Strain through sieve before serving.

Thick Soup-Like Mashed Potatoes

⅓ cup (75ml) mashed potatoes
¼ cup (50ml) warm milk.

Combine the mashed potatoes with warm milk. Mix well. Strain through sieve before serving.

Thick Soup-Like Pureed Vegetables

1 jar baby pureed vegetables or blended cooked vegetables

¼ cup (50ml) strained cream soup or broth

Combine baby pureed vegetables or blended vegetables with the strained cream soup or broth. Mix well. Strain through sieve before serving.

Cooked Cereal

When making oatmeal, farina, or other cooked cereals, add extra protein and calories by using fortified milk or half-and-half instead of water. Top cereal with a pat of butter and serve with fortified milk or half-and-half.

1 cup (250 ml) fortified milk adds 220 calories, 14 g protein.

1 cup (250 ml) half and half adds 324 calories, 8 g protein.

1 tbsp. (15 ml) butter adds 100 calories.

Other Foods That May Be Served

- Very thick refined cereal, e.g., Cream of Wheat, Cream of Rice, Malt-O-Meal, or Farina.
- Plain tapioca pudding.
- Finely ground meat: grind cooked meat using fine attachment of a meat grinder. If no fine attachment is available, you can grind the meat twice using the regular attachment. Serve with hot broth or gravy, if desired. A meat grinder is required to produce proper consistency. A blender will not produce correct consistency.
- Thick mashed potatoes: serve well-mashed but very thick mashed potatoes.
- Riced vegetables: using a spoon, mash cooked vegetables through coarse sieve or ricer. Carrots, beets, wax beans, green beans, or turnips are the only vegetables that will produce the desired consistency using this recipe. No other vegetables should be used.
- Thickened cream soup: combine equal amounts of strained cream soup and well-mashed potatoes. Mix well. Strain through sieve before serving.
- See also recipes for Fortified Milk and Fortified Skim Milk (p.265)

Cooking with Nutritional Supplements

Ideally, you can receive all your nutrition from whole foods. However sometimes nutritional supplements may be necessary to achieve greater calorie and protein intake. The following recipes use commercial high-calorie and high-protein supplements for added nutritional value. Ask your dietitian about these supplements.

Ensure and its equivalent, Boost, add both protein and calories. They are lactose free so you can use them even if you are lactose-intolerant. Use Ensure Plus or its generic equivalent for an additional calorie and protein boost.

Polycose is a tasteless and odorless source of calories. It can be added to foods and drinks without significantly changing their flavor or volume. You can increase the protein and calorie content in recipes calling for milk by using fortified milk or cream in place of regular milk. If you must restrict the fat content of your diet, you can use skim milk or fortified skim milk instead of regular milk. If you are lactose-intolerant, use a milk substitute such as Mocha-Mix or Dairy Rich, or you can make milk lactose-free by adding Lactaid. Ensure and Polycose recipes below from *Nutrition: A Helpful Ally in Cancer Therapy*, courtesy of Eaton Laboratories.

Ensure Pancakes

1 cup (250ml) flour

1 tbsp. (15ml) baking powder

½ tsp. (2ml) salt

½ tsp. (2ml) cinnamon (may be irritating)

1 egg, lightly beaten

1¼ cups (300ml) vanilla Ensure

2 tbsp. (25ml) vegetable oil

½ cup (125 ml) finely chopped apple

In a bowl, combine flour, baking powder, salt, and cinnamon. In a small bowl, mix together egg, Ensure, and oil. Stir liquid ingredients only until moistened. Fry pancakes on dry griddle.

Serves 2.

429 calories, 10 g protein per serving

Polycose Shake

1½ cups (375 ml) ice cream
¼ cup (50 ml) whole milk
6 tbsp. (90 ml) Polycose powder
2 tbsp. (25 ml) sundae topping

Combine all ingredients in a blender and blend to desired consistency.

Serves 2.
358 calories, 6 g protein per serving

Fruit Eggnog

1¼ cups (300 ml) whole milk
½ cup (125 ml) drained canned peaches
1 cup (250 ml) Polycose powder
¼ cup (50 ml) sugar
1 egg
1 tsp. (5 ml) fresh lemon juice

Combine all ingredients in a blender and blend until smooth and creamy. Chill before serving.

Serves 3.
363 calories, 7 g protein per serving

Fortified Fruit Juice

½ cup (125 ml) fruit juice
¼ cup (50 ml) Polycose liquid

Stir ingredients together.

Serves 1.
180 calories per serving

High-Calorie Chocolate Pudding

1 cup (250 ml) Polycose powder
9 tbsp. (140 ml) chocolate pudding powder
11 tbsp. (165 ml) nonfat milk powder
2 cups (500 ml) half-and-half
1 cup (250 ml) chocolate syrup
1 cup (250 ml) whipping cream

In a saucepan, blend all dry ingredients in half-and-half. Stir in chocolate syrup. Heat until thick and creamy,

stirring frequently. Cool completely. Whip cream and fold into cooled pudding. Chill before serving.

Serves 8.
365 calories, 6 g protein per serving

High-Protein Rice Pudding

2½ cups (625 ml) whole milk
⅔ cup (150 ml) Polycose powder
3 tbsp. (45 ml) sugar
¼ cup (50 ml) hot water
¼ cup (50 ml) nonfat milk powder
¼ cup (50 ml) cooked rice
2 tbsp. (25 ml) margarine
pinch salt

Put milk in top of double boiler. Mix Polycose powder and milk powder with hot water. Stir into milk. Add remaining ingredients and cook over simmering water until thick and creamy, stirring frequently. (Pudding also may also be baked in a casserole for 2 to 2½ hours at 275°.)

Serves 3.
438 calories, 11 g protein per serving

Macaroni and Cheese

½ cup (125 ml) milk
1 tbsp. (15 ml) margarine
1 tbsp. (15 ml) flour
½ cup (125 ml) shredded Cheddar cheese
salt and pepper to taste
½ cup (125 ml) Polycose powder
½ cup (125 ml) macaroni

Mix Polycose powder with 2 tbsp. (25 ml) milk and set aside. In a saucepan, melt margarine over medium-low heat. Stir in flour and cook, stirring constantly, for 3 minutes. Whisk in remaining milk and cook until thickened, stirring constantly. Remove from heat and stir in cheese, salt, and pepper. Return to low heat, stirring until cheese is melted. Remove from heat and beat in Polycose mixture. Cook macaroni in boiling salted water until tender. Drain well. Stir macaroni into cheese sauce and place in a casserole. Sprinkle with additional shredded cheese, if desired. Bake 30 minutes at 350°

Serves 1.
742 calories, 16 g protein per serving

Grocery Shopping

Sttock up on nonperishable foods and foods with a long shelf life. A supply of canned, frozen, and packaged foods will save you shopping trips and offer you a variety of foods to meet whatever your taste preference may be at the moment. Many of these products now come in a one-serving size and are especially good for between-meal snacks to increase your calorie and protein intake.

Grocery List

Beverages

- ❏ Canned and dry milk
- ❏ Carbonated drinks
- ❏ Fruit and vegetable juices (nectars, low-salt V-8, etc.)
- ❏ Fruit-ades (Kool-Aid, Gatorade, etc.)
- ❏ Instant beef and chicken broth
- ❏ Instant breakfast mix
- ❏ Instant cocoa mix
- ❏ Tea, regular and herbal
- ❏ Soy beverages
- ❏ Supplements (Ensure Plus, Boost Plus, etc.)

Breads, Grains, and Cereal Products

- ❏ Bread-machine mixes
- ❏ Crackers (saltines, grahams, etc.)
- ❏ Dry cereal
- ❏ Packaged grain mixes (rice, couscous, lentils, or risotto)
- ❏ Instant pancake mix
- ❏ Muffin mix
- ❏ Regular and instant hot cereal as oatmeal

Fruits and Vegetables

- ❏ Canned fruit, frozen fruits
- ❏ Canned vegetable soups
- ❏ Vegetables, frozen and canned
- ❏ Creamed spinach
- ❏ Dried fruit
- ❏ Pureed baby foods
- ❏ Vegetables that keep well, such as sweet potatoes, citrus, and apples

Meat and Other Protein Foods

- ❏ Canned meat, poultry, and fish
- ❏ Canned pasta, noodles, rice, macaroni, or bean entrées
- ❏ Canned soups
- ❏ Grated cheeses such as Parmesan and Romano
- ❏ Peanut butter, almond butter, and other nut butters
- ❏ Canned beans, dried lentils, and other beans

Desserts

- ❏ Cake and cookie mixes
- ❏ Pudding and custard
- ❏ Instant pudding
- ❏ Ice cream
- ❏ Applesauce

Snacks and Sweets

- ❏ Granola bars
- ❏ Crackers and cheese
- ❏ Hard candy
- ❏ Honey
- ❏ Instant breakfast bars
- ❏ Jam and jelly
- ❏ Nuts
- ❏ Plain chocolate
- ❏ Power bars

From the Freezer Case

- ❏ Burritos
- ❏ Blintzes
- ❏ Frozen vegetables and fruits
- ❏ Lasagna/ravioli
- ❏ Macaroni and cheese
- ❏ Pancakes
- ❏ Pot pies
- ❏ Quiches, soufflés
- ❏ Soups
- ❏ TV dinners
- ❏ Waffles
- ❏ Whipped topping

Sauces and Seasonings

- ❏ Canned gravy
- ❏ Canned sauces
- ❏ Gravy mixes
- ❏ Seasoning mixes

Nutrition Supplement Resources

Ross Products Division
Abbott Laboratories
Columbus, Ohio 43215-1724
(800) 986-8502 to order products
www.ross.com
  Products:
  Ensure, Ensure Plus, Ensure Pudding, Polycose, Promod

Mead Johnson Nutritionals
Evansville, IN 47721
(800) 247-7893 to order products
www.meadjohnson.com
  Products:
  Boost, Boost Plus, Boost High Protein, Boost High Protein Powder, Boost Pudding

Scandipharm, Inc.
22 Inverness Center Parkway
Birmingham, AL 35242
(800) 472-2634 to order products
www.scandipharm.com
  Products:
  Scandishake, ScandiCal

Nestle Clinical Nutrition (formerly Clintec)
Three Parkway North, Suite 500
P.O. Box 760
Deerfield, IL 60015-0760
(800) 776-5446 to order products
  Products:
  Carnation Instant Breakfast, NuBasics Drinks, Peptamen, Nutren

Novartis Nutrition (formerly Sandoz Nutrition)
5100 Gamble Drive
Suite 200
Saint Louis Park, MN 55416
(800) 999-9978
  Products:
  ReSource, ReSource Plus, ReSource Fruit Beverage, ReSource Yogurt Flavored Beverage

30

Choosing a Multivitamin

Bernadette Festa, M.S., R.D.

Who May Need a Multivitamin (MVI) Supplement

Ideally, you will work with a Registered Dietitian (R.D.) to meet your needs through proper food choices. However, the following conditions may make it advisable for you to take a supplement:

- If you experience loss of appetite, taste, smell, or difficulty with swallowing resulting from surgery to the head and neck area, you may not be able to meet all of your nutritional needs by eating.
- If you're a postmenopausal female and not on hormone replacement therapy or tamoxifen, you may need to supplement your diet with calcium and vitamin D to protect against osteoporosis.
- If you have cancer of the digestive tract—such as intestinal, pancreatic, liver, and gallbladder—you may have impaired digestion and absorption of nutrients.
- If you eat fewer than 1,000 calories per day or your diet is limited because of food intolerance.
- If you follow a special diet that eliminates certain food groups, eat a vegetarian diet that omits all animal products, or have been told that you have poor wound healing due to nutrient deficiencies, you may need additional vitamin B_{12} or calcium.
- If you are over fifty years of age, your nutritional requirements may not be met if you have loss of appetite or eliminate food groups. Consult your dietitian about changes in your nutritional needs.

How to Choose a Multivitamin

Reading the Label

Check the Daily Value—The daily value (DV) is a government standard which specifies the amount of a nutrient required daily in order to prevent a deficiency disease in a healthy person. The DV is based on intake of at least 2,000 calories per day. You may need more or less than 2,000 calories per day. A dietician will help you determine the amount of calories you need.

Check the serving size—Be sure to verify how many tablets are needed to provide the stated nutrients. You may need to swallow up to six tablets a day to get the amounts listed on the label.

Skip the iron in a multivitamin— If you are a cancer patient, ask your medical team whether or not you should take iron in a multivitamin. Usually, unless you have iron-deficient anemia, are at risk of anemia, or have had recent surgery, you may not need to take extra iron. When using erythropoietin (Procrit, Epogin) for anemia, you may already be taking an iron supplement and may not need the extra iron in a multivitamin. If you have anemia, you should consult your physician about iron dosage. Iron supplements can cause constipation, so if you take iron you will need to increase your fiber and fluid intake.

Don't pay more for "timed-release" medications. This has no meaning for a multivitamin. To improve absorbability, take your supplement with food. Chelate (pronounced key-late) minerals may be better absorbed because they are protected from substances in foods that can bind with them. For example, the phytic acid in grains or the oxalates in spinach can bind with minerals like calcium and decrease the amount absorbed. Multivitamins containing chelated minerals may cost twice as much as regular ones. Evaluate the price of the chelated mineral to determine if it is worth the additional cost.

Ask your medical team about any specific vitamin or mineral interactions with your particular chemotherapy. Many practitioners recommend stopping any high-dose supplements during a window of time while receiving chemotherapy or radiation therapy.

Always read the labels and avoid added agents like coloring, such as Yellow #5, and additional fillers.

Read specialized formulas (those for women, men, seniors, etc.) carefully. Because these claims are not regulated by the government, each vitamin company determines what formula each group needs. For example, most formulas for women have additional calcium but may lack the daily value for vitamin D, which aids in calcium absorption and utilization. Formulas for seniors may not contain the appropriate amount of daily value for vitamin B_{12}.

Check the expiration date on all supplements and medications. Be sure that each is stored according to its instructions, for example, some need to be refrigerated, some need to be kept at room temperature, and others need to be kept away from light. It is advisable to take the vitamin with food to assist with absorption. Generally, multivitamins work better when taken with food.

Avoid megadoses—especially with the fat-soluble vitamins such as vitamins A, D, E, and the minerals iron and selenium, or when taking any supplements long-term. The fat-soluble vitamins can be stored in your liver, putting extra demands on this organ which already is working overtime when you are receiving chemotherapy.

What to Look for in a Multivitamin

- 100 percent of the Daily Value (DV) for vitamins B_1 (thiamin), B_2 (riboflavin), niacin, vitamins B_6, B_{12}, C, D, E, and folic acid. If you need additional antioxidants, such as vitamins C or E, you should take these separately. Most of the multivitamins do not provide adequate supplemental amounts of these antioxidants. However, more than 1000 mg of vitamin C per day may cause diarrhea, gas, or stomach upset. To prevent diarrhea, you should take smaller doses more often.
- Two other antioxidants, beta-carotene and vitamin A, are in most multivitamin supplements. Beta-carotene is converted into vitamin A, but it will not cause vitamin A toxicity. Beta-carotene use is controversial with lung cancer.
- Minimize or avoid iron unless your medical team recommends additional amounts.
- Most people get enough phosphorus from their diets; too much can prevent calcium absorption. Look for minimal amounts of this mineral.
- There is no evidence that supplements of substances such as iodine, manganese, molybdenum, chloride, or boron are beneficial.
- Look for "USP" on a label. This specifies that the supplements meet the standards of the U.S. Pharmacopoeia. These supplements have been tested for dissolvability with a procedure that mimics what happens in your body.
- Supplements are available in tablet, caplet, capsule, liquid, and chewable forms. Determine which form is easiest for you to take.

Tips for Taking Multivitamins

- Treat nausea prior to taking a multivitamin.
- Take the multivitamin with meals rather than on an empty stomach.
- Multivitamins come in many forms; if you have problems swallowing, try taking a liquid or chewable multivitamin.

- Be aware that liquid forms may not meet the daily value for minerals since some minerals may not remain dissolved in solution.
- Remember, a good multivitamin is just a supplement, not a substitute for eating well.

Special Consideration

Chemotherapy agents—Use of certain chemotherapy medications may require additional supplementation. Be sure to ask your medical team before supplementing.

Those people receiving cis-platin may require additional magnesium and potassium. Good food sources of magnesium include whole grains, nuts, legumes, dark green leafy vegetables, and meat. Potassium food sources include bananas, oranges, potatoes, and apricots. Most multivitamins do not contain potassium, but some have 100 percent of the daily value or more of magnesium. You may need more potassium and magnesium than the amount in your multivitamin. Your medical team will determine this based on your blood levels. Chronic illness can lead to poor eating habits or deplete your nutrient stores. Extra supplements may be needed if you have a long-term digestive problem or have liver or gallbladder problems. Be sure to consult with your medical team on your individual needs before taking supplements.

Antioxidants

Antioxidants, such as vitamin A, caroten, vitamin E, vitamin C, and selenium, act by destroying harmful molecules called free radicals that form in the body naturally. Free radicals can damage DNA, RNA, and fat and protein molecules, and may be involved in the development of cancerous cells. Antioxidants decrease DNA damage and may also help prevent the transformation of normal cells into malignant cells, thus acting as protective substances. However, there is no conclusive evidence that a diet rich in antioxidants reduces the incidence of cancer or cures it.

Reliance on Fast Foods or Processed Foods

These food groups contain an unusually high amount of sodium and possibly phosphorous. Too much phosphorous will interfere with calcium absorption. If fast foods comprise the majority of your diet, be sure to look for lower amounts of phosphorous in your multivitamin. Daily Values reflect the recommended levels of intake for most vitamins and minerals, and you will see these on a multivitamin label. If you take multivitamin and other supplements, keep the amounts that you take within the safe upper limits.

DAILY VALUES

Micronutrient	Daily Values	Safe Upper Limits
Vitamin B_1 Vitamin B_2	1.5 mg (mg) 1.7 mg	While high intake of vitamin B_1 and B_2 may not be harmful, consult your dietitian
Niacin	20 mg	No more that 35 mg
Vitamin B_6	2 mg	No more than 100 mg
Vitamin B_{12}	6 micrograms (mcg)	While high intakes of these B vitamins may not be harmful, consult your dietitian.
Biotin	0.3 mg	No more that 2.5 mg
Pantothenic Acid	10 mg	Consult your dietitian.
Vitamin A	5,000 international units (IU)	No more than 10,000 IU, no more than 2,000 Retinol equivalents or mcg
Vitamin C	60 mg	No more than 500mg
Vitamin D	400 IU	No more than 2,000 IU or 50 mcg
Vitamin E	30 IU	No more than 100 mg or IU while on anticoagulant therapy, no more than 800 mg or IU generally.
Folate	400 mcg	No more than 1,000 mcg or 1 mg
Calcium	1,000–1200 mg	No more than 2,500 mg
Iron	18 mg	Iron supplementation is not recommended unless your medical team advises it.
Selenium	70 mcg	No more than 200 mcg
Phosphorus	1,000 mg	No more than 1,200 mg (age dependent)
Iodine	150 mcg	1,000 mcg
Magnesium	400 mg	700 mg
Zinc	15 mg	30 mg
Copper	2 mg	9 mg

Adapted from Fred Hutchinson Cancer Research Center—Professional Guidelines for Supplement Preparations During Transplantation and High Dose Chemotherapy

ABC'S—MAIN FUNCTIONS AND FOOD SOURCES OF MAJOR MICRONUTRIENTS

Vitamins	Functions	Food Sources
B_1 Thiamin	Helps body cells obtain energy from food. Needed for normal functioning of the nervous system and muscles, including the heart muscle.	Lean pork, wheat germ, sunflower seeds, organ meats, lean meats, poultry, fish, legumes, whole grain, enriched breads, cereals.
B_2 Riboflavin	Necessary for the production of energy within cells of the body. Helps with red blood cell formation.	Milk, cheddar cheese, cottage cheese, yogurt, organ meats, lean meats, eggs, green leafy vegetables, enriched breads, cereals.
B_3 Niacin	Necessary for release of energy from foods and tissue respiration.	Brewers yeast, peanuts, peanut butter, organ meats, lean meats, fish, poultry.
B_6 Pyridoxine	Involved in metabolism of protein and fat, and in synthesis of hormones and red blood cells.	Yeast, oatmeal, other whole grain cereals, wheat germ, pork, bananas, potato, legumes, glandular meats.
B_{12} Cobalamine	Required for blood formation, and healthy nervous system.	Animal protein food such as liver and kidney, muscle meats, milk, eggs, fish, cheese, sea vegetables.
Vitamin C	Collagen formation that acts to bind cells together; wound healing and tissue repair; plays a critical role in the immune system; antioxidant.	Citrus fruits such as oranges, lemons, grapefruit; tomato, peppers, broccoli, berries, cantaloupe.
Folic Acid	Normal growth, development, and formation of red blood cells.	Dark green leafy vegetables, brewers yeast, kidney beans, lima beans, fortified whole grains, orange juice.
Vitamin A	Promotes growth and repair of body tissues, bone formation, healthy skin integrity, and has a role in night vision.	Sweet potato, carrots, spinach, liver, butternut squash, cantaloupe, apricots, fortified milk.
Vitamin D	Promotes the absorption of calcium.	Fortified milk, fish liver oils, herring, salmon, sardines. *Sunlight* is also a good source.
Vitamin E - tocopherol	Antioxidant, protects cellular and subcellular membranes, enhances the activity of vitamin A.	Wheat germ oil, corn, soybean and safflower oils.
Vitamin K	Blood clotting.	Green leafy vegetables such as turnip greens, broccoli, cabbage, lettuce; also made in our intestinal tract.

Minerals		
Selenium	Antioxidant, especially in association with vitamin E. May reduce risks of certain cancers.	Brazil nuts; seafood, meat, poultry; vegetables — depending on the selenium content of their growing soil.

(Continued from page 277)

Vitamins	Functions	Food Sources
Iron	Red blood cell formation and transport of oxygen through the blood, an active part of enzymes involved in the oxidation of fat and carbohydrates.	Liver, lean meats, poultry, seafood, whole or enriched grains; legumes, dark green vegetables especially when vitamin C is present.
Magnesium	Functions in a number of biochemical processes, nerve and muscle function, component of bone.	Whole grain cereals, nuts, green vegetables, legumes, meat.
Calcium	99 percent is in bones and teeth, gives structure and strength; blood clotting; muscle contraction and relaxation.	Milk and milk products such as yogurt; fortified tofu and soy products; dark green leafy vegetables such as kale, collards, turnip greens, broccoli; legumes like black beans.
Zinc	Functions as part of more than 200 enzymes. It is abundant in the cell nucleus, stabilizes RNA and DNA.	Oysters, shellfish, whole grains especially wheat bran, dry beans, nuts, red meat.

31

Complementary Medications and Chemotherapy
Antioxidants and Herbal Medications

Sharya Vaughn Bourdet, Pharm.D.
Robert Ignoffo, Pharm.D.

Antioxidants

The use of complementary and alternative medicine for the prevention and treatment of various diseases has become more popular in recent years. A treatment is considered complementary when it is taken in conjunction with accepted mainstream medical therapy, but the same treatment may be considered alternative when taken instead of accepted medical therapy. For more information and a more detailed definition, see Chapter 12. With the growth of the Internet, consumers now have more accessibility to information and advertising about complementary and alternative products.

Some people are reluctant to take prescription medications because of fear of unwanted effects. Thus, they turn to dietary and herbal supplements to treat their illnesses because they feel these products are "natural" and safe. Some individuals may choose to take both mainstream and complementary medicine to treat illnesses. This practice is especially common among those patients receiving treatment for cancer. Surveys indicate that 7–64 percent of cancer patients use complementary medicine. However, as many as 50 percent of patients who take complementary therapies do not tell their physicians.

Several types of alternative and complementary therapies exist, including herbs, vitamins, and dietary products. Many of the benefits from these products result from their antioxidant properties. Antioxidants have received much media attention in recent years regarding cancer prevention. A diet rich in fruits and vegetables, which are good sources of antioxidants, has been reported to lower a person's risk for some types of cancer. Antioxidant supplements, which contain larger amounts of antioxidants than contained in food sources, have also been reported to decrease a person's risk of developing certain types of cancer. Specifically, studies have shown that vitamin E and selenium supplements may reduce the incidence of prostate and colon cancer.

Antioxidants are also used by some patients during cancer treatment in the hopes of reducing the side effects of chemotherapy. Two prescription antioxidants, Mesnex (mesna) and Ethyol (amifostine), are used to prevent side effects of chemotherapy agents such as ifosfamide, cyclophosphamide, and cisplatin. Because these two antioxidants are for prescription use only, they have been evaluated in human studies by the Food and Drug Administration (FDA) and have been found not to reduce the effectiveness of cisplatin, cyclophosphamide, or ifosfamide in the treatment of cancer.

The FDA considers nonprescription antioxidant supplements to be dietary products and does not regulate them. Human studies showing the impact of dietary supplements on chemotherapy effectiveness are not required for these products to be sold in the United States.

There are many different chemotherapeutic agents used to treat cancer. Most of the agents can be grouped into classes based on how they work against cancer cells. Several classes of chemotherapy work by producing a reactive oxygen compound called a free radical. Free radicals can damage proteins or other structures within a cell, cause the death of that cell, or prevent that cell from dividing and making new cells.

There are three classes of common chemotherapy agents that work by producing free radicals: alkylating agents, which include cisplatin (Platinol), carboplatin (Paraplatin), chlorambucil (Leukeran), carmustine (BiCNU), cyclophosphamide (Cytoxan), busulfan (Myleran), and ifosfamide (Ifex); anthracyclines, which include doxorubicin (Adriamycin, Doxil), daunorubicin (Cerubidine), epirubicin (Ellence), Mitomycin (Mutamycin), and bleomycin (Bleoxane); and podophyllum agents, which include etoposide (VP-I6, Vespid) and teniposide (Vumon). While cancer cells are the main target of chemotherapy, normal cells may be affected as well, causing side effects such as hair loss, low blood cell counts, and mouth sores.

Antioxidants are compounds that bind and inactivate free radicals. Free radicals are normally produced from many of the body's everyday stresses such as inflammation, exercise, alcohol, ultraviolet light, and fatty diets. A healthy diet complete with fresh fruits and vegetables provides enough dietary antioxidants to inactivate the normal production of free radicals. Antioxidant supplements, which contain mega-doses of antioxidants, are available in many health food stores and pharmacies. Some common antioxidants that may be found in dietary supplements include: alpha lipoic acid, grape seed extract, proanthocyanidins, beta-carotene, lutein, vitamin A, lycopene, vitamin C (ascorbic acid), selenium, vitamin E (alpha-tocopherol), zinc,

and coenzyme CoQ_{10}. Antioxidants may decrease chemotherapy-induced damage of normal cells by inactivating free radicals, but the same damage may also be decreased in cancer cells. Therefore, doses of antioxidants that are larger than those provided in a normal diet may potentially interfere with the effectiveness of certain chemotherapy agents by reducing their action in cancer cells.

The combination of antioxidants and chemotherapeutic agents may present some potential problems to the patient and health care provider. First, many patients do not tell their physician that they are taking antioxidants because they fear disapproval from the physician or because their physician has never asked about such therapies. Second, the use of antioxidant supplements during chemotherapy has not been studied to assess long-term effects of these supplements on patients' safety or survival. Because no such scientific studies have been conducted, the potential interactions between antioxidants and chemotherapy must be predicted from the knowledge currently available.

Patients should fully understand the possible consequences of combining antioxidant supplements and chemotherapy. Based on the current knowledge, there is the potential of reduced effectiveness of certain chemotherapeutic agents when combined with antioxidants. This means that patients may not receive the full benefit of cancer treatment. Whether a reduced benefit corresponds to therapy failure, including a lack of clinical response, continued progression of the cancer despite therapy, or decreased long-term survival, has not yet been determined. Patients and physicians should be aware that combining antioxidants with chemotherapy may improve side effects in the short-term, but may hinder long-term survival or clinical response. Patients and physicians should decide on a course of action that ensures maximum clinical benefit yet embraces the patient's wishes regarding therapy. This plan may include the decision not to take antioxidants and chemotherapy at the same time, to find chemotherapeutic agents that have no possible interaction with antioxidants, or not to take antioxidants at all during cancer treatment.

It is important that patients and health care providers be informed about all possible interactions between dietary supplements and medications. This means that health care providers should ask patients about the use of complementary therapies and that

CONTRAINDICATED HERBALS

Herb	Toxicity/Side effects
Chinese/oriental herbs	Unknown active ingredients
Chaparral	Hepatoxicity
Cleansing Herbal Dietary Supplement	Contains digitalis glycosides
Ephedra or Ma Huang	High blood pressure
Jin Bu Huan	Hepatitis
Laetrile	Carcinogenic, cyanide poisoning
Mistletoe Extract (Iscador)	Nausea, bradycardia, gastritis, hypertension
Pau d'arco	Anticoagulant bleeding
Pennyroyal	Hepatoxic
Plantain Extracts, Nature Cleanse tablets	Contaminated with digitalis
Botannical Cleanse Tablets	Glycosides
Blessed herbs, Siberian ginseng	Contains male hormone-like chemicals

ACCEPTABLE HERBALS

Herb	Therapeutic Use
Blackberry, raspberry tea	Diarrhea
Fenugreek seeds	Diarrhea
Ginger tea, cookies	Nausea or vomiting
Cinnamon	Nausea
Peppermint tea	Diarrhea
St John's wort	Depression
Saw palmetto	Urinary obstruction or enlarged prostate
Valerian	Insomnia
Kava	Insomnia

From Cassileth: *Cancer Nursing*, 22:85-90, 1999

patients should be open and honest with providers when asked. Patients and physicians should jointly decide a plan of action for using complementary and mainstream therapies that will achieve the goals of both the physician and patient. New information concerning complementary and alternative therapies is continually becoming available. Possible interactions between therapies such as antioxidants and chemotherapy should be reevaluated once more information is available and long-term clinical studies have been conducted.

In the meantime, the following are specific recommendations for those cancer patients who are taking antioxidant supplements or herbal medications:

1. Inform your doctor(s) that you are currently taking dietary or herbal products. In order for your doctor to keep an accurate list of medications, it may help to bring the products or a list of ingredients and doses with you to your office visits.

2. Keep your doctor(s) updated if you start taking any new dietary or herbal products.

3. As a general rule, do not take antioxidants the day before, during, and the day after receiving chemotherapy.

4. Antioxidants are available in many forms including vitamin, mineral, and herbal supplements. If you are not sure if a dietary supplement that you are taking contains an antioxidant, ask your doctor or pharmacist.

Herbal Medications

The use of herbal medications is a common practice of patients being treated for cancer. Herbs are touted for their medicinal properties and may be useful for treating some of the side effects associated with chemotherapy. However, because they are derived from botanicals, some herbal products may have impurities (bacteria, fungi, or parasites) that could put patients at risk for infections during periods of decreased white blood cell counts. In addition, some herbal preparations have adverse effects of their own that may worsen toxicities from high-dose chemotherapy. These herbal treatments are not recommended because of their serious side effects. Thus, many institutions advise patients to discontinue herbal and nutrient supplements before and during chemotherapy.

References available upon request.

Chinese herbalists claim that many of their preparations may be helpful in minimizing side effects of chemotherapy. These herbal treatments may work through the same antioxidant mechanisms described for the vitamin preparations. Further study is necessary to determine if herbal treatments affect the effectiveness of some chemotherapy regimens. Many studies are underway in the United States to determine whether traditional Chinese herbal medications are beneficial in improving patient quality of life while receiving chemotherapy.

32

Rehabilitation and Fitness Exercises

Francine Manuel, R.P.T.
Ernest H. Rosenbaum, M.D.
Jack LaLanne
Eric Durak, M.Sc.
Isadora Rosenbaum, M.A.
Kathleen Dzubur, M.S.
Gary Abrams, M.D.

Editor's Note: Demonstrations are by Jack LaLanne, Jennifer Green, Lisa Glassberg, Dr. Don Bornell, and Jennifer Hackworth, R.N.

Physical fitness is a matter of movement. In everyday life, people undertake many activities that use and maintain normal muscle tone. When a person is healthy, he or she needs no special training or assistance for such common activities as walking, making the bed, shopping, climbing stairs, or running for a bus.

People with an acute or chronic illness, however, can't take even minimal exercise for granted. Prolonged bed rest, which is often essential or unavoidable, can lead to muscular weakness, tissue breakdown, and poor functioning of vital organs. To preserve these vital functions during and after your treatment, you must make regular physical activity, including supplemental exercises aimed at maintaining muscle tone, normal joint motion, and physical strength, part of your routine, starting as early as possible. Many forms of exercise can improve your fitness, circulation, stamina, muscle strength, and endurance, including:

- isotonic exercises (moving a limb through a full range of motion);
- isometric exercises (resistance against a nonmoving object); and
- rhythmic repetitive movements and activities of daily living (ADLs) which include household tasks, moving the body through space, and other functional chores.

If you exercised regularly before you became ill, you will probably be open to the idea of getting involved in an active program all through your recovery. But if you have never been involved in an organized exercise routine, you may need some encouragement and instruction. Welcome this encouragement if you get it. If you don't get it, seek it out, because becoming and staying physically fit should be one of your primary goals. Many cancer patients say that regular exercise was one of the most effective means for improving their health during and after their oncology treatments.

While you should think of your program as being as much a part of your recovery as visits to the doctor, try to enjoy yourself. Exercise can be a lot of fun and it can be very stimulating. If you have days when depression and boredom get you down and exercising seems like too much of a burden, just remind yourself of all the benefits of exercising regularly. The more you exercise, the better you will feel. Don't say you're too tired and wait for tomorrow. Tomorrow may be no better than today. Start now, and keep up a reasonable exercise schedule for better health.

The Benefits of Exercise

Physical fitness is healthy for everyone, but it is essential for cancer patients. Even though it's harder to find the energy to exercise when you are sick, the benefits of keeping active are great. Participating in a daily exercise program will help you in several important ways:

1. You will improve your prognosis. If you are in good physical condition, you may be better able to tolerate cancer therapy. This, in turn, may allow you to have more aggressive treatments, thus standing a better chance of remission or cure.

2. You will improve your quality of life. Exercise can help you tolerate pain more readily, recover more quickly from surgeries and medical procedures, and feel more in control of your situation. Exercise also reduces fatigue and nausea, and increases appetite. Having the energy to remain functionally independent and to continue to fulfill social roles is important to quality of life. Most of our recent medical reports state that exercise improves many quality of life scores, such as mood, self-esteem, depression scores, and anxiety.

3. You will prevent your muscles from wasting away. When we are healthy, we usually exercise our muscles by walking up and down stairs, doing housework, shopping, taking part in athletic activities like golf and tennis, or performing weight training exercises. Even a low level of activity helps maintain muscle tone and strength. But during an acute or chronic illness, prolonged bed rest is often necessary. When muscles aren't used, they shrink (atrophy) and lose strength. Muscles can atrophy after only 96 hours (four days) of disuse. Moderate exercise aimed at strengthening the large muscles, as described later in this chapter, will prevent this from happening to you, so that you can return to active living more quickly.

4. You will recover faster. If you do not exercise after surgery or while you're undergoing radiotherapy or chemotherapy, the tissues that may get broken down by therapy will not repair as quickly as they should. Exercising can help your tissues rebound and minimize any deterioration in your joints. It may also help prevent complications such as bone softening, blood clots, and bedsores. And you'll get some welcome relief from the boredom and depression that often come with being confined in bed. Recent research states that even patients who are on high doses of chemotherapy or having stem cell transplants may improve their recovery process by performing conditioning. Therefore, exercising can become a vital part of your fight for your life.

Regular exercise also offers many general health benefits. Exercise decreases stress, controls weight by burning calories, and generally promotes a greater sense of well-being. Keeping body weight normal may have an influence on the development of certain types of cancers. Flexibility exercises alleviate general aches and pains, including those from arthritis. Strengthening your abdominal muscles can also help relieve back pain.

Resistance training and other activities can maintain and increase your bone density, thus reducing your chances of developing osteoporosis (weak bones). Impact exercises such as jogging or strenuous aerobics are also believed to play a part in preventing this disease of gradual bone loss. In cases of fatigue, weakness, severe osteoporosis, or progressive illness, high-impact exercise programs such as jogging can be detrimental. Gentler activities, such as brisk walking, can help maintain bone density and health. Remember, although activity is good, moderation is essential. Overdoing exercise—going beyond your limits—can actually reverse your progress.

The most important benefit of all is that you can live longer if you exercise. Many studies have shown conclusively that an inactive (sedentary) lifestyle leads to an appreciably shorter life. In fact, recent reports from the Cooper Institute in Dallas, Texas, state that being sedentary increases the risks for developing lung cancer and premature death from all cancers. Exercise has been shown to maintain youthfulness, promote longevity, and help prevent heart disease as well as certain types of cancer. Along with the general health benefits, studies on prevention and survival rates in cancer patients have shown that regular moderate physical activity can help protect against some cancers, such as breast and colon, while also improving the clinical course, at least in the early stages of the disease. Several studies conclude that in the late stages of cancer, exercising improves quality of life right up to death. In one study, cancer patients who included moderate exercise in their routine reported decreased discomfort; after five weeks of moderate exercise, there was a strict connection between improvement and frequency of exercise. These patients also reported that exercise enhanced their quality of life. There is strong evidence that even beginning exercise late in life is beneficial, whereas stopping exercise is harmful. Having exercised as a child has no effect, but more recent activity in life definitely has an impact on the risk for developing cancer.

Physical Attributes of Exercise

White blood cells are believed to have a powerful inhibiting effect on tumor growth and to be able to destroy cancer cells. Studies have shown that intense exercising, such as the heavy training of professional athletes, has a negative effect on the immune system, but that moderate exercise actually enhances the immune system. Low-intensity exercise (e.g., walking) has also been shown to have positive effects on the body's ability to fight infections. So moderate exercise programs, such as walking, using aerobic machines, tai chi, etc., may be the best way to enhance general fitness and may have an impact on the development of cancerous tumors.

Several studies have shown that people with more active lifestyles experience fewer breast, ovarian, prostate, and colon cancers. Researchers believe that exercise may decrease breast and ovarian cancer by affecting ovarian hormonal levels and the percentage of body fat. Female athletes who have decreased estrogen levels and low percentages of body fat also have a decreased incidence of breast and ovarian cancers.

Incidence of colon cancer is also lower among more active people. Again, the mechanism may be associated with decreased adipose (fatty) tissue, especially in the abdomen, or the fact that exercise tends to decrease constipation and increase the speed with which waste (and therefore toxins) passes through the intestines. One study compared "highly active" people (defined as those whose activities burn more than 2,500 calories a week above resting metabo-

lism) with inactive people (those who expend fewer than 1,000 calories a week above resting metabolism). The highly active people had an estimated 40–50 percent reduced risk of developing colon cancer. Here are some sample activities that produce this result:

Activity	Duration	Times/week
Aquajogging	40 minutes	3–4
Biking	40–60 minutes	3–4
Jogging	1.5–2 miles	3
Swimming	2,000 meters	3–4
Tennis	2–3 sets	2
Weight lifting	1 hour	3–4

Recent studies have also found an association between exercise and decreased risk of prostate cancer. Lower testosterone levels are believed to be one mechanism behind these results. Of course, a proper diet may also play a role.

How Much Exercise Is Necessary?

Fortunately, you don't have to be a marathon runner to achieve the active lifestyle that experts recommend. The Centers for Disease Control (CDC) and the American College of Sports Medicine (ACSM) have endorsed a prescription for "moderate activity" developed by Dr. James M. Rippe, an associate professor at Tufts University. This approach calls for thirty minutes of accumulated exercise per day. You do not need to go to a gym: a brisk walk at a speed of between three and four miles an hour can do it, and so can many common activities of daily living, such as climbing stairs, raking leaves, gardening, or dancing.

Although evidence shows that a person needs to exercise a minimum of only five days out of the week to reap the health benefits of physical fitness, the CDC and ACSM recommend that every American should engage in thirty minutes or more of some type of physical activity daily.

Many cancer survivors benefit from two to three days of exercise per week with a program including both aerobic and strength training. Studies from the Cancer Well-fit Program in California demonstrated that patients improved 30–50 percent in physical fitness from three days of exercise per week. The participants in this exercise program also improved their quality of life scores in as few as ten weeks of exercise. Their program consists of a few minutes on aerobic machines or group walking for cardiovascular fitness, overall strength training for muscle strength, and stretching exercises to improve any surgical scar tissue and the general suppleness of muscles. Results like these have also been reported from the University of Michigan and the Rocky Mountain Cancer Institute in Colorado, where aerobic and strength exercise programs performed three days per week had similar effects. These programs show that even moderate exercise every other day can have tremendous benefits on fitness and quality of life.

Designing the Right Exercise Program for You

How do you decide which activities to pursue if you want a well-planned fitness program? To answer that, you should first be aware of the three different types of exercise:

- *Activities that increase your flexibility.* The older you are, the more important stretching is, especially if you tend to be inactive. Simple stretches, such as reaching to touch your toes, will keep you limber. Other activities that can improve your joint mobility include yoga, tai chi, and any type of dancing. You can purchase books or videos with specific stretching programs.
- *Activities that build strength and endurance in your muscles.* Strength building requires working against progressive resistance, whether with weight machines or other workout equipment at a gym, dumbbells, elastic tubing, or even your own body weight. When applied to specific parts of your body, these kinds of activities increase the size of your muscle fibers and give your muscles definition.

To increase strength, you should lift a heavier weight no more than ten repetitions, and increase the load as you decrease the repetitions to eight, six, and sometimes to four. This challenges the muscle to constantly push a heavier resistance. To build muscle endurance, you can decrease the load and increase the number of repetitions to twenty or thirty times. You can also boost your endurance by going through your general exercise routine with two-pound to five-pound weights strapped onto your legs or arms. This type of strength training is often used by patients as they are just beginning their exercise program.

- *Activities that improve heart and aerobic endurance.* Exercises in this category involve the body's large muscles (those in the hips, thighs, chest, back, and shoulders). Walking, swimming, jogging, bicycling, aerobic dancing, and ballroom dancing all enhance the ability of your heart and lungs to deliver nutrients and oxygen to your body, as well as to remove waste products via the blood. You can, however, train in any combination of these activities.

Although you can concentrate on any one of these three exercise types, you might want to try a workout program that draws from each category. You can start on a standard workout routine, or be creative.

When to Start

Become physically active as soon as possible after your cancer surgery or other treatment. At first you may have some restrictions on your level of activity (see "When to Avoid Exercising"), but it is now the general practice to get patients out of bed and at least sitting in a chair within one day of surgery. Even this minimal activity helps to reduce the loss of muscle mass and to increase strength. Many therapists recommend starting your formal program after your second cycle of chemotherapy so you don't feel overwhelmed by all of your life changes.

Pain can limit physical exercise after a mastectomy, bowel surgery, or some other major operation. Depression, brought on by changes in your body image, may also make you feel like not doing anything. You may need help to get going. Get a family member, friend, coach, or trainer to help you. For some people, exercising alone is boring. Using music or a videotaped program may help.

Begin a gentle exercise program while you are still in the hospital. This may involve simple muscle tightening while you lie in bed. As your strength returns, different forms of physical activity—isometric and isotonic exercises, and rhythmic repeated movements for various muscles—will help get you on the path to improved fitness.

Making an effort while you're still in the hospital may seem difficult, but you will feel much more confident when you go home if you have already started to regain your strength. You will also be less prone to falls or other accidents that might result from being in a weakened condition.

Before you leave the hospital, your physical therapist can assess your physical condition and help you develop an appropriate set of exercises. Everyone has different wants and needs, so such programs are usually customized. One sample progressive program is described later in this chapter (see "A Sample Progressive Exercise Program" on page 290). The physical therapy staff or exercise specialist can also instruct you, your family, and other caregivers on how to proceed with your program at home. Their recommendations on an appropriate program may be essential to your recovery.

Once you leave the hospital, you have many options to choose from. If you aren't comfortable with a formal program, you can choose something as simple as walking every day or every other day. (Ask your physical therapist about the Winningham program, a simple exercise routine based primarily on walking, either alone or in a group. Designed for patients at all stages, it encourages the use of a walking diary to help make exercise one of your prescriptions for medical treatment.) You can also exercise by going up and down stairs at home or at work for fifteen to twenty minutes every other day.

On days when the weather is forbidding, you can exercise on a treadmill, stationary bike, rowing machine, elliptical machine, or stair climber in your home. Home equipment is worthwhile if you want to exercise at your own pace and convenience. Each year, *Consumer Reports* magazine lists the top exercise machines on the market, and gives information about their durability, safety, and costs. You can join a health club if you want a variety of equipment to choose from and to be with people who are also exercising. Also, visiting websites such as www.bodytrends.com can assist you in purchasing home exercise equipment, as they are the largest exercise equipment website and have medical product lines.

If you like classroom-type aerobics, you could join a group, attend a class, or purchase an exercise video. These videos offer an ideal way to work up to a full routine: some show a slower group on one side of the screen and a more athletic group on the other, but you can also stop the tape or limit the number of times you repeat an exercise. A variety of TV shows (such as *ESPN Workout, Body by Jake*, etc.) can also take you through an aerobic workout. To avoid boredom, you may even alternate programs.

When to Avoid Exercising

Discuss your exercise plans with your physician. If you are ill or are in the first phases of recovery, your physician should instruct you about your limits and about the medical effects of exercise. The following are good criteria for avoiding exercise completely, but always check with your physician before beginning a program:

- Karnofsky Performance Scale under 70 (100 is best).
- Bone density scan less than 8 gr/cm^3.
- White blood cell counts less than 1,000 mg/dl.
- Excessive fatigue (Epstein-Barr virus or other pathogen is present).
- Multiple chemotherapy regimens.
- Presence of shunt catheters.
- Pulmonary or cardiac abnormalities relating to treatments.
- Gait or balance problems associated with treatments.
- Peripheral neuropathy associated with treatments.
- Abnormal electrolytes (sodium/potassium) or protein blood counts.
- Blood platelet counts less than 30,000.
- Metastatic bone cancer patients with less than 50 percent bone cortex involved should NOT be doing any weight-bearing exercise.

Many breast cancer patients who have lymph nodes removed find that the nerve endings to this tissue are still active. The electrical impulse that is generated after surgery can cause pain in certain movements, especially when lifting the arms over the head. This pain may occur because an exercise program was not instituted after surgery. If you have had surgery for breast cancer, discuss range-of-motion limitations with an exercise professional, especially if you experience shooting pains. Several options are available to avoid causing further pain, including massaging ice on the affected areas after exercising. Using a modified cardiac support hose (stretch wrap) over the length of the arm may help with blood supply, reducing stimulation to the nerve, and reducing the swelling in the hands that often happens after exercise. Physical exercise also plays a role in reducing the symptoms of lymphedema, chronic swelling of the arm that has had lymph nodes removed during breast cancer surgery. Keeping the upper body strong and being aerobically fit are important in reducing lymphedema symptoms.

Determining Your Fitness-for-Activity Level

Karnofsky Scale	
100 percent	No evidence of disease
90 percent	Normal activity with minor signs of disease
80 percent	Normal activity with effort; signs of disease
70 percent	Cannot do normal activity, but cares for self
60 percent	Requires occasional assistance
50 percent	Requires considerable assistance and frequent medical care
40 percent	Disabled; requires special care
30 percent	Severely disabled; hospitalization may be indicated
20 percent	Very sick; hospitalization necessary for supportive treatment
10 percent	Moribund
Zubrod Scale	
0	Asymptomatic; normal activity
1	Symptomatic but fully ambulatory
2	Symptomatic; in bed less than 50 percent of the time
3	Symptomatic; in bed more than 50 percent of the time; not bedridden
4	100 percent bedridden
Approximate Relationship of Karnofsky Scale to Zubrod Scale	
0 Zubrod = 100 percent Karnofsky	
1 Zubrod = 85 percent Karnofsky	
2 Zubrod = 65 percent Karnofsky	
3 Zubrod = 40 percent Karnofsky	
4 Zubrod = 15 percent Karnofsky	

Knowing When to Stop

If your physician decides that you may begin an exercise program, you will still need to pay close attention to how you feel during an exercise session. Be aware of the following alarm signals:

Shortness of breath (difficulty breathing, either when resting or when exercising). If an exercise is hard to perform without your becoming short of breath, exercising for even a minimal amount of time can be hazardous. See your physician before continuing with your exercise program.

Dizziness. This is usually a sign of pushing too hard, but it can have other causes, including fatigue, low blood pressure, or dehydration. If you become dizzy, check with your physician. He or she may suggest that you back off exercise until the symptoms have subsided for a few days.

Chronic muscle soreness that interferes with daily routines. If your muscles are sore, you should stop exercising for a few days in order to rest your muscles.

Bruises or swelling. These may be caused by chemotherapy, but bruises and swelling may signal that a bacterial or viral infection is not healing well. Check with your physician.

In general, when you exercise it's important not to get too tired or to hurt yourself. Here are some rules for safe, comfortable exercising:

- When doing exercises for flexibility and muscle strength, try to repeat each exercise three to five times at first. If you feel too tired or too weak, do only one or two repetitions. Gradually increase to between ten and twenty repetitions.
- Try to exercise at least twice a day, and more often if you like it.
- Keep a daily record of your progress, using an Exercise Progress Chart similar to the one on page 290. The repetitions and periods will vary for each person, depending on the person's strength and medical problems.

With any exercise program, always warm up a little before starting, and cool down when you finish. When engaging in aerobic exercise, stay within the following recommended heart rates during exercise, and monitor your perceived exertion (how hard you feel the exercise is) during the activity. The chart below gives ranges for each, based on your age.

Always take your pulse before, halfway through, and at the end of any aerobic routine. During aerobic exercise you should aim to roughly double your resting heart rate if you can, unless your physician sets a specific rate that you should not exceed. The rule is: moderation—take it easy.

If your pulse is slow and you become short of breath, your heartbeat becomes irregular, or you develop chest pain, stop and consult your doctor soon. Have a medical evaluation to prevent harming yourself from exercise.

Breathing

Proper breathing techniques are essential to exercise and can be both therapeutic and relaxing. The techniques have been around for thousands of years and are practiced in the martial arts and used for meditation purposes. Breathing affects the parasympathetic nervous system—the part of the central nervous system that controls our relaxation responses.

Perhaps the best way to breathe is in and out through the nose. This produces a sensation of "fullness" of breath and does not dry the throat. If you can breathe in or out only through your mouth, go ahead—just keep a glass of water handy.

Breathe with as much relaxation as possible. Try to let go of any tension in all the muscles in your neck and shoulders, and fill your lungs all the way. It is important to keep inhaling and exhaling as you perform any exercise. Many people tend to forget to breathe, especially when doing muscle-strengthening or endurance exercises. Never hold your breath during an exercise: holding your breath increases pressure on the heart and may cause dizziness or fainting.

In our culture, only babies breathe correctly. After years of being told to "sit up straight" and "suck in your stomach," many of us develop the bad habit of shallow chest breathing: inhaling by lifting our chests instead of by pushing down our diaphragm. A good relaxation routine centers on slow breaths. The easiest way to make sure you're doing this slow breathing correctly is to press your hand over your abdominal region when you inhale and concentrate on pushing the air into your belly. This will cause distension and a feeling of fullness in the abdominal region. This "diaphragm" breathing also results in inhaling and exhaling more air than chest breathing.

Bed-bound patients risk collecting mucus in their lungs, which can cause pneumonia. Deep breathing followed by coughing can help prevent this complication.

Deep-breathing exercises can help you improve your breathing habits so that you use your entire lung, not just the upper part. Begin each exercise session with a deep-breathing exercise. Deep breathing is also a good way to rest between exercises.

Here are two exercises that help promote breathing and relaxation:

Slow, deep breaths. Using the technique described above, breathe in for a count of four seconds and breathe out for a count of eight seconds. When your capacity improves, you may be able to breathe in for a count of ten seconds and out for a count of twenty seconds. For more information on relaxation cassette tapes, see the "Resources" section in Part VI.

Short, fast, deep breaths. This exercise helps you learn the rhythm of using your diaphragm instead of your rib muscles to breathe with. Concentrate on pushing the air out through your nose from the diaphragm, and then relax and allow your lungs to fill back up with air, making sure that your belly expands at the same time. Aim for a rate of one push every second.

Deep-Breathing Exercise

The following deep-breathing exercise may be done standing up or lying down:

1. Leave your arms at your sides, keeping your hands loose.
2. Slowly take in a deep breath through your nose while raising your arms over your head.
3. Slowly breathe out through your mouth while bringing your arms back down to your sides.

Breathing (Incentive Spirometer) Blow Bottle

The following exercise uses a breathing blow bottle (also called a breathing incentive spirometer) to increase your lung capacity and help avoid pulmonary complications. If you do not breathe deeply, especially after lying on your back for prolonged intervals, you become increasingly susceptible to bronchitis and pneumonia, because fluid tends to collect in the lungs. Coughing is also good for you; take a deep breath and cough three to five times to clear your lungs.

EXAMPLE OF EXERCISE PROGRESS CHART

Date	Exercise Stage	Repetitions Each Exercise	No. of Exercise Periods per Day	Total Minutes Exercised
10/5	1	3	2	3
10/6	1	3	2	5
10/7	1	5	3	10
10/8	1	5	4	10
10/9	1	10	4	20

Increasing Lung Expansion

1. Blow out your breath (exhale).
2. Inhale through the breathing tube, causing the ball to rise as high as possible.
3. Repeat steps 1 and 2 from five to ten times.

A Sample Progressive Exercise Program

The exercise program described in this chapter (see "Sample Exercises" below) has been devised to increase your strength and endurance. The program, which takes you from your bed to being up and around in three stages, can be started as soon as your physician says you are able to exercise.

The exercise programs outlined in this chapter have been done on videotapes for better clarification. The tapes are available through the Stanford Complementary Medicine Clinic Library website at healthlibrary.stanford.edu/resources/videos.html. Stage I is on one tape and Stage II and III are together on another tape. The demonstrations include warm-up and full-exercise programs with relaxation session at the end. An exercise kit includes weights, elastic stretchers, theraband, theraplast, a breathing bag, and other helpful toys.

- Stage I exercises are simple exercises to help you maintain and increase your range of motion. They require little exertion and can be done in bed.
- Stage II exercises use a small added weight to increase resistance and can be done when you are spending part of the day out of bed. Once you have gotten back to your normal activities, you will need to establish an exercise routine that includes exercises like these to build up your body's reserves so that temporary bouts with bed rest will not deplete your energy stores.
- Stage III exercises provide you with a strengthening and maintenance program for when you are able to spend the whole day out of bed. This series of exercises is a progressive and comprehensive physical rehabilitation program for people with acute or chronic illness. With your doctor's permission, you can begin these exercises even while you are recovering from surgery or undergoing cancer therapy.

Start with light warm-up exercises several times a day, gradually increasing both the difficulty of the exercises and the number of times you repeat them. Your maximum physical capacity will improve with time and with use of the program. When you reach the level of more advanced exercises using muscle resistance, you will also need to add a deceleration or "cool down" period to your program. Suddenly stopping exercise after a ten- to twenty-minute period can be dangerous. (On the other hand, if you experience irregular heartbeats, chest pain, lightheadedness, or nausea while exercising, stop immediately. Do not continue until you have clearance from your doctor.) These exercises will need to be modified for each individual. Often, you will

Age	Target Heart Rate	Perceived Exertion Ceiling
20–29	140–148 bpm	6–8 (out of 10)
30–39	132–140 bpm	6–7
40–49	125–132 bpm	6–7
50–59	115–122 bpm	5–6
60–69	108–116 bpm	5–6
70+	(consult with your physician)	

have limits dictated by your physical condition. Your physician and your physical and occupational therapists can help you set up a program that matches your abilities. In addition, you may need to adjust your exercise program daily, depending on how you feel and your medical treatment and testing schedule. It can be done at times convenient to you. You can do only part of the program if your energy level is low, or change the pace several times a day so that by the end of the day you have accumulated several one- to ten-minute periods of exercise for various parts of your body.

The Medi-Gym

Some of the exercises in Stage I and Stage II require simple items of exercise equipment to help you increase your muscle strength by making you work against a slight resistance. These items may be purchased together in the Medi-Gym kit described below, or you can make your own kit using the substitutions suggested.

- Elastic tubing: items such as the Iso-Band, which is available in different strengths and colors. Some of the exercises using this elastic band are shown on the following pages.
- Breathing incentive spirometer: a breathing appliance with a mouthpiece. Used in Stage I exercises to increase lung capacity and to avoid pulmonary complications. You can substitute a soft balloon or a surgical glove with a mouthpiece.
- Exercise putty (Theraplast): elastic putty. Used in Stage I to strengthen and coordinate hands and fingers. You can substitute clay or Silly Putty.
- Sponge ball: a lightweight sponge ball, about 4 inches (10 cm) in diameter. Used in Stage I's general limbering, strengthening and coordination exercises. You can substitute a small Nerf ball, available in toy stores.
- Clothespin: an ordinary wooden clothespin. Used in Stage I to coordinate hands and fingers. For added resistance, wrap a rubber band around the clothespin's tip.
- Ankle weight: a 3-pound (1 kg) ankle weight with

a Velcro closure, used for added resistance in Stage II's general strengthening exercises. You can purchase ankle weights at most sporting goods stores or you can substitute moderately heavy household products in a bag or purse.
- Exercise stretcher: an elastic rope with looped handles. Used in Stage II exercises for stretching and strengthening the large muscles. You can construct a stretcher from elastic cord, such as an Iso-Band bungee cord, available from MII Technologies, or you can substitute a piece of surgical rubber Penrose drain. Make loops at the ends by tying knots.
- Jump rope: any type of rope will suffice. If you are bed-bound, you can tie the rope to the foot of the bed and use it to pull yourself up to a sitting position. Also used in jump rope exercises. You can substitute a piece of rope or clothesline.

Sample Exercises

This section offers some sample progressive exercise programs. Some of the exercises use equipment described earlier (see "The Medi-Gym"); some use equipment (such as an over-the-bed trapeze) that may be provided by the hospital while you are recovering from surgery. In Stage II, some exercises call for a cane or broom handle, and several require a chair.

Stage I: Beginning to Move

Stage I exercises are simple range-of-motion exercises that require little exertion and can be done when you are bedridden. Even if you are very ill, you will probably be able to do some or all of these exercises. Remember, it is important to exercise in order to maintain your muscle tone and joint mobility.

Begin by taking ten deep, relaxing breaths. Remember, do not hold your breath while you do any exercise. Breathe rhythmically in and out.

Shoulders and Chest

The following exercises increase the mobility of your shoulder joints and strengthen your chest muscles.

Straight Arm Lifts

1. Lie on your back and place your arms down by your sides.
2. Keeping your elbows straight, lift your arms up and as far back over your head as you can.
3. Keeping your elbows straight, lower your arms to your sides.

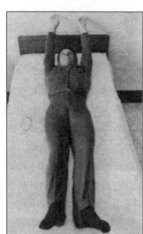

Elbow Touches

1. Lie on your back and place your hands behind your head with your elbows flat on the bed.
2. Bring your elbows together in front of your body.
3. Lower your elbows back down to the bed. (This exercise can also be done sitting up.)

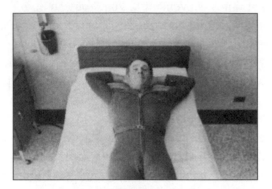

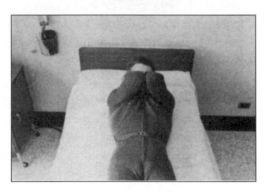

Side Arm Lifts

1. Lie on your back and place your arms down by your sides.
2. Keeping your elbows straight, bring your arms out to the sides and up over your head until your hands touch.
3. Keeping your elbows straight, lower your arms back to your sides again.

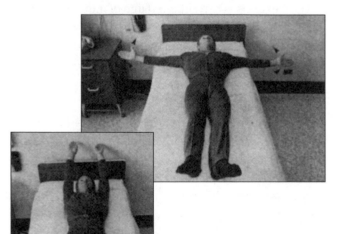

Straight Arm Crosses

1. Lie on your back and put your right arm straight out to the side at a right angle to your body.
2. Keeping your elbow straight, bring your arm across your chest to your left side.
3. Keeping your elbow straight, return your arm to its original position.
4. Repeat steps 1 to 3 with your left arm.
5. Try using both arms at once, crisscrossing them in front of you.

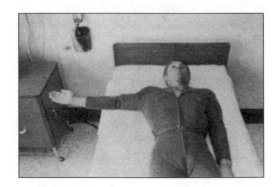

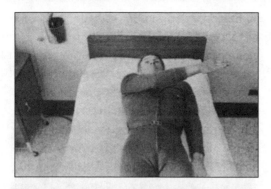

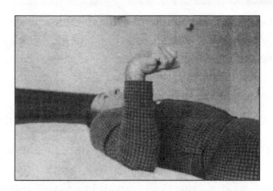

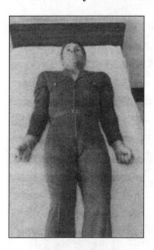 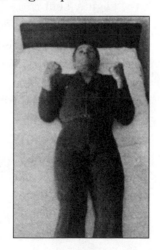

Elbows and Wrists

The following exercises help preserve the mobility of your elbow and wrist joints.

Elbow Bends

1 Lie on your back, place your arms down by your sides, and make a fist with each hand.
2. Bring your fists up to your shoulders, bending your elbows.
3. Lower your fists to their original position.

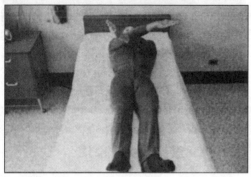

Wrist Rotation

1. Lie on your back and make a fist with each hand.
2. Make small inward circles with your fists.
3. Reverse direction, and make small outward circles with your fists.

Now is a good time to stop and rest. If you are tired, pause and take ten to twenty deep, relaxing breaths. Try to relax your neck and shoulders. If you let tension build up, you'll get tired more easily. Place your hand on your stomach and try to make it rise when you breathe in. Blow out as long as you can.

Hips, Knees, and Ankles

The following exercises mobilize and strengthen your walking muscles.

Knee-to-Chest Lifts

1. Lie on your back, placing your legs together and flat on the bed.
2. Bend your left leg and bring your knee up toward your chest.
3. Straighten your knee while lowering your leg slowly to the bed.
4. Repeat steps 1 through 3 with your right leg.

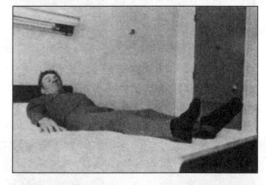

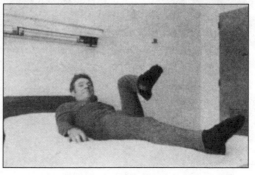

Remember to breathe; do not hold your breath. Breathe in when you lift your leg, and blow out as you lower it back down.

Straight Leg Lifts

1. Lie on your back, placing your legs together and flat on the bed.
2. Keeping your knee straight, lift your left leg as high as you can.
3. Keeping your knee straight, lower your leg slowly to the bed.
4. Repeat steps 1 through 3 with your right leg.

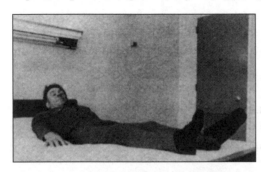

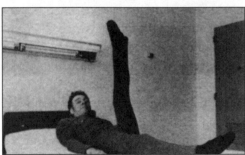

Knee Touches

1. Lie on your back with both knees bent, keeping your feet flat on the bed.
2. Relax and let your knees fall slowly outward as far as they will comfortably go.
3. Bring your knees back up together.

Ankle Rotation

1. Lie on your back, lift your right heel a little off the bed, and make small inward circles with your foot.
2. Reverse direction, and make small outward circles with your foot.
3. Repeat steps 1 and 2 with your left foot.

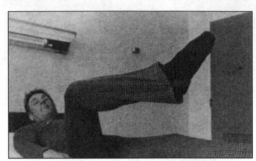

Now is a good time to stop and rest. Take ten to twenty relaxing breaths before starting the next series of exercises.

Trunk

The following exercises strengthen your trunk.

Side-to-Side Rolls

This exercise helps prevent bedsores.

Caution: If you are in a hospital bed, do this exercise with the bedrails raised. If there are no bedrails, have someone stand beside the bed to make sure you do not roll out of bed.

1. Lie on your back, with your knees and elbows slightly bent.
2. Lift your left shoulder and roll to the right, reaching with your left arm for the bedrail or the side of the mattress.
3. Roll back.
4. Repeat steps 1 through 3 on your other side.

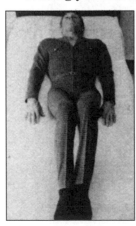
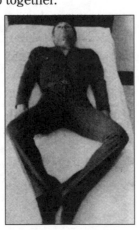
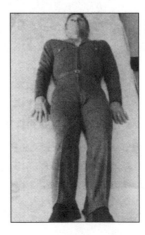
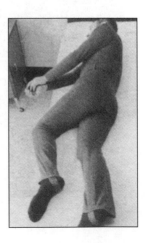

Trapeze-Bar Pull-ups

1. Lie on your back and place both hands upon the trapeze.
2. Lift your buttocks up off the bed.
3. Try to get your nose or chin up to the bar.
4. Lie back again, and repeat steps 1 through 3.

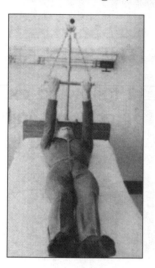 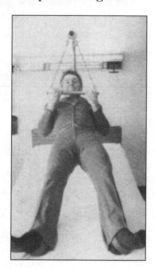

Partial Sit-ups

1. Lie on your back with your hands clasped behind your head.
2. Try to lift your head off the pillow.
3. Now try to lift your head and shoulders up.
4. Lie back down and repeat steps 1 through 3.

The next set of exercises uses the Medi-Gym equipment for added resistance. If you are tired, take a rest before proceeding. Breathe deeply ten to twenty times.

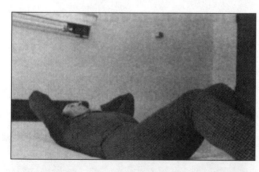

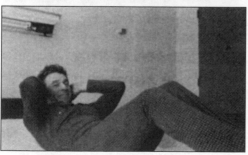

STAGE I MEDI-GYM

In the following exercises, you will use the clothespin, rubber band, exercise putty, sponge ball, elastic sheet, and breathing incentive spirometer from your Medi-Gym.

Clothespin and Rubber Band

These exercises use a clothespin and a rubber band to strengthen your hands and fingers. They can be done lying down, even if you have an intravenous feeding tube in your arm.

Finger Squeeze

1. Squeeze the clothespin between your thumb and your first two fingers. If this is too difficult, squeeze the clothespin between your thumb and all four of your fingers.
2. For added resistance, wrap a rubber band around the tip of the clothespin and repeat step 1.

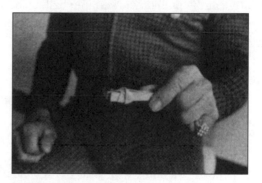

Advanced Finger Squeeze

1. Hold the clothespin between your thumb and first finger, trying to keep your thumb and finger in a circle.
2. Open the clothespin as wide as it will go, and hold it open for a few seconds.
3. Repeat steps 1 and 2 with your thumb and each of your other fingers.
4. For added resistance, wrap a rubber band around the tip of the clothespin and repeat steps 1 through 3.

Finger Spread

1. Place a rubber band over the fingers of one hand, stretching the rubber band.
2. Spread your fingers apart.
3. Repeat steps 1 and 2 with your other hand.

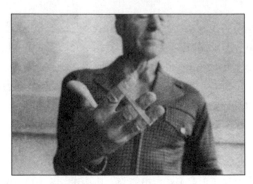

Wrist Pullups

1. Place your left forearm on a table and hold a piece of putty in your left hand.
2. Hold the other end of the putty in your right hand.
3. Pull the putty up with your right hand.
4 Repeat steps 1 through 3, starting with your right forearm on the table.

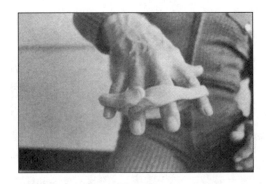

Exercise Putty

The following exercises use exercise putty to strengthen your hands and your coordination control. The putty can be pulled, worked in a ball, or bounced. Use your imagination to invent your own exercises in addition to those described here.

First-and-Second-Finger Pinch

1. Place a ball of putty between your thumb and your first finger.
2. Squeeze through the ball until your thumb and finger meet.
3. Repeat steps 1 and 2 with your thumb and each of your other fingers.

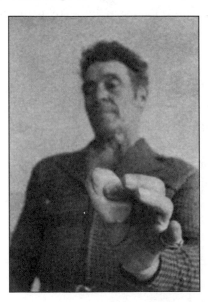

Finger Spread

1. Make a loop out of putty.
2. Place the loop around the fingers of your left hand, between the top two joints.
3. Spread your fingers apart against the loop.
4. Repeat steps 1 through 3 with your right hand.

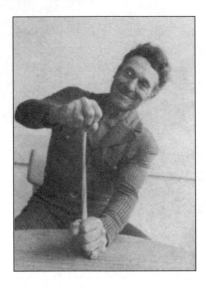

Finger Opening

1. Smash the putty flat with the palm of your hand.
2. Stick your thumb and first finger into the putty, close together.
3. Push your thumb and first finger apart.
4. Repeat steps 1 through 3 with your thumb and each of your other fingers.
5. Change hands and repeat steps 1 through 4.

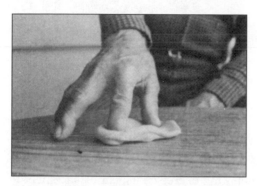

Hand Squeeze

Squeeze the putty in your hand like a ball, moving it around at the same time.

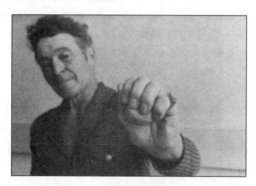

Sponge Ball

The sponge ball is light, easy to handle, and safe–it won't bruise your skin if it hits you. Some of the following exercises are done lying down; for others, you will sit up.

Knee Squeeze

While either lying down or sitting up, put the ball between your knees and try to hold it there.

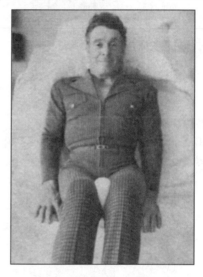

Leg Lift

Lie down, put the ball between your feet, and try to lift it off the bed. (Breathe in when you lift. Blow out as you lower the ball back to the bed.)

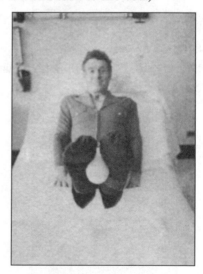

Hand Squeeze

Squeeze the ball in your hand, moving it around at the same time.

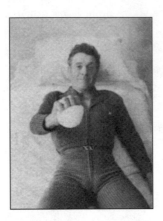

Up-and-Down Toss

Sit up (make sure your bedrails are raised); throw the ball up and catch it.

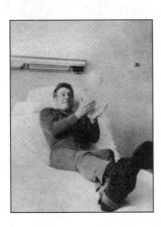

Side-to-Side Toss

Toss the ball from one hand to the other, leaning from side to side to catch it.

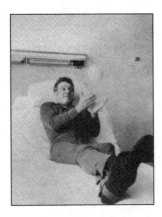

Clap and Catch

Toss the ball back and forth with a friend. For more coordination practice, try clapping your hands just before catching the ball.

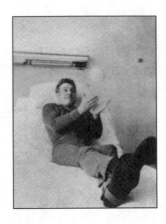

Elastic Sheet

The following exercises use an elastic sheet for resistance. The sheet is very thin and easy to stretch. All of these exercises may be done either lying in bed or sitting up.

Caution: Never use the elastic sheet close to your face. If you lose your grip on it, it could injure your face or eyes. Do not do these exercises if you have any weakness or tremor or if your grip has been injured.

Arm and Chest Stretch

Grab both ends of the elastic sheet and stretch it sideways.

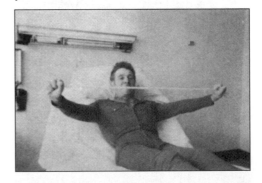

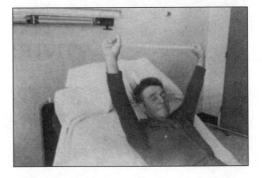

Chest and Shoulder Stretch

With the sheet held behind your head, grip each end and stretch the elastic sheet apart.

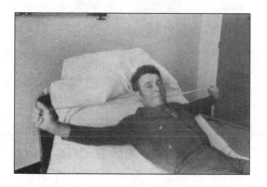

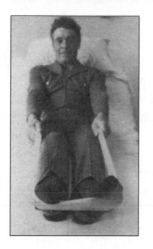

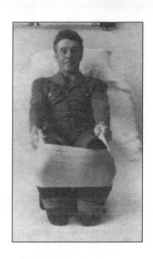

Wrist Stretch

1. Hold both ends of the elastic sheet in your left hand.
2. Loop the sheet around your right wrist.
3. Push your right wrist against the elastic sheet.
4. Repeat steps 1 through 3 with the elastic sheet looped around your left wrist.

Leg and Thigh Stretch

1. Hold one end of the elastic sheet in each hand.
2. Loop the sheet over the bottom of your left foot.
3. Bend your left knee toward your chest.
4. Push your left leg straight out against the elastic sheet while pulling the sheet up with your hands.
5. Repeat steps 1 through 4 using your right foot.

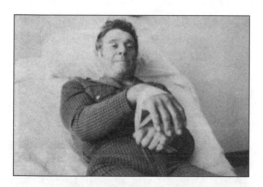

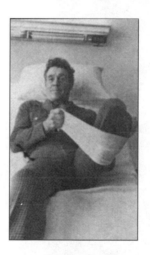

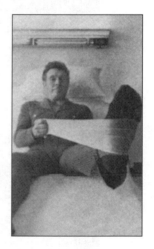

Thigh Stretch

1. Hold one end of the elastic sheet in each hand.
2. Loop the sheet over the bottom of your feet.
3. Try to spread your legs apart against it.

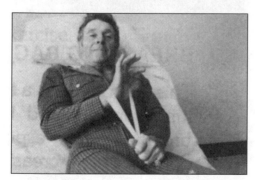

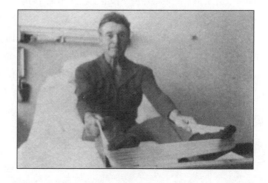

Calf Stretch

1. Hold one end of the elastic sheet in each hand.
2. Bend your knees and loop the sheet over the bottom of your feet.
3. Push the sheet down with your feet while pulling the sheet up with your hands.

Stage II–Bed/Chair with Resistance
Neck

The following exercises strengthen your neck muscles. If you have had surgery or treatment to the head and neck area, either omit these exercises or check with your physician before trying them.

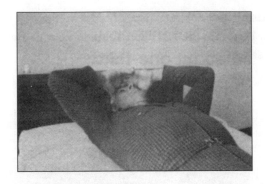

Chin Tuck I

1. Lie on your back and place your hands behind your head, with your elbows bent and pointed out to the sides.
2. Holding your hands behind your head, bring your chin up to your chest.
3. Push your head back against your hands.
4. Lower your head back against your hands.

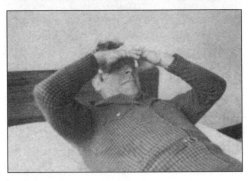

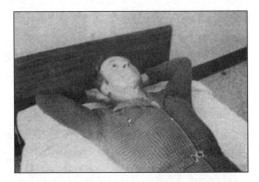

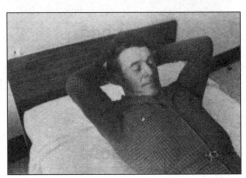

Side Neck Bends

1. Lie on your back, bending your right elbow and putting your right hand on the side of your head.
2. Bend your head to the left.
3. Bend your head to the right while pushing against your head with your right hand.
4. Repeat steps 1 three 3 with your left hand.

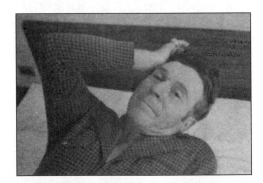

Chin Tuck II

1. Lie on your back and place your hands on your forehead, with your elbows bent and pointed out to the sides.
2. Pushing against your head with your hands, bring your chin to your chest.
3. Relax and lower your head back down to the bed.

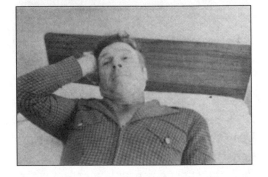

Shoulders and Chest

The following exercises strengthen the muscles of your shoulders and chest.

Straight-Arm Cane Lift

This exercise uses the 3-pound (1 kg) weight to strengthen the shoulders, expand the rib cage, and exercise the chest muscles. Lifting your arms over your head greatly expands your rib cage, giving you an excellent opportunity to breathe deeply as you raise your arms.

1. Loop the 3-pound (1 kg) weight around the middle of a cane or broom handle.
2. Lie on your back and take the cane in both hands.
3. Keeping your elbows straight, lift the cane up and as far back over your head as possible.
4. Keeping your elbows straight, lower the cane slowly to the original position.

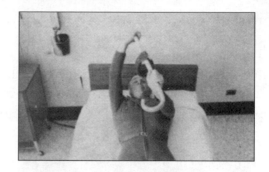

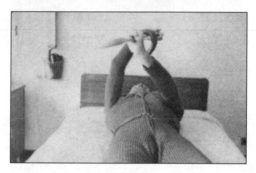

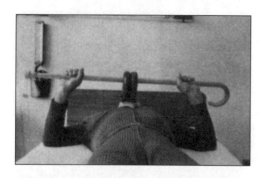

Side Arm Stretch

This exercise uses the exercise stretcher from the Medi-gym kit to strengthen your chest muscles.

1. While either sitting up or lying down, take the ends of the exercise stretcher in your hands.
2. Stretch your arms out to the sides, pulling against the exercise stretcher.

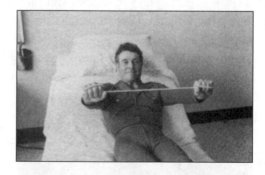

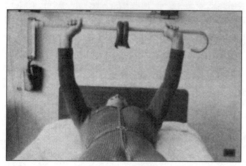

Straight-Arm Cane Twist

This exercise uses the 3-pound (1 kg) weight to strengthen the shoulder muscles.

1. Loop the 3-pound (1 kg) weight around the middle of a cane or broom handle.
2. Lie on your back and take the cane in both hands.
3. Keeping your elbows straight, hold the cane up over your head.
4. Twist the cane slowly to the left and then slowly to the right.

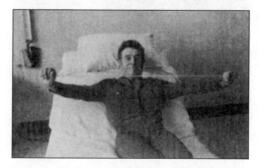

Overhead Arm Stretch

This exercise uses the exercise stretcher to strengthen your shoulder muscles.

1. While either sitting up or lying down, take the ends of the exercise stretcher in your hands.
2. Holding your arms over your head, stretch sideways.

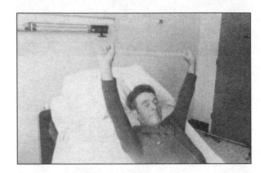

Stop and rest before proceeding. Take ten to twenty deep breaths. If you are not too tired, start the next group of exercises.

Walking Muscles

The following exercises strengthen your walking muscles.

Straight Leg Lifts

This exercise strengthens your knees and thighs.

1. Strap the 3-pound (1 kg) weight around your right ankle.
2. Lie on your back. Keeping your knee straight, lift your right leg straight up as far as you can.
3. Keeping your knee straight, slowly lower your leg to the bed.
4. Repeat steps 1 through 3 with your left leg.

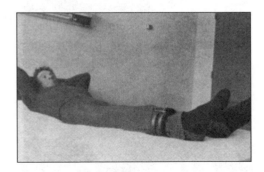

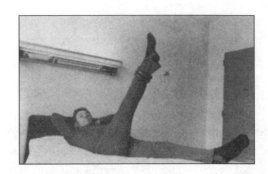

Backward Leg Lifts

This exercise strengthens your buttocks.

1. Strap the 3-pound (1 kg) weight around your right ankle.
2. Lie on your stomach, with your abdomen on the bed and your feet touching the floor.
3. Keeping your right knee straight, lift your right leg up and back.
4. Repeat steps 1 through 3 with your left leg.

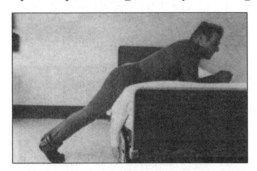

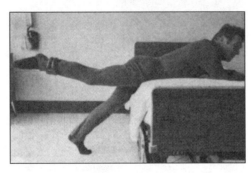

Sideways Leg Lifts

This exercise strengthens your thighs.

1. Strap the 3-pound (1 kg) weight around your left ankle.
2. Lie on your right side, with your right arm under your head. Brace yourself against the bed with your left arm in front of your chest.
3. Keeping your knee straight, lift your left leg up.
4. Keeping your knee straight, lower your left leg slowly to the bed.
5. Repeat steps 1 through 4 on your other side.

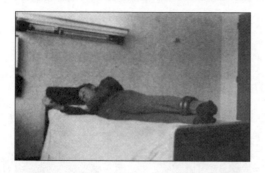

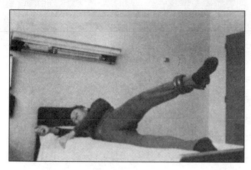

Arms and Legs

The following exercises strengthen your arms and legs.

Elbow Bends I

This exercise uses the exercise stretcher to strengthen your arms and back.

1. Sit on the bed, placing the loops of the exercise stretcher around the bottoms of your feet and holding the middle of the exercise stretcher in your hands.
2. Sit up with your legs straight out and your arms straight out in front of you.
3. Bending your elbows, bring your arms to your chest.
4. Relax, allowing your arms to return to their original position.

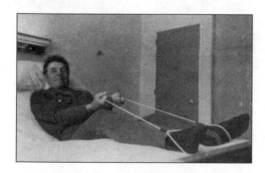

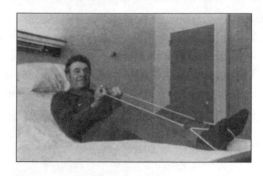

Upward Arm Stretch

This exercise uses the exercise stretcher to strengthen your upper arms.

1. Lie on your back with the exercise stretcher underneath your back.
2. Holding the ends of the stretcher in your hands, extend your arms straight up, pulling the ends of the stretcher toward the ceiling.

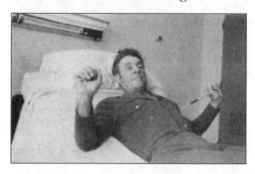

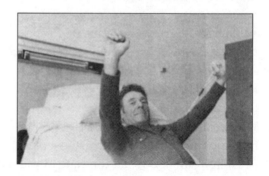

Trapeze Arm Stretch

This exercise uses your bed trapeze to strengthen your upper arms.

1. Loop the exercise stretcher over the trapeze.
2. While sitting up, take the ends of the exercise stretcher in your hands and pull down as far as you can.
3. Raise your arms and repeat step 2.

Downward Arm Stretch

1. While sitting up, place the exercise stretcher around the back of your neck like a scarf.
2. Taking the ends of the exercise stretcher in your hands, pull down until your arms are straight.

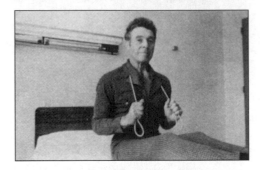

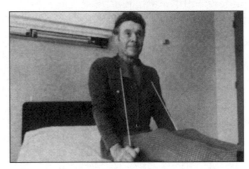

The following exercises are done sitting on the side of the bed or in a chair. If you are not used to standing up and walking around, be sure to have someone with you to help if you get dizzy.

Elbow Bends II

This exercise uses the 3-pound (1 kg) weight to strengthen your arms.

1. Loop the 3-pound (1 kg) weight around the middle of a cane or a broom handle.
2. While sitting in a chair or on the edge of a bed, hold the cane in both hands, palms up.
3. Bending your elbows, lift the cane to your chest.
4. Lower the cane to your knees, straightening your elbows.
5. Repeat steps 3 and 4 while holding the cane in both hands, palms down.

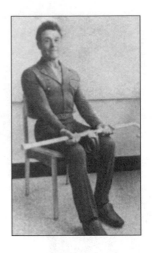
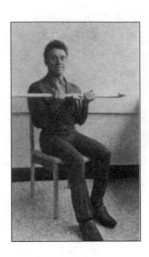

Knee Lifts

This exercise uses the 3-pound (1 kg) weight to strengthen your knees.

1. Strap the 3-pound (1 kg) weight around your left ankle.
2. While sitting in a chair or on the edge of a bed, extend your left leg, straightening your knee and lifting your foot off the floor.
3. Repeat step 2 with the weight strapped around your right ankle.

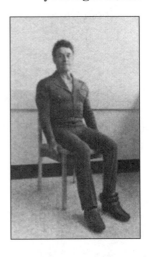
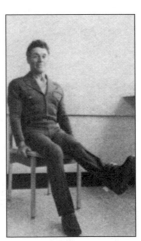

Stand Up–Sit Downs

This exercise strengthens your whole set of walking muscles and your hips, knees, and buttocks.

1. Sit on the edge of either a bed or a chair that has arms.
2. Stand up slowly.
3. Sit down slowly.
4. Use the arms of the chair at first; then try to rise without using the arms.

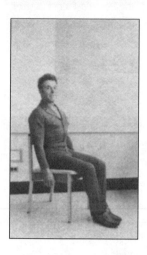 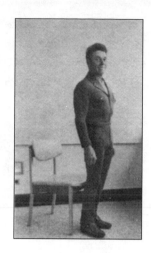

Stage II Exercises

The following program is appropriate when you are able to spend more than half of your day out of bed or when the Stage I exercises have ceased to be challenging. Cancer treatment and physical inactivity results in a decrease in the size of muscle fibers, therefore reducing their ability to generate force. In this stage of exercise, you will apply the principle of overload by placing a greater than normal physical demand on your major muscle groups. You can use the Iso-Bands, or some other elastic exercise product, to accomplish this.

Your goal is to increase muscle strength, which requires exercising against a force (Iso-Band or weight) that asks your muscles to call upon approximately 40–60 percent of their maximum strength. Generally this is accomplished by choosing the appropriate tension. You should be able to perform ten repetitions of each exercise with proper form, but by the ninth repetition it should become moderately challenging.

Overload is a dynamic process. With training, the muscles worked will increase their absolute strength so that 40–60 percent of this strength translates into a higher force needed to produce changes, or in other words, to become stronger. If you are exercising in this program two times per week, you will probably need to increase the intensity of your work every two to three weeks. Start with the lightest tension (white Iso-Band). If you cannot perform ten repetitions with proper form, do as many as you can and with regular performance you will increase the muscle strength sufficiently to allow more repetitions. If you cannot perform any repetitions without sacrificing your form, just do the exercises without the band until you increase your strength

enough to start using it. Conversely, if the work seems so easy that you are not challenged, increase the intensity of your work. There are two ways to accomplish this. Either choose a band with more tension or shorten the band you are using by making a loop at the top of the band. Important changes occur in muscles with this type of training. These changes include increases in the size of muscle fiber and increase in the size and strength of tendons and ligaments that may have become weakened by chemotherapy. Additionally, muscle-strength training improves the ability of your nervous system to get messages to and back from your muscles, allowing you to respond more quickly. This is very important if your reaction time or balance has suffered during treatment or if you have neuropathies (nerve damage) from chemotherapy affecting your nervous system. Additionally, your muscles will be able to store more energy, in the form of glycogen, thus allowing you to be more active without fatigue. Regular training can also increase your appetite so that eating can become pleasurable again.

Instructions and Precautions

1. Your chair should be sturdy and free of armrests that might impede your movement. Make sure that the height of the chair is such that your feet can be placed firmly on the floor with a ninety-degree angle at the knee joints. The spine should be firmly against the back of the chair.

2. Focus on the muscle or muscle groups that you are working and try to relax the rest of your body. For example, if you are exercising your biceps (bicep curl), keep your neck long and shoulders down. Keep your movement confined to the elbow joint.

3. Perform each exercise through your full range of motion. Don't shorten the movement. For example, in the bicep curl, your arm comes up as close to your shoulder as possible and then lengthens so that it is straight. Do not lock the elbow joint.

4. Do not hold your breath because this can raise your blood pressure too much. Take a breath in and then breathe out with the first part of the movement. Breathe in again with the second part of the movement.

5. Start with one set of ten repetitions for each exercise, two times per week. After two weeks, perform two sets. After four weeks, work yourself up

to three sets. If you cannot initially perform ten repetitions, do as many as you can and try to add one repetition every week until you reach ten comfortably. Then proceed as discussed earlier in this article.

The Program

It is important to warm up your working muscles with gentle movements before starting the muscle strength portion of this program. Perform eight repetitions of the following movements. Follow the warm-up with the stretches illustrated.

1. Move head from side to side.
2. Move ear toward shoulder then back to other shoulder.
3. Bring chin toward chest and then look forward.
4. Shrug your shoulders up toward your ears and down again.
5. Roll your shoulders in forward circles.
6. Roll your shoulders in backward circles.
7. Bring both arms straight out in front of you and relax again.
8. Rotate your wrists.
9. Bend your elbows and bring your hands, palms facing up, toward your shoulders.
10. Tilt your pelvis so that your lower back presses firmly against the back of the chair, then relax until the normal curve in the low back returns.
11. Lift your knees up toward your chest, one at a time. (Keep the spine long).
12. Straighten each leg one at a time so that you are tapping your toe on the floor in front of you.
13. March your legs quickly on the floor.

Your muscles should be warmed up now. Perform the following stretches now and after completion of the strength exercises. Research has shown that doing stretching exercises three times per day, with each stretch held fifteen to thirty seconds, provides gains in joint range and motion without compromising safety. Try to progress slowly until you can do these stretches three times per day. Pay attention to your form. Do not take any stretch beyond the point of slight resistance. Use a mirror to make sure that your position is correct. For example, when performing the seated posterior thigh stretch, do not slump your shoulders. Keep the spine long.

Upper Chest and Shoulder* (Anterior) Stretch

For the most effective stretch, roll your shoulders back and then down your back. This stretch is very important for you if you have had a mastectomy.

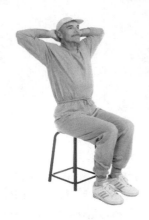

Upper Back and Shoulder (Posterior) Stretch

Do not twist your torso or hips. Do both sides.

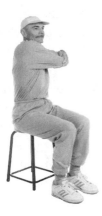

Anterior Thigh Stretch

If you experience balance problems, do this stretch on your side on the floor.

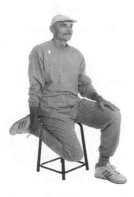

*Illustrations are used with permission of MII of Santa Ynez, CA. Donald G. Bornell, Ed.D. and his wife Cecil Jean Bornell have developed numerous stretching exercises using the Iso-Band.

Seated Gluteal Stretch

To activate more of the muscles in the lower spine, straighten the opposite leg.

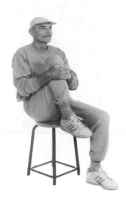

Seated Posterior Thigh Stretch

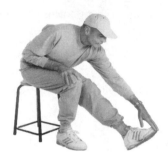

Strength Exercises

Caution: if you have had a mastectomy with nodes removed, these first four exercises are specifically important for you. If you have bone metastasis, do not use the Iso-Band or any other resistance tool. Just perform the movement with your limbs.

Chest Muscle Strength Exercise

1. Place the band around the middle part of your back. Hold the plastic handles comfortably.
2. Push arms forward; gently pull back to starting position.
3. Keep the shoulders down and the spine long.

Caution: if you find that you are lifting your shoulders or if there is movement in your lower back, the resistance might be too great. Put the band aside and just use your limbs until your muscles get stronger.

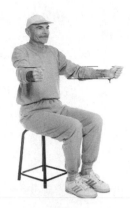

When you are ready for an advanced exercise, alternate the forward movement with the following:

1. Start with straight arms out to the side, shoulders relaxed, palms slightly below shoulders.
2. Bring the band in front of your chest, with your elbows slightly bent, then slowly move back to starting position.

Anterior Shoulder Muscle Strength Exercise

1. Place the bottom of the loop securely under your feet.
2. Hold the plastic handles and lift the arms up and forward without lifting your shoulders.
3. If you are not yet strong enough to execute the movement with the arms straight, they can be slightly bent, but make sure you then get an adequate biceps stretch following the exercise. Biceps stretch: place your straight arms behind you, lacing your fingers together with palms facing the wall behind you. Roll your shoulders back and then down the back and lift gently until you feel the stretch in the front of the arms.
4. If you find yourself moving your torso or head, the resistance is too great. Use just your limbs.

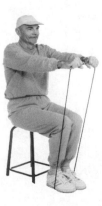

Middle Back and Shoulder (Posterior) Strength Exercise

1. Hold the band in front of your chest, elbows slightly bent.
2. Pull the band back, pulling your shoulder blades together.

Precaution: do not lift your shoulders and keep your neck long.

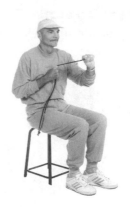

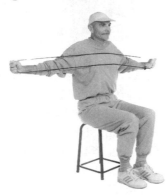

Biceps Curl

1. Place the band looped securely under the feet.
2. Hold the plastic handles in both hands and pull your hands up toward your chest.

Precaution: do not lift your shoulders. Do keep your wrists straight.

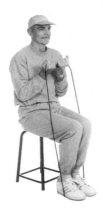

Triceps Extension

1. Secure the band at the chest as shown.
2. Hold the band with the opposite hand, palms facing downward.
3. Gently extend the arm toward the floor.
4. Repeat with the other arm.

Note: You can increase the intensity of the exercise by shortening the band.

Precaution: keep your wrist straight.

Seated Leg Press Exercise

This exercise is especially important for strengthening the walking muscles.

1. Place your back securely against the back of the chair.
2. Loop the band on the bottom of the foot.
3. Lift the thigh up for a count of three. The knee should have a ninety-degree angle.
4. Straighten the leg out for three seconds.
5. Bend the knee back to ninety degrees for a count of three.
6. Lower the thigh, placing the foot on the floor for a count of three.

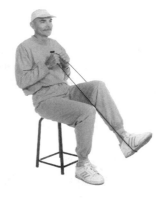

Stage III: Up and Around

Once you start spending the whole day out of bed, walking around the house, and resuming your normal daily activities, you are ready for Stage III activities. These are vigorous exercises, and safety precautions should be observed when using a chair. Take your pulse when you begin and after you finish. Your pulse should return to its resting rate within five minutes. Try to exercise four to five times a week. As with Stages I and II, begin with three to five repetitions of each exercise; try to work your way up to between ten and twenty repetitions.

Once again, especially with vigorous exercise routines like the following ones, proper breathing is very important. Be careful not to hold your breath. Inhale and exhale regularly during all the exercises.

Outlined below are two types of exercise routines, one for aerobic conditioning and the other for improving strength. You may perform one or both types of activities, depending on your medical condition and exercise goals.

Sample Program I: Aerobic Conditioning

Goals: Modest improvement of cardiovascular capacity and improved functional abilities (enhanced energy, reduced fatigue, better breathing capacity), with possible improvement in the immune system over time.

Sample Program II: Strength and Conditioning

Goals: Improve posture, strength, range of motion, and flexibility.

A typical strength-training program for cancer patients should consist of a specific exercise routine. One such routine is detailed below:

Resistance Band and Fit Ball Exercises for Home-based Programs

These exercises are for persons who want to have a basic exercise program for their home, performing some basic stretching, elastic band, and fitness ball exercises that help to prepare the muscles for walking programs, or performing daily living activities more efficiently. Below are some basic stretches and exercises that can be performed in the home using a pair of slippers or tennis shoes as the only equipment you may need.

Front Shoulder Stretch

Body Part Worked: back and shoulder

Exercise Comments: Interlace the fingers and pull the arms straight in front and upward, keeping the palms facing outward.

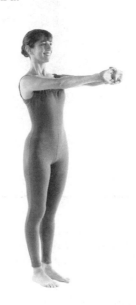

AEROBIC CONDITIONING ACTIVITIES

Exercise	How Performed	Times/week	Length/Intensity
Aqua aerobics	self/class	2–3	20–40 min., 50–70%
Aqua deep-water walking	self	2–4	10–25 min., 50–70%
Breathing/slow	self	daily	5 min.
ITP (interval training program) walking		1–2	Slow walk 30 sec. Fast walk 10–15 sec. Repeat 5 sets of slow and fast walking
Qi gong, with tai chi centering	1-on-1	daily	depends on style
Stationary bike (treadmill, rower, upper-body arm crank, etc.)	self	3–6	10–40 min., 50–70%
Tai chi	self	daily	depends on style
Walking	self/partner	3–6	20–60 min., 50–60%

Back Shoulder Stretch

Body Part Worked: shoulder and chest muscles

Exercise Comments: Interlace your fingers behind the waist and gently move them up and back.

Hamstring Stretch

Body Part Worked: back of thigh and calf muscles

Exercise Comments: Place your feet about eighteen inches apart and point your left foot in front. Place your hands on your knees, bend the right knee, and rotate your body over the left knee for the stretch. Repeat with your right leg.

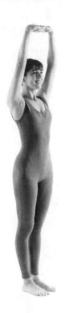

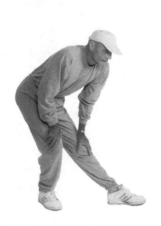

STRENGTH AND CONDITIONING ACTIVITIES

Exercise	How Performed	Times/week	Length/ Intensity
Individual body parts: work on movements in postsurgery areas that have pain and decreased motion.	self/partner	3–6	10–15 min.
Elastic bands: increase isotonic strength and range of motion in major muscle groups; learn principles of progressive resistance.	self/1-on-1	2–4	10–20 min.
Light dumbbells: increase strength in upper body.	self/1-on-1	2–4	10–20 min.
Manual: perform resistance movements with instructor, to improve function postsurgery.	partner/1-on-1	2–4	10–15 min.
Weights: improve general strength through specific ranges of motion.	self/class	2–4	20–60 min.

	Sets	Repetitions
Warmup, 5 minutes		
Resistive exercises:		
Bench press, lateral pulls	2–4	10–8–6*
Shoulder press, T-rows	1–2	10 each
Biceps, triceps, abdominals	1–2	10 each
Leg press, extensions	2–3	10–8–6*
Leg curls, calf raises	1–2	10 each
Stretching component, 5–10 minutes		

*Increase weight as you become comfortable at each weight level and are ready to increase the weight by a fixed amount (e.g., 2, 5, or 10 pounds [1,2 or 3 kg]) to provide progressive resistance with major muscle groups.

Calf Stretch

Body Part Worked: calf muscle, Achilles tendon

Exercise Comments: Stand with one foot behind the other—three feet from the wall. Place both hands on the wall, lean forward, and keep the back heel firmly on the floor.

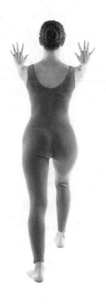

Elastic Band Hip Extendor

Body Part Worked: hip gluteals, low back

Exercise Comments: Loop the band under the extension arch of the right foot and secure the hands out in front of the waist about twelve inches. Keep the knees straight while you extend the right leg to the back against the resistance of the band. Repeat with left leg.

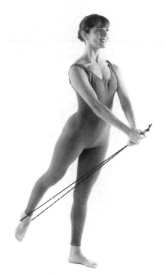

Elastic Band Front Pull

Body Part Worked: chest, shoulders

Exercise Comments: Hold the handles with both hands, palms facing down. Step on the band so it is under the arches of both feet. With your elbows straight, raise the band until your arms are extended in front of you.

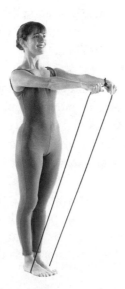

Elastic Band Bicep Curls

Body Part Worked: biceps muscles

Exercise Comments: Hold the band with both hands facing outward. Drop the band down and step on it so that the band is under the arches of both feet. Bend both elbows and bring the hands up to the chest against the band resistance.

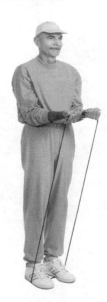

Elastic Band Half Squats

Body Part Worked: gluteals and thigh muscles

Exercise Comments: Holding the band in both hands, step on the band so that it is under the arches of both feet. Starting with your knees bent, try to straighten up to a standing position against the band resistance.

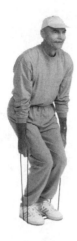

Fit-Ball Abdominal Curls

Body Part Worked: abdominals

Exercise Comments: Begin from a sitting position on your ball. Roll down so your middle back is pressing against the top of the ball. Cross your arms across your chest. Keep your feet at a wide width apart and your eyes in a fixed position straight ahead. Inhale before initiating your exercise. Exhale as you squeeze your abdominal muscles and bring rib cage closer to your pelvis. Hold this contraction for about one second.

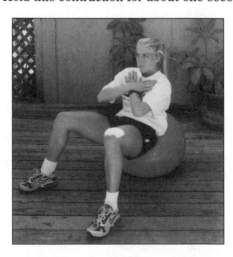

Circulation Enhancers

Vertical Arm Swings

1. Stand with your feet apart.
2. Clasp your hands together, keeping your elbows straight.
3. Swing your arms up over your head, and then bring them back down toward the floor again.

Finish up your exercise session with ten to twenty deep breaths.

Note: not all patients should perform all types of strength exercises. If you have had surgery for breast cancer in the upper chest/armpit area, you may use rubber tubing for the chest pulls and rowing exercises. Your goal is to progress to light dumbbell or hand-weight exercises for chest work and flies (pendulum exercises moving the arms to the front and sides). Rubber tubing allows you to experience the feel of progressive resistance and to control how much force you exert. Over time, you will increase your upper body strength enough to move on to other strength training.

Sports and Recreation

When you are able to do Stage III exercises comfortably, think about adding some sports and recreational activities to your exercise program. You can work up to these gradually: climb stairs four or five times daily, take walks. Pace yourself; go one block the first time and try to increase your distance daily. Gardening is an excellent exercise if you enjoy it. At first, someone may have to assist you with the heavier work. Even a small plot will provide you with exercise as well as fresh air, sunshine, and a sense of accomplishment.

- Bicycle: plan your routes to be more or less strenuous to fit your needs.
- Jump rope: this vigorous exercise gives overall muscle toning and coordination.
- Swim: if you feel energetic, join a health club and use the saunas and steam rooms as well as the pool. You may find it easier to exercise in the pool because water supports your limbs.

Post-Mastectomy Rehabilitation

You can enhance your physical and psychological recovery following a mastectomy by returning as quickly as possible to the normal activities of your daily life.

Your first step is to better understand post-mastectomy problems by talking about your concerns with members of your medical team, family, and friends, and, if possible, a volunteer from the American Cancer Society's Reach to Recovery program.

Your next step is active participation in a structured exercise program, such as the American Cancer Society's Reach to Recovery post-mastectomy exercise program, the YWCA's ENCORE (Encouragement, Normalcy, Counseling, Opportunity, Reaching Out, and Energies Revived) program, or a similar exercise program, such as the one given here. (For information about Reach to Recovery and ENCORE, see the Resources section in Part VI.)

This section describes the Reach to Recovery and ENCORE programs and presents a series of post-mastectomy exercises to help you increase your muscle strength and range of motion. In addition, Chapter 39, "ADL–Self-Care and Activities of Daily Living," gives suggestions on coping with the activities of daily living and using them as helpful exercises.

Research shows that beginning a regular exercise program like the one presented in Stage III or the Winningham walking program is effective in overall disease control.

Reach to Recovery

Reach to Recovery's approach offers strong support immediately following surgery. The program's volunteers have also experienced a mastectomy and have returned to their normal activities. They offer their personal experience and emotional support to help you to maintain your self-esteem and self-confidence and to reduce your fears.

Volunteers supply the Reach to Recovery booklet, a temporary breast (prosthesis) and helpful hints about self-image, sexuality, and clothing. They also provide a free demonstration of exercises with necessary tools so that you can begin exercising as soon as you have permission from your physician, usually a few days after surgery. A member of your health care team can help you contact your local Reach to Recovery chapter. There is no charge for this volunteer visitor program.

ENCORE

The ENCORE program complements Reach to Recovery and is available in approximately twenty-four YWCAs across the United States. You may enroll in ENCORE about three weeks after surgery, with your doctor's permission. The program includes group exercises and discussion groups, where you can share your concerns.

Post-Mastectomy Exercises

The following program of standard exercises is similar to the Reach to Recovery program. You can use this program along with videotapes, cassette recordings, and the Medi-Gym (see the Resources section at the end of the book). The most important thing is to involve yourself in a program on a regular basis. Appoint yourself your personal health instructor and go to work. You can gain satisfaction in your achievement. You know best how hard to try, how hard to push, and how much pain you can tolerate.

The following exercise program will help initiate your recovery and you can use it in conjunction with the Reach to Recovery or ENCORE programs. If you underwent breast reconstruction at the same time as your mastectomy, do not begin this program without your surgeon's approval.

Post-Mastectomy Stage I: Beginning to Move

The following exercises are done with your affected arm and do not require much motion.

Upper-Arm Isometrics

1. Start with shoulder shrugging, ten repetitions, holding for a count of six.
2. Tighten the muscles of your upper arm by slightly bending the elbow and pulling the arm in toward your body.
3. Hold for a count of six; relax for one to two seconds before repeating.

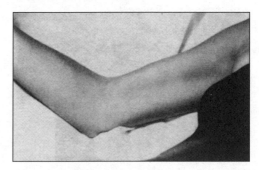

Lower-Arm Isometrics

1. Turn your hands palms up.
2. Make a fist and curl up your wrist.
3. Hold for a count of six; relax for one to two seconds before repeating.

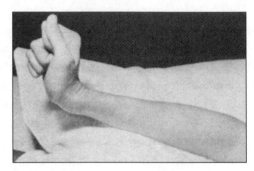

Hand Squeeze

In your Medi-Gym kit you will find some exercise putty and a sponge ball. Squeeze them in your hand.

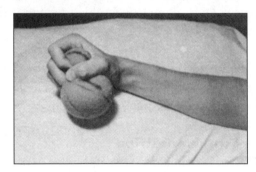

Fingers

Use the exercise putty, the sponge ball, and the clothespin from your Medi-Gym kit for gentle finger work.

Post-mastectomy Stage II: Increasing Physical Activity

Crawling the Wall

1. Stand facing a wall, about six to eight inches away from it.
2. Reach toward the wall and "walk" your fingers up as far as you can. Mark the place where you stop each day to encourage you to go higher the next time.
3. Repeat steps 1 and 2, but begin by turning so that the side of your body faces the wall.

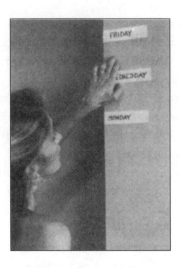

Pendulum Exercise

1. Begin by sitting in a chair. Bending forward, let the arm hang straight down. Move it in small circles, the way a clock's pendulum moves.
2. Progress to a standing position. (Hold onto a chair or place your hand on a counter or table for stability.) Swing your arm forward and out to the side, as well as making circles.

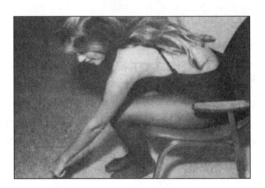

Elbow Touches

1. Lie on your back, placing your hands behind your head with your elbows flat on the bed.
2. Bring your elbows together in front of your body.
3. Lower your elbows back down to the bed. (This exercise can also be done sitting up.)

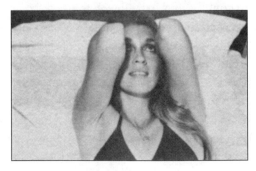

Cane Exercises

1. Put a cane (a broom handle or a yardstick is also good) behind your back and put both hands on it. Pull from side to side.
2. Put the cane behind your neck, and repeat as above.

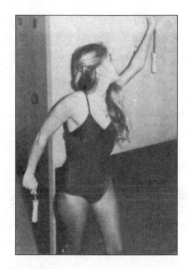

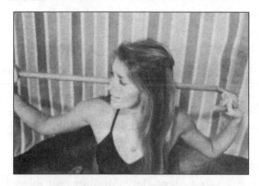

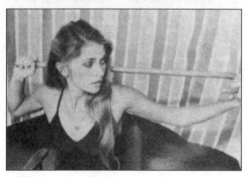

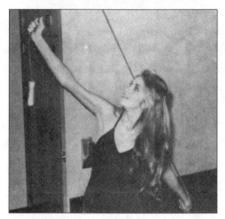

Pulley Exercise

1. Place the exercise stretcher from your Medi-Gym, or a jump rope, over a door. (You can hammer a nail at the top of the door to keep the rope from falling off.)
2. Stand with your back to the edge of the door. (You can also face the edge of the door. This exercise can also be done sitting down.)
3. Use your good arm to pull your affected arm as high over your head as possible. Go only slightly into the painful range.

Conclusions

There has been an increase in the recent medical publications on the topic of exercise and cancer. Now more than ever, results from studies on the benefits of regular physical activity are more available to doctors, nurses, therapists, and patients. Regular physical exercise is important for cancer recovery, and with new research and reports of its health benefits, we hope that many survivors can participate in a structured program that will help in their own recovery process.

The Cancer Well-fit Program was started by one of the authors, Eric Durak. He is the Director of Medical Health and Fitness in Santa Barbara, CA, and a leader in a movement encouraging health clubs to set up post-rehab programs that offer ways to continue exercising in groups and in a cost-effective manner. Many patients are interested in maintaining or improving their physical function beyond that of acute care. Such programs are designed to create a link between medicine and fitness. Special instruction is given to trainers about the medical aspects of working with cancer patients as well as patients with other diseases. If none of your local gyms have a program, you can speak with them about starting a group for cancer patients. Or contact Eric Durak at (805) 692-9929 or at medhealthfit.com.

Exercise websites for cancer survivors:
- **bodytrends.com** offers home exercise equipment and a medical products line.
- **cancerwellfit.com** is the Cancer Well-Fit exercise website.
- **fitcare.com** is an integrative health and exercise site with cancer and exercise section.
- **medhealthfit.com** offers monthly exercise articles for cancer survivors, plus products and books.

References

Barlow, C.E, Kampert, J.B., Wei, M., Blair, S.N. "The effect of low cardiorespiratory fitness on the association between BMI and cancer mortality." *Medicine and Science in Sports and Exercise.* 32;5:S293, 2000.

Courneya, K.S., MacKay, J.R., Jones, L.W., "Coping with Cancer: Can Exercise Help?" *The Physician and Sports Medicine.* 28:5:1-17, 2000 www.physsportsmed.com/cover.htm.

Dennehy, C.A., Bentz, A., Stephens, K., Carter, S.D., Schneider, C.M., "Prescriptive exercise rehabilitation adaptations in cancer patients." *Medicine in Science in Sports and Exercise.* 32;5:S234, 2000.

Dimeo, R.C., Tilmann, M.H.M., Bertz, H., Kanz, L., Mertelsmann, R., Keul, J.R., "Aerobic exercise in the rehabilitation of cancer patients after high dose chemotherapy and autologous peripheral stem cell transplantation." *Cancer.* 79:1717-22, 1997.

Durak, E.P., Lilly, P.C. "The Application of an Exercise and Wellness Program with Cancer Patients: A Preliminary Report." *Journal of Strength and Conditioning Research.* 12;1:3-6, 1998.

Durak, E.P., Wollitzer, A.O., Lilly, P.C. "Reporting the Results of a Breast Cancer Exercise Program: A Two Year Follow-Up Survey." *Journal of Rehabilitation Outcomes Management.* 3;4:53-57, 1999.

Kramer, M.M., Wells, C.L. "Does physical activity reduce risk of estrogen-dependent cancer in women?" *Medicine in Science in Sports and Exercise.* 28;3:322-34, 1996.

Miller, L.T. "Exercise in the management of breast cancer-related lymphedema." *Innovations in Breast Cancer Care.* 3;4:101-06, 1998.

Segar, M., Katch, V.L., Garcia, A., Haslanger, S., Wilkens, E. "Aerobic exercise reduces depression, and anxiety, and increases self-esteem among breast cancer survivors." *Oncology Nursing Forum.* 20:317-21, 1998.

*References for the studies cited in this chapter are available on request from Keren Stronach, Cancer Resource Center, UCSF Comprehensive Cancer Center, 1600 Divisidero, San Francisco, CA 94143-1705.

33

Massage and Compassionate Touch for Persons with Cancer

Francine Manuel, R.P.T.
Lee Daniel Erman, N.C.T.M.
Ernest H. Rosenbaum, M.D.
Isadora Rosenbaum, M.A.

One of the most relaxing and enjoyable experiences for a person with cancer—or for any other human being—is to receive gentle, compassionate, accepting touch from another person. This can range from a one- or two-hour massage from a trained massage therapist to something as simple as having your hand stroked by a friend. Touch is fundamental. It is the first sense we develop—indeed, all infant mammals require touch to survive and thrive—and it may be one of the last senses to be lost in the dying process.

With appropriate precautions, touch or massage can be helpful to all persons with cancer with little risk of injury. Some people are concerned that the increased circulation promoted by massage might help spread the cancer. However, there is no substantive evidence for this belief, and many of the most prominent cancer medical centers support massage for their patients. General guidelines include not doing any deep work in known or suspected cancer areas; avoiding deep pressure for leukemia patients or if platelet counts are low; and being careful in cases of bone metastases or osteoporosis. An overriding guideline: if any massage or touch technique does not feel right to you, do not allow it to continue–the goal should be to foster well-being with delightful touch, and "no pain/no gain" does not apply.

Compassionate touch, or massage, can be extremely helpful to cancer patients for several reasons. First, being sick can be lonely, and being touched provides an antidote to the probing, uncomfortable, manipulative touches that all too frequently are part of modern medicine. Second, a patient can take what he or she needs most, without needing to ask and without the toucher, or perhaps even the patient, needing to know what that is. These benefits and emotions include hope, human contact, affirmation, release of anger, relief from pain, relaxation, playfulness, love, acceptance of bodily changes, or a reminder of something important.

The following have all been shown to be physical benefits of touch/massage under some conditions:

- relaxation
- increased blood and lymph flow
- endorphin release

- release of tight muscles
- toning of flaccid muscles
- edema (extra fluid in tissues) reduction and relief
- normalized blood pressure
- stress reduction
- increased immune function
- improved balance
- pain reduction
- sleep improvement
- better digestion
- softening of scar tissue
- increased energy and cognitive performance
- communication without the need for words
- communication without the need for energy, or even consciousness, of the receiver

Hints for Providing Compassionate Touch

For effective, focused, therapeutic massage, a skilled and experienced massage therapist is needed. All humans, however, are capable of providing loving and beneficial compassionate touch. Although we all have innate touching skills, many of us have not practiced those in our often touch-deprived culture. Before you begin, it may be helpful to review the following list of reminders.

- First, center yourself.
- Pay attention to the verbal and nonverbal cues of the person you're touching.
- Open yourself to the sensations you feel while touching. Remember that you can directly sense only yourself—everything else is interpretation.
- Enjoy touching. No matter how extreme the person's condition, revel in the miracle and beauty of him or her as a living human being.
- Relax. Any tensions or apprehensions you have will be conveyed to the other person.
- Don't do anything that makes you emotionally uncomfortable.
- Don't do anything that makes you physically uncomfortable. Do what you need to find a comfortable position. Shoulders down. Back straight. Work from the center of your body, not from your hands or arms. Keep breathing smoothly.
- Use your full hands, including your palms. Let your hands mold to fit whatever you're touching. Use and feel your own wonderful living fleshiness.

- You don't have to rub, especially on thin or tender skin or on weak or meager muscles or bones. Squeeze gently, or just hold.
- Move your hands slowly. Even slower. Even slower than that. Just hold.
- Good candidates for compassionate touch: hands, feet, back and shoulders, scalp.
- Keep the person warm.
- Be gentle, but firm and definite.
- Breath is central to all life. Breathe smoothly. Be aware of the person's breath. Try synchronizing your breathing.
- Listen for and trust your intuition.
- Give up any agenda or expectation of results— just experience the touch in the moment.

In addition to the benefits for the recipient, indicated above, studies have shown that the person providing the touch also benefits. So, if you are receiving compassionate touch from a friend, caregiver, or another person with cancer, turn the tables on them and provide them with some loving compassionate touch—you'll both love it!

Basic Massage Strokes

There are four basic massage strokes: effleurage (light or deep stroking), petrisage (kneading), tapotement (hacking or slapping), and friction.

Effleurage. Effleurage is the very slow stroking with which you begin and end every massage. The two types of effleurage are light stroking, which is used to relax the patient, and deep stroking, which empties the blood and lymphatic vessels.

Begin by placing your hands very lightly on the area to be massaged. With the lightest pressure you can apply, run your hands slowly over the area. Make full contact with the skin with both hands. All strokes should be done with a continuous motion. After five minutes of light stroking, begin to deepen the strokes in the direction towards the heart. Lighten the strokes going away from the heart.

Petrisage. Petrisage can be done in two ways: with the palms or heels of your hands or with your fingertips. In this stroke, you actually pick up the muscle tissue away from the bones and work on the affected areas to decrease muscle spasms.

Tapotement. Tapotement is done by hacking with the sides of your hands or by cupping your hands and using them to percuss (tap sharply) an area of the body. This stroke, while pleasing to most muscle-bound athletes, is usually not pleasing to a seriously ill patient; it should never be used without a physician's approval. It can be dangerous to anyone with kidney disease.

Friction: Friction is done with one or two finger-tips. Apply pressure in a circular manner over bony prominences, such as the pelvic bones, shoulders, vertebrae (backbones), and kneecaps. Do not move around with this stroke; stay in one spot for a prolonged time and then move on to another spot.

Finding a Massage Therapist

If you do wish to receive massage from a trained professional, make sure to find one who is compatible with you and your needs. As with any other kind of skilled personal service, one of the best ways to find a qualified massage therapist is by referral from someone whose judgment you trust. Another way is via the American Massage Therapy Association's "locator" service, which can be reached toll-free at (888) THE-AMTA or (888) 843-2682 or via their website www.amtamassage.org. (The website contains a wealth of other information about massage, including questions to ask of a therapist you are considering engaging.) In any case, make sure that the massage therapist feels right to you—do not hesitate to ask questions, explain what you want, and go elsewhere if you cannot get what you want or feel dissatisfied or concerned with the service you are receiving.

Types of Massage/Bodywork

Swedish/Western Massage

Based on the Western concepts of anatomy and physiology, Swedish massage employs the traditional strokes of effleurage, petrissage, vibration, friction, and tapotement (percussion). Swedish/Western massage is the most widely used system in Europe and the United States. However, most massage therapists are trained in and utilize a wide variety of other techniques blending them with Swedish/Western into a treatment tailored to your needs.

CranioSacral Therapy

A gentle, hands-on method of evaluating and enhancing the function of the craniosacral system—the physiological body system composed of the membranes and cerebrospinal fluid that surrounds and protects the brain and spinal cord.

Cross-Fiber Friction Massage

Friction massage applied in a transverse direction across the muscle, tendon, or ligament fibers. The stroke is only long enough to cover the intended tissues. The fingers do not move over the skin but move the skin and superficial tissues across the target tissue.

Deep Tissue Massage

The term refers to various massage techniques that are directed toward enhancing or correcting particular, focused structures of the muscle and fascia (connective tissue). Most deep-tissue massage techniques aim to affect particular areas within the various layers of fascia that support muscle tissues and to loosen bonds between the layers of connective tissues. Although some deep-tissue techniques do press "deeply," they do not necessarily produce pain or discomfort.

Feldenkrais Method

A form of body movement education that teaches how we can improve our range of movement through repeating slowly evolving exercises. The method teaches us to be comfortable at our current level of movement and simultaneously expand those capabilities to function better in our daily lives.

Lymphatic Drainage Massage

This method uses light, rhythmical, spiral-like movements to accelerate the movement of lymphatic fluids in the body.

Myofascial Release (Connective Tissue Massage)

Slow, focused stretching through one or more body planes. This can also include ischemic compression (the application of progressively stronger pressure) to release the tenderness of trigger points. A trigger point is a hyper-irritable spot, usually within a taut band of skeletal muscle or within the muscle's fascia, that is painful on compression and can give rise to characteristic referred pain, tenderness, and body dysfunction.

Neuromuscular Therapy

Identifies soft-tissue abnormalities and manipulates the soft tissue to normalize its function. Addresses the neuromuscular dysfunctions created by trauma, improper body mechanics, poor posture, and other stressors.

Reflexology

This method originated with the Chinese and is based on the idea that stimulation of particular points on the surface of the body has an effect on other areas or organs of the body. Today's techniques focus mainly on the hands and feet.

Rolfing

A systematic program developed out of the technique of structural integration. Rolfing reshapes the body's physical posture and realigns the muscular and connective tissue through manipulation of the fascia (connective tissue).

Sports Massage

A method of massage especially designed to prepare an athlete for an upcoming event and to aid in the body's regenerative and restorative capacities following a rigorous workout or competition. It is also designed to reduce the athlete's risk of injury.

Shiatsu

A Japanese system of acupressure based on the Oriental concept of *chi* (life force energy) and *tsubos* (energy points). When pressure is properly applied to the energy points (via finger pressure), energy circulation is improved and the body is thought to be better able to heal itself.

The Trager Method

This method uses movement exercises, called *mentastics*, along with gentle shaking of different parts of the body, to eliminate and prevent tensions.

Zero Balancing (ZB)

A hands-on body/mind system to align body energy with the body's physical structure. It represents the integration of Eastern views of energy with Western views of science and teaches how to use energy as a working tool in relation to body structure.

Conclusion

Massage therapy is an easy, practical method to relax not only the muscles but the entire person. It is also a method of nonverbal communication that gives reassurance and bridges the gap between caring and therapy. If you have a willing family member or friend, massage can be a pleasant way for others to participate in your recovery and gain satisfaction from being able to help.

34

Self-Care and Activities of Daily Living

Judy Bray, O.C.
Mary Godfrey, O.T.

Activities of daily living (ADL) are all the little things we do throughout the day for self care, such as bathing and dressing, household tasks like washing dishes, doing the laundry, planning and preparing meals, home/personal management, correspondence, scheduling, and other tasks.

Performing self-care tasks provides overall muscle toning and increases your range of motion. Performing as many self-care tasks as possible will also help you regain independence and self-esteem. Feeling dependent on others can be defeating, while setting objectives in life and accomplishing them can be deeply satisfying. Recovering from an illness or injury is certainly one of these accomplishments.

As you begin your recovery, consider the degree of physical effort required for each self-care task in terms of how much mobility and energy it requires. Begin with those activities which are easiest for you to accomplish. For example, feeding yourself is probably one of the first activities you'll be able to do, because it requires the least amount of effort. When you are stronger, you will be able to do some hygiene and grooming activities; still later, you'll be able to bathe and dress yourself. Your overall goal is to return to your former activities as fully as possible. Use the Self-Care Progress Chart at the end of this chapter to keep track of your progress. Make a list of all the activities you perform daily in caring for yourself, and then add each new accomplishment to the list along with the date on which you achieve it.

Many assistive devices or gadgets, which make certain tasks easier to accomplish, are available to help you achieve greater independence. It is important that you conserve energy, using it appropriately to achieve both short-term and long-term goals. In addition, you should consider safety in the home. When you are tired and weak, it is all too easy to have an accident that could slow your recovery or even reverse your physical status dramatically.

Assistive Devices

An assistive device compensates for loss of function and enhances your ability to take care of yourself comfortably and safely. Such devices can be as simple as a long-handled bath brush to scrub your own back, or as complex as a wheelchair. Assistive devices can be obtained from the medical and surgical supply stores listed in your telephone directory yellow pages. Your local hospital will also have the names of supply companies in your area. Some commonly used devices are described below; many can be improvised at home.

Homemaking Aids

- one-handed bread and cutting board
- one-handed vegetable basket for straining cooked vegetables
- one-handed electric can opener
- one-handed "Spill Not" bottle and jar holder
- rubber twister for unscrewing lids of bottles and jars
- multipurpose clamp that provides good leverage for small items and for turning knobs (e.g., on a TV or radio)
- electric plugs with handle
- one-handed suction nail brush (you attach it to a surface and move your hand to clean your nails)
- one-handed suction nail file (you attach it to a surface and move your hand to file your nails)

Eating and Drinking Aids

- Special cups with lids to avoid spilling liquids.
- If you have poor coordination or trouble swallowing with a cup, a cup with a lidded spout may be helpful. A sport water bottle may also be used.
- The Wonder-Flow vacuum cup (Figure 1) allows you to drink while lying flat on your back or on your side. These cups can be used with straws. Use extra-long (18 in./46 cm) straws if you tire while trying to hold a cup. You can also improvise with foam cups that have plastic lids, such as those used for take-out food.

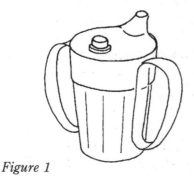

Figure 1

- Serve soup in a cup for ease and safety.
- If you have trouble swallowing, a plastic glass with a cutout for the nose (Figure 2) will allow you to drink without tipping your head back, as a precaution against choking.

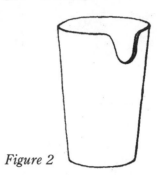

Figure 2

- If your grasp is weak, a stretch-knit coaster clipped around a glass (Figure 3) will give you a firmer grip. You can also use adhesive-backed bathtub safety treads or similar rubber decals wrapped in a spiral around the glass.

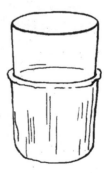

Figure 3

- The Mac Mug (Figure 4) has an easy-to-grasp T-shaped handle that is insulated to protect heat-sensitive skin. Two-handled cups, similar to children's cups, are also helpful.

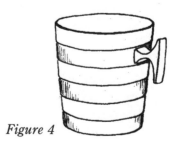

Figure 4

- Built-up handles on knives, forks, and spoons (Figure 5) will help if you have difficulty in grasping. You can improvise these by using foam-rubber hair curlers, sponge rubber, or washcloths.

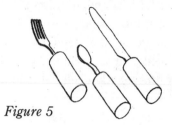

Figure 5

- If you have difficulty with coordination, a plate guard (Figure 6) will prevent food from being pushed off the plate. The guard clips onto the edge of the plate and acts as a stable surface to push against. You can also use a dish with a high edge, such as a pie plate, or a special plate that is raised on one side.

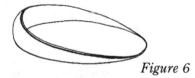

Figure 6

- If you must have your meals in bed, a firm, wedge-shaped cushion (Figure 7) behind your back will place your body in a more comfortable position, especially for swallowing.

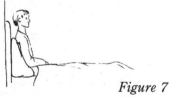

Figure 7

- Use a breakfast tray with legs (Figure 8) or a serving tray, or improvise with a cardboard box with spaces cut out on the long sides for your legs (Figure 9). Cover the tray's surface with a damp towel or some other material to keep dishes from sliding.

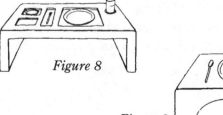

Figure 8

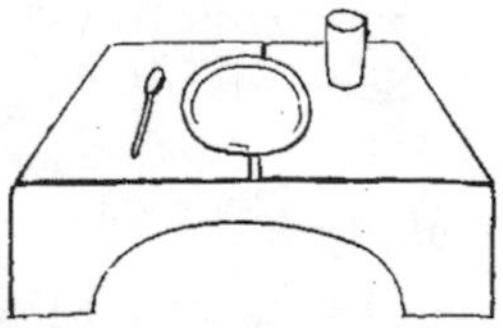

Figure 9

Bathing Aids

- Grab bars (Figure 10) can be fastened to the bathtub or attached to the wall to make it easier and safer to get in and out of the tub or shower.

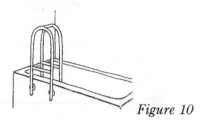

Figure 10

- A bath seat (Figure 11) will help you get in and out of the bathtub and allow you to sit in the shower.
- A combination grab bar and bath seat (Figure 11) is available in many styles to fit all needs and types of bathroom fixtures.

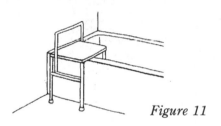

Figure 11

- A portable, hand-held showerhead can be used with a bath seat to shower in the bathtub.

Toilet Aids

A three-in-one commode can be used over the toilet to increase the height of the toilet seat and provide arms or rails to assist in coming up to stand. A raised toilet seat (Figure 12) makes coming to a standing position more comfortable (especially if you are bothered by hip pain). Easy-to-clean padded vinyl toilet seats are also available (Figure 13).

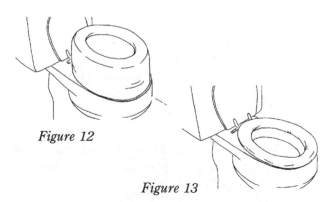

Figure 12

Figure 13

Energy Conservation

Conserving energy in small tasks will help you have enough stamina to manage your daily self-help tasks. By eliminating extra steps or movements or combining tasks, you are able to pace your day and build up your energy reserves. Analyze your day and pace yourself so the tasks you do are in accordance to your energy level. Do heavier or more demanding tasks when you are feeling stronger and your energy level is high. Save the lighter tasks for later on.

Dressing

- Try to do the major part of this task while seated in a chair, preferably one with arms.
- Long-handled reachers (Figure 14) will eliminate having to bend over and will help you get garments started over your feet.

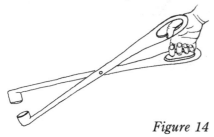

Figure 14

- It is easier to put your weak arm or leg in first when dressing and to take your strong arm or leg out first when undressing.
- Loose-fitting tops with front-closing zippers, ties, or buttons are the most convenient.
- A buttonhook (Figure 15) may help you with manipulating small shirt and trouser fastenings.

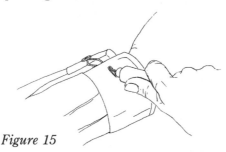

Figure 15

- If you are not ready to dress in street clothes, an attractive sweat suit or lounging outfit will give you and those around you a boost in morale.

Housework

- Where possible, sit rather than stand. A seat that is bar stool height is a compromise between standing and sitting.

- Have work in front of you rather than at the side.
- Move slowly and do not lift heavy objects.
- Slide objects rather than lift them.
- Maintain good posture when standing, bending, or sitting.
- To reduce fatigue, use fitted bed sheets to make bed-making easier.
- To decrease the need for bending, use long-handled dustpans and self-wringing mops.
- Store frequently used items in an easily accessible area.
- Put everything you need for a particular task in a basket or box. For example, group together items for morning care (Figure 16).

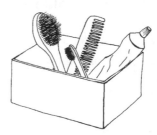

Figure 16

- Wear a cobbler's apron (Figure 17) or similar garment for carrying small lightweight items to reduce unnecessary trips about the house.

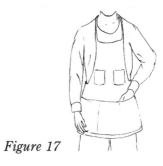

Figure 17

- Use a wheeled cart for moving items from one room to another.
- Alternate work and rest periods.
- Plan a basic schedule each day in order to reduce unnecessary motions and steps.
- Pace your work schedule. Don't try to complete all tasks in one day. Have a weekly plan for scheduling major tasks such as washing, ironing, shopping, and cleaning, so that one task can be done each day.

Cooking

- Plan ahead—write out menus for a week's meals

at a time. Shop for staples once a week and for fresh produce twice a week, or have your groceries delivered.

- Assemble all ingredients and utensils before beginning to prepare a dish.
- Make larger quantities, and freeze portions for later use.

- Plan how to use leftovers when cooking.
- Don't be reluctant to use frozen or convenience foods. You can add your own seasonings.
- A slow cooker will allow you to cook a one-pot meal with minimal preparation time and effort. Your dinner will cook safely in it throughout the day, allowing you to rest.

YOUR SELF-CARE PROGRESS CHART		
Activity	**Date Initiated / Notes (how much help)**	**Goal**
EATING		
Drinking from straw		
Drinking from glass		
Using napkin on face and hands		
Eating finger food		
Eating with spoon or fork		
Cutting with knife		
Opening and pouring liquids		
HYGIENE		
Using handkerchief		
Brushing or combing hair or putting on wig		
Shaving		
Brushing teeth or dentures		
Using bedpan or urinal		
Sponge bath—face and upper body		
Sponge bath—lower body		
Make-up, nail care, etc.		
DRESSING		
Assisting with putting on sleepwear		
Putting on robe		
Putting on slippers		
Putting on street clothing (sitting)		
Putting on street clothing (alternating sitting and standing)		

- Use small tabletop appliances, such as an electric frying pan or rice cooker, to eliminate standing or bending at the stove.
- Use lightweight cookware to conserve energy.
- Use nonstick cookware for ease in cleaning up.
- Use paper plates or plastic cups for snacks or lunches to eliminate dishwashing.

Home Safety

- Remove throw rugs so you do not trip or slide on them.
- Disengage the self-closing mechanism on a door if you can't get through it without it hitting you.
- Clear floors of all small objects, such as bathroom scales or doorstops, to reduce the risks of slipping or tripping.
- Install additional phones, especially a cordless phone that can be kept by you in any room.
- Avoid loose or floppy slippers or shoes. Use slippers and shoes with a rubber sole to prevent slipping.
- Check all stair treads, thresholds, and banisters for loose hardware and slippery surfaces.
- Falls are common on stairs, especially on the last step. Make sure the stairwells are well-lit. Paint the bottom step a contrasting color.
- Install railings on stairs if you do not have them and always use them.
- Use a night light.
- To prevent dizziness when you first get out of bed, sit and dangle your feet for a moment before standing up.
- Check the bathroom for safety. Use a rubber bath mat or adhesive-backed strips in the tub or shower. Use liquid soap so you do not need to worry about dropping the soap.
- When in the kitchen, do not reach across a hot burner.
- Survey your own living situation and take precautions that would benefit you.
- Have a large, easy-to-read list of emergency numbers, including fire, police, personal physician, relatives, and friends, near your telephone.

Activities of Daily Living for Post-Mastectomy Patients

Specific daily living and self-care skills should be incorporated into your exercise program. Your goal is to resume your normal way of life by gaining progressive independence in daily personal care, household responsibilities, work, active hobbies, and exercise. You can help yourself reach that goal by steadily increasing your range of motion, strengthening your muscles, and decreasing pain and swelling.

Initially, you may need to adapt some tasks to your range of motion, energy level, and comfort. Pace yourself to accomplish a task, and then work on gradually increasing your strength and range of motion. The most difficult daily living activities will be those requiring you to reach up, out, and around (especially a two-handed task).

The following suggestions will help you cope with activities of daily living; you can also use them to gradually increase your range of motion and muscle strength.

- Continue to use both hands as you did before the mastectomy. It is often tempting to avoid using a sore limb. To encourage yourself to use your sore arm, wear a cotton glove on your opposite hand to decrease its ability to feel accurately. If you have had surgery on the left side, wear the glove on your right hand. If you have had surgery on the right side, wear the glove on your left hand.
- Towel drying with both hands after bathing will help you increase your range of motion.
- When blow-drying and styling your hair, initially it may be more comfortable to support the affected arm on a telephone book or other prop until your range of motion and strength have been restored.
- To fasten a bra, begin by fastening it in front and then turning it around. Progress to reaching behind your back to fasten it, first with the straps off, and then with straps on your shoulders.
- When putting on a blouse, shirt, or sweater, put the affected arm in first. When undressing, take the affected arm out last. To remove slip-on clothing, draw it over your head first, and then slide it off your arms.
- When closing a zipper at the back of a garment, use a zipper pull. As you achieve more active arm motion, you can discontinue using the pull. Hanging up your clothes in a closet will provide you with movement similar to that obtained when using a pulley. Begin by hanging up a lightweight garment using your affected arm. As you gain strength and range of motion, try hanging up heavier garments, such as slacks or a coat.

- When cooking, do the stirring with your affected arm. At first, you may prefer to slide rather than lift cookware off the stove or counter; then try lifting and reaching, using both hands, as soon as you are able.
- Plan your shopping to eliminate heavy lifting or carrying.
- Use general household activities as exercises to increase your range of motion, including sweeping; making the bed; mopping; polishing mirrors, silver, etc.; turning doorknobs and keys; folding laundry; washing walls and windows; vacuuming; and reaching up to high shelves.
- When watering plants, use both hands to hold the watering can. As your strength increases, try using your affected arm, especially for watering plants in high spots.
- Gardening offers many opportunities to help you increase your range of motion, such as raking, hoeing, cutting, and planting. Caution: wear gloves to avoid cuts or injuries to your hands or fingers, because your affected arm is more susceptible to infection after surgery.
- Sports that offer more vigorous exercise, such as swimming, tennis, bowling, and Ping-Pong, may be attempted when you have already achieved a good range of motion. Remember to reach up, out, and around.

35

Sexuality and Cancer

Jean M. Bullard, R.N., M.S.
David G. Bullard, Ph.D.
Ernest H. Rosenbaum, M.D.
Isadora R. Rosenbaum, M.A.

Sexuality can sometimes be affected by a serious illness, such as cancer, and its treatment. By "sexuality," we mean the feelings we have about ourselves as sexual beings, the ways in which we choose to express these feelings with ourselves and others, and the physical capability each of us has to give and experience sexual pleasure. Sexuality can be expressed in many ways, including how we dress, move, and speak, as well as by kissing, touching, masturbation, and intercourse. Anxieties about survival, family, or finances, along with changes in body image and the ability to tolerate different levels of activity, can place a strain on the expression of sexuality and create concerns about sexual desirability.

It is important to understand that even healthy adults often report difficulties with sexual satisfaction. Recently, the *Journal of the American Medical Association* reported a survey of thousands of men and women that found that more than 40 percent of the women and 30 percent of the men regularly had no interest in sex, were unable to have orgasm, or suffered from some other form of sexual dysfunction. Other researchers felt that these statistics might actually understate the problem, which is often thought to relate to lack of time, job pressures, money troubles, and emotional or health problems.

So, having an enjoyable sexual life is not easily attainable for many people. The good news is that if you were comfortable with and enjoyed your sexuality before your illness, chances are excellent that you will be able to keep or regain a healthy sexual self-image despite the changes brought about by cancer. Many people who have cancer or who are the partners of persons with cancer may experience no change in sexual feelings or behavior. Others may find that increased closeness and communication resulting from the experience of illness enhances their sexuality. Still others may never have considered sexuality to be of great importance in their lives, or may consider it less important now than previously.

If, however, you are experiencing some changes or stresses in your sexuality because of cancer or its treatment, the material presented here is designed to help you explore ways to deal with these changes. We do not intend to present a course in sex counseling, or a list of "how to's" about sexual functioning. Nor do we intend to suggest that everyone with cancer will have sexual problems. Sexual problems frequently arise not so much from changes imposed by a medical condition or its treatment but from how we feel about and deal with those changes.

We will present concepts and principles that many people who have handled changes in sexuality have found useful. We hope that this information will help you become more aware of your attitudes about your sexuality; that it will form a basis for you to begin to communicate your sexual feelings and needs more directly to people important to you, including those responsible for your health care; and that it will help you decide how sexuality fits best into your own life at this particular time.

Remember, you are the expert on your own sexuality. We hope that the material presented here will validate your sexual concerns and stimulate your thinking about how best to handle them. For more information on specific concerns or questions, see the Resources in Part VI.

Sexuality Issues for Patients and Their Partners

Sexuality has long been a matter of great interest and concern in our culture. We have moved from one extreme—in which our puritanical views made public discussion about sexuality totally unacceptable—to the current extreme, in which explicit sexuality is commonplace and is exploited in popular advertising and as the main theme of many books and films. Feelings about sexuality tend to be intense ones, closely tied to moral and religious beliefs, as well as to deep feelings about self-esteem and desirability. Sexuality has different meanings and importance for each of us, and we each have our own ways of expressing ourselves as sexual beings.

Until recently, little accurate information about sexuality has been available. Most of us have been exposed to a wide assortment of myths and misinformation about sexuality handed down through generations or gained from discussions with our friends. The popular media (books, magazines, television, films, etc.) have "told" us what sexuality is and have set many standards for being "sexually attractive."

Unfortunately, these ideas tend only to reinforce much of the misinformation we grew up with and make it difficult for us to feel secure about our own unique sexuality. There are as many different ways of expressing sexuality as there are people, and most people experience concerns about their sexuality at some time during their lives. Consequently, health care providers are beginning to recognize that addressing sexuality is an important part of health care.

"We are all sexual beings." This simple statement makes the important point that sexuality is part of who we are, not just what we do. Sexuality is expressed in many ways—how we dress, how we talk, how we work, and how we play. Furthermore, each of us is uniquely sexual in the sense that we choose whether or not to be actively sexual, and in what ways, how often, and with whom. If sexuality were something people could easily discuss, we would no doubt discover that the importance of sexuality varies tremendously from person to person.

One problem that can get in the way of a comfortable discussion of sexuality has to do with the words we use. Some "labels" that supposedly describe sexual problems are demeaning and embarrassing. It would be difficult to feel good about being described as "impotent" or as a "premature ejaculator." One of the more degrading ways to describe a woman with sexual concerns is to label her "frigid." These labels say nothing about what someone is actually experiencing and may in fact lead to false assumptions about that person's specific problems.

Anxiety about sexuality often comes from trying to make ourselves fit a stereotype of what is supposed to be "normal," "super sexual," "masculine," or "feminine." One problem that may arise from comparing our sexuality against some external standard is that expectations about how we should be, feel, or act sexually may prevent us from discovering and enjoying what is right for us. Trying to live up to the pressure of these expectations can lead to fear of failure or of not being as "sexual" as someone else.

Our ideas about the "right way" to be sexual, which often stem from the myths or expectations we grew up with, may hinder the expression of our sexuality.

Common Myths about Sexuality

Myth 1: "Sex is only for the young and able-bodied." We seldom see older people or physically disabled people in "sexy" commercials or movies. We are thus led to believe that the only way to be attractive to others is to have a young and "perfect" body. Although most of us know that this is not true, we can still be influenced by the myth. We are sexual beings from birth to death, capable of sexual pleasure regardless of our age or our body's condition.

Myth 2: "Sex means intercourse." This myth makes it difficult to enjoy the special pleasures of touching, kissing, and stroking for their own sakes. If we view them only as steps toward the goal of intercourse, we may not consider them as options for sexual expression and satisfaction when intercourse is not desired or is difficult because of fatigue, illness, or anxiety. If we avoid touching for fear that it must lead to intercourse, we may cut ourselves off from forms of sexual affection that can be warm, comforting, and satisfying.

Myth 3: "The goal of sexual activity is orgasm." While many people enjoy orgasm, every sexual experience does not have to include it. In fact, trying too hard to have an orgasm can create pressures that prevent orgasm from happening. Satisfaction can come from a variety of pleasurable experiences, and it is usually enhanced when the expectation and the goal of orgasm are removed.

Myth 4: "Sexual performance equals love." You don't have to prove your love with sexual prowess. (Moreover, being able to perform sexually with someone does not necessarily prove anything about your feelings for that person.) Sharing your sexuality in a variety of ways can be an important part of loving, but there are many other ways of expressing love as well. Showing how much you care in these other ways can help take the pressure off sexual activity.

Myth 5: "Sexual activity is natural and spontaneous." "You shouldn't have to talk about it," is a phrase we often hear. When sexual activity feels good, there is often no need to talk about it. But when questions or concerns arise, as they do at some time for most people, it is important to be able to communicate feelings and needs, likes, and dislikes. No one is a mind reader. No matter how well we know another person, talking about what makes us feel good is usually necessary to prevent incorrect assumptions from being made. Assumptions are built on the past; it is important to be able to find out if your partner wants to try something new or different. Talking about sex can also help to reduce anxiety, and it can be one more way of sharing.

Myth 6: "Masturbation is harmful." Many people have grown up hearing warnings about the "evils" of masturbation or self-stimulation—an activity that has been humorously described as "the world's worst-kept secret." Although most of us don't talk about our masturbation patterns, many of us, including people in happy relationships, continue masturbating throughout our lives. It is not surprising that people continue activities that they have found pleasurable in the past. Whether or not masturbation is an acceptable practice for you, is, of course, a personal choice based on your own values and preferences.

The important thing to remember is that medical evidence has shown that masturbation is not only harmless, but it can be a very healthy part of sexuality. It provides an opportunity to learn about how our bodies respond—information that can be important for sexual pleasure with a partner. For example, research has found that women were more likely to have orgasms with intercourse if they had previously had orgasms through other means, such as masturbation.

Read through some of the above myths again to see if any are important for you, and spend a few moments thinking about or talking with your partner about other expectations that you are aware of that were not mentioned. Do your expectations help you enjoy and feel more comfortable about your sexuality, or do they hinder your enjoyment and comfort? Answering that question for yourself can be useful in beginning to make positive changes.

The Sexual Response Cycle

How do our bodies respond sexually? Sexual response is a natural total-body response involving more than just our genitals. With stimulation from thoughts, touch, or other sources, general muscle tension begins to build up, and blood begins to flow toward and accumulate in the genitals and other sensitive areas. If stimulation continues and we are relaxed, comfortable, and able to focus on our pleasurable body sensations (rather than on anxiety or worry), the level of body tension and blood flow continue to increase, and orgasm may then occur.

Orgasm is a reflex. It happens by itself under the right circumstances—much like a sneeze. We can't directly will an orgasm to happen any more than we can will a sneeze to happen. If orgasm does occur, blood then flows back from the genitals to the rest of the body, muscle tension diminishes, and our bodies return to their preexcitement state. If orgasm does not occur, these same changes do eventually happen, but more slowly.

The natural sexual response cycle can be interrupted in a number of ways. If, for example, a man becomes anxious about his "performance," he may lose his erection or climax sooner than he wishes. If a woman is worried about being able to have an orgasm, her anxiety may make it impossible to have one.

Each of us has particular conditions that are necessary if we are to enjoy sexual activity. The more aware we are of what is right for us, the greater are our chances of enjoying sexual pleasure. Most of us have learned one way of obtaining sexual satisfaction or orgasm—through various kinds of genital stimulation such as masturbation, intercourse, and oral or manual stimulation.

Many people, however, are able to experience sexual excitement, even orgasm, through stimulation of other sensitive body areas. Because it is the brain, rather than the genitals, that interprets and experiences this stimulation as pleasurable, it has been said that the brain is the real "sex organ." This means that we do not have to depend on our genitals for our sexuality. Our options for sexual pleasure are as varied as our imaginations.

Many people with serious illnesses find that the circumstances they need in order to enjoy their sexuality have been altered in some way because of the illness and its treatment. Under the stress and worry of a life-threatening illness, expression of sexuality frequently takes a back seat. It is difficult to feel sexual when you are fighting to survive, are in pain, or are constantly tired. Treatment for cancer may involve lengthy hospitalizations and separations from those you love. Hospitals or convalescent facilities usually do not provide much privacy, and hence there may be little opportunity for sexual expression.

Being in a hospital may mean separation from sources of feedback about your worth and desirability. Wearing hospital gowns and being deprived of familiar means of enhancing your appearance, like makeup, aftershave lotion, and your own clothes, can temporarily lower your self-esteem and make you feel uncomfortable in the presence of others.

Physical examination and diagnosis often involve exposing portions of your body that you normally consider private. Feelings of shame and embarrassment can result if hospital staff neglect to ensure adequate privacy during these procedures. The attitudes of staff, numerous examinations and procedures, and lack of privacy may make you feel asexual: that is, they may temporarily deprive you of any sense of yourself as a sexual person. Many hospitals are beginning to encourage ways of minimizing this depersonalization and are providing space and opportunity for people to have privacy. If your hospital has not yet addressed these issues, there are some things you can do to make your stay there more comfortable. If you want time alone or with someone special, ask for a "Do Not Disturb Until __ o'clock" sign or make one yourself to place on your door. Ask the staff to knock before they enter your room. A "Please Knock" sign may help remind them. If you request it, many hospitals will provide an extra cot in your room for an overnight visitor. If you are on a ward and share a room with other patients, your doctor may know of a way that you can get some private time in another room, a private lounge, or on a sun porch. You may bring special items from home, such as pictures for the wall, plants, personal items, family photos, or pillows, to create a more comfortable atmosphere. Wearing your own pajamas, nightgown, or robe can help, too.

During an illness, the control you usually have over your body may be lost, and you may feel inadequate and helpless. Serious illness may change the way you experience your body, or actually change the way you look, through surgery, amputation, scarring, weight loss, or other events. These changes may create painful anxiety about whether you will be able to function in your accustomed social, sexual, and career roles, or about what people will think of you. This anxiety, the depression and fatigue that may accompany it, and the numerous other worries that can occur with serious illness understandably make sexuality assume less importance.

Once the immediate crisis of serious illness has passed, however, sexual feelings and how to express them may become important to you again. Feeling anxious about resuming sexual activity is normal and natural. It is easy to "get out of practice" when you are away from any activity. You may have questions about whether sexual activity will hurt you in any way or whether you will be able to experience sexual pleasure. Your partner may share the same worries and may be especially concerned about tiring you out or causing you pain.

Starting a new relationship is a task we all face at one time or another, but it can be made more difficult by worries about our worth and attractiveness. If your body has undergone changes as a result of your illness and treatment, you may have questions about whether you are still desirable, how to please your partner, or what dating will now be like. Whether you are looking for a new relationship or already have a regular partner, you may find yourself in the position of having to share your feelings about these changes with someone, perhaps for the first time.

This sharing may feel awkward at first. Learning how and when to start talking about sexual issues may not come easily. You may feel shy or nervous about exploring new and different ways of experiencing sexual pleasure. You may be waiting for your partner to make the first move toward sexual activity, while your partner is waiting for you to make the advances. This waiting game is often misunderstood as rejection by both people. To think of breaking the silence yourself may be frightening. Yet the payoff for making the first move—greater understanding of each other's needs and concerns—is usually worth it.

Although health care personnel are now more aware of sexual concerns, many people continue to receive little or no information about sexuality during their treatment for and recovery from illness. You may have no opportunity to ask important questions about these matters. If your health care provider has not discussed sexuality with you, or has avoided your questions, you may feel that your worries and questions are foolish, unimportant, or inappropriate. Don't let these feelings prevent you from seeking answers. Ask questions of your doctor, nurse, social worker, or other staff person with whom you feel comfortable. He or she should be willing to listen to your questions and either answer them or refer you to someone who can. Help is available. Some university medical centers offer sexual counseling specifically for people with medical illnesses or physical disabilities. Your doctor or social worker will know whether such resources are available near you.

The kinds of changes in and concerns about sexuality that we have just discussed are general ones. The next section outlines some of the specific ways that cancer and its treatment can affect sexuality. For information on self-help organizations for specific kinds of cancer, see the Resources in Part VI.

Body Image

Cancer and its treatment frequently bring about body changes. For example, surgery may entail removal of a breast (mastectomy); creation of an artificial hole in the abdomen for the evacuation of wastes (ostomy); removal of part or all of the reproductive organs, or removal of a body extremity (amputation). Chemotherapy or radiation therapy may cause side effects, such as hair loss or weight loss.

Some people adjust to these changes relatively soon, some take a longer time, and some may never accept them. But acceptance need not mean total comfort with the situation. For some, a sense of outrage and loss may always remain to a certain extent. It is natural to have feelings about these changes, including anger, grief, mourning, and anxiety.

Body image—the mental and emotional picture we have of our bodies—may also be altered. Anxiety can arise when there is a conflict between what we think our bodies should look like, or what they previously looked like, and how they actually look now. This anxiety can influence our interactions with others and affect how we view ourselves sexually. If we see ourselves as less attractive or less lovable, we may avoid social or sexual situations so as not to experience the rejection we may expect from others. Unfortunately, such avoidance may also deny us positive experiences that could contribute to feeling better.

Dealing with feelings about body changes may be difficult. The support systems we have available to us, our social and career roles, and the meanings we attach to a particular loss or change will all influence our ability to cope.

Mastectomy and Sexuality

Sexual issues after treatment for breast cancer may include lowered desire, difficulties with physical arousal, and concerns about body image. Chemotherapy, by causing premature menopause due to lowered estrogen and androgen levels, may lead to lowered desire, problems with arousal, or reduced lubrication. Some women report improvement in these difficulties after topical application of testosterone or estrogen cream to the labia and vulvar areas, although the long-term safety of such hormonal creams has not yet been studied. Problems with lubrication and physiological arousal may be helped with artificial lubricants and vaginal moisturizers.

Body image concerns are normal and are especially understandable in view of the overemphasis that our culture places on the sexual significance of breasts. Undressing in front of your partner or sleeping in the nude may feel awkward and uncomfortable. With time and patience, many women are able to overcome their self-consciousness and again feel secure and comfortable with their bodies. Some women have found it helpful to explore and touch their bodies, including the area of the scar, while nude in front of a mirror. You may want to try this alone first and then together with another person—a spouse, lover, or close friend—while sharing your feelings about these changes. Others prefer to wear sexy lingerie such as a teddy or bra during sex until they become more comfortable.

After surgery, your partner may not know what to say or how or when to bring up the topic of sexuality, and may wait for you to bring it up while being afraid of hurting or embarrassing you. Sometimes this "protection" may feel instead like rejection. Although it will probably feel risky to break the ice and broach the topic of sex, most people feel relieved once they've done this.

When you first resume sexual activity, you and your partner may worry about pain. If your incision or muscles are tender, minimizing pressure on your chest area is important. Lying on your unaffected side may give you more control over your movement and reduce irritation of the incision. Don't hesitate to stop if you feel pain. Be sure to let your partner know why you are stopping.

If your partner trusts that you will speak up if something is painful or uncomfortable, you will both feel more relaxed and less inhibited in exploring and experimenting. Taking a rest or changing position may help you to relax, and relaxing will usually decrease any pain that you are experiencing. With communication and cooperation, you and your partner can work together to find the positions and activities that will give you the most pleasure.

Experimentation and time seem to be key factors in finding satisfactory ways of adapting sexually after breast cancer. Talking with other women who have had mastectomies—with support groups and with volunteers in the American Cancer Society's Reach to Recovery program, for example—can provide support and encouragement as well as suggestions about clothes and prostheses.

Ostomy and Sexuality

An ostomy may represent a new start in your life, removing pain and worry along with the diseased body part, but some new concerns may arise, such as wondering how a partner will react to the stoma or how the risk of odor or spilling during sexual and other activities can be minimized. In the past, our society has treated bowel and bladder concerns as taboo subjects (like the topic of sexuality). With very little open discussion in general about bladder and bowel functions, and even less opportunity to talk with other people with ostomies, it is easy to see how people felt that there was something shameful about having an ostomy. Although we may still hear and feel those negative messages, today people do have access to more supportive attitudes if they seek them out. As a society, we are beginning to increase our realization of how negative social stereotypes and silence about important body functions can be destructive. Concerns about hygiene and cleanliness are natural, but as experience with your ostomy increases, so will your comfort and confidence in social and sexual situations.

Sharing information about your ostomy with certain people may be a way for you to become more comfortable. If the fact of an ostomy is a "secret" that you have felt would be painful to reveal to anyone, you may find that talking about the ostomy for the first time with someone you trust is a real relief. The support and caring you receive will help you feel less alone. It is also true that when you share something intimate about yourself, other people quite often feel more comfortable talking about things that are meaningful to them. Being vulnerable and showing your feelings about important things can lead to greater closeness and intimacy.

Talking with other people who have ostomies—such as members of the United Ostomy Association—may be especially helpful in understanding that you are not alone and that you can learn to be more comfortable with the fact of your ostomy. Having someone who can listen to you and understand your questions can be of real benefit. Similarly, talking openly with your partner about your feelings and encouraging him or her to do the same is often the best way to decrease any anxiety that might surround the topic.

Experimenting with the timing of your ostomy management and with different types of appliances may help you to discover when your ostomy is most and least active. Learning about your individual patterns and how best to regulate your elimination may take a month, six months, or longer. There will probably be some spilling or accidents during this learning stage, until your pattern and schedule of evacuation are more regular. Laughing about, crying over, or just accepting these occurrences as inevitable in the beginning are important for both you and your partner.

Laryngectomy and Sexuality

After a laryngectomy, the surgical removal of the voice box, you may worry about odor from the stoma or about the noises you make while breathing through the stoma. These worries can be distracting and may make it difficult to enjoy sexual activity. Keeping the area around the stoma clean and using perfume or aftershave lotion can help. Wearing a stoma shield or a T-shirt will muffle the sound of your breathing and minimize the amount of air your partner feels being pushed through the stoma. Sharing your feelings with your partner will help you both adjust to the changes that have taken place and will create the best ground-work for a pleasurable sex life. Communication with other people who have had laryngectomies can also be helpful.

Cancer of Genital or Reproductive Organs and Sexuality

Surgery or radiation therapy for cancer of the genital or reproductive organs can bring about intense concerns with body image. For some people, such treatments may also directly affect their physical ability to get an erection, ejaculate, have intercourse, or reach orgasm. Other people may experience little or no change in sexual functioning after the same treatment. As a result, it is generally impossible to predict the effects of treatment for any one individual. Sexual problems that may appear to stem from physical results of treatment may in fact be due to anxiety and concern about body image and sexual functioning.

Discussing potential problems and possible solutions with your doctor or other members of your health care team before treatment will reduce worry and reassure you that if problems do occur, there are ways of handling them. In most situations, there are no totally reliable means of sorting out physical from emotional causes of sexual problems, so your exploration of and experimentation with what you can do is most impor-

tant. Your diagnosis does not dictate what is possible for you sexually.

Energy Level

Life after cancer treatment may be exhausting. Fatigue, depression, and generally feeling sick are common. Treatments for cancer, such as chemotherapy and radiation therapy, may in themselves create unpleasant and tiring side effects. The amount of energy you have available for the activities of living, including sexual activities, may vary from day to day or week to week. Some people learn to cope with these variations in energy level by planning their activities to coincide with times of the day they feel best. If you are experiencing some of these difficulties, being sexually active may not always be important to you. But for times when it is, planning to have sex when you feel least tired may be helpful.

Remember, too, that sex does not necessarily mean intercourse or orgasm. If you can expand your view of sexuality to include other ways of being close—such as holding, caressing, touching, and quiet talking—your options for sexual expression, even when you feel tired, are greatly increased. Talking openly with your partner will help you both to be flexible in dealing with the variable course of your illness. Many people find that, as they become more skillful in communicating about their feelings and needs, their options for sexual satisfaction increase as well.

The important thing is to be patient, both with yourself and with your partner. Adjustment will not occur overnight. Give yourself time—time to explore and share your feelings about your body's changes and time to begin seeing yourself as a desirable sexual being again. When you can grant yourself some acceptance of your body and recognition of your potential for sexual pleasure, it will be easier to imagine someone else doing the same. Sharing feelings about and exploration of a changed body have brought many couples closer together and enriched their relationships in surprising ways.

If there has been an interruption in your accustomed sexual interaction, it is important to realize that there are no set guidelines or timetables for resuming sexual activities. You are unique in your sexuality; only you can decide when and what is right for you. If you need help, ask your doctor to refer you to a competent sex counselor, or contact a nearby university medical center or community mental health center for a list of local resources.

Painful Intercourse

After treatment for genital cancer, some women find intercourse painful. If intercourse has become painful for you, it is important to visit your physician or gynecologist for an examination to determine the cause of the pain. It may be related to surgery, radiation therapy, or chemotherapy, or it may be the result of a simple problem such as an infection. If the cause is insufficient lubrication, try using an artificial lubricant, such as Astroglide, Gyne-Moistrin, or K-Y Jelly; a vaginal moisturizer such as Replens; and vaginal and vulvar application of estrogen creams.

Exciting new research is pointing to the potential benefits to both men and women from the use of Viagra (sildenafil) and the soon-to-be-available Cialis. Both have shown to help men and women by increasing blood flow to the genital area, resulting in enhanced erection in men and greater lubrication, arousal, and orgasm in women.

Shortening of the vagina, or stenosis, a condition in which the vagina loses its elasticity, can result from surgery or radiation therapy and may make intercourse difficult. If this is a problem for you, a physician may recommend the early use of dilators to exercise and stretch the vagina. Early resumption of intercourse can also help to prevent these problems. Different positions during intercourse, especially sitting or lying on top of your partner, may enable you to move in ways that are pleasurable rather than painful.

The most important thing to remember is to stop when you first feel any pain. If you let your partner know ahead of time that you will immediately communicate any experience of pain, he or she will probably feel less worried and more able to enjoy experimenting with you. Stopping to rest, slowing your movements, breathing deeply, and sharing your feelings will help you to relax. By exploring together what feels most pleasurable, you and your partner will eventually discover the kinds of sexual activity that suit you best.

Getting and Maintaining Erections

Some men who have trouble getting and maintaining erections may suspect that this problem may have been caused by cancer or its treatment. Because some drugs can temporarily interfere with the ability to have erections, you may want to ask your physician about any possible side effects from drugs you are taking. If you get an erection with masturbation or if you wake up in the middle of the night or in the morning with one, it is most likely that anxiety or "trying too hard," rather than a physical problem, is keeping you from having erections.

In trying to deal with erection problems, it is important to explore the sensations in and around your penis. Exploring these sensations when you are not distracted by trying to please or perform for your partner will help. Spend some time alone in a comfortable place, such as the bedroom or bathroom, at a time when you will not be interrupted. Undress and begin to explore your entire body, focusing especially on and around your genitals. Touch your penis, scrotum, abdomen, thighs, perineum (the area between the scrotum and anus), and anus. Try different kinds of touch—soft and light, firm and strong. Pay attention to the different kinds of sensations you feel, and notice which touches are most pleasurable. You may find that moistening your hand with oil, lotion, or soap makes your touch more pleasurable. Learning about what feels good to you is valuable, because doing so allows you to show your partner what pleases you most. Trying some of the exercises described in *The New Male Sexuality* (see Resources in Part VI), either by yourself or with a partner, can help you explore your potential for erections.

The more options you have for sexual expression, the less emphasis there is on having erections; this lack of pressure, in turn, makes it more likely that erections will occur. There are many kinds of sexual expression and stimulation of your partner that do not require an erect penis. Knowing that many women need or prefer direct stimulation by hand or mouth on or around the clitoris in order to have an orgasm may be reassuring. This is stimulation that even an erect penis in a vagina usually cannot provide. If you explore other kinds of sexual touching and expression for a while, you may discover that erections will return with time. You may also find that the increased variety of sexual options satisfies both you and your partner, making an erection less important. Patience, communication, and time are critical factors in developing pleasurable sexual experiences.

If erections have not returned and you feel that this is important to you and your partner, you may consider asking your doctor to refer you to a sex therapist for brief counseling. If, after counseling, you are still not getting erections, your counselor may refer you to a urologist, who, together with you and your counselor, can make a careful assessment of whether one of the following medical treatments would suit your particular needs and those of your partner.

Medications to Enhance Sexuality

- Viagra (sildenafil) is the first oral medication developed and approved to help erections in both men with organic and with psychological-based erectile problems. Taken one hour prior to sexual activity, Viagra has been found to be highly effective and safe, although it is not appropriate for men with certain cardiac problems or who may be taking organic nitrate medications, such as nitroglycerin, for heart disease. Additional medications that will enhance erection are currently being tested and may be available soon. A similar medication, Cialis, may have some advantages to Viagra and may be available as early as 2002.

- Yohimbine tablets (taken three times a day for four to six weeks) can stimulate desire and improve erection. It is often suggested for men with a suspected nonphysical cause, and may help 15–20 percent of such patients. Side effects may include headaches, dizziness, and nausea. This drug is probably contraindicated for men with ulcers or hypertension.

- Antidepressant medication, especially Trazodone, can be effective in treating erectile disfunction. However, some antidepressants may contribute to erection difficulties.

- Low-dose beta-blocker therapy (such as Inderal) before sex for men whose performance anxiety is very high can be helpful.

- Urethral suppository treatment, such as MUSE (alprostadil) has helped some men.

- External penile vacuum devices. A tension ring is placed around the base of the penis after it has become erect with the aid of a vacuum cylinder. These devices may work better for men who clearly have a major organic component to their erectile difficulties, such as severe diabetes, multiple sclerosis, or a spinal cord injury. While this approach does create erections that are functional for intercourse, men whose erection difficulties may be more emotional or psychological may be disappointed when the results are not as firm as they had been expecting. Side effects may include bruising of the penis.

- Intracorporeal penile injections. These were originally used diagnostically in urologists' offices, but patients can now be taught to inject themselves prior to sexual encounters, resulting in firmer erections that often do not disappear at orgasm or ejaculation. Side effects are pain, a persistent and painful erection (priapism), and scarring.

- Penile implant surgery. A variety of implants with semirigid silicone rods or inflatable cylinders are available. Costs are high (from $6,000 to $15,000). Complications are device failures, which require additional surgery, and infection.

Orgasm

After a serious illness, an interruption in your usual ability to experience sexual pleasure can be perfectly natural. For some women, this interruption may make having orgasms more difficult. If this is a problem for you, learning to reexplore pleasurable body sensations may be helpful. Do this at a time when you can be alone and are not distracted by having to please or perform for your partner.

Find a comfortable place where you can be alone, such as in your bedroom or bathroom, and a time when you will not be interrupted. Undress slowly and stroke your entire body gently. Then focus on the most sensitive areas. These may include your neck, breasts, thighs, genitals, or any area that feels good to you. Use different kinds of touch—soft and light, firm and strong. Try touching your body after moistening your hands with oil, lotion, or soap. Pay attention to the different kinds of sensations you feel, and notice which ones are most pleasurable. Learning which kinds of touch feel best will help you heighten your sensations and will give you information to share with your partner about what pleases you most. The discussion and exercises in *For Yourself* (see Resources in Part VI) may help you continue to explore your potential for sexual pleasure and orgasm.

Orgasm is a reflex that results when the right amount of physical and psychological stimulation occurs. It can be felt as a somewhat mild and pleasurable sense of relaxation or as a stronger, more intense sensation, depending on many factors, such as your level of energy, the source of stimulation, and the setting. From research and from the reports of many people, we know that men and women can experience orgasm even when the genitals have been removed or when there is no genital sensation (as with some spinal cord injuries), because orgasm and other sexual pleasures are actually experienced in the brain. With exploration, you may discover that other body areas, such as arms, breasts, neck, ears, and underarms, can be highly sensitive. With practice, stimulation of these areas may lead to orgasm. Some people have reported that orgasms from these sources feel different, but they are pleasurable and satisfying.

Changes and Your Sexuality

Survival overshadows sexuality. Remember that stress, depression, worry, and fatigue may temporarily lower your interest in sex. It is normal and natural for someone who loses good health to experience such feelings. When you are ill, just coping with basic, everyday decisions may seem like a burden. Taking one day at a time and being patient with yourself are important. Sexual interest and feelings generally return when the immediate crisis of an illness has passed.

Expect the unexpected. The first time you have sexual relations after being treated for cancer may be a new and different experience. Physical limitations or fears about performance, appearance, or rejection may initially prevent you from focusing on the pleasure of your sexual contact. On the other hand, you may be surprised by enjoying unfamiliar pleasurable sensations. Such new experiences are often reported by people who have recently divorced, lost a job, or weathered a family crisis, as well as by people recovering from an illness. If you expect some changes as a natural part of your recovery, they will be less apt to distract you from sexual pleasure if they do occur.

Give yourself time. It can be natural at first for you or your partner to be frightened of, perhaps even repulsed by, physical changes such as scars or unfamiliar appliances. Such feelings can be temporary, and talking about them—as frightening as they may be—is usually the first step to mutual support and acceptance. Becoming comfortable with changes in yourself and your sexuality will probably not happen overnight. Take the pressure off yourself about having to "work on

sex." Reaching a satisfactory and enjoyable sex life will happen gradually, one step at a time. At first you may want to spend some time by yourself, exploring your body, becoming familiar with any body changes that have occurred, and rediscovering the unique textures and sensations of your body. Once you feel relaxed doing this, move on to mutual body exploration with a partner, if you wish. (More specific ideas for such exercises are described in Resources in Part VI, particularly in *For Yourself* and *The New Male Sexuality*.)

Communication is all-important. The more talking and sharing you can do, the more your awareness of what feels good to you sexually will increase. It is rarely easy for anyone to begin talking about sex. You might initially try sharing with your partner some of the myths or expectations you grew up with about sexuality. Discussing this topic is often humorous and may break the ice in starting a frank conversation about your sexual needs and concerns. Make "I" statements about what is important for you and how you feel. Rather than general statements, try something like this: "I would really like to experiment with different positions that would be more comfortable for me. How would you feel about that?" Then ask your partner to try these statements also.

Take the emphasis off intercourse. When you first resume sexual activity, try spending some time in pleasurable activities such as touching, fondling, kissing, and being close without having intercourse. Reexperience the pleasure of playing, holding, and being held without having to worry about erections and orgasms. Once you feel comfortable with this, you can proceed at your own pace to other ways of being sexual, including intercourse if you wish. Intercourse is only one of many routes to sexual satisfaction. Your own experimentation and exploration can help you discover what feels best and what is acceptable to you.

Don't let your diagnosis dictate what you can do sexually. Your sexuality cannot be "diagnosed." You will never know what you are capable of experiencing in terms of sexual pleasure if you don't explore being sexual—new positions, new touches, and above all, new attitudes. You are the sexual expert about yourself; your brain is your best sex organ, and its ability to experience sensation is virtually limitless.

You are loved for your total worth, not just for the appearance of your body. Try not to make the mistake of placing so much importance on the way you used to look or feel that you can no longer appreciate your unique worth. Your partner and friends will continue to love and value you as long as you let them. The crisis of illness often brings people who love each other even closer together and it can enrich their relationships in ways they never expected.

You don't have to do it all yourself. Don't hesitate to seek counseling or information if problems arise. Help is available from a wide range of sources. If you have questions about sexuality or are experiencing some difficulties you wish to discuss further, we strongly urge you to bring them up with your health care providers or to ask them to recommend competent sex counselors or therapists in your area. Other resources that may be available near your home include persons or groups of people who themselves have had cancer and who have had experience in talking about sexual concerns with others.

36

Sleep Problems and Solutions

David Claman, M.D.

The medical community and the lay public have become increasingly aware of sleep issues and sleep disorders. This chapter discusses current knowledge and approaches to sleep and sleep disorders.

Sleep issues have evolved dramatically over the last one hundred years. When electricity was not ubiquitous in America, the average person probably slept about an hour more per night than the average person sleeps today. It is clear that human beings have not evolved so much in the last hundred years as to need an hour less of sleep—and there are many sectors of society where people are sleeping even less or have disrupted sleep schedules.

Medical conditions that cause pain or discomfort may disturb sleep. Cancer patients may have their sleep disturbed not only by physical pain or discomfort, but also by psychological issues such as anxiety or depression regarding their condition or prognosis.

Several centuries ago, Cervantes said, "Sleep, it covers a man all over like a cloak, it is meat for the hungry, drink for the thirsty, heat for the cold, cold for the hot. It makes the shepherd equal to the monarch and the fool to the wise. There is but one evil in it, Between a dead man and a sleeping man there is but little difference." This is a very old view of sleep as a passive state where it was assumed that nothing active was going on. Since Cervantes, we have learned a lot of information about sleep and sleep stages. It was only in the 1950s that dreaming sleep or rapid-eye movement sleep was described as a different type of sleep from other sleep stages. Now we see sleep as a highly regulated physiologic state, with multiple activities of different kinds and sleep stages. It is no longer viewed as a passive state.

Stages of Sleep

A normal night of sleep consists of different stages of sleep. People go through wakefulness, stages 1, 2, 3, and 4 of non-REM sleep, and then REM (rapid eye movement) sleep. When you go to sleep, you will be awake for a few minutes, and then go through the non-REM stages of sleep. The deepest sleep is in stages 3 and 4 of non-REM, and the longest periods of stages

3 and 4 occur during the first one to two hours of sleep. This is the time when young kids are likely to have night terrors or sleepwalk. After this period of deep sleep, the first period of dreaming, or REM, sleep occurs. At one to two hour intervals, more REM periods occur such that most people have between four and six separate dreaming periods a night. People usually remember the dreaming episodes if they wake up right afterward. A normal sleep pattern goes through the various REM and non-REM stages of sleep.

A review article in *The New England Journal of Medicine* about sleep in the elderly showed the normal patterns of sleep as the population ages. In the first few years of life, there is a much larger number of hours slept per day, but this slowly decreases through the age of twenty, by which time most people have settled in to a stable pattern of sleep hours and sleep stages that persists for many decades. In fact, the amount of REM sleep as a percentage of sleep time stays pretty constant for many decades and may have only a slight decrease in the elderly. Typically, the total time in bed increases around sixty to seventy years of age, which is when many people retire from work. At this time, people frequently go to bed earlier and tend to be awake in bed for longer periods of time. These sleep stages stay pretty constant over time and sleep duration does not change significantly during later years.

The More Common Sleep Disorders
Purposeful Sleep Deprivation
Many of us undervalue sleep and make shortcuts about when we go to bed and when we get up, so that we're not getting a full seven-and-a-half or eight hours of sleep per night. The most common cause of sleepiness during the daytime is purposeful sleep deprivation because people are not making enough of a priority of getting a full night's sleep.

Insomnia
Insomnia is far and away the most common sleep disorder reported in the population. From a survey done for the National Sleep Foundation back in the early 1990s, we know that approximately 36 percent of the U.S. population has reported either occasional insomnia or chronic insomnia, and of these 9 percent reported chronic insomnia.

Insomnia means different things to different people; it is a very subjective complaint. People may say they have insomnia when they have trouble getting to sleep at bedtime, if they wake up frequently during the night, or if they wake up at 3 A.M. and cannot get back to sleep. An insomnia complaint can be a combination of these different issues.

If you can't get to sleep at bedtime, it may be that you're having coffee after dinner and that the caffeine is keeping you awake. Or perhaps you're worried or tense about different issues related to work or family. If you're waking up frequently at night, there may be physical or emotional issues causing your wakefulness. If you're waking up early in the morning, again, that could be stress or depression. Emotional causes are less common than physical problems, but it really depends on the individual person, the issues involved, and the medications he or she is taking.

There are four main categories of causes of insomnia: (1) medical, (2) psychiatric, (3) situational, and (4) pharmacologic causes. The more medical problems people have, the more frequently they complain of insomnia. This is an important area to focus on for patients, who may be waking up with shortness of breath from lung problems, or with ulcer pain, or with chronic arthritis in the hips or knees or hands. Hopefully, treating these medical problems will improve the problems involving sleep.

Psychiatric issues are common causes of insomnia; psychiatry as a general discipline has become more interested in insomnia over the years because people with depression, anxiety, and schizophrenia frequently report insomnia. It is estimated that about one-third of the patients with chronic insomnia may have some problem with depression or anxiety disorders, and this is an important clinical association.

Situational issues, such as tests, lectures, or job changes, can also cause insomnia. Most people with stressful situations that cause insomnia don't seek medical attention for it and hope that when the situation resolves, their sleeping patterns will return to normal.

Pharmacologic causes of insomnia include many medications, both prescription and nonprescription, that have sleep-related side effects. The two most common pharmacologic causes of insomnia are caffeine and alcohol. If you drink caffeine in the evening, it may keep you awake at bed time and be a cause of insomnia. If you drink alcohol at bedtime to get to sleep, and the alcohol wears off two or three hours later, you may find yourself waking up and not being able to get back to sleep. Prescription drugs also have sleep-related side effects. You should ask your doctor about any medications you are taking.

Cancer patients have multiple reasons to develop insomnia, as they may be affected by physical, psychiatric, and pharmacologic issues related to their diseases. Patients may not receive adequate sleep due to anxiety in anticipation of a doctor's visit or treatment. Patients awaiting surgery or chemotherapy tend to suffer from insomnia. Chemotherapy has also been shown to disrupt brain chemistry and some cognitive functioning that, in turn, interferes with sleep. Pain, which can be related to the underlying cancer or to the treatment, may be present. Pain can make it more difficult to get sleep, or to stay asleep, or it may interfere with sleep quality, therefore making sleep less restful. Effective relief of the pain may improve all of these sleep issues.

Breathing issues are frequently important to cancer patients. Breathing may be more difficult due to either the underlying cancer or to treatment of other conditions such as asthma, emphysema, or congestive heart failure. Treatment focused on improving breathing should improve sleep quality and help a cancer patient feel more rested. Anxiety and depression can seriously disturb sleep, and these issues can often complicate the sleep of cancer patients. Fear of dying during sleep also prevents many cancer patients from getting adequate sleep. Most commonly, the issues that cause depression can be treated by medications, but improved sleeping habits (see later discussion) may improve sleep without need for medications. Lastly, medication side effects can disturb sleep, and cancer patients are frequently treated with multiple medications. Examples of this would include pain medicines causing daytime drowsiness and antidepressants causing insomnia. Caffeine and alcohol may also disturb sleep quality. Medications such as Decadron (a stimulant) or Tamoxifen (an antiestrogen) make changes to brain chemistry and often will interfere with sleep patterns. A detailed review of medications and potential side effects is a good first step when sleeping patterns have become disrupted.

The factors that affect the development of insomnia can be broken down into three different groups: (1) predisposing factors, (2) precipitating factors, and (3) perpetuating factors.

Predisposing factors include personality type, sleep/wake cycle, and age. As the population ages, insomnia is very frequently a subjective complaint. All of us struggle with occasional precipitating factors, such as changes in our personal lives or environments, medical or psychiatric illnesses, or new prescription or nonprescription medication. But most people will struggle with some amount of predisposing and precipitating factors, have a brief episode of insomnia, and then slowly improve over time and never develop chronic insomnia or the need to see a doctor about the problem. Most people who have chronic insomnia have some perpetuating factors that reinforce the insomnia problem. Negative conditioning about sleep is particularly common. For example, people say "I'm so tense about my sleeping problem that as soon as I go into my bedroom, I'm worried sick that I'm not going to sleep that night, and I lie awake for hours." Situations like this are quite striking, and you can easily imagine how people with that kind of negative conditioning about sleep can lie in bed and sleep poorly. How can you relax and get to sleep when you are filled with tension and worry? Substance abuse, whether it's sleeping pills, caffeine, alcohol, or illicit drugs, can precipitate sleeping problem. And performance anxiety, for example, "If I'm not asleep in the next ten minutes, I won't be able to do my job tomorrow," can also result in sleeping problems. Last on the list of perpetuating factors is poor sleep hygiene.

Sleep Hygiene

The best intervention for insomnia is a behavioral approach termed "sleep hygiene." Sleep hygiene is a somewhat awkward term that refers to sleeping habits—both good and bad. The goal is to practice good sleeping habits so you sleep better, and to avoid bad sleeping habits, which will make you sleep more poorly. So, for good sleep hygiene, here is a list of recommendations:

- Maintain a regular schedule for going to bed and waking up. The most common problem people have is that they get up early on weekdays and late on weekends. Then Sunday night, because they woke up "late," they have trouble going to bed at their weekday time, so they're up late and then can't get up early Monday. By the time they've straightened their schedule out, it's another weekend and the cycle starts again. Keep the same schedule seven days a week, and you'll head off a lot of sleep problems.

- Avoid excessive time in bed. If you spend too much time in bed, you end up being frustrated that you can't sleep and that will add to your overall sleeping problem.

- Avoid taking naps during the day. If you sleep poorly, you will usually feel as though you need a nap to catch up. If you take a nap to catch up during the day, that night, you won't need to sleep as much and that reinforces the bad sleeping pattern at night. However, if you're sleep deprived for other reasons, naps can be very beneficial. But I always tell people, if you have a lot of problems with insomnia, napping may be detrimental to you.

- Use the bed and bedroom for sleeping and sex only. Make your bed a pleasant place to be, not one filled with anxiety. Hopefully, people think of sleeping and sex as pleasant activities, which will be associated with positive conditioning.

- Do not watch the clock while you are in bed, because it reinforces how much time has gone by and may add to your concerns about not sleeping.

- Make the bedroom quiet and comfortable, so that it's conducive to sleep.

- Avoid taking the troubles of the day to bed with you. You want to be relaxed when you go to bed. Do something relaxing before going to bed so that you don't go to bed tense.

- Avoid alcohol and caffeinated beverages.

- Try to get regular exercise, but not within two hours of bedtime.

If you have insomnia, focus on your good sleeping habits and try to avoid the bad sleeping habits, in order to improve your chances of sleeping well at night and feeling rested in the morning. This behavioral approach of sleep hygiene measures is the best way to try to treat insomnia. Avoid using sleeping medications, if at all possible, unless it's really and truly necessary. Most people can make significant improvement by focusing on their sleep hygiene.

Obstructive Sleep Apnea

Obstructive sleep apnea is estimated to affect between 2–4 percent of the general population as estimated by a fairly large study performed in Wisconsin in the early 1990s. Apnea means not breathing. Sleep apnea is peri-

odically not breathing while you're sleeping. In the vast majority of instances, while people are sleeping, they have no idea of whether they have breathing problems or not. Sleep apnea is usually identified when a sleeping partner or family member reports that the person stopped breathing. In adults, sleep apnea is almost always obstructive, which means that the airway closes off and blocks breathing. When a patient with sleep apnea goes to sleep, the airway closes and the person stops breathing. The chest is still trying to breathe and makes bigger and bigger efforts at breathing. Finally, the mind interrupts the sleeping pattern to restart the breathing. The airway opens and the breathing resumes, but this causes a disturbance in the brain wave sleeping pattern so that the person is not rested in the morning.

Generally, when you have a period of apnea, there is a reduction in the blood oxygen level as an outcome of the absence of breathing. The body continues to do all its normal metabolic activities and uses up oxygen during the time that you're not breathing. Obstructive sleep apnea is a fairly common disorder, and one that is diagnosable and treatable. The expert witness in cases of sleep apnea is often the sleeping partner, and it's very important for a physician to talk to the sleeping partner. The patient is usually unaware of the sleep apnea issues, and the sleeping partner can often provide reliable information about the presence of snoring and episodes of interrupted breathing.

Treatment for Obstructive Sleep Apnea

There are a number of different treatments that can be given for obstructive sleep apnea:

- If the sleep apnea patient is overweight, weight loss is commonly recommended. Weight gain causes deposits of tissue in the neck. This accumulation makes the airways smaller and predisposes patients to sleep apnea. Patients who lose weight will generally reduce the severity of their sleep apnea.

- It is also recommended to avoid alcohol and sedatives near bedtime. Alcohol relaxes the muscles in the windpipe, making it more likely that your airways will close off and block breathing. That's why a lot of people will say, "I don't seem to snore much on the weekdays, but when I go out and have a few drinks on the weekend, that's when I snore the most." Many people have made the connection that alcohol leads to snoring being much louder.

- Postural training, involving retraining yourself to sleep on your side instead of sleeping on your back, can also help sleep apnea. Many people with sleep apnea have more breathing problems when they sleep on their back; most of the time, this is something a sleeping partner can tell you. "Well honey, when you sleep on your side, everything sounds nice and quiet, and then when you're on your back, that's when you stop breathing." Postural training can help those people with significant differences in apnea based on sleep position changes. If sleeping on your side does help, try sewing a tennis ball into the back of an old T-shirt. If you roll over onto your back, you'll feel the tennis ball and, hopefully, roll back over on your side.

- Allergies, a runny nose, or congestion will cause more breathing and snoring problems at night, so allergy treatment may be helpful. Also, if there are polyps or swollen tissue blocking nasal passages, you may with to consult with an ENT (Ear, Nose, and Throat) doctor, who may recommend surgery to correct the problem.

- CPAP, which stands for Continuous Positive Airway Pressure, is a relatively recent treatment that involves strapping on a mask that covers the nose. The mask connects to an air hose, which connects to a small air compressor that sits at the side of the bed. The compressor gently blows positive airway pressure into the windpipe, which keeps the airway open and enables you to breathe normally.

- Oral appliances are plastic bridges that fit the upper and lower teeth to hold the jaw in a more forward position to keep the airway open. They are worn during sleep on an ongoing basis to lessen episodes of sleep apnea. Your doctor can prescribe that an oral appliance be made for you.

- On rare occasions, antidepressants such as Protriptyline or Prozac can be used for two beneficial effects. First, they are nonspecifically energizing so that for people who are tired during the daytime, these medications may give you a little more energy. Second, antidepressants seem to increase the muscle tone of the airways dilating muscles, which may help keep the airway open and reduce sleep apnea. Antidepressants are not

recommended as a first approach to sleep apnea but may be used as a last resort.

- Last, surgery can be done for sleep apnea. Surgery for sleep apnea raises a complex set of issues, which depends on the severity of the sleep apnea and the patient's anatomy. Despite the risks and potential failure of surgery to cure apnea, as a last-ditch effort surgery is clearly an appropriate option for some patients.

Circadian Rhythms and Sleep Disorders

Circadian (from the Latin *circa dia*, which means "about a day") rhythms have been clearly described over the last few decades. They are rhythms of behavioral and physiological processing that occur approximately every twenty-four hours. All of us have normal circadian rhythms, and the strongest stimulus for circadian rhythms is sunlight—which makes sense from an evolutionary point of view, although social cues and exercise can also have an affect. This is why, when you have a regular sleep schedule, your mind and body know when to lie down and go to sleep. After you sleep around eight hours, if you've had a restful sleep, then your mind and body feel rested and know that it's time to wake up.

Our circadian rhythms do get confused in two situations: air travel and shift work. When we travel, the physical stimuli of bright sunlight and social interactions encourage adjustment to the new time zone and most people can adjust their circadian rhythms one to two hours per day. For example, if you go to New York City and have a three hour time change, typically you can adjust to the time change in one, two, or three days. When you "jump" more time zones, however, the difficulty you will experience adjusting is in direct proportion to the number of hours of adjustment.

Shift work is a different problem. In shift work, if you are not working a day shift, physical stimuli—including natural light and the social stimuli of family and friends—are oriented to keeping you awake during the daytime. Most people who work late-afternoon or night shifts try to sleep during the daylight hours several days per week, but many then sleep at night on the weekends. Such irregular sleep patterns resist realignment of the circadian rhythms. The most effective way to perform shift work in terms of your sleeping pattern, is to sleep at the same time seven days a week. Most people say that during their twenties and thirties they can handle shift work and irregular sleep patterns, but by the time they get into their fifties or sixties, it's too difficult and challenging.

Jetlag and shift work are a nice contrast to each other in terms of the different issues they pose to realigning circadian rhythms and sleeping when your body is going to be able to rest the most effectively. Your need for sleep will vary, depending in part on your activities and habits (not all people require eight hours of sleep nightly).

Prolonged lack of sleep reduces efficiency and the ability to function. How you sleep is important too. A good night's sleep is "as good as gold." If sleeping pills or tranquilizers are helpful in obtaining an adequate night's rest, they should be used. Resolving any perplexing and annoying emotional problems helps immeasurably. The use of relaxation techniques, meditation, self-hypnosis, and biofeedback is often invaluable. If behavioral treatments are not effective, sleeping medications may be available through your doctor.

This is a brief overview of an exciting and developing field that affects many people in our society. The most important points are: (1) get enough sleep to feel rested, and (2) sleep disorders are diagnosable and treatable.

Part IV

Supportive and Social Services for Life and Death Issues

37

In-Hospital Routines and Health Care Support Teams

Ernest H. Rosenbaum, M.D.
Isadora R. Rosenbaum, M.A.
Diane Craig, R.N. Onc, B.S.H.S.
Carol Viele, R.N., M.S.

Today we are witnessing many changes in medicine, including new diagnostic techniques not even conceived of ten years ago, as well as new methods in surgery, radiation therapy, chemotherapy, immunotherapy, and other areas of patient care. Physicians and other members of the health care team—registered nurses (RNs), licensed vocational nurses (LVNs), nurse's aides, residents, interns, medical students, nursing students, social workers, clergy, therapists, mental health consultants, and translators—are changing their attitudes toward the ethical and medical responsibilities of the practice of medicine. Training has become more specialized; in many areas, responsibilities are delegated to various members of the health care team. Changes have continued to occur in patient financial payment for third-party medical and office services as well.

Patient's Rights

Nearly everyone who has been in a hospital for even the briefest time knows how demoralizing and upsetting the hospital routine can be. Until recently, the patient's position has been one of extreme frustration. Feeling trapped, the patient could do little about this because the hospital routine tended to be inflexible, except in emergencies.

These days, the patient has much more control over the situation. We are seeing an increasingly humanistic approach to patient care. Members of the medical team recognize that they are there to serve the patient and to help them get well, and that, no matter how advantageous a smoothly running routine may be, it should be modified to meet the patient's needs.

A hospital has many functions: the prevention of disease, the pursuit of clinical research, the education of health professionals, and, increasingly, the education of patients and their families. But all these activities must be conducted with an overriding concern for the patient. Recognizing the patient's dignity as a human being will help ensure that his or her rights as a patient are respected. The complete text of the Patient's Bill of Rights, recognized by many hospitals, is printed in Chapter 3.

Admission to the Hospital

Admission procedures may vary depending on the type of insurance coverage or managed-care plan you have. Health Maintenance Organizations (HMOs), Preferred Provider Organizations (PPOs), and similar providers may require you to obtain authorization prior to being admitted unless it is an emergency, and some of these third-party payers also control the length of your stay.

In an emergency, you may have little to do with the details of your admission. A friend or family member may be asked to go through the admitting procedure for you. This person should be familiar with the necessary information about you. In addition, he or she should remember to bring any personal items you'll need.

In a scheduled admission, your first stop is the hospital's admissions office. You will need identification and health insurance cards. An admissions clerk will ask you questions about your insurance—the reason you are being admitted, your next of kin, and so on—to fill out the admission forms required by the hospital.

Your doctor, or his or her staff, will usually have reserved a bed for you. The admissions office may offer you a choice between a private room and a semi-private room. The clerk will discuss these options and their cost with you. (Unfortunately, in some hospitals, particularly county or city hospitals, limited availability and cost considerations often restrict choice.)

You should bring necessary personal items—such as a brush and comb, a toothbrush and toothpaste, your bathrobe and slippers—as well as any special items that will make your stay more comfortable or cheer you. You should not bring anything of substantial value or more than five to ten dollars in cash. If you are admitted through the Emergency Department, you may check your valuables with the cashier.

You may not be allowed to keep any medication you bring with you. To help your doctor evaluate your medication program, bring a list (as shown below) of the names and dosages of the medications you normally take.

Coping with Hospital Routine

Being admitted to the hospital and becoming a patient are extremely stressful events. You are suddenly placed in a strange environment, with few or none of your familiar supports. Though your role has changed, you do not need to give up everything that is important to you—your independence, control over your own life, or the handling of responsibilities.

It is the message of this book that you can best help your recovery by becoming an active participant in your own medical care. But how can you adjust to being a patient? How can you participate in your medical care?

1. Accept that a hospital stay is a difficult time. You can reduce your stress and fear of the unknown

Medication Name	Dosage	Frequency

by learning what to expect in the way of hospital routine, understanding the roles of the nurses and other members of the health care team, and knowing what to do about problems.

2. Be aware of your rights and communicate your needs.

3. Offer your own suggestions.

4. Do not hesitate to ask questions.

Here are some practical suggestions for dealing with common hospital situations. Learning the roles and procedures of the various staff who will be caring for you can reduce your fear and frustration.

Patient-Staff Relationships

The Nurse Staff

After you have been admitted and taken to your hospital room, one of the first people you will meet is the nurse. Your nurse will greet you, introduce him or herself and check your weight, blood pressure, temperature, and pulse. (In some hospitals, a LVN or nurse's aide will check these vital signs.) He or she should see that you are comfortable, show you how to operate the "call" buttons, ask questions about allergies to medications, and ask whether you have any questions or requests.

Nurses are the direct line to the doctor in his or her absence and are a vital link between doctor and patient. They are the primary people to whom patients regularly communicate their needs, frustrations, fears, and delights. The principal nurses assigned to each patient within a twenty-four-hour period try to communicate to one another all the things each has learned about the patients in their care. They meet as each shift changes to ensure that patients' needs, desires, medical history, and status are communicated from one nurse to the next.

Nurses are responsible for approximately 80–90 percent of patient care in the hospital. In most other areas of patient care, the doctor relies on the nurses' knowledge and judgment, along with input from the patient, to make patient care decisions.

Doctors

While you are in the hospital, your doctor will visit you during the day. This is the time for you to make requests or discuss problems. Nurses also communicate with the doctor about your condition during the doctor's rounds.

For practical reasons, the doctor's visits cannot be regularly scheduled and often occur at different times. Surgeons often see their patients in the early morning (that is, between 6 and 7 A.M.). If the doctor arrives unexpectedly or awakens you, you may forget important questions or requests. It therefore may be helpful to make a list of questions to have ready when the doctor sees you. Keep a pad of paper at your bedside, and jot down things you would like to discuss as they come to mind.

The Clergy

One of the many functions of the clergy is to comfort the sick, at home or in the hospital. Clergy visits in a hospital are not necessarily limited to members of one congregation or even one religion. Some patients may have no religious affiliation. Yet the clergy still can be welcome figures, sympathetic listeners, and sources of emotional and spiritual sustenance. Have a family member or friend notify your own church that you are in the hospital. If you would like to be visited by one of the hospital chaplains, ask your nurse. Similarly, tell your nurse if you do not want to be visited by the clergy.

Loss of Independence

With illness comes varying degrees of dependence on family, doctors, nurses, friends, strangers, machines, and medications. For many, the idea of dependence may be accompanied by fear. Feelings about dependence are learned patterns that cannot easily be changed; becoming aware of them may help you decide what areas of life you are willing to delegate control of to others, so that you can expend your energies on what is important to you.

Waiting

Having to wait is a frequent problem in the hospital. Waiting can produce anxiety, frustration, exhaustion, and anger. Some waiting cannot be prevented, because certain activities or procedures take a long time to complete. At other times, waiting is just one of those inexplicable mysteries of large institutions. Sometimes reminding those in charge that you are waiting can eliminate the waiting: you can often help by keeping yourself and others informed.

But you must also put reasonable limits on what you demand of your health care team. Sometimes answers or help cannot be given immediately. Emergencies must take precedence over routine ward care and may cause delays. Your understanding, patience, and cooperation during medical emergencies, or when more time needs to be spent on a critically ill patient, makes good sense; another time, you may be the person needing special emergency care and you can then expect to be given whatever additional time and efforts are necessary.

Fear of Staff

Patients often are afraid to complain, fearing that they may alienate the very people on whom they ultimately depend to give them comfort or to help save their lives. But, within reasonable limits, you should communicate your feelings and problems. To help you, your nurses must know both your positive and negative reactions to the care and services you receive. You are in the hospital to help yourself get well, not to please the doctor or the nurses.

Unfortunately, some people you meet during your hospital stay may be rude, unsympathetic, or otherwise not the kind of people you usually like or respond to positively. You can help both yourself and other patients by registering a complaint about these people and any problems you encounter with them. Hospital staffs need your help in monitoring themselves and in improving the quality of the care they provide. Please speak up.

Doctor's Admitting Orders

When you are first admitted to the hospital, your doctor writes admitting orders. These go in the front of your chart, which is kept at the nursing station. The orders are a formal list of directions and precautions that will be the basic guide for your care in the hospital. The format for admitting orders is as follows:

- Admit: "to Ward ____" or "to Room ____"
- Diagnosis: the name of your disease (e.g., "lung cancer")
- Condition: "good," "fair," "stable," "poor," "gravely ill," etc.
- Vital signs: the schedule for checking your temperature, pulse, blood pressure, and respiration rate (usually "every four hours"; but if your condition is unstable—for example, after surgery—the order may be for "every hour" or even "every 15 minutes")

- Allergies: any that might be known from your experience (e.g., codeine, penicillin, sulfa drugs, adhesive, etc.)
- Activity: "ad lib" (i.e., as you seem able to accommodate it), "restricted to bed with bathroom privileges," "commode use only," etc.
- Diet: "regular," "low fat," "low salt," "high protein," "high roughage," etc., and the number of calories you should be ingesting
- Nursing orders: "daily weights," "intake and outputs" (measure all fluids in and out), check for blood in stools, schedule for changing dressings, etc.
- IV orders: information about any intravenous fluids you should be receiving
- Medications: information about any medications you should be receiving
- Labs: orders for blood tests, X rays, etc.
- Notifications: when the doctor should be notified because of a change in your condition that would indicate a problem (e.g., "call house officer for temperature over 100° F," "...for pulse over 120 or less than 60," "...for respiratory rate greater than 30 or less than 10")

The doctor signs the orders, and they become the legal flow sheet for your care; you cannot receive any care or medications not specified or allowed in the orders, but your doctor will change or adjust them as the need arises, usually in consultation with the nursing staff. Nurses are allowed to add or change orders only with the doctor's permission.

Your Own Admitting Orders

Your List

The best way for you to be comfortable and to maintain control over your life in the hospital is to think about what you like and about what you want to continue to do for as long as you are able, and then do those things. Much is possible if you know what you want and remember to ask for it. If possible, before you go to the hospital, make a list of your likes and dislikes and ask that these be considered in making up your orders.

Diet

As a patient, you might consider these important matters: When do you like to eat? Do you like a bedtime snack? Are there foods you do not like?

In most hospitals, the dietary department is willing to be flexible in accommodating your desires. Ask to see the dietitian and let your wishes be known. (Your diet must, of course, conform to your medical needs as determined by your doctor.)

You may be more comfortable with the idea of eating foods prepared at home and brought in for you. Occasionally, a meal ordered from your favorite restaurant could be a pleasant change.

Bathing

Do you prefer to take baths or showers? If you are able, continue your bathing habits; the exercise you get is a bonus. Ask for help if necessary. In some hospitals, a doctor's order is necessary for a bath or shower, so be sure to include that need on your list of things to discuss with the doctor.

Hospital Room

Hospital rooms can be bleak and dreary, their odors and sounds foreign and sometimes offensive. For a prolonged stay, you may want to bring in a poster for the wall, photographs of your family, a religious picture, or a portable tape recorder or radio with earphones. Sometimes, bringing your own bed pillow from home is comforting. If you have a roommate, be as considerate of his or her needs as you would expect him or her to be of yours.

Visiting

A special stay with a family member or friend beyond the usual visiting hours is an item you may want to include on your list of needs. A long wait in the X-ray department, for example, or a particularly difficult period during your illness, can be made easier by the presence of someone who provides company and comfort. Ask the nurse what the visiting hours are, but do not hesitate to ask for exceptions if your needs do not fit into the prescribed hours. You have certain rights; again, though, you must also be reasonable and try to work within the structure of your hospital's rules.

Many hospitals will provide a cot for a relative or friend to spend the night, particularly when the patient is critically ill. Children are not the only ones who sleep better with someone close by. Cots are provided only for patients in private rooms.

Sleep Problems

Everyone who faces an illness and its treatment has certain fears—fears of surgery, therapy, pain, and death. These are very real fears to the patient and must be dealt with; some can even be eliminated.

Nighttime, in particular, can be frightening. In unfamiliar surroundings, many people have trouble relaxing and falling asleep. You may be kept awake by the noise of nurses at work, machines operating, or voices or TV sounds coming from another patient's room or from a roommate's portion of your room. After the distractions of the hospital's busy daytime activities have diminished and visitors are gone, patients are left with their own thoughts. The perception of pain sometimes becomes more intense because there is nothing else to think about.

A hospital functions twenty-four hours a day. At night, the health care team's members are awake, caring for their patients, and are as available to patients for physical and emotional needs as in the daytime. Nurses are always about; they will try to disturb you as little as possible, but they will check on you because they need to care for patients and carry out the doctors' orders. If you feel you are being disturbed unnecessarily, or if you have nighttime problems you need help with, talk things over with your nurse or doctor.

We often do little things at home before retiring that help us get to sleep more easily—for example, you may drink a cup of warm milk or read a few pages of a book. Try to continue these patterns while in the hospital. If you are accustomed to taking a sleeping pill, tell your doctor or nurse to ensure that the appropriate order will be written. Your doctor may prescribe a sleeping pill for you to take as needed; do not hesitate to use it if you feel the need. A good night's sleep can help you feel physically refreshed and better able to cope with the stresses of the day ahead.

Before the lights are off, be sure you know how to get the nurse's help if you need it during the night. Know where the nurse's call button is. All hospitals have some system for calling the nurse—use it if you need it. You will be helping your nurse to help you. You might want to ask that a night-light be left on in your room so that you won't be disoriented by darkness. If you are able to get up, be careful: bedrails are raised at night for your protection unless otherwise specified by the doctor.

Hospital Tests

We can all identify with fear of the unknown. Patients have often said, "If I had only known what to expect, I could have relaxed, or at least tried to cope." Unfamiliar tests and examinations by consulting physicians, residents, interns, or even your own doctor can cause fear and anxiety.

The doctor usually will tell you what tests are being scheduled. Ask your nurse what time they are scheduled for. If your doctor has not already made the following things clear, or if you remain unsure about any of them, ask the nurse:

- the purpose of the test;
- what will be done to you;
- what you will be asked to do;
- how you will feel, both during and after the test;
- how long the test will last; and
- any other questions you may have.

You may simply want to know what is likely to hurt and what probably won't, or whether the test has potential risks or side effects. Again, your doctor probably will have answered these questions, but the nurse also knows and can reassure you further. Some hospitals provide literature about tests such as X rays, scans, and so on.

When you understand and appreciate a diagnostic test's nature and purpose, as well as how the test is performed, much of the fear is dispelled. Not knowing what will happen is what causes the most fear. Once a test is performed, an explanation of the results of the test and how they relate to your therapy also will help alleviate your fears.

Patients often are afraid of receiving test results. Ask to learn about your test results early in order to reduce your anxieties and worries. These are subjects about which you should ask your doctor, but after that, you may need to talk about the results numerous times with a nurse or another member of your health care team. They want to help you understand what is happening to your body.

They also understand that there may be times when you are too afraid to discuss the specifics of a painful or embarrassing subject. What you should know is that someone will be available for you when you are ready to talk.

Common Problems

It would be impossible for this book to cover all the problems you might encounter while in the hospital. Whether a specific problem arises depends on the individual, the illness, and how these relate to one another.

But we can discuss some of the more common problems that a hospital stay can cause or make worse.

Fears and Anxiety

Sometimes you may not know exactly why you are afraid; you simply have an overwhelming sense of anxiety. It can be fear of the unknown or fear about your future. Talking with someone is a step toward dealing with your fears, known or unknown.

No matter how silly or uncomfortable you feel, consider asking your doctor or nurse for a few minutes of time. Not every nurse or doctor will be the right person for you to talk with; so as soon as possible, start thinking about the people on your health care team with whom you feel most comfortable. Have a conversation with one of these people and discuss your specific fears if you have identified them, or simply admit that you feel scared. Nurses are familiar with patient fears and often can help relieve them.

Constipation

Lack of activity, a different or significantly changed diet, intravenous feeding, or certain drugs (such as narcotics) can produce constipation in hospital patients.

Sometimes constipation occurs from stress because your environment has changed, because you have to use an unfamiliar bathroom (perhaps with a roommate not far away), or because someone else is doing the cooking. And having to use a bedpan has caused the system of many a patient to rebel.

Do not suffer. Ask about receiving bran or a glass of prune juice for breakfast. A glass of hot lemon water works for some people. You may add these items to your menu if they are not listed; you will be told if your condition would not tolerate particular foods. Drink lots of fluids of all kinds, and try to keep your level of activity up: take walks in the hall or ask whether you can have some physical therapy sessions. Tell your nurse that you are constipated so that your doctor may prescribe laxatives or enemas if needed.

Nausea

The medications you receive can cause nausea or an upset stomach. To reduce or relieve this common problem, the medications can sometimes be given late at night (so that you can sleep through the nausea period) or early in the morning on awakening (to help eliminate morning nausea). Tell your nurse or doctor that you are nauseated. Your doctor can order an antinausea medication. Taking antinausea medicine about thirty minutes before meals will help reduce mealtime nausea.

Skin Problems

Having a chronic illness and being confined to bed can cause skin problems such as pressure sores (bedsores) or rashes due to the roughness of bed linen. The nursing staff will be working to prevent and care for pressure sores, but you can help too. Good hygiene is extremely important at this time. If you can, take a shower or a tub bath daily. Try to change your position in bed as often as possible to get the blood circulating to the affected area. Accept the back rub that is offered you at night; not only will it feel good, it also helps prevent and treat skin problems.

Pain

Pain is sometimes the main reason for admission to the hospital. It can be both physical and mental. Severe, chronic pain can be a most destructive problem that affects many functions of your life. It often prevents a person from expending energy in personal relationships with loved ones at a time when those relationships are most important.

Pain is often accompanied by anxiety. You may worry about whether the pain will go away; if you have received medication and the pain is ebbing, you may feel anxious about the return of chronic pain. Reducing anxiety often makes it possible to achieve better or complete pain control.

Some patients prefer taking pain medications only when pain occurs. But for others, pain control cannot be achieved by treating the pain only when it comes. They do better with a regular schedule of pain medication throughout the day, with additional doses as needed. In all cases, treatment must be individualized.

Finding an effective pain relief measure can reduce anxiety about pain. Knowing that your pain medication will be available on request will also reduce fear of suffering. Medications are also available to help decrease anxiety. Thinking positively and trying to relax will help your pain medication give maximum relief. Medications are also available to help decrease anxiety. We often teach patients how to give their own pain shots so that they can get faster relief and can be in control of their pain when they go home.

Many patients feel that they are "acting like a baby" if they complain of pain; as a result, they suffer needlessly. It is all right to say that you hurt. The best pain control can be achieved when pain is treated before it becomes severe.

Pain medications that contain narcotics commonly cause side effects; usually these affect the gastrointestinal tract and can be managed. Side effects should therefore not prevent the use of narcotics if the narcotic is working to control pain. Constipation is a common side effect. Daily stool softeners, laxatives, and enemas may be needed as long as you are receiving the narcotic. Close attention must be given to treating constipation in order to prevent more serious complications, such as stool impactions (severe constipation with stool accumulation and blockage in the rectum).

Many pain medications are available today. They come in pill, liquid, and injectionable forms. It is extremely important to tell your doctor and nurse the location of the pain, what it is like, under what conditions it gets worse, and whether the medication you are taking gives relief. Only you can provide them with this important information.

Because pain medications are often effective only when they are given before the pain gets out of control, it is your responsibility to tell your health care team about the pain early, before it hurts too much. It also is important for you to know that there are stronger and variable forms of medication. Pain control without heavy sedation is possible. Local pain blocks, or neurosurgery to cut the nerves that carry pain fibers, may sometimes help.

Remember that the team wants to see that your pain is relieved before it reaches a high level, because severe pain is devastating and can precipitate other problems. It is your responsibility to communicate your needs to the medical staff. Only by knowing your problems can they help you.

The Role of the Family

Traditionally, the patient's family has been overlooked as a resource in care and recovery planning. The idea that health status is a private matter has long been accepted without question. Originally, the family was asked to "wait outside"; the patient was expected to keep the family informed, letting them know "what the doctor said"—an approach that eliminated communication between the family and the health care team.

That concept of the family's role is becoming as archaic as that of the passive patient. Just as patients must take more responsibility for helping themselves get well, so too must the patient's family. Having the family "wait outside" wastes a great deal of valuable "people power" that could be available to facilitate a patient's recovery. Also, many family members want or need to do something to contribute actively to the patient's healing.

Becoming Familiar with the Environment

Here a few examples of the many things a family can do to help:

- Know the nurses and doctors in charge of the patient's care, and help the patient remember them.
- Learn how to work the bed and how to call the nurse.
- Find out what supplies are in the room and where to get others.
- Locate the visitors' room, sunrooms, televisions, and kitchens nearest the patient's room.
- Locate the bathrooms, phones, and cafeteria; ask about cafeteria hours.
- Learn how to reach the nursing station by phone so that family members can call in for updates.

Family Communication with the Nurse and Doctor

Tell the nursing staff that as a family member, you wish to participate in the patient's care; otherwise, they will assume that you do not choose to help. Sometimes family members want to help, but fear that they will be in the way. Others may believe that they would not be allowed to help. Be assured that the nursing staff can use all the help they can get: let them know that you want to actively participate in caring for your loved one. Family members often can serve as spokespersons for patients who are either reluctant or unable to speak for themselves.

Here are some questions the health care team might like answered by the family:

- Is the patient likely to be outspoken or passive about expressing needs?
- Does the patient have any habits or characteristics that might easily be upset by the hospital stay—e.g., difficulty in sleeping, or attitudes about illness?

- Does the patient have any fears or anxieties about illness, pain, or body image that might not be revealed to a stranger?
- Are there outside influences, such as specific worries or joys, that might affect the patient's drive to get well?

The answers to such questions help the health care team understand the patient more fully and to take a realistic and more personal approach to the patient's care. The family usually knows how the patient reacts under stress; the nurse does not. Nurses do know that illness and hospitalization are stressful situations for most people, but they need the family's help in minimizing this problem for specific individuals.

Conversely, the nurse can tell the family the following useful information:

- when the doctors make rounds, and the best time and place to reach them
- how to help the patient meet special physical needs for therapy, such as nutrition, exercise, or mental diversion
- the reasons for tests and treatments
- where to find help about financial, disability, or insurance matters

We strongly encourage families to share their feelings with the doctor and the rest of the health care team as much as possible. It is sometimes difficult to be hopeful about a patient's recovery in the face of a life-threatening illness.

When recovery is expected to be limited, or to take a long time, it is normal to become disappointed and discouraged. The nurse's job includes listening to the family's as well as the patient's fears and anxieties. Nurses may help to dispel doubts. More often, they can reassure families that their feelings are appropriate. No one is ever completely positive or without doubts. Talking with the nurse can be helpful, if only to get these feelings out into the open.

It is difficult for family members as well as patients to ask a question about something they know little about. Because of its terminology, medicine can seem like a foreign language. If for any reason you have failed to ask the doctor to explain unfamiliar words, ask the nurses for help. Let them know what you do or do not understand.

Some people prefer to know only the barest details, while others want to know everything. Remember, no question is unimportant or ridiculous. If you take unanswered questions home with you, your anxieties and fears will increase.

When a patient is questioning the doctor, it is often easier if two or more family members are present. Making a list beforehand can help the family remember what they were concerned about and get many questions answered at one time. Patients can benefit greatly from having a family member present at these question-and-answer sessions.

For example, many couples prefer to be seen as a team when one is hospitalized or receiving outpatient therapy. When both are present, the healthy partner can take responsibility for much of the information received by both, recalling it for the patient and communicating it to other family members at a later time.

Some patients do not want their families involved and do not want their physicians to discuss their case with family and friends. The patient has the right to request this and to have the request respected.

A word of caution to the family is important here. Some patients may become completely passive, letting their families give and receive all information. This can lead to two problems:

- It is important for the medical staff to hear the patient's own account of symptoms and of how he or she views the illness. If the family takes over the entire process, understanding and insight into the patient's attitudes and feelings may be lost.
- Active participation in all areas of treatment is necessary for early and optimal recovery. Involvement in their own care helps patients generate the energy needed for their recovery. Family members can help, but doing everything for the patient will inhibit the patient's recovery.

Family Responsibilities

Sometimes, another family member falls ill during a patient's long or difficult hospitalization. Whether through caring for the rest of the family in the patient's absence or through expending much of his or her energy on the patient's behalf, the relative may have neglected his or her own health.

Sharing patient responsibilities with other members of the family is essential. If you as a family member wish to undertake all the responsibilities, that may be fine. If you do not, or if you need to rest or must be absent from the patient, ask the nurse or the hospital

social worker for help. They can contact you should the need arise and can, if necessary, explain why you are away taking care of yourself.

When dealing with patients who show anger or resentment because their support person is away, the doctor, nurse, or social worker can be helpful. These health care team members always should remember that understanding the other patient's needs and point of view is essential if they are to deal rationally with both their own feelings and the feelings of others.

Patients must be realistic about their expectations of others. A lot of positive energy is often mobilized within a family by focusing on getting the patient well. But that is not always the case, and patients should neither expect it nor be disappointed if it does not take place. Remember, too, that the family's life goes on outside the hospital, and many family members are at times either totally unavailable or available only at limited times.

Resentments should not be allowed to build up. It is still the patient's responsibility to understand the family's position and to know when to lean and when to stand alone. If necessary, the patient can have a family conference with the health care team.

Discharge Planning

It is natural to feel some anxiety when you anticipate release (discharge) from the hospital to go home; there are significant differences in the two environments. You will be leaving the security of the hospital support team—the nurses and physicians, who provided physical care and support; the physical therapist, who began an exercise program and whose firm assurance enabled progressive ambulating; the occupational therapist; the nutritionist, who provided diet instruction; and the medical social worker, who helped you and your family deal with the practical problems relating to your illness, as well as fear and anxieties. But proper discharge planning can assure you of a continuing support system at home, and your rehabilitation will be enhanced by all the additional advantages, both physical and psychological, of being at home.

Discharge from the hospital represents a crucial move and a progressive step in your rehabilitation. Many patients become more alert and better oriented after returning home. You can expect your appetite to improve and your interest in becoming active to increase. As you become physically able, you will find enjoyment in taking up favorite activities once again. Gradually resuming some of your particular roles in the home, as your health allows, will have noticeable effects on your physical rehabilitation, as well as on your attitude about yourself. Even small accomplishments are important in bolstering your sense of being able to cope and your motivation toward as full a recovery as possible. As you mobilize your strength, your accomplishments may surprise you, your family, and your health care team.

The transition from hospital to home can be smooth if it's facilitated by early discharge planning, involving the health care team, you and your family, and the discharge coordinator. The discharge coordinator—usually a medical social worker or a discharge planning nurse—is the key professional who arranges for any needed home care and acts as a liaison with the patient, the family, the health care team, and home health care agencies.

Discharge planning should begin shortly after admission to the hospital, as soon as a diagnosis is made and therapy initiated, even though there are still many unknowns. While you are in the hospital, your health care team will work together to anticipate what your medical and physical needs will be in the home and will discuss these needs with you and your family. You will need to participate in planning your home care by providing information regarding the physical setup at your home (stairs, bathroom facilities, etc.), the availability of people to help you, and whether special equipment can be accommodated.

Your doctor, assisted by other members of your health care team, will outline your required at-home plan of care, what side effects to expect following treatment, what limitations to expect because of physical weakness, and what problems may result from chronic illness. They will establish guidelines to enable you to handle both temporary and long-term problems. The health care team will help you and your family set realistic goals and suggest ways to obtain assistance when needed.

A call by the discharge coordinator to your insurance company or to your county's social services department will reveal many at-home services that can be provided free to you. These services may include visiting nurses, attendant care, meal preparation, and equipment rentals. Certain organizations, such as the American Cancer Society, also provide some services

and equipment. You and your family should become aware of the services available in your community as early as possible in your illness, by meeting with the medical social worker or discharge planning nurse.

Discharge planning is simply a continuation of your in-hospital program. Generally, by closely observing the nursing care you receive in the hospital, you and your family will gain valuable clues about areas of concern. When you participate in organizing and carrying out your hospital care, you also learn how to care for yourself at home. Patients who are most involved in their hospital care will make the most effective transition to home care.

Your medications will already be familiar to you from the hospital. Making a written schedule of the amounts and times prescribed by your doctor will prove helpful while you settle into a routine at home. You also should already be aware of the vital importance of good nutrition and regular exercise in your recovery. Planned programs in both these areas should be continued at home. While you are in the hospital, ask the dietitian and the physical therapist to talk to you and your family to help set up your home programs.

Unfortunately, sometimes discharge planning may be sketchy, and many needs may be overlooked. Make it your responsibility to initiate plans for your home needs. List questions to discuss with your doctor, your family, your nurse, the dietitian, and the physical and/or occupational therapist. A poorly planned discharge can cause much anxiety for you and your family, and can result in an unnecessary readmission to the hospital.

Even with a well-planned discharge, certain limitations in your home setup or in your own or your family's abilities to cope may not become apparent until you have been home for a while and tested things out. If you have been discharged recently, you can call on the medical social worker or discharge planning nurse for further help in planning your home care. Your doctor and his or her office staff also will be able to help you reevaluate your home situation and arrange for needed care.

It is reassuring to know that when you are home, help and support are just a phone call away. If you have questions or need reassurance, or if a troublesome situation arises, phone your doctor. In private medical practice, a physician or a member of the office team is available twenty-four hours a day to give medical care and advice and to meet your emergency needs. Restrict routine questions and problems to regular office hours, though: evenings and weekends are for emergencies only.

If you cannot reach your doctor, your questions or problems may be solved by someone who knows you and your medical situation. Do not be reluctant to call your hospital ward and speak to one of your nurses. Take their names and the ward phone number with you when you leave the hospital; a nurse is always on duty there. He or she can answer many of your questions, direct you to the appropriate person to call, or reassure you just by talking to you. A problem that could wait until morning also can keep you and your family awake all night with worry. Nurses do remember patients and their families, and too often this resource remains untapped after the patient goes home. In an emergency, you can always request an ambulance and go to your hospital's emergency room.

38

In-Home Services and Support Programs

Ernest H. Rosenbaum, M.D.
Isadora R. Rosenbaum, M.A.
Eugenie Marek, R.N.

The concept of home care, which is as old as medicine itself, reflects the belief that health care begins at home. Today, interest in home care has been renewed. Hospitals are discharging patients earlier—not only because of new government and insurance company guidelines but also because healing occurs more rapidly when a patient is most comfortable, surrounded by what is familiar.

For the more chronic levels of illness, earlier discharge means that skilled services are needed at home. Home care agencies, nurses, and other health care professionals with increased expertise have expanded the range of services available in the home. Patients' needs are looked at from a perspective of providing for the person, rather than just solving a problem or performing a task. Patients feel more secure exercising their choice to return home sooner or to remain home as long as possible.

Having been hospitalized is not always a prerequisite for in-home health care. Services are available at any time during your illness. If you have a chronic illness, the assistance and support provided allow you to continue your recovery in your own familiar environment and to adapt your daily life to coping with physical limitations.

Hospital-Based Programs

Many hospitals have developed home care programs that allow the patient to remain at home instead of being institutionalized. The hospital's home care team and the physician establish the home care plans, in conjunction with the patient and family. Services available through such programs may include those of a public health nurse, home health aide, medical social worker, physical therapist, occupational therapist, speech pathologist, and home care intern.

Community-Based Programs

Depending on the type of insurance plan you have, there are numerous reputable, accredited home care agencies that now can supervise a patient's home care program. The range of services provided by home health agencies includes nursing; physical, occupational, and speech therapies; dietary consultation; medical social work; and home health aide and homemaker services. These services are all delivered under your physician's instructions.

Payment

Insurance companies are glad to explain their benefits for in-home services. Your discharge planner may be of assistance here. Policies vary greatly in the number of visits, degree of illness or disability required to qualify, and type of equipment paid for. If you anticipate that you might need such services, find out about them in advance, when you feel well. This will help you prepare for future decisions that might come with a price tag (See Chapter 43, "Paying for Cancer Care").

Home Visits

When service is requested, it is usually the home health agency nurse who makes the initial assessment visit. On the first home visit, the nurse will interview you and your family members for information on your health history, recent illnesses, present symptoms, and any concerns that you or your family may have. Your ability to manage, the required care, family and neighborhood resources, and the areas in which a home health agency can assist will be explored.

With this information, the nurse will work with you and your family to determine whether continued nursing service is needed or whether the main need is for another therapeutic or paraprofessional service, such as physical therapy or a home health aide. Sometimes nursing or other skilled services are not required—only bathing or housekeeping help. If the home health agency from which the nurse comes does not provide such services, there are other agencies that do, and the visiting nurse will make the arrangements for such care.

Although the home care nurse will be performing specific procedures as needed, his or her efforts will focus on instructing you and your family in managing your care, on providing assistance and support as you learn, and on professionally assessing your response to the care. Home care nurses have experience in managing problems involving safety, nutrition, elimination, mobility, skin care, medications, and pain, and in adapting procedures performed in the hospital to the home.

Just as the discharge planner in the hospital was the essential liaison between the hospital and the home health agency, the home health professional now assumes this role between the patient and the family

unit and members of the health care team and other community agencies that may be involved. The visiting nurse or other home health professional will stay in close contact with your physician to provide information on your progress, response to treatment, and changes in condition.

You can help the home care agency by designating a place to keep information and items related to your care. Be sure to have a list of telephone numbers, a calendar for appointments and home care visits, and a list of medications with a schedule for refills. You also might want to keep a log of how you respond to various treatments. Keeping medications and supplies in the same place will give you a sense of control and organization at what might feel like a chaotic time.

Emergencies

The home care nurse will help you make your home as safe as possible to help prevent any falls. But if you do fall, you may need assistance, so you should identify strong neighbors or nearby family members, or local agencies that can help. Find out how to reach your physician in an emergency, what to do if you are unable to reach him or her, and whether house calls may be made. Keep emergency numbers near your telephone; if you have a programmable phone, program it with these numbers and post the list of numbers and names or service in a prominent place.

Medications

Check to see whether you have all the medications you are supposed to be taking. If you have questions, ask. A good method of ensuring that medications are taken on schedule is to set out each day's pills in a pill organizer. Be sure to double-check your medication schedule for the prescribed amounts and times.

It is wise to keep a list of all current medications (especially because you may have prescriptions from several physicians), in addition to a list of allergies and poorly tolerated or ineffective medications. If a new medication is to be ordered, you might ask your physician to prescribe a small amount to try initially, until its effectiveness and your tolerance is determined.

Safety caps on your medication containers may be a problem. If you have no children or grandchildren around, you may not want safety caps. If you do not want them, when you order your prescriptions, tell the pharmacist you want regular (nonchildproof) caps.

Pain Control at Home

One of the biggest concerns for patients who are about to go home is often pain management. If you have been in pain while in the hospital and have been receiving medications administered by the nursing staff, you may wonder who will give you the medicine at home? What if you run out of medicine? What if you need an injection? What if you're alone and the pain gets worse?

Fortunately, you will not have to suffer needlessly. There are many medications available that can help relieve pain very effectively by themselves or in combination. Often, all it takes to get pain under control is some careful observation by your family or other caregivers, some accurate feedback from you, and some minor adjustments in medication or schedule by your physician.

So, the first important point to remember is that your pain can be relieved. If one medication or schedule does not work, there are always others. If your pain persists, call your physician or his or her nurse for a program that will control your pain. Your home care nurse can help you gather and communicate this information to your physician to ensure prompt, efficient pain control.

The second thing to keep in mind is that there are two types of pain: chronic and acute.

1. *Chronic* pain is pain that is with you most of the time. Your medicine may relieve it for a while, but it usually returns. Because it is continuous, chronic pain needs continuous treatment. Your doctor probably will prescribe medicine for you to take around the clock, much the way you would take an antibiotic.

2. *Acute* pain is any pain that is either new to you or more severe than it has been. Acute appendicitis, for example, is characterized by sudden, sharp pain in the abdomen. Any time you have acute pain, you should notify your physician.

Acute pain needs investigation. It does not necessarily mean that your cancer has spread or that something is seriously wrong with you. It may be your body's way of coping with extra tension, or it may be caused by a minor problem, such as constipation. In any event, remember that it is important to let your doctor know about any new pain.

Whether you are experiencing acute or chronic pain, you need to become familiar with your pain and its management. Pain is a very complex phenomenon.

It has both a physical and a psychological component. Often, it is made worse by anxiety or fatigue. Yet some patients with severe pain are able to be very functional, particularly if they have worked out a good schedule for their medications and know how to administer them themselves or have someone dependable administer them.

Remember that you are the expert. Pain is a very private and personal thing, but it is vital that you learn to share this information with your family and physician. Start by asking yourself these questions:

- Where is the pain now?
- What does it feel like? (Is it sharp? Burning? Dull?)
- What relieves the pain?
- After I take the medication, how long does it take for the pain to disappear?
- After I take the medication and the pain is relieved, how long does it take for the pain to return?
- Does the pain interrupt my sleep?

The answers to these questions will be extremely valuable to your physician. Often, it is helpful to write down your observations as you make them. Telling your doctor that "the medicine doesn't work" is the first step, but try to be more specific when you report on a medication's effectiveness. The more information you can provide, the easier it will be for the doctor to make the necessary adjustments in your medication. Your home care nurse can help you in this important process.

Medications come in different forms: pills, skin patches, rectal suppositories, liquids, and injections, as well as through IV systems that can be used at home. Before you leave the hospital, ask your physician about the type of medication you will be taking home with you. Then become familiar with how to take the medicine, or have your family or home caregivers learn how to give it to you.

Usually, your doctor will send you home with the same pain medication that you have been taking in the hospital. If you are going to be taking a different type of medicine, your doctor will start to give you this medicine before you are discharged to see how effective it is or whether you experience any side effects. It is better to have this trial in the hospital, where you can be observed by the nursing staff, treated for any adverse reactions, and get comfortable with the medicine.

If you are going to be taking pain pills home with you, ask the nurse about pill organizers—boxes with compartments that let you set out your doses in advance. This will help you stay on schedule and be more comfortable. They also are handy if your family wants to be able to leave a nighttime dose out for you.

If you are having difficulty swallowing, pills may be crushed by placing them in a plastic bag and pounding the pill with a butcher mallet or by gently crushing them with a teaspoon. They then may be added to a spoonful of soft food, such as applesauce or oatmeal. You also may dissolve the crushed mixture into a small amount of water or juice.

Small plastic medicine cups are useful for taking liquid medications. The markings on the cup's side make it easy for you to measure out the correct amount. Some liquid medications may be mixed into juices to make them more palatable, but sometimes this may cause bad reactions. Ask your doctor if it is okay to mix your medications with liquids.

Rectal suppositories also are easy to use. Simply remove the foil wrapper, lubricate the tip of the suppository (the smaller end) with K-Y jelly or water, and insert it into your rectum using your index finger. It must be pushed up past the rectal sphincter or muscle, usually as far as your finger will reach. You might want to use a disposable rubber glove (available at your pharmacy) or a plastic bag to cover your finger. Wash your hands thoroughly when you've finished.

Injections usually pose more of a problem for patients and their families. Many people fear injections and are horrified by the thought of giving one to themselves or to someone that they love. If you ask nurses how they felt the first time giving an injection, they probably will relate similar feelings, or perhaps tell humorous stories about those first injections. Keep in mind that injections often provide excellent relief from pain, and the technique is easily learned if you are patient and willing.

If you are willing to learn how to give yourself injections, ask your doctor to arrange for you to learn the technique. Have either a family member or the person who will be caring for you at home learn along with you. It is important that someone else know the technique: you should not have to worry about who will give your injections at home.

You and the others who are going to be responsible for your injections will probably need a number of prac-tice sessions before you all feel comfortable giving an injection. The nurse will help you with your practice sessions, providing you with syringes and an orange to inject. After you have practiced on the orange, you will get help with your first self-injection. Remember, you *can* learn to give an injection—even to yourself!

One of the most important advances in pain relief has been patient-controlled IV pump systems. This method provides better pain management by releasing small doses of medication at short intervals. A patient experiencing acute pain also can be instructed to give occasional extra medication through the pump. Using such a system is often easier than giving an injection, and it eliminates the inconvenience of being "attached" to an IV line. An IV pump system can offer pain relief that is not available from some of the other methods.

You will be instructed in using IV medication before you leave the hospital. Your home care nurse will then ensure that you and a caregiver are comfortable with this system. He or she will be available by phone or visit, if you have additional questions or need further instruction

Pain medication skin patches that are changed every three days, and long-acting morphine pills (lasting twelve or twenty-four hours) are other alternatives for pain management.

Pain medications that contain narcotics commonly cause side effects; these usually affect the gastrointestinal tract and can be managed. Side effects should therefore not prevent use of narcotics if the narcotic is achieving pain control. Constipation is a common side effect of taking narcotics. Daily stool softeners, laxatives, and enemas may be needed as long as you are receiving the narcotic. It is very important to start early to prevent constipation and thus avoid more serious complications, such as stool impactions (severe constipation with stool accumulation and blockage in the rectum).

Another common side effect is nausea; this, too, can be managed. If you experience any unpleasant side effects from your pain medication, be sure to tell your doctor. Your home care nurse will ask you about side effects. Be frank. It will help you stay comfortable. Never discontinue your medications without checking with your doctor first.

Do's and Don'ts of Pain Medications

Whatever type of medications you are taking for pain,

there are certain important considerations to keep in mind. Here is a brief list:

Do:

- Know the names, dosages, and side effects, if any, of your medications.
- Have a responsible member of your family or someone in your home learn how and when to administer your medication.
- Follow the instructions on the label carefully. Many medicines for pain are ordered "PRN." This means that you are to take them "as needed." Take these medications *before* your pain gets severe: they are more effective at the start of pain.
- Reorder your medication before your supply runs out. It is best to reorder on weekdays as your doctor's office has your record.
- Remember that narcotics require a "triplicate" form from your physician. Call during office hours if you need to have your prescription refilled.
- Know the name and phone number of your pharmacy.
- Triple-check all your medications before taking them. If your eyesight is poor, use a magnifying glass to read the label. Use a pill organizer or have someone with better sight put out the medication.
- Keep a list of all the medications and the dosages that you are currently taking. Include on this list any past medications that gave you unpleasant side effects and any medications to which you are allergic.
- Make a copy of this list to carry in your wallet or purse, and bring the list with you when you visit your doctor or if you return to the hospital.
- Keep a careful record of each time you take your medicine, including the date and time (and whether the time is A.M. or P.M.).

Don't:

- Transfer medication from one container to another.
- Leave medications in reach of children.
- Stop taking medications, or change your medica-

tion schedule, without checking with your doctor.
- Neglect to notify your doctor if your medication is not relieving your pain.

Activities of Daily Living

Beds or chairs may need to be elevated to reduce the strain of changing positions from sitting to standing and vice versa. To provide elevation and arm support for standing, you can place a commode over the toilet or install a raised toilet seat and supporting rails. Your home care nurse or physical or occupational therapist will suggest equipment that could be useful. Your primary goals are safety and independence. It is wise to call several equipment agencies and to compare the costs of renting or purchasing. Some of these expenses may be covered by your insurance company. Some equipment may require a doctor's prescription for insurance reimbursement.

Continuing Care: Regaining Independence

Home visits may be needed daily at first, then gradually less often as you and your family develop skill and confidence. You may reach the point at which you can follow your rehabilitation program independently. If you have a progressive chronic illness, though, the relationship between the home health professional and the family will be ongoing, marked by the need to reevaluate the care program and make changes as necessary.

Even if your health cannot be fully restored, rehabilitation is most important. Fears associated with some progressive illnesses are often reduced if rehabilitation continues whenever you face new disabilities. In-home health services can enable you to maintain dignity and control and can help you keep functioning at an optimal level despite limitations. Goals must be constantly and sometimes rapidly readjusted to meet your changing needs.

In-home health services may be crucial in allowing you to continue rehabilitation, prevent deterioration, and avoid institutionalization. Home support lets you remain with your family and friends, continuing to live and love in your own familiar surroundings.

39

The Doctor's Office and Ambulatory Clinics

Ernest H. Rosenbaum, M.D.
Isadora R. Rosenbaum, M.A.
Catherine Coleman, R.N.
Paula Chung
Betty Lopez, C.M.A.
Regina Linetskaya
Dominique Davis, M.A.
William Wong, M.A.

The managed-care trend of insurance plans and HMOs is causing the practice of medicine and health care delivery to change rapidly. But much of the primary and continuing care of patients still takes place in the doctor's office. Initially, you may be seen and thoroughly evaluated as a hospital inpatient, but your follow-up care will involve regular appointments as an outpatient.

The doctor's office differs from the hospital in that there is an ongoing one-on-one relationship between the patient and the same health care team. The resulting familiarity and rapport can be an important factor in therapy and recovery. It is also the basis for building trust, confidence, and security.

As supportive relationships develop, it will seem easier to discuss physical, emotional, vocational, or financial matters that contribute to your total sense of well-being. The medical office team strives to maximize your independence and to minimize the fragmentation of your care.

The Role of Office Personnel
The Receptionist
In most offices, when you phone or come in for an appointment, the first contact you make is with the receptionist. Receptionists can assist you in many ways, for they are the link between you and the rest of the office team. They will give you certain forms for insurance and medical information which will be important to your physician, the accounting department, and the appropriate department in your HMO or managed-care organization.

You or your family and friends often may find it necessary to phone the doctor's office for information or to report a problem. It is extremely important to be open about your reason for calling and to communicate this to the receptionist. One of the receptionist's chief duties is to direct incoming calls to the person best equipped to resolve your concern or problem. It is impossible for the doctor to talk to every patient who calls in, so the receptionist is trained to answer questions whenever possible and to refer your medical problems to the nurse or doctor, according to the need.

When a new patient calls for an appointment and cannot be accommodated immediately, disappointment and sometimes even panic may result ("I'm desperately ill, my life is at stake, and you can't take me until *when*?"). It is helpful to have your medical records faxed to the office so the doctor can review them and rescheduling can be accommodated in an urgent situation.

Another function of the receptionist may be to help you schedule any laboratory tests or X-ray procedures the doctor orders. These tests often must be done at inconvenient times (such as early morning) or may involve specific instructions (such as fasting or taking time for a "prep" for an X ray or a CT scan). If you discuss your personal needs with the receptionist, he or she will make every effort to arrange tests around your schedule. Remind the receptionist of your insurance provider so that tests can be scheduled at the location through which your insurance company delivers services.

The receptionist also may need to call you sometimes. Don't panic. Some patients report being terrified when they receive a call from the doctor's office, anticipating that they're about to receive bad news from a lab report. But most such calls are made just to change an appointment date or time.

The Laboratory Technician

The laboratory technician is another important member of the medical team (though some offices do not do their own lab work, but instead have you visit an outside lab for your tests). Usually, the patient sees the lab technician before seeing the doctor. Often, you will have blood tests at each visit, as the results may be needed to establish the progress (improvement or regression) of the disease as well as to provide clearance for chemotherapy or radiation therapy. Other times you will have blood tests every few visits, depending on your treatment plan.

Since even the simplest blood count takes time to complete, ask the lab technician or the doctor's receptionist how much time you should allow so that your lab values will be ready before your visit with the doctor. Most labs require at least half an hour to produce results, even for urgent tests.

The Doctor

During your initial consultation concerning your diagnosis, your doctor will try to give you a basic understanding of your disease, the reasons for diagnostic and staging tests, and the potential outcomes of various kinds of treatments. The doctor will also want to listen to your questions and apprehensions so that he or she may allay unnecessary fears and offer help with any practical problems you may face because of your disease.

This first interview may be highly charged emotionally. Faced with a serious, possibly life-threatening illness, you may be shocked, frightened, and unable to exercise your normal capacity to express your feelings, ask questions, or take in new information. We have found it helpful for patients to tape record consultations. You will then be able to review your doctor's explanations and recommendations later when you may be better able to absorb the information.

You may find it helpful to bring the person or persons on whom you will most depend for emotional support with you to the consultation. Family and close friends will be able to be more supportive if they are included from the beginning and understand the intricacies of, and possible side effects from, the tests and treatment you will undergo. They also may assimilate information that you miss, and help you articulate questions and concerns of which they are aware. If those close to you are unable to be present during a consultation, a tape recording will help you share with them what has been discussed.

The Nurse/Medical Assistant

Physicians choose office nurses and medical assistants carefully, making sure that their attitudes, philosophy, and outlook complement the doctor's. The office nurse works with the physician and is responsible for direct delivery of medical care under the doctor's supervision. He or she serves as an important communication link between the patient/family unit and the doctor, and as a key resource in patient education, counseling, and coordination of hospital or home care needs.

In a clinic setting, you will see the nurse for a shorter duration of time than if you are in a hospital setting. If you are to receive chemotherapy or any other supportive treatment such as a blood transfusion or intravenous hydration, once the nurse receives the order from the doctor, you will spend the remainder of your time with the nurse. He or she will assess your vital signs and other functions depending on what activity is going to take place. This assessment time provides a great opportunity to verbalize how you feel, any concerns, questions, fears, or anxieties you may have. Many patients develop a close and trusting relationship with their oncology nurse. This kind of relationship can help minimize anxiety and decrease the overall stress a visit to the clinic can entail. In partnership with your doctor and nurse, your needs for activity, comfort, diet instruction, elimination aids, equipment, pain relief, safety, skin care, and so on, will be addressed. Individual and family needs vary depending on the stage of the disease, the goals of the treatment, and the emotional state of the patient and family.

Many treatments that were once given only in the hospital are now administered in the outpatient setting. Usually, your doctor's office or ambulatory clinic will have comfortable chairs or even beds you can relax in while you receive your treatment. Many outpatient treatments are very short in duration, taking only five to ten minutes. Other treatments may take up to eight hours. Knowing the duration of your treatment before starting can help you plan your stay. If you are receiving a longer treatment, you may want to bring a good book or an audio tape to occupy your time. Also, bringing a lunch or snack item from home is a good idea.

Before starting any outpatient treatment, ask to see the infusion area. Taking a short tour and meeting some of the infusion nurses can do much in reducing stress during that first chemotherapy visit. Outpatient oncology nurses also will refer you to community-based services and to rehabilitation and home health agencies for assistance with transportation, escort service, financial aid, social services, and locating support groups.

During your visit, the nurse will update medical records as needed and check your weight, blood pressure, and pulse. He or she also may assist with certain types of physical exams. Preparing and administering chemotherapy and immunotherapy are the nurse's job in some offices, as well as reviewing medications, side effects, and physician instructions.

Open lines of communication between you, your doctor, and your nurse are vital in planning your care. Please feel free to voice your concerns, questions, fears, and anxieties. Together, your doctor and nurse will assess your individual needs for activity, comfort, diet instruction, elimination aids, equipment, pain relief, safety, skin care, and so on. Individual and family needs vary depending on the stage of the disease, the goals of the treatment, and the emotional state of the patient and the family.

When you have a problem at home and need to speak with your doctor, it is likely your call will be turned over to the nurse. Because of their busy schedules, oftentimes it is difficult to talk directly to the doctor. Remember that the nurse is your direct line to the doctor. Your questions or concerns may be adequately addressed by the nurse or he/she may be able to communicate your needs to the doctor in a timely fashion. Always be clear and concise with your concerns. If you need to be seen by the doctor, the nurse can arrange to schedule a sick-call appointment for you.

Remember—the office is just a phone call away. If problems arise, the nurse and other office staff can help find solutions.

The Bookkeeper/Accountant

Continued visits to a doctor's office, particularly if special tests and lab work are required, are often costly. When you first visit the office, speak to the bookkeeper/accountant about your insurance coverage, and ask any questions you may have about office policy. Many patients have little or no knowledge of what their insurance benefits cover. To help the bookkeeper/accountant with your insurance claims, do the following:

- If you have private insurance coverage, give the office the specific form provided by your insurance company—after completing your information—and let the office know where the completed form should be sent.
- If you have point-of-service coverage, give the office your card so that they may either make a photocopy of it or make a notation of the necessary identification numbers and coverage. Find out whether your insurance company has a contract with your doctor; if so, you may expect to pay a co-payment amount.
- If you are on Medicare, discuss with the bookkeeper how the office handles Medicare claims. Some offices bill the Medicare carrier directly; others ask patients to submit their own bills. When completing a Medicare form, be sure to list, in addition to your name and address, your Medicare number and the nature of your illness in the proper place on the form. You do not need to describe your illness in medical terminology. Put in your own words why you had to see the doctor. If you don't know what to say, ask the

nurse or receptionist to help you. Sign the form, attach a copy of the doctor's bill, and mail it to the proper address given at the top of the Medicare form. When this information is listed correctly, it will hasten your reimbursement.

- If you have a financial problem or are running out of funds and would like some assistance, most cities have social service agencies that help patients who need financial aid. Most doctors' offices also are willing to make financial adjustments when circumstances make it necessary to do so. Contact the bookkeeper to discuss your particular situation.
- If you belong to an HMO or a managed-care insurance plan, know what your co-payment is and where your lab work, X rays, and other tests can be done. You usually need a referral from your primary doctor for each specialist visit. The primary doctor's assistant or secretary usually does the referral.
- Notify staff of any change in your insurance.

Your Responsibilities

The Medical Care Plan

No matter what illness you are confronted with, you must assume the responsibility of being a partner with your doctor. Your doctor and nurse will explain why you are being given certain medications and what side effects you can expect. They will give you other instructions concerning diet, exercise, etc., that will hasten your recovery. If your memory is not sharp at that moment, ask your doctor to write everything down so that you won't forget. Be sure to let the doctor know of any herbal medications you are taking.

Your Medications

- Know the name, dosage, and directions of all your medications.
- *Never* stop taking any medication unless given specific orders by your doctor to do so.
- A responsible person should handle your medications if you cannot. The visiting nurse will be able to assist you as needed, under your doctor's direction.
- Count your pills. When your supply runs low, reorder in time, and on a weekday—not on a weekend.
- If you are taking a new medication, before the

doctor reorders, she or he may want you to report the effects of the drug and whether it was successful.

When you reorder medications from your pharmacy, you should know the following:

- The pharmacy's name and phone number.
- The name of the medication, dosage, directions, amount, and prescribing physician, all as listed on your current bottle. Never expect to order by color! Accurate information will save time and energy. The prescription will state the number of renewals (refills) for your medication, and whether the drug is an over-the-counter item.
- The reason for reordering during the doctor's regular office hours is that the pharmacist may have to call your doctor's office for approval.
- If your doctor cannot be reached for verification, and you absolutely need your medication over a weekend, the pharmacist may give you enough to last until Monday, except in the case of drugs for which a special written or triplicate prescription is legally required (such as sleeping pills, narcotics, and certain tranquilizers). If you keep proper track of your medications, you won't let them run out.
- If you have a language barrier, have a friend serve as your interpreter.

Consulting the Doctor

Write down complex questions or problems before consulting the doctor. Have necessary information available when you call your doctor. For example:

- Constipation, diarrhea, or bloody stools?
- Pulse: regular or irregular (skipping)?
- Heart: normal rate, racing beat, thumping?
- Nausea or vomiting?
- Numbness?
- Lightheadedness or dizziness?
- Fever? (Take your temperature—own a thermometer and know how to read it. The nurse will teach you, if you do not know how.)
- Chills: How long did you shake? What time of day? How often?
- Any unusual swelling, redness, or evidence of an abscess?
- Pain: Where? How long? What intensity? Does it move in different directions? What makes it worse? What seems to alleviate it?

Consulting the Doctor "On-Call"

A patient may call the office when another doctor is covering for that patient's regular physician. Your chart is usually available to that doctor so that he or she can make the right decisions about your care. Occasionally, the chart is not available because it is on loan to the hospital. To obtain the best help, except for an emergency, always call during hours when your doctor's office is open. The office may provide you with a self-care card, which lists valuable information for you to relay in case your doctor is not available and another doctor is taking his or her calls.

Being Prepared for Emergencies

List emergency telephone numbers on a card and keep it near the phone. Here is a sample Emergency Phone Numbers Card:

Emergency Phone Numbers

Police: Tel: (____) _____

Fire Department: Tel: (____) _____

Physician: Tel: (____) _____

Pharmacy: Tel: (____) _____

Ambulance: Tel: (____) _____

Nearest relative or friend: Name _____

Relationship _____

Tel: (____) _____

Self-Care Card

Name: _____

Diagnosis: _____

Treatment: _____

Drugs: _____

Allergies: _____

Name and Telephone Number of Oncologist: _____

Advance Directives: _____

IF YOU HAVE AN EMERGENCY—CALL 911 FIRST!!!

40

Social Services in the Hospital, Home, and Office

Irene Harrison, L.C.S.W.
Lee L. Pollak, L.C.S.W.
Isadora R. Rosenbaum, M.A.
Ernest H. Rosenbaum, M.D.

This chapter describes the special hospital and community social services available to cancer patients to supplement medical care and rehabilitation services. Cancer brings with it many practical and emotional problems in addition to medical ones: problems of financial assessment (Who will pay or help with hospital or home bills?); transportation (Who will bring the patient to the doctor's office or hospital for therapy?); home help (Who will plan and carry out medical care and make the practical arrangements?); and emotional crises. The support and guidance of social services can be critical for finding feasible solutions to acute problems and as a pathway to maximum rehabilitation.

The Medical Social Worker

Many hospitals have a Social Services Department with medical social workers available to all patients.

You may have never needed the services of a social worker. You may even feel that you don't need anyone else to talk with. But cancer brings extraordinary challenges for you and for your family. You will need to marshal all of your emotional energy so that you can participate most effectively in your treatment and rehabilitation. That's why the medical social worker is there: he or she has known many patients who have faced these same emotional and practical problems, and understands what you and your family are going through.

It is the social worker who can best assist with the nonmedical aspects of patient care and support, as well as locating community services to help with home care. Community service agencies can provide professional social services in conjunction with medical teams, adapting services to each patient's situation. They can help solve such typical problems as who will pay or help with mounting bills, work, or other activities; how the patient will get to and from medical appointments and treatments; how the practical needs of at-home care will be managed (what might be needed and who will arrange for it); how unexpected crises will be handled; and the how the patient and family will handle the intense emotional issues that often arise from a diagnosis of chronic or end-stage disease.

Traditionally, oncology social workers have been found in medical settings, and were available through the hospital social service departments. Today, as medical and inpatient health care are experiencing changes, some services formerly provided within hospital social service departments are being provided by hospital discharge nurses, discharge planners, and case managers, and, outside the hospital, by community social service agencies.

Though this may be your first involvement with cancer, the social worker will have worked with many patients and families facing the problems you are now addressing, and will understand what you are all going through. Because you need to marshal your own individual strength to face the challenges ahead, the social worker can provide pertinent information, support, and services.

Learning to compensate for and live with disabilities is one of the compromises you must make when you have a chronic illness. The medical social worker can help you adjust while being sensitive to your emotional needs, family obligations, and decisions about future goals.

Specific Support Services the Social Worker Can Provide

Initial Diagnosis

When they first receive a diagnosis of cancer, many people feel overwhelmed. This may be a time in which you feel least able to reach out for help. Information is coming in too fast to be assimilated. You want to understand your illness, prognosis, and treatment choices, yet you don't want to deal with them. During this period, you need to allow yourself time to deal with your illness, your reactions, and your understanding at your own pace. Your social worker can be your sounding board and also can help you resolve many practical concerns and determine priorities.

Here are some common practical questions:

- What is this going to cost me?
- How can I support myself or my family while I am being treated?
- How will I manage at home after I leave the hospital?
- How can I get back and forth for treatment when I am feeling so weak?
- I live out of town, but need to come in to the hospital daily for the next several weeks for treatment; where can I stay?
- What do I do about my work?

All of these concerns are real, and the social worker can help with information about insurance coverage; private and government medical and financial benefit programs; and community home health agency, rehabilitation, and cancer service programs.

Many cancer patients have difficulty talking about their cancers. Your social worker can help you find ways of talking about it that will put you and others more at ease. Being able to talk with your family about your fears and concerns can result in greater understanding and intimacy and will help you and them to feel less alone. Your friends also need you to be able to talk to them honestly and openly; when they don't know what to say, they may stay away.

The goal for you, with the assistance of your social worker, should be to maintain open communication with all the people on your medical team, as well as with people in your personal and professional lives. This will help you feel respected and supported, and also will let you offer respect and support to the people who care about you—who, like you, are undergoing intense responses to your cancer diagnosis.

Social workers on cancer teams have found that one of their most important tasks is to help you deal with some of the myths and misconceptions we all have about cancer, and to help you get past the shock or "not hearing" stage. You may have had some contact with cancer before, either directly in your family or through friends or the media. There is an urge to swap information and compare medical experiences and treatments with others who have cancer, but doing so can result in confusion. There are many different types and stages of cancer: it is not just one disease, but can take many forms. You need all the information you can get about your specific illness.

Cancer does not inevitably lead to death, it is not contagious, and it is not a punishment for previous sins. These may seem like strange ideas, but they come up repeatedly among the feelings of people at the beginning of learning to deal with their cancer diagnoses. And all of us have heard about "alternative" cancer treatments, some of which are pure quackery. Discuss any questions you have about these matters with the hospital medical social worker.

Surgery

Some treatment options, including surgery, may require hospitalization and outpatient care.

The period while you are waiting for surgery is often one of heightened anxiety. Common concerns include fears about anesthesia, survival, loss of control, pain, mutilation, and general impact on lifestyle. These fears are often not discussed with anyone. You will find it helpful to talk to a social worker before surgery to prepare yourself for the operation and its consequences. Talking about your anxieties will help you cope with the actual event. Your social worker also can help you if you need to make practical arrangements before your surgery.

The post-surgical period requires you to make many adaptations, which are often accompanied by mood swings. You may need to mourn something lost or changed. How you react to your surgery will depend on the meaning it has for you. Talking about it can help you understand its unique meaning for you and how you can deal with it.

Post-surgical changes in self-image and fears of rejection may lead to an unnecessarily restricted life. Supportive services can help you adjust; in particular, involvement in programs with other cancer patients will make it easier for you to live a better life with your cancer.

Radiation Therapy

The beginning of radiation therapy is another crisis point. Once more, the fear of the unknown has to be confronted. It is frightening to go into the subterranean quarters where most radiation therapy departments are located.

Common fears and feelings are:

- Will the radiation cause cancer?
- Will I be radioactive (overexposed or contaminated)?
- I feel alienated and abandoned.
- What if the radiation machine fails?
- Has the technician forgotten me?
- I'm worried about side effects: nausea, vomiting, hair loss, appetite loss.
- Will I be able to have children?

As a cancer patient, you have to absorb a great deal of new information. You may misinterpret or distort information that you are not able to assimilate emotionally. To plan realistically for your own care, you need to ask questions repeatedly and learn what you need to know about radiation therapy and about its anticipated side effects, duration, and outcome.

Hospitals and radiation therapy centers frequently offer group counseling that can help patients share their concerns and cope emotionally with treatment.

Chemotherapy

If you are receiving chemotherapy, it is difficult for you to get your mind off your cancer; your life must now accommodate a treatment schedule, and you may often have to deal with uncomfortable side effects, such as hair loss, weight loss, and nausea. Feelings of frustration and anger need an outlet. Group therapy programs have proven supportive in helping people participate in their chemotherapy programs; the social worker can advise you about the possibilities.

Recurrences

If your cancer recurs, you will be disappointed—and perhaps feel desperate and/or hopeless. You may frantically search for miracles. During this period, you may need special help to mobilize your efforts to participate in further treatment. You may be angry, depressed, weepy, or demanding. Individual or group counseling sessions with your social worker can give you a safe and acceptable place to express those feelings.

Remission

It is logical to feel joyful when you are in remission. However, many patients find their joy is held in check by the persistent fear that the disease will recur and become uncontrollable. It is common to experience a letdown as it becomes necessary to invest your energy somewhere else besides just dealing with your disease.

Family Support and Counseling

A medical social worker can help your family understand the ramifications of your disease and treatment. Family members often experience crises relating to the changes and concerns brought about by a loved one's illness. Because they are healthy, they may find it particularly difficult to think of their own needs and may need to be encouraged to find an outlet for their feelings.

Common feelings experienced by family members are:

- What have I done to make my loved one get cancer?
- Why me?
- What can I do to make him well?

- I have to devote myself to her needs, and my needs are not important.
- I feel so alone, because he doesn't really tell me how he feels.
- I am scared that she may die, and I don't know how I will manage without her.
- I am worried about expenses.
- I am ashamed to take city or state aid.
- I am ashamed because I feel so angry at her.

All of these feelings are perfectly normal, but they often go unexpressed, either because the relative fears making the person with cancer more ill, or because the relative feels ashamed of having such concerns.

Your family members need to know that they too are active participants in your treatment program. But they may need help recognizing their own needs as they cope with the changes in family life brought about by your illness. Many hospitals and community agencies have family groups or individual counseling services available to assist family members.

Job-Related Assistance

Often, patients find it easier if a third party informs their employer that they will not be able to return to work as early as planned or will be unable to return to work for an extended period of time. The medical social worker can help you explain to your employer your present health status and prognosis. If a formal letter is required, that too can be arranged. If you can no longer work at your previous occupation, the medical social worker may also help you learn about vocational-transition resources.

Discharge Planning

One of the roles of the medical social worker is to help the patient and family with discharge planning. The medical social worker acts as the coordinator of collaborative future health planning, as outlined by the attending physician and other members of the health care team. It is the function of the medical social worker to see that the transition from hospital to other community care facilities is smooth. He or she can arrange for home care, special equipment, meal services, friendly visitors, and so on.

Financial Aid

You may be unfamiliar with your medical insurance or HMO or PPO managed-care coverage and with the various financial support systems that are available. The social worker is trained to evaluate, investigate, and advise you about insurance and financial aid programs.

Transportation

Many patients need specialized transportation to the doctor's office, to special therapy centers, and to rehabilitation facilities. The medical social worker can provide information or arrange service through the many volunteer organizations in your community.

In certain instances, you may have to travel out of the city or state for consultation or treatment. The medical social worker can arrange for transportation and housing as well as hospitalization.

Support through Crisis Periods

Everyone responds differently to cancer. The impact varies with age, sex, personal history, and the severity of the illness. But you can expect to encounter at least some changes in how you experience your life; at such times, the social worker can be immensely supportive to you.

The changes aren't necessarily obvious; in fact, they are more likely to involve subtle shifts in your self-image, priorities, and attitudes. In some instances, you may experience major disruptions in your lifestyle. These will differ depending on the effect of your illness. Such changes need not be sad, for they can offer new opportunities for you to make changes in your life and to make active choices about how you want to live.

Ironically, it is the points of intense crisis that may offer the greatest opportunities for personal growth and positive changes in your family relationships. During such crossroads periods, cancer patients are often able to make considerable progress in taking control of their situations and in finding new ways to communicate with their loved ones. By acting together in unison, many find tremendous support and connection with important people in their lives. Other cancer patients have identified these same stress periods as times when they felt most insecure and alone and wished they had had professional help for themselves and their families.

Cancer can have its stages of medical necessity, periods of hospitalization, and serious outpatient issues. It can also have many long periods of stability. Acute crisis periods force people to face situations as they arise. Dealing with cancer as a chronic illness requires other skills, such as insight, patience, and attention to ongoing emotional and practical needs.

Social services can significantly help you to cope with—even grow from—such crossroads and crisis points. In addition to the social support services and other support services provided by your local hospitals and community agencies, you can obtain information, counseling, and practical services from a host of national, regional, and local institutions. Your social worker will be your best single resource for information about what is available in your community. The Resources in Part VI contain the names of some of the organizations that are best known for providing the essential services described in this chapter.

41

Dealing with Death If Cancer Becomes Terminal

Ernest H. Rosenbaum, M.D.
Isadora R. Rosenbaum, M.A.
Sabrina Selim, B.A.
Irene Harrison, L.C.S.W.

Death is a part of life. We all must die sometime—we just don't know when. Yet we persist in thinking of death as something that happens to other people. We do not accept our mortality until a crisis forces us to contemplate nonbeing. Even then, we may fight, bargain, and connive to gain more time. Life, however, is elusive as well as precious. It may be snuffed out at a moment's notice or drain away slowly with disease or old age. And, although physicians fight to preserve life at almost any cost in time, money, or effort, we also know that a day will come when the time is right to let a person die.

In partnership with their physicians, cancer patients face many difficult issues. Throughout treatment they share in medical decisions and, if the cancer becomes progressively worse, they will, at some point, discuss with their physician matters concerning their dying. For example, people often ask that no extraordinary measures be taken to keep them alive when there is no longer any hope of being restored to a good quality of life. Other decisions involve a choice of where to die—home, hospital, nursing home, or hospice. Funeral arrangements also are often discussed between patients and physicians.

We are all concerned with maintaining dignity in life as well as in dying, and we share certain standards as to what constitutes an acceptable level of dignity. The cancer patient may gradually feel that level recede as he or she experiences diminishing control over personal destiny. A loss of privacy and of the ability to influence one's present or future may become more of a concern than dying. Sometimes people begin to question whether life is worth living under the circumstances, and whether euthanasia might be the best solution. Implementing such a request is neither ethical nor legal, but under the current official guidelines of medical practice, maximum comfort with a minimum of suffering can be promised. A physician also can promise not to interfere with a natural death by keeping a patient alive with special life-sustaining equipment and procedures. A patient has a right to die and to direct the physician to see that this wish is honored.

Several forms of hospice units have emerged, helping to ease some of the problems associated with both home and hospital care. In some communities, a hospice unit is a segregated ward in the hospital with an associated staff of physicians, bedside nurses, home-coordinating nurses, and social workers, managing inpatient care and supporting at-home care by interacting with other community resources. Most units in the United States have developed as out-of-hospital home care agencies, coordinating inpatient services through a loose affiliation with neighboring hospitals.

In some settings where a separate hospice unit has not been created, a group of hospital-based personnel that includes a physician, a nurse, a social worker, and a chaplain is available for consultation and support to patients throughout the institution.

A few freestanding hospices also have been constructed. These low-technology, inpatient facilities admit only terminal patients and often are associated with a home care program.

The hospice movement is beginning to fill a void in the medical and psychological care of the terminally ill. But the hospice team should not replace the concerned physician. Patients and families need continuity of care, and physicians should not relinquish their involvement when a patient is admitted to a hospice service. They should remain as physician-of-record, working with the terminal care staff.

Hospice Care

Irene Harrison, L.C.S.W.

Hospice is derived from the Latin word *hospitium*, "hospitality," an inn for travelers, especially one kept by a religious order. The hospice movement was started by Dr. Cicely Saunders in England in the 1940s, when St. Christopher's Hospice was opened to provide a quiet place where people could die in peace and dignity. It was staffed by nuns who had a sense of commitment to service.

Hospice care was introduced in the United States in 1974 at Yale in New Haven, Connecticut. Since then, the movement has expanded rapidly, with programs based on several organizational models: all-volunteer, hospital-based, integrated with home health agencies, or freestanding community hospices. Though diverse, these programs share a philosophy.

Philosophy

Despite all the advances in diagnosis and treatment, a cure is not always possible. Continued treatment, even if available, may compromise a patient's quality of life. After discussion with the physician and consideration of treatment options and the potential outcomes, it may be appropriate to consider palliative (comfort) care. Some patients and families are frightened by the word hospice, believing that all treatment will be discontinued and the patient is being sent home to die. But many kinds of treatment may be continued to provide comfort and relief of pain.

The hospice philosophy embraces a holistic approach that encompasses physical, emotional, and spiritual concerns. The patient and family are seen as the unit of care. Care has to be individualized to meet the patient's and the family's needs, as well as being responsive to differences in lifestyles. The hospice philosophy:

- affirms life;
- promotes self-determination, as patients and families participate in their plan of care;
- provides education to help patients and families provide appropriate care;
- promotes understanding and accepting that the journey of life eventually leads to death, and encourages people to view this experience as an opportunity for growth; and
- emphasizes palliation, which includes physical, psychological, and spiritual comfort delivered by a multidisciplinary staff.

Why Choose a Hospice?

When medical treatments have been exhausted or the burden of treatment outweighs the benefits, it may be time to consider hospice care. Most people would like to end their lives surrounded by family and friends. By bringing services into the home,

(Continued from page 374)

hospices help patients and families provide the necessary care. Patients and families are able to retain a greater sense of control at home than in the hospital. Hospices also will provide services in convalescent homes to ensure pain and symptom management and to provide support to families. The hospice experience can foster spiritual and personal growth as the hospice team empowers patients and families to manage difficult situations.

Members of the Hospice Team

Medical Director

The director is a physician who is committed to the philosophy and goals of hospice care for the terminally ill. She or he attends team meetings and provides consultation to the staff. The medical director also helps educate other physicians about hospice care, encourages them to make appropriate referrals, and may consult with primary physicians to assist them with pain management.

Nurses

Hospice nurses are highly skilled in effective pain management, which is a primary concern to patients and families. Family members are included in education about pain management, because they are the ones providing the daily care at home. Seeing a person in his or her own home is quite different from an office visit. Hospice nurses can thus obtain additional information that lets them collaborate more effectively with the physician.

Medical Social Worker

Medical social workers are trained to understand the emotional and social needs of patients and families and how best to help them in this end-of-life stage. They facilitate communication between family members, provide advocacy, and teach problem-solving skills. Social workers are aware of cultural diversity and of the belief systems that affect how people respond to hospice services. Social workers link clients to community resources.

Home Health Aides

Home health aides are very important members of the team. They provide hands-on care and perform intimate tasks like bathing and grooming. Patients and families may feel more at ease with home health aides than with other personnel. Nurses supervise the home health aides.

Chaplain

Because one of the goals of hospice care is to acknowledge and tend to a person's spiritual needs, some hospices have a chaplain on their team. Spirituality goes far beyond identifying religious affiliation and where someone worships. It involves the exploration of fears, values, and beliefs—especially those relating to what awaits us after death. At this time, many people experience a strong need to review their lives and to seek meaning and purpose. Ethnic and religious differences need to be appreciated. Rituals can be helpful in coping with the unknown. Patients may hope for reunification with God or family members, an idea that provides comfort and reduces fear. Even patients who are not affiliated with any specific denomination often wish to get in touch with their spirituality or their existential search for meaning. Life reviews are helpful, and reconciliations help patients "let go" of life. If the team does not have a chaplain, other team members address these issues and can also refer the patient to community clerical support.

Volunteers

Volunteers are the backbone of many hospice programs. They are trained prior to working with patients, and their supervision continues after their formal training ends. These individuals give willingly of themselves to enhance the quality of life for hospice patients and their families. They may, for example, assist with transportation or stay with patients to give caregivers a break. Sometimes they visit patients in the hospital or nursing home, helping to reduce feelings of loneliness or abandonment. Some volunteers specialize in supporting the bereaved. They make follow-up telephone

(Continued from page 375)

calls and, if they note any problems, they arrange for a team member to assess the situation. Volunteers are great people with a real commitment to service. They are essential to the success of the hospice program.

Nutritionist

A patient's eating habits are of great concern to the family. Often, a patient's appetite and tastes change, and family members may be at their wits' end to find something to prepare. Weight loss affects body image and worries families. The nutritionist can help with information and suggestions that might help to improve appetite. The nutritionist works closely with families and is sensitive to ethnic preferences. Education helps patients and families adjust their usual eating habits. Medications also may affect appetite. Families get particularly upset when their loved ones are no longer able to take food or fluid by mouth, worrying that the patient will die of starvation. Some request tube feedings or intravenous hydration. It is crucial to have a calm discussion with the patient and family to determine the stage of illness and to weigh the advantages and disadvantages of these procedures. Each case needs to be examined individually, keeping in mind that comfort is the goal of hospice care.

Pharmacist

Pain control, one of the primary goals of hospice care, is also the patient's main worry. Pharmacists contribute their knowledge of drug potencies and of interactions among drugs to attain maximum pain control and symptom relief while minimizing side effects.

Physical Therapist

Physical therapists help patients maximize their ability to move around and to get in and out of bed, chairs, and transportation. The therapist teaches families techniques that will prevent them from injuring themselves while assisting the patient. The therapist also will recommend some exercise to encourage the patient's independence.

Occupational Therapist

Occupational therapists help improve the patient's ability to perform the activities of daily living, teaching people how to conserve energy and how to adapt the living environment.

Speech/Language Pathology Services

Speech therapists consult with team members in cases where the patient's ability to speak has been compromised. They help to develop alternative communication systems.

Psychologist

Psychologists consult on difficult cases. Depression and preexisting psychological problems may affect how people cope. Psychologists make recommendations for improving the management of care for patients and families.

How Are Hospices Financed?

Some hospices are supported by the community with their own fundraising and donations; other programs have a large volunteer component. Hospices may be incorporated with home health agencies or hospitals, or they may receive funds from foundations and grants. Private health insurance and Medicaid are some other forms of reimbursement. In 1982, Medicare began reimbursing certified Medicare hospices, which must adhere to specific guidelines. Part A of Medicare covers most of the costs.

Medicare Hospice Benefit

- To qualify for the hospice benefit, patients must be eligible for Medicare.
- A physician must certify that the patient has a prognosis of less than six months.
- Patients who elect the hospice benefit must waive their rights to traditional benefits.
- Patients are entitled to two ninety-day periods and then sixty-day extensions, which can be extended if the physician certifies the need for further care.
- Patients and families receive services from the core hospice staff according to an

(Continued from page 376)

interdisciplinary team plan.

- Patients and families have access to a twenty-four-hour advice line that is answered by a nurse who prioritizes problems and arranges for appropriate care.
- Equipment for home use is rented and supplies are furnished.
- Medication for symptom management and pain relief is covered.

Bereavement services are included in hospice care. Some hospices have very comprehensive programs, with staff assigned solely to provide bereavement services; others use their core staff and specially trained bereavement volunteers. Services typically include:

- attending funeral services
- making home visits
- telephoning at regular intervals
- contacting the bereaved on birthdays, anniversaries, and holidays, which tend to be especially sad times
- providing nonthreatening educational programs that offer practical information
- hosting social events, often combined with an informative speaker or fund-raising component
- facilitating bereavement support groups.

Bereavement support groups are most com-monly facilitated by a professional, and are semistructured and time-limited. Bereaved children may need additional intervention. Hospice staff members help teach families how to deal with a child's grief. Children's groups, such as Good Grief, are a great resource. Your hospice care provider can make a referral to a child specialists.

Euthanasia or Physician-Assisted Suicide

To hasten a person's death by active euthanasia is inconsistent with the hospice philosophy of providing quality care at the end of life; but attaining effective pain control may in some cases hasten death. The hospice will focus on helping patients differentiate between giving up and accepting death as a natural progression in the life cycle.

Making End-of-Life Decisions

With the current emphasis on patients' rights, self-determination, and informed consent, people are encouraged to make decisions before they become terminally ill. Advance directives are documents that allow individuals to specify their wishes. A person must be mentally competent to complete an advance directive. Chapter 44, "Decisions for Life," provides details on living wills, durable power of attorney for health care, and do not resuscitate (DNR) forms.

Communicating Your Wishes to Your Physician

A person can sign a directive to the physician and choose the place where he or she will die. The only thing one cannot dictate is *when* one will die.

Most people know when they are dying and are sensitive to the suffering of those around them. Yet sometimes when they express a desire for peace, they are made to feel guilty by relatives who prefer to keep them alive under any conditions. To prevent such conflicts, many patients agree in advance with their physician to sign a document or directive called a "living will" that states their request not to be kept alive by artificial means or heroic measures when there is no reasonable expectation of recovery. Living wills also can stipulate other conditions under which the patient wishes either to be freed from, or remain on, life support.

For some patients, there is a preterminal phase before descending into a coma. At this time, a patient is still alert enough to take comfort in talking with his or her family or with the medical staff. During this phase, anything or anyone especially dear to the patient should be made available. He or she may want to spend time with a particular relative, friend, child, or pet. This may be an appropriate time to complete an ethical will. But we must remember that physicians aren't capable of predicting when a person is going to die. We have only clinical judgment as to the time remaining for any patient. Moreover, no health care professional can prejudge the value of extra days or hours. Some time ago, a patient was dying of a massive malignancy that was obstructing his liver. Not wanting him to suffer any longer, the doctor left a verbal order with the interns and the resident that when he died, no efforts at resuscitation should be made. About half an hour later, the patient went into cardiac arrest. Neither the intern nor the resident were in the room, and the nursing staff had changed for the morning shift; the nurse naturally sent for the cardiac resuscitative unit, and the patient was revived. He lived another forty-eight hours, and during that time several relatives arrived from the Midwest and were able to visit with him. In addition, a brother, from whom he had been estranged for twenty years, arrived at his bedside, and they were reunited. He also had warm, emotionally satisfying talks with his wife and children about their lives together.

Such communication is invaluable. It is natural for a dying person to experience a heightened sensitivity to the meaning of life and to want to convey special messages to those close to him or her. But these thoughts are not always expressed, either because of awkwardness at expressing deep feelings or because of a reluctance to talk about death. So survivors are often left without a final communication.

Patient-Family Good-Byes

Saying good-bye before death can be a comfort to everyone concerned—family, friends, and patient. As healthcare professionals, we often have participated in such a farewell to life by encouraging patients and key family members to make a tape recording together while the patient is still alert. The recording may include a family history or anecdotes, or it may be a philosophical conversation on life and death. A physician or nurse can often be instrumental in helping people to break their silence by initiating similar conversations.

People who find it difficult to speak of their feelings sometimes write a letter expressing their thoughts and love. Such a letter often contains hopes for the future happiness of their loved ones, in effect giving them permission to seek joy and fulfillment in the next phase of their lives.

For example, we recently received a copy of a letter sent by a young woman to her husband several months before she died. She wrote of their life together, her happiness with him, and her sadness that it would end soon. She also told him that he would need to return to active living and that he should marry again when he met the right person.

It doesn't matter how eloquently or awkwardly such thoughts are expressed. This conscious, deliberate communication can relieve the stress of silence between two people and bring them closer together. Remorse and guilt may be lessened in both people. The person who is dying may gain peace of mind, while the survivor experiences a bond that can be a solace during mourning.

Death is never easy to accept, no matter what the cause. Family members need special attention throughout the ordeal, but especially in those final days. Help may come from within the family or from friends; but physicians, nurses, clergy, social workers, and hospital volunteers also are available and ready to listen. We always hope that families will find solace in the knowledge that their loved one received good medical care and sensitive emotional support; that he or she lived as long and as well as possible under adverse conditions; and that all possible comfort was provided to ease the process of dying.

42

Grief and Recovery

Ernest H. Rosenbaum, M.D.
Isadora R. Rosenbaum, M.A.
Sabrina Selim, B.A.
Lee L. Pollak, L.C.S.W.

"The value of life depends on the impact on others."
—*Jackie Robinson*

Grief is a normal, necessary psychological process that helps a person adapt to the loss of a loved one. The survivor is depressed and often withdraws from former interests, activities, and even friends. Grief is a very personal experience. Even among members of a family who lose the same person, the experience of the loss will be different for each person. The closer the relationship to the deceased, the greater the loss.

For an adult, the psychological work of grief is connected with remembering and reliving the experiences shared with the person who has died. Grief is not a consciously determined task; rather, it is set in motion automatically and proceeds at the rate that is bearable for the individual. Grieving is painful because, as we remember good times as well as bad, the very process of remembering requires a continuing recognition that the person we loved is no longer present.

Grief involves intense mental anguish, remorse, and sorrow. The outward signs of grief are identical to those of depression. But these are mere words, and can in no way suffice to describe the deep burst of emotional pain and shock experienced by a person who mourns. He or she has lost love, goals, friendship, and/or security—none of which are immediately replaceable.

The depth of grief is unpredictable because it reflects so many factors, including the availability of support from family, children, and friends; one's culture or religion, and the degree of preparation for the event. And there is no universal approach to the process of grieving, although in our society many people follow specified religious procedures. Each of the major religions observes a degree of ritual, quite similar in format, when dealing with death.

Because doctors deal with these problems frequently, we try to prepare a patient's family and friends as well as possible for an anticipated death. We do this by providing medical information and by holding family conferences on the patient's progress. Yet no matter how thoroughly we have prepared them, families still experience shock and momentary disbelief when the death occurs. In addition to dealing with their grief, family members will need to make a number of decisions and answer questions: "Will there be a autopsy?" "What funeral arrangements must be made?" The doctor can be helpful at such a time, because those who were close to the patient are typically not thinking or remembering clearly. If the disease was chronic, funeral arrangements may already have been completed, or at least initiated, by the family.

When the funeral is over, the family, as well as members of the medical team who have been involved with the patient, need time for their sorrow to abate. At this time, we usually write the family a letter expressing both sympathy and hope for the future. A review of the patient's medical problem and the therapy is provided, along with pertinent autopsy information if one was performed. These steps help to clear up any questions or misunderstandings among family members about what actually occurred, especially in the final days, when their comprehension may have been clouded by concern for the patient. We have found this approach very helpful for the grieving process.

During the first few weeks, phone calls, visitors, and cards of sympathy distract the attention of the grief-stricken. Then suddenly the attention diminishes and one is left alone with the problem of the future. Often there is a denial of mourning, an attempt to hold back tears and suppress grief. Crying is believed by some people to be a sign of weakness, but it is merely a means of releasing pent-up emotions.

Sometimes grief occurs simultaneously with unremitting depression in which the survivor becomes obsessed with loss. When this happens, the crisis has become chronic and debilitating for the survivor, whose persistent loneliness, helplessness, guilt, shame, and anger may lead to a regressed state. Professional help may be required to alleviate these problems. Grief may seem endless and recovery may seem impossible, but grief must be allowed to run its course.

One Family's Story

We invited Mary, whose husband had died one year previously, to our monthly conference with the patient service volunteers at Mount Zion Hospital. The topic was grief and recovery. After opening the meeting with remarks on the mechanisms of grief and adaptation to loss, we asked Mary to describe her experiences since Howard's death.

Mary: It's hard to know where to start. During this last year, I have had wildly fluctuating moods and attitudes and have been better or less able to handle what my life is now compared to what it was before. Howard and I were married almost ten years and had a blessed and easy life. Neither of us, by personality, lived in the future, and so our life together didn't end with many regrets about things we hadn't done or were waiting to do. So I would keep thinking about all the good things that had happened. But each time I did this—and it is still true today—I would have to face the fact that Howard is gone and will not be back. Our children, Noah and Semantha, are now four and six; and the fact that they won't have the influence of this most remarkable man is still, and probably always will be, hard for me to accept.

I feel guilty because I complain. What we had in a relatively short time was probably a whole lot better than many people experience all their lives. It seems ungrateful to complain, but I do. I had thought I would go through a maturing process in my grief and reach a point where I would face the fact of Howard's death and accept it graciously. It was just in the course of the last week, while talking to a friend, that I realized I'm not ever going to accept it. Never, never, never!

The last year has not been a completely sad year for me. I don't feel that my life ended with Howard's death or that good things won't happen, because they have, and I expected they would. Of course, there were the circumstances at the end of his life. All that he was going through, his suffering, was finished, and that was a relief. But, you know, I may live to be 120 years old and have some wild life beyond anything I could imagine in the future—I think that's perfectly possible—but I will never—no matter what happens in the future—I will never be able to accept graciously that Howard died when he did, and the way he did.

(Continued from page 380)

In the course of the last year, I have been through different phases of grief. The phases seem to be repetitive and very short. At times, I can be overcome and almost nonfunctional with grief, sad thoughts, resentment, and anger. I wonder what I would be like if I didn't have the children to spur me to action, decisions, and all the other things.

I might otherwise have apathy or become one of those people who sit in the corner and put the drapes over their head, and everyone would have to work to get me to move. The children saved me from that. They've also had a year of grieving and also have a lot of pleasant memories of Howard. Noah has always been able, without any concerted effort, to talk about Howard or refer to him, because Howard was a big person in our lives and is just naturally a part of our conversations, or record or reference.

Noah will say, "Was that a car like Howard's?" or "Remember when Daddy took us here?" or "That's Howard's book." For me, this has been helpful.

Ernest Rosenbaum: The effect of a parental loss on children is deep. A few months ago, when I said good-bye to Noah after a visit, he replied accusingly, "Ernie, you're not going to come back, just like my daddy."

Mary: One thing I wonder about is my decision that the children should not see Howard after he died. They saw him the morning he died, and he was able to recognize them and talk to them and joke a little. Then they went out of the room, and an hour later Howard died.

I did not have them come back and see Howard, and that is out of my childhood. I went to wakes with open caskets and remember thinking, "That's not what Grandma looked like," and for me that image remained.

I felt this particularly for Noah and Semantha. I did not want that image of Howard to be their most vivid memory of him, and I was concerned that it would be. They had known him such a short time and wouldn't have a store of images to draw on.

They have had a lot of questions since then, and I don't know, but maybe they would have felt better if they had seen him. But I made the decision for them. I still think it was right, but there is one step they can't quite put together. The last time they saw Howard he was alive: and the next time, after I told them he had died, there was the funeral and his body was in a casket.

They have asked me the same questions many times since then. "Was Daddy's whole body in the box? Was he wearing clothes?"

Noah became very angry immediately after Howard's death. He had always been a friendly type, but then he was positively furious. His anger manifested itself with physical displays—throwing things and so forth.

Semantha knew Howard better. She reacted in a more "adult" way. She would be overcome with sobbing and want to talk, but was unable to talk because she just could not get the words out. As the months went by, she became more able to say the words that Howard was dead and that she would never be able to touch him again.

Noah would, on occasion, say things like, "I wish I were dead, because if I were dead then I could see Daddy. Then I would be with Howard." I still don't think the children have accepted it either.

I had a lot of preparation before Howard died, because we knew it was going to happen, and both of us talked about things and did some reading. What I'm trying to say is, I was better able to handle it because of the preparation.

Grieving is a selfish experience but, I guess, a necessary one. Grief is more intense the closer you are to the person who has died. You may have various parts of that relationship filled by other people, so that instead of one person or one source, there are many sources. In that case, the sum of the parts still doesn't equal the whole. Nevertheless, I've had a lot of support, and for that I am very grateful.

The people who have helped me most through the grieving period are those who knew Howard, his complexities and his interests, because they

(Continued from page 381)

know what he was really like. The support that comes from someone who knew the person—the talk, the conversation, the reminiscing, or whatever—is most helpful. In the grieving thing, it is sort of hard for me to hold myself together. It has been hard some of the time. Right now, I don't think I have a lot left to give to someone else who is grieving.

Ernest Rosenbaum: We all grieve after personal tragedies and losses. We progress from shock to recovery and, with time, move toward a new life. Anger and disbelief subside. Throughout the period of mourning, the concern and support of friends help the bereaved until a time comes when grief lessens. Life goes on and the bereaved person joins in.

The Duration of Grief

To the survivor, grief may seem endless and recovery impossible. Nevertheless, a process does begin whereby grief and recovery occur simultaneously, in alternating patterns and moods. Of course, nothing is ever quite the same again. The survivor's attitudes may be permanently altered by the long acquaintance with illness, suffering, and death; quite likely he or she will emerge from the ordeal a stronger, more mature person.

The means and length of time required for recovery will vary. Those who are alone will have a more difficult time and may need additional and continuing support from clergy, social workers, or the medical team to help them through their period of grief.

Slowly, a new pattern of life evolves. At first, the bereaved may feel guilty when experiencing brief episodes of enjoyment. To feel happiness may seem inappropriate, like being a traitor. Yet it is these interludes of enjoyment that gradually create new hope. As they accumulate, they coalesce into a vision of the future, and the survivor becomes able to acknowledge emotionally what he or she always knew intellectually: that vitality and involvement with others will return.

Little by little, the painful memories of the departed person's suffering and illness become less poignant, and it becomes easier to relive and enjoy thoughts of earlier, happier times. From these cherished memories, the bereaved also may derive courage by identifying with the positive qualities of the person who is gone. At the same time, the survivor begins to recognize with diminishing guilt that his or her own needs continue. This is the turning point.

There is no prescribed time that elapses before a grieving person begins to mobilize his or her interests toward the present and the future. There is no line of demarcation between grief and recovery. Old memories are kept alive while new ones are continuously being created.

Acute and Chronic Loss

The way a person dies can affect how that person's survivors grieve. There is a major difference between grieving an acute loss (a sudden death) and grieving a chronic loss (a death that is expected). Grief is more acute with a sudden death—for example, one that results from an auto accident or from an unexpected post-surgical complication. An unexpected death allows no time for planning. On the other hand, when a person has a chronic illness such as cancer, kidney failure, or heart disease, people know that death is coming. One is often given a lot of support from friends, family, and clergy about what to expect where death is concerned.

While someone we care about is dying, we often feel anticipatory grief. We may begin to fear the loss and may go through phases of depression, anger, or just difficulty in coping with the situation, knowing that death is near.

This is a time for compassion, where people often put their trust and faith in their belief system or religion. They may also get helpful support and advice on how to cope from friends, neighbors, and relatives. There is a feeling of sorrow throughout this chronic process; on behalf of the patient who is suffering, we may often wish for mercy—that the process would end. This sometimes leads to feelings of guilt. Accepting that the shortening of life is not fair often results in anger when the impending death occurs.

There are great vicissitudes or changes during the course of illness. With a sudden, unexpected death, there is no time for preparation; suddenly, one

A Grandson Remembers

Another person wrote the following about the death of his grandfather:

One of the many things that I learned from my grandfather while he was alive was something he taught me in his death from myasthenia gravis.

I had been pretty much living in the intensive care unit with Grandfather for about three weeks. During that time, I spent as much time with him as I could, usually sleeping in a chair in the ICU with him. Throughout the time that he was in the hospital, he had a tube sticking down his throat that made it impossible for him to talk. He was too weak to write, so he couldn't communicate at all. He was also very confused and disoriented. Whenever he was conscious, I would ask him if he knew where he was and why, and he would always shake his head "no." I would then explain everything to him as best I could and sit there holding his hand until he went back to sleep. Each time he woke up, the same thing would happen.

All I wanted to be able to do for him was to help him prepare for his death, which (to me) was obviously close at hand. He was frightened, confused, and in a fair amount of physical discomfort. And there was not a damn thing that I could do about it.

After the drugs and treatments had wound their way down and the doctors decided that there was really nothing further that they could do for him, it was time to allow him to die.

So they took away the medication, and they took him off the breathing machine. I was with him when he began to be aware that it was difficult for him to breathe. He looked into my eyes and mouthed, "Help me, please."

For the entire time that I'd been there, he had been really disoriented because of all the drugs. I'd wanted to talk to him, to help him consciously prepare for his death, but he hadn't been there enough to even start. But this morning there he was, looking right out at me through his eyes and asking me to help him. I started to cry. I held his hand, I looked into his eyes and I told him, "There's nothing else we can do, Grampa. The doc-

tors have tried everything they can, and your lungs just aren't working right."

I sobbed and had difficulty speaking. But for some reason, I suddenly had no difficulty at all in reading his lips. He mouthed, "Does this mean that I am going to die?" He looked right into my eyes. I looked back into his. "Yes, Grampa, you are."

"When is this going to happen?"

"I don't know, Grampa; it could be a few hours, or it could be a few days."

He nodded his head and closed his eyes. He understood. It's a pretty simple matter when you get to the point. There aren't really a whole lot of questions or much to be said.

He squeezed my hand and mouthed, "I want to go outside."

I repeated it back to him in the form of a question: "You want to go outside, Grampa?"

He nodded and mouthed, "Please."

I went to ask the nurse how I could take him outside, but she said I couldn't. There was no way to take him out in his bed, and there was no way to take him out of his bed without him dying right then and there. And it was snowing and raining and very cold outside, on top of everything else.

I felt trapped. My grandfather made his dying request—something so simple. He just wanted to go outside. But we were stuck in a context of death so complete, a place that kills you so fully, that it doesn't even let you die the way you want to.

The rest of the family arrived. He was still fairly alert. Everybody exchanged a lot of love: holding his hand, telling him that everything is OK, that he doesn't have to worry, that he can just rest peacefully. My grandmother asked me why they don't just give him something to knock him out. I explain that I asked them not to unless it seemed like he was really suffering. I asked my grandfather several times during the early part of the day whether he was suffering, whether he wanted some medication to knock him out. He kept shaking his head no.

(Continued from page 383)

The day went on. His breathing got shallower. His extremities got colder. His skin got paler. I'd been awake for thirty hours or so, hardly having left his room at all in that time. The family left for the night. It was sort of a shock to me, but at the same time, not too surprising. They all told me that I should call them if anything "happens," but it was clear to me that they didn't want to have to watch him die. It was probably better that way anyway. I was prepared for this. I spoke to him, telling him that I love him, and he squeezed my hand a little bit.

His breathing got shallower and faster. He was breathing forty breaths a minute, but he couldn't keep that up for long. It slowed down. His oxygen saturation began to drop, and so did his heart rate. The breaths were very shallow then and very slow, but still regular. I held his hand and his head, telling him that it's OK for him to stop breathing, that he doesn't have to fight anymore, that it's okay to end his association with this body and this world and that his experience will continue in another place.

His breaths were almost nonexistent, and there was a fair amount of time between them. His heart rate went down to about twenty. He stopped breathing. He was completely still. I held his head and his hand. His heart continued to beat for a minute, and then he flat-lined. I knew that his brain was still active, so I kept talking to him softly, my lips close to his ear, telling him that it's OK to leave, that he doesn't need to hold on to the body anymore, that he will find people who will help him.

The nurse quickly and carefully helped me dis-connect the body from all the machines and turn everything off. I did a little puja [a Hindu prayer] with some incense and asked the nurse to keep anyone from coming into the room for about an hour, and I just sat there in the room with him and meditated.

Aside from the horrible hospital surroundings, it was really an incredibly natural, graceful event. My grandfather lived his life a loving man, and that's the way he died.

The reason that I'm telling you all this is because in his graceful death, my grandfather showed me much "will to live." More, if I'm perfectly honest. Let me explain.

What I kept thinking was how important it is to make the distinction between the "will to live" and the "fear of death." I think that it would be very easy to mistake fear of death, a craven need to hold on to experience in a particular form, for such concepts as "fighting for life." But I think that the true will to live is a matter of love, life, and experience in all its forms and transformations. It is an openness to experience of all kinds, a gesture of full-ness and love. And death, and whatever lies beyond death, is very much a part of life.

This is no longer a theoretical issue for me. When I sat with my grandfather as he died, the thing that became so perfectly obvious to me was the naturalness of it. Death was very obviously a specific transformation in the course of life, similar to birth. The continuity of consciousness beyond that transition was completely obvious to me. But again, this is a matter of feeling and not intellect. It can be talked about, but not really communicated in words.

experiences a grievous loss. The death of a loved one in war might be expected, yet people on the home front constantly pray and do many acts, often of kindness, aimed psychologically at helping "prevent" that death. When the dreaded telegram arrives, it is therefore such a crushing blow and shock that it totally alters the recovery process. Recovering from an acute death is often difficult and slow. When shootings or assaults result in a sudden death, survivors may suffer psycho-logically for years.

Visits from family, friends, and the clergy to offer compassion and support during a chronic illness can prepare the family for death. The family members of a patient who enters a hospice program also have more time and built-in support; after death, they can get addi-tional counseling.

People try to keep hope alive through the realiza-tion that life continues during the many crises one undergoes during a chronic illness—and also in preparing for the eventual death. In Part V of this book,

"Planning for the Future," we describe many ways to prepare for death and provide forms and sample documents. Having such documents in place can avert suffering and pain, and help family and friends honor the patient's wishes.

We also discuss ethical wills, in which people transmit their thoughts either verbally or with an audio or video recording. An ethical will communicates a person's thoughts, love, and philosophy to survivors, providing a chance to say good-bye and to leave a legacy of encouragement and support, as well as to give instructions on how the estate and possessions should be distributed.

Frequently, we have participated in conversations where a dying person tries to alleviate feelings of guilt in his or her partner by advising the loved one to become romantically involved again if the opportunity presents itself. We believe grieving can be shortened and eased when the survivors receive explicit permission to continue living, and strong advice that although memories of the deceased will always be alive, life must go on.

The ethical will is a great avenue for recording such thoughts. When curing or controlling a person's cancer is no longer possible or practical, an ethical will can provide the patient with a continuing sense of hope that although he or she may not live longer, he or she will live better. Peace of mind comes with having shared important events in our life and knowing that we will live what remains of our life without pain and suffering.

The ethical will also allows people to acknowledge that their lives have been successful: for example, having raised a family, or leaving a moral or financial inheritance that reflects their values. This often gives a patient a sense not only of the value of life but also of continuing hope for the future—that family and friends will continue to grow and mature, emulating the moral standards and patterns of the patient. This hope can comfort a dying person, strengthen his or her beliefs and faith, and provide a sense of inner peace despite the most stressful circumstances.

In ethical wills, patients often express hopes that "my family will be all right when I am gone." Some hope for some extra time that has meaning; others, for a peaceful death that will not traumatize their family. Those whose religious faith includes a belief in life after death hope that at some time in the future they'll be reunited with their loved ones.

Patients have expressed such feelings as, "I hope that I die peacefully and painlessly, and that my memory will linger," and "I hope that my life has had meaning that will give strength to my survivors, and that I have served others in a way that has enhanced my feeling of what I term a successful and happy life." Such expressions not only give solace and comfort to the family but are very helpful to remember in the grieving process to come.

Those who have had angry relationships or discord within their families may try to "mend their fences," so that when death does occur, they will have achieved better peace of mind for themselves and their families. People who have not talked to a particular relative or friend for years—angry because of an incident that occurred a long time ago—have made calls to and met with the other person so that they could make peace. Others have sought forgiveness for deeds they have come to regret. Reaching out in this way can be very helpful for the survivors, softening the grieving process.

Expressions of what a dying person perceives as the meaning of his or her life can also be a touchstone for survivors. Though patients may see no hope for themselves, they may still hope that recalling the events that made their life meaningful will provide their survivors with hope for the future. Often during such a period, religion can play a role through the belief in God who has shown them a path of righteousness and a way of life. They know that when God "takes" them, their family will be comforted by the faith that although their body is no longer present, their spirit will continue on and will be remembered.

Some have remarked that their illness has brought back old religious feelings, giving them reassurance. This can also give strength to the family. We have also seen the reverse. A priest came to see a dying patient, who refused the "last rites" with the statement, "I'm not going to die." The patient was subsequently discharged from the hospital and went home, but he returned to the hospital a few weeks later. For some people, the idea of receiving the "last rites" increases their fear of death, and this practice has now been renamed "sacraments for the ill."

Religious beliefs can give people a lot of strength to face life's inevitable changes and to prepare for death. As we approach this event, we often reconnect with our beliefs, even if they have not been present for some time. This can improve the quality of life for whatever time remains, and can transmit strength to the survivors. The patient and the survivors have put their faith in God's hands for comfort, and know that it is not up to them alone. We have often heard people say—after either giving a final confession or receiving the sacraments—that they are now at peace and are no longer worried.

Receiving absolution helps not only the dying but also the survivors to continue their anticipatory and subsequent grieving process. This often requires an acknowledgment that the dying no longer have control over their lives or their cancers, and that even though they will not receive a remission or complete healing, they are now ready to continue living as best they can. This can give strength to the family.

Those who do not have strong religious convictions can experience similar peace by reaffirming their faith in humanity. Others, even those who have strong religious faith, who are angry and hostile about being afflicted by an illness that is costing them their life, may not attain any peace and may die without absolution. This is often devastating to survivors, and can accentuate and prolong their grieving.

Intimate Conversations

Saying good-bye to family and friends is hard, and may be one of the most difficult aspects of dying. One always hopes to live a little longer, to attend another event, to take another trip—but this is now being denied. One may appreciate how illness has affected everyone's lives, including its emotional and financial costs.

Discussing and implementing ways to assist survivors, as described in Part V, "Planning for the Future"—by signing living and ethical wills, and by trying to answer difficult questions for relatives, such as "How has living with cancer affected your life?"—can be very helpful to those around the patient. It also can allow them to interact with one another in loving, supportive ways that can be a touchstone to help in the grieving process. But there are times when such an approach will not work: the dying person may be denying reality, or may not be interested in or able to have such sensitive discussions.

This type of anticipatory grief session or conversation can cause great anxiety as well as sadness, because it accentuates the fact that the loss of life will

soon occur. Even so, we have found that it gives great strength to the survivors. It can involve admitting some inadequacies—for example, that one has not prepared enough to provide well for one's survivors. It can also involve expressing guilt. But an honest approach to the reality of life can be consoling, and the advice that is given can often be helpful and supportive for family and friends.

There is no "right time" to have such a conversation. Often, though, having it weeks or months before death occurs can help in the anticipatory grief process, as well as lay a foundation for support during the actual after-death grieving. Speaking frankly and setting future standards for the family's expectations, as well as compassionately discussing and revealing the inadequacies of life, can be very meaningful during this difficult and serious time. Such a somber experience may help renew faith in beliefs and give a sort of breath of life, not only to the dying person (because it may relieve anxieties) but also to his or her survivors (to whom it may give future strength). This is a recognition of the frailty of life and humanity, but it is also an expression of the meaning of one's spirit and philosophy.

Some people hope for a miracle, putting great effort into treatments—whether conventional or alternative—only to experience disappointment and depression when those treatments fail. Talking about one's concerns, one's fears, and even one's death can be a strengthening experience that gives people a bridge to the future.

The ability to confide one's thoughts, which may not have been possible for many years, and also the ability to listen nonjudgmentally, can help a dying person acknowledge and reaffirm the feelings of sadness and acceptance, reflecting the resilience of the human spirit, and reducing some of the shock, pain, and ongoing feelings of loss in the grieving process.

Ways to Help with Grieving

1. Engage in conversations about what should happen after death. Prepare an ethical will; leave instructions for what kind of funeral you want—for example, who should officiate and whether it should be private. Such information can relieve the guilt that survivors often feel after a loved one's death, when decisions must be made while grief clouds the mind. It can also prevent

unnecessary expense, since many people do not wish to have an elaborate funeral. Those who wish to be remembered in a more elaborate way, with a special public memorial, can make this clear. (See Part V)

2. Use a memorial service to try to consolidate the survivors' feelings about the person who has died. This formal means of expressing feelings can initiate and accelerate grieving. Often, survivors talk about their feelings and express their love at such a service, which can be a positive, reaffirming experience.

3. During the mourning period, make use of visits from family and friends. Most religions go through rituals and periods of observance that aid in the grieving process. For example, a wake—a party to celebrate a person's life—is a Christian custom. In Judaism, during a week of intense mourning (called *shiva*, "seven"), mirrors are covered, the immediate family sits on the floor or lower than visitors, and meals are provided by friends and members of the extended family. After this week, the family gradually progresses back toward living. The setting of the headstone, approximately eleven months later, is supposed to end the period of mourning so that life can go on.

Emotional counseling and support from clergy, family, and friends is more available during the first week or two. As time goes on, friends and family return to their homes and their lives. Calls and letters come less frequently, and the grieving person is gradually left more alone to face the finality of the loss. This loneliness can be so devastating that many people have great difficulty in functioning. Periodic letters and telephone calls give continued support, but in reality, the grieving person has to take over, regain control of his or her destiny, and resume taking care of self, family, and friends. Life will go on at its own pace.

We often tell people that this is the time when they need courage, fortitude, and strength, and that, in part, they could take such strength from their lost relative or friend, who exemplified strength in going through the illness. The survivors now need to emulate that person, calling on a similar strength to continue living in a way that honors the person's memory.

If grief persists without abating over six to twelve months or becomes the dominant force in a survivor's life, spiritual or psychological support becomes essential in order to help the bereaved return to an active and productive life. There is a need for a purpose in life and for setting new goals.

There are clearly many things on a person's mind during life's final episode. Expressing these concerns can be an effective part of palliative care, improving the quality of the remaining time. It also provides a unique opportunity to help family members bond in a way that fosters both current and future faith and hope, enhancing their courage and giving them strength to face the future.

How a person dies also makes a difference, because survivors will remember many events from the final days, hours, and minutes. Compassion shown by the medical team, clergy, psychologists, and social workers can reduce the chance that grieving survivors will feel angry that not everything possible was done. There are always questions along the lines of whether a person could have lived longer had the medical team only kept him or her on the respirator, or the feeling that this death is not fair. Feelings that "my life is now ruined" and "now I have to fend for myself" are normal and natural, but can often be lessened through appropriate guidance during the final episode in life. Attacking the psychosocial problems as well as the medical problems can reduce or eliminate many of the emotional crises common to grieving.

In facing your own death by taking the steps described in this chapter, you may help your survivors live better and lessen their grief of loss. Not everyone can provide this type of help, though. In part, our resistance to doing so may relate to Freud's suggestion that "the unconscious mind does not recognize its own death, and regards itself as immortal....It is indeed impossible to imagine our own death; and whenever we attempt to do so, we can perceive that we are, in fact, still present as spectators."

Often, even near death, people act in an unknowing way. A sudden death, which denies the dying person a chance to express helplessness, abandonment, or fear of death, presents a more difficult situation. The difficulty, in part, relates to one's ego when the final event is taking place. There may be a sudden shudder, as when one has a sudden awareness that death is going to occur and that nonexistence is probable. This realization causes strong reactions that are different for everyone.

In the hospital, the approach of death is often denied until the time it occurs. Media revelations of magical cures and new treatments give false hope. Elisabeth Kübler-Ross reports that only 2 percent of dying patients reject the chance to discuss their dying, but many staff members become so emotionally upset that they cannot participate in helping a dying patient share the experience with staff, family, or friends. Such discussions are usually less upsetting to the dying person than to those around him or her. The fear of death can provoke withdrawal, depression, or a heroic transcendence into a more giving and gracious attitude. The dying person can provide a touchstone for the survivors and future generations by reflecting on the meaning of life and by giving hope that his or her spirit and thoughts will continue.

The care of the dying provokes a pervasive fear in many people—that they themselves will die and be extinct, helpless, abandoned, and lose their self-esteem. People who wallow and struggle in their own mortality during the final episode of the dying process may be detaching themselves from reality. This is one of the normal mechanisms of escape, but such repression of death and anxieties about the future, although normal, can affect not only how the dying person copes but also how the survivors cope.

This leads to what has been termed "appropriate grief," where the mourning resolves around recognizing and integrating each person's feeling of love or hate for the person they are mourning. Our attitudes toward life and death play a role not only in how we live and how we die but also in how we grieve. The process of death and grieving is thus different for each person. Preparing for death through physical means (such as arranging for funerals, buying burial plots, and deciding on code status) and through emotional means (such as making an ethical will) can alter the grieving process.

Courage

It takes a lot of courage and compassion to stand and act with others during times of distress. The virtue of courage in approaching reality can be an expression of our inner feelings and philosophy on how to live as well as our emotional capacity to endure difficult crises. This can provide a springboard for thoughts and acts toward relatives and friends, as well as a chance to share strength and support with companions during times of great stress and woe. Benevolent acts, no matter how small, such as doing kind deeds or giving friendship, compassion, and support, can infuse confidence and hope.

Philosopher David Hume stated, "Compassion is a natural feeling which, by moderating the violence of love of self in each individual, contributes to the preservation of the whole species. It is this compassion that hurries us without reflection to the relief of those who are in distress."

By giving compassion, we share our emotions and our philosophy with another, supporting the hope not only that life is worthwhile but also that it will have meaning. This process supports the desire and will to live. Like birth and marriage, death is a turning point for the dying person and for those around him or her. It is only through kindness and giving that one extends oneself.

This is well stated by Emily Dickinson in her poem "If I Can Stop One Heart from Breaking":

> If I can stop one Heart from breaking
> I shall not live in vain
> If I can ease one Life the Aching
> Or cool one Pain
> Or help one fainting Robin
> Unto his Nest again
> I shall not live in vain.

Grief Counseling

Lee L. Pollak, L.C.S.W.

Grief affects people in many ways, and impacts their physical, emotional, social, spiritual, and practical lives. Grief care, therefore, must address all of these aspects. Time alone is not a sufficient healer. We have learned that the mourner who is quickly "doing well," who is back at work, socially active, emotionally stable, and outwardly fine, is often the person who has done inadequate grief

(Continued from page 388)

work. This person may be taking a detour around grief rather than finding a way to move through it. It is not unusual for such grievers to exhibit symptoms in other areas, often in declining physical health, an increase in ailments, accidents, and/or emotional ups and downs, and to have no idea that such responses may be grief related, and not unexplainable. These, too, are often the people who suffer an emotional backlash in later life, or in the face of later loss experiences.

Due to current societal norms, as well as the fast pace at which most of us live, most individual grief work is necessarily addressed privately and internally. It is generally unacceptable to express or dwell in an openly grieving mode beyond the formal services of funerals, memorials, and some brief religious ritual time periods. Family and friends, though caring, have their own lives to lead, and may be moving at a different pace or grieving in a different style. They may also just not be inclined to see the pain of someone they love. It may make them uncomfortable enough to stay away, get angry, or pressure their loved one to get back to normal. A grieving person is pressured by society to internalize their grief, tough it out, and get on with life within a given time period. There is a customary reliance on a one-year marker for bereavement. The grieving person hears the familiar formula that time heals all. Add to this the complications imposed by a society where families rarely live in close proximity and communities are often diverse and varied, and it is not surprising that the griever is hurried through the bereavement process. It is only the aware griever who knows that the customary work provision of three days off for grief is ridiculous. It is in response to such societal expectations that community services have evolved to support the bereaved among us. There now exist a number of helpful options for grief care.

Through individual grief therapy, the bereaved can gain support and be professionally guided in acknowledging grief, expressing emotions, managing detachment from the deceased, and, finally, in integrating the loss. Such progress enables a mourner to manage his or her grief, and ultimately to move forward with life. It is only by recognizing feelings and identifying them that one can cope with them. Accepting that grief is basically an individual experience, and that unacknowledged feelings can be very isolating, bereavement counseling is an important step in bringing the mourner back into human relationships and experiences. The bereaved may obtain this kind of focused psychotherapy from professional grief counselors, whose licenses may be as clinical social workers, family therapists, psychiatrists, Ph.D.'s, psychologists, or members of the clergy.

Peer support is another important form of grief care. Sharing feelings provides opportunities to explore them, acknowledge their import, and deal with them. Sharing promotes access to the ideas of others with similar feelings and validates the commonality of many aspects of grief responses. Most importantly, sharing helps to make the invisible visible, and reduces the incredible isolation often described by mourners in our society. Widowed Persons Services, a national organization, is only one of many such support groups. Others can be found within communities, sometimes as follow-ups to professionally led groups that have ended, and in today's technological world, on specific websites and in chat rooms.

Professionally led groups can be highly useful as mourners begin the journey back from an intense focus on individual loss into the broader concerns of the community at large. Composed of a varied population, some groups are time-limited while others are long-term, and still others are ongoing, drop-in gatherings. All are facilitated by care specialists who guide group members in addressing grief issues in a safe environment for disclosure and expression of feelings. Some groups are organized according to the specific loss relationship (e.g., Parental Loss, Spousal Loss, etc.) and some according to the specific cause of death (e.g., Survivors of Suicide, etc.). Some are specific to families, and others specific to kids, adults, or seniors. Many have no membership restrictions on age, stage of grief, gender, or type of death.

(Continued from page 389)

These psychosocial groups offer a broad range of support and guidance, and are often labeled as psychoeducational. They can be located through grief care professionals, doctors, local hospitals, social service agencies, religious institutions, and hospices, and accessed through a variety of customary intake procedures. Some have minimal charges or donations requested, while others have higher fees commensurate with local fee structures for private group therapy work.

Medication is another option for grief care. Best used in conjunction with psychosocial grief work, it can be prescribed by a medical doctor or therapist. Used alone, medication may provide immediate respite from overwhelming feelings of intense sadness and pain. Medication used in conjunction with other grief care options promotes temporary respite and can also enable the mourner to develop long-term coping and adjustment strategies.

Some communities provide alternative options for grief work with conferences, educational programs, workshops, and/or regularly scheduled healing services. These are usually offered through local religious institutions, schools, agencies, or as part of other grief care services. The National Hospice Organization provides a Grief Teleconference on an annual basis. This is only one of a variety of sporadically offered media, radio, and television programs. Some communities offer residential retreats that focus on loss and grief work; typically these are staffed by professional clinicians and organized around clinical grief issues. All of these programs can help ease the mourner through the debilitating shock and isolation of early grief back into their community of family, colleagues, and friends. All rely on the belief that a relationship with the deceased does not end in death, and that it is the survivor's task not to forget but to transform and manage that relationship as life goes forward. Towards this end, much grief work is directed towards addressing unfinished business with the deceased. Other common aspects of grief work involve working with the common feelings generated by loss, such as guilt, anger, sadness, and fear—and even the feeling of relief that sometimes accompanies a death.

Professional care helps with such grief-related tasks and provides guidance and a safety net while the mourner remains open and vulnerable. Grief support can be a tremendous source of strength and opportunity. It empowers the individual to openly seek health and recovery, and it does not require that the bereaved remain a secret griever. Long after the relatively short-term supports of ritual, recognition, and acknowledgment have diminished from the bereaved's personal, social, and work life, professional grief care options remain. More and more mourners are taking advantage of these options and are finding comfort in learning that they are not alone in their feelings, that there is help available, that healing takes more than time, and that grief work does not mean pushing away or forgetting the deceased.

You can access any of these options, and learn about others as a mourner, or as a friend, colleague, or family member of the bereaved. Such outreach can be a useful solution for those who just do not know what to do for themselves or their loved ones, and an important answer to the question of, "What can I do to help?"

Part V

Planning for the Future

43

Paying for Cancer Care

Joseph S. Bailes, M.D.
Barbara Quinn
Malin Dollinger, M.D.
Joel Pollack, C.P.A.

Newly diagnosed cancer patients are suddenly confronted with critical questions about their insurance coverage. Paying for medical care is complicated. Managed care has introduced new rules and methods of operation. There is a new vocabulary of words and initials that is confusing even to health care workers.

The health insurance industry—both public and private—has its own policies, guidelines, and methods of payment specific to cancer care. Each company's rules may be different. It is important for you to understand how your insurance company's payment system works so that you will get the care you need at a cost you should be able to pay. It is especially important to know your policy restrictions.

Group health care plans are often available through employers, labor unions, and other associations. As a rule, group plans do not discriminate against preexisting conditions, including cancer. Individual (nongroup) health insurance plans are also available. In contrast with most group plans, individually purchased plans almost always preclude or at least limit coverage for preexisting conditions. Some individual plans reject people with serious preexisting conditions.

If you are a newly diagnosed cancer patient, you may be uncertain about the scope of your coverage, as well as about how you can obtain the benefits you are entitled to under your insurance contract. Not being fully informed can put you at great financial risk, particularly since you may end up paying for services that should have been covered by your insurance. This chapter is designed to help cancer patients understand some of the issues both regarding both public and private health insurance. If you have specific questions regarding your health insurance, refer to your policy or call your insurance company.

Types of Health Care Coverage

There are many types of payment plans, insurance plans, and medical groups.

Medicare

This government-sponsored health insurance program is for people aged sixty-five and older. It also covers people who are permanently disabled, provided they have received Social Security disability benefits for at least two years.

Medicare is divided into two parts:

- *Part A—Hospital Insurance:* This part of the program covers inpatient hospital stays, limited skilled nursing care, part-time home health care, and hospice care for those who are eligible. It is available without payment of a premium, although some services require a deductible or co-payment. Medicare Part A is administered by the Health Care Financing Administration (HCFA) through insurers called intermediaries.
- *Part B—Medical Insurance:* This part of the program covers physician services and hospital outpatient care, such as blood transfusions, X rays, and laboratory tests. There is limited coverage for medical equipment, such as wheelchairs and walkers. Enrollment is optional, and the payment of a premium is required. Medicare Part B covers 80 percent of allowed charges. You are responsible for the other 20 percent of allowed charges, called coinsurance. You also must meet a yearly deductible before Medicare Part B coverage applies.

Medicare Part B is directed by the federal government through the HCFA and is funded through a monthly premium, which comes out of your Social Security check. It is administered through contracts with insurers (called carriers) throughout the United States.

If you need additional information or want to receive a free handbook describing the Medicare program, contact your local Social Security office.

Medigap

This insurance is sold by private carriers and traditionally covers the 20 percent coinsurance you are responsible for under Medicare Part B. Federal law stipulates that there be only ten standard types of Medigap policies available. These policies vary widely in their scope of coverage. You should thoroughly familiarize yourself with the particular Medigap policy you are considering purchasing, so that you will have the coverage appropriate for your situation.

Medicaid

This is a joint federal- and state-funded program for low-income individuals. It provides coverage for inpatient care, outpatient services, diagnostic testing, drugs, skilled nursing facility care, and home health care. Each state has its own rules about eligibility for the Medicaid program. Your local social service or welfare department is the best place to obtain information about Medicaid.

QMBE

This is a program in which the state pays coinsurance and premiums for certain low-income Medicare Part B beneficiaries even if they don't qualify for Medicaid.

Traditional Indemnity Insurance

Sometimes called Major Medical Coverage, this type of insurance is sold by numerous private insurance companies. It is the most common type of insurance coverage for people not eligible for Medicare or Medicaid. Such insurance plans typically pay the usual fee for service each time you see your doctor.

There is usually a deductible and/or co-payment associated with traditional indemnity insurance. This means, for example, that you might pay the first $250 or $500 in covered charges each year and/or pay 10 or 20 percent of all fees. There may be limits in the policy (a maximum dollar amount that will be paid); these often apply to hospital room and nursing costs and to treatment for psychological problems. Commonly, reimbursement to a physician is based on the "usual and customary" amount, not on the physician's actual fees.

An employer will often have a plan for general insurance coverage for each employee.

Managed Care Plans

Managed care usually requires individuals either to pay a fixed fee for a certain set of services or to see only certain physicians, who have agreed to discount their fees for particular services. There are many variations of managed care plans.

Health Maintenance Organization (HMO)

An HMO is a prepaid health plan that requires you to use a specific network or group of provider physicians, hospitals, and labs. For a fixed fee each month, HMOs provide care specified by your contract. This care may or may not be all-inclusive, so it is important to read and understand the contract of your particular HMO. For instance, some HMOs have no outpatient prescription drug benefit. In an HMO, you are usually required to select one physician as your primary or family doctor. This individual coordinates all of your care.

Examples of HMOs include Kaiser Permanente, Cigna Health Plans, and Blue Cross HMO plans. HMO members aged sixty-five and older should remember that the HMO plan replaces Medicare coverage, and you must stay within your HMO plan in order for your claims to be paid by Medicare.

Preferred Provider Organization (PPO), Exclusive Provider Organization (EPO), or Independent Practice Association (IPA)

Traditionally, PPOs, EPOs, and IPAs are groups of physicians and other participating providers who have agreed to offer a discount from their usual fees in order to participate in a particular group. Such groups function as "old-fashioned private practices" in that the physician or other provider receives a fee each time a service is performed or each time you see the physician. There are usually deductibles and/or co-payments for which you are responsible. You do have a choice of using providers or physicians who are not in the plan, but if you do, you will have to pay a larger portion of the cost.

What Does Your Plan Cover?

Your health benefits manual, insurance representative, or the health plan manager at your place of employment should be able to answer the following questions. Because cancer treatment can be quite expensive, it is absolutely essential for a cancer patient to be familiar with both the benefits and the restrictions of his or her coverage. Here are some key questions to consider:

- *What is the effective date of the policy?* In other words, when does your coverage begin?
- *What is your deductible?* This is the amount you need to pay before your insurance plan starts paying the rest. Only medical care received as a benefit under your policy is calculated against your deductible. Uncovered services that you pay for do not count toward the deductible. Typically, deductibles must be met on an annual basis.
- *Do you have a stop loss?* This is the annual amount you must pay out of your own pocket before your

insurance pays at 100 percent. Stop losses can be very beneficial when diagnosis and treatment are expensive.

- *What percentage of billed charges is paid by your insurance?* Some policies pay 80 percent or 90 percent of some costs but pay only 50 percent of other costs.
- *Do you have coverage for home care, nursing visits at home, private duty nursing (twenty-four-hour care), and care at a skilled nursing facility or convalescent hospital?*
- *Do you have coverage for custodial care?* Most insurance companies cover only skilled care. Custodial care—such as housekeeping, bathing, doing laundry, and assistance in getting to the bathroom or in preparing meals—is typically not covered.
- *Does your plan cover hospice care?*
- *Does your insurance provide coverage only if you go to specific providers?*
- *Is a referral or a plan authorization required for doctor's visits, hospital admissions, or outpatient testing?*
- *Are there any waivers that would preclude payment for treatment for your condition?* This might include prior treatment (within one year, for example) for the same or a similar condition.
- *What is your lifetime maximum?* This is the maximum benefit your insurance will pay in your lifetime. It can be $25,000 or $1 million or more.
- *How do you get care after hours or in an emergency?*
- *If you have group coverage through your employer, does coverage end if you are fired or laid off?* If so, is there a way to continue coverage? (Ask your employer about COBRA, the federal law that requires certain plans to extend your group employer coverage up to eighteen months after you are terminated from a job—though you must usually pay the entire premium yourself.)

Why Claims May Be Denied

Even though your policy may appear comprehensive, denials for medical care claims are common. Sometimes a denial reflects only a practical problem, such as missing information or incorrect documentation. Sometimes the policy does not cover certain types of care. This is often a matter of interpretation. If your policy has such exclusions, you may need to advocate with your doctor or other health care provider to establish that your care should be covered even though the insurance company's agent interprets the policy as appearing to exclude it. An explanation of common reasons for denial follows, along with recommendations for responding to any denials.

Preexisting Condition

Your claim may be denied if your medical condition existed before you became eligible for or bought your policy. Be absolutely sure about how your particular plan interprets the term "preexisting condition."

Uncovered Benefits

Most policies have a section that lists illnesses or services that are excluded from coverage. Because of the possibility of uncovered benefits, it is a good idea to check your insurance plan *before* any treatment or tests are ordered. Some treatments are covered only when given or administered in the hospital, for example.

In such cases, you or your physician's office may be able to make arrangements for outpatient coverage in lieu of hospitalization. Services may actually be cheaper that way.

Not an Authorized Provider

Many insurance plans require that you use providers who are part of their network. Seeing a specialist usually requires that you be referred by an authorized provider for a consultation and for all subsequent treatment. Failure to go to contracted providers with a written referral can result in a complete denial of payment for all treatment provided.

Investigational Treatment

Virtually all health insurance plans cover standard cancer diagnosis and treatments (e.g., chemotherapy, radiotherapy, surgery), but many insurers will deny claims deemed to be investigational (experimental), unnecessary, or inappropriate. Bone marrow transplants and certain other new treatments often fall into this category. While there is no guaranteed way to prevent denial of such a claim, try to receive preapproval in writing for the treatment from your insurance carrier. To do this, you should have a "letter of medical necessity" from your physician documenting that the proposed treatment is medically appropriate, along with supporting clinical literature and a full description of the procedure or services to be provided. The anticipated cost and duration of the treatment should also be included.

Off-Label Treatment

Your insurer may deny a claim if the drug your doctor has prescribed is used for any reason other than its labeled indication or the use listed on the drug company's package insert. The claim may also be denied if the drug is used in a new dosage or according to a new schedule, given by a different route, or combined with other drugs.

You should be aware that fully half of all uses of cancer drugs are not listed on the drugs' official package inserts or labels. Such uses reflect advances in cancer treatment that occurred after the drug was released onto the market and are, in fact, the ordinary, proper, and accepted uses of such drugs. Using drugs for established "off-label" uses is perfectly appropriate.

When your health insurance plan uses "drug use is off-label" to deny a claim, it is very important to appeal this denial to the insurance carrier. Such denials are usually reversed, especially if the use of the drug is standard in the medical community and is a necessary and effective treatment for your illness. Most pharmaceutical companies will provide clinical literature, if needed, to help support your claim. In fact, they often provide reimbursement "hotlines" to provide assistance. Your oncologist's insurance or billing staff is usually familiar with ways to help you with this problem should denial occur. In many states, cancer physicians have formed organizations to advise insurance companies about effective new treatments for cancer, especially established drugs in off-label uses.

Nonpayment of Premiums

It is very difficult to obtain another insurance policy once you have a preexisting condition. Keep your current policy up to date to ensure that your insurance policy is not canceled.

Submitting Claims

You must bring proper insurance plan identification on your first visit to your oncologist's office. Your insurance provider—whether it is Medicare, Medicaid, a PPO, an HMO, or a private indemnity plan—should give you an identification card. This card will have your subscriber identification number (often your social security number), group number, office co-pay amount, and the address to which any claims should be submitted. If your insurance requires submission of a claim form, also bring a fully completed and signed claim form to the office.

Always inform your physician's office of any changes in your address, phone number, employment, or insurance information. Notifying the office immediately will prevent unnecessary delays in claim submission, avoid the need for resubmission, and reduce possible denials of payment. It will also result in quicker payment of claims.

Your physician's office will submit the claim for some plans. This may also be true for hospitals, laboratories, and other kinds of service providers. Most oncology offices have an insurance or finance department. Their patient representatives will explain the billing procedures to you before you begin treatment. Find out whether they will submit your claim or whether you are expected to submit the claim yourself.

Always request a copy of your charges, which should include an itemization of all services and the diagnosis (including its code) for your visit.

Common Terms and Abbreviations

To better understand the procedure for submitting and processing claims, you should understand the terms and abbreviations used by most insurance carriers. Here are the most common ones:

- *ICD-9 (International Classification of Diseases, 9th Edition) Code.* This code identifies your illness. All claims submitted to your insurance carrier will require the correct code. Carriers will not pay your claim if this code is not provided.
- *CPT (Current Procedural Terminology) Code.* This code identifies the medical, surgical, and diagnostic services rendered by your physician. It is used by most insurance carriers to identify what services were performed. Claims are paid using these codes.
- *Deductible.* This is the amount you have to pay before your insurance starts paying the rest. Only medical care that is a covered benefit under your policy is counted against your deductible. Uncovered benefits, which you must pay yourself, do not count against your deductible.
- *Co-payment.* This refers to the amount of your bill that you are responsible for. The co-payment is usually a specific dollar amount rather than a percentage of the bill. Prescription drug programs, for example, often have a co-payment, usually a fixed dollar amount per prescription. Co-payments are generally associated with HMOs.
- *Co-insurance.* This is the percentage of the bill you are responsible for after you have met your deductible. If your policy has a $100 deductible and a 20 percent co-insurance, for example, you would pay your $100 deductible and 20 percent of all covered expenses. You are also responsible for paying for all services not covered by your policy. Co-insurance provisions are most commonly associated with PPO-type plans.
- *EOB (Explanation of Benefits).* This is the statement you will receive from your insurance carrier when your claim has been processed. It will show the provider of services, the place of service, and how the benefits were paid. If you have a deductible or co-insurance, this also will be stated on your EOB. If you have a secondary insurance carrier, that company will need a copy of your EOB in order to pay its portion (see "EOMB" below).
- *EOMB (Explanation of Medicare Benefits).* This statement, similar to an insurance carrier's EOB, is sent to you as soon as your claim has been paid. It will state the provider of any service, the amount allowed under Medicare's fee schedule, the amount paid, and what charges were applied toward your deductible. If your physician is a Medicare provider, the check will be sent directly to his or her office. You will need this explanation of Medicare benefits in order for your secondary insurance company to pay your claim.
- *Assignment of Benefits.* This is required by most physicians' offices. It means that you give written permission for your insurance company to send payments directly to the service provider. An assignment-of-benefits form is usually provided by the physician's office for you to sign. There is also a place for your assignment-of-benefits signature on your claim form.
- *Medicare Assignment.* Any physician may accept the fee schedule set by Medicare in an individual case. A participating provider in the Medicare program has agreed to always take the set fee schedule ("assignment").

If your physician takes Medicare assignment (fees), you are then responsible only for uncovered services, for your deductible, and for your co-insurance. However, if the physician is *not* a participating provider in the Medicare program, it is possible for you to end up being responsible for *more* than the 20 percent co-insurance. If the physician's charge is more than the Medicare allowable charge, for instance, the physician will receive only 80 percent of the Medicare allowable fee, while you will be responsible for the rest of the bill. So if you are eligible for Medicare, make sure you *ask ahead of time* whether your physician participates in the Medicare program and will accept assignment of Medicare benefits for your care.

- *UCR (Usual, Customary, and Reasonable).* This is the fee determined by your insurance carrier to be the usual fee charged for the same service by the average provider with similar training in your geographic area. This may be different from the fee your physician charges.

- *Preauthorization.* This is a requirement by your insurance carrier that certain services be authorized before the services are rendered. If your insurance contains this requirement, make sure your physician's office is aware of it.

- *Superbill.* This is a standard, itemized "checklist of services" in widespread use. It will contain all the required codes (CPT and ICD-9) that will enable you to submit your claim.

- *COB (Coordination of Benefits).* When you are enrolled in two separate group insurance plans, those plans will coordinate their benefits so that your claim is paid at no more than 100 percent of the covered benefits. If you have more than one insurance plan, make sure you notify your physician's office so that the office can submit both claims for you.

New Ways of Paying for Medical Care

Our society is engaged in a great effort to reform the health care payment system. For example, despite all the numerous types of health insurance and managed care plans, many Americans have no health coverage.

There used to be only two players in the system: the doctor and the patient. Now there are several others: the health insurance industry, various federal and state regulatory agencies, employers (who often provide employee health care plans), and the federal government. New rules and regulations are being proposed and implemented that will change the basic concepts and practices of health care.

The patient's need for skillful, dedicated, and considerate care by the physician has never changed. From the viewpoint of the physician—now called a health care provider—what has changed is that other parties and agencies have taken over some of the decision making that used to belong to the physician alone. Consequently, physicians and hospitals and their staff must now interact continually with these other decision makers. Many decisions now require outside approval. These can include the decision to hospitalize, where to hospitalize, which consultants may be called, what types of treatment may be used, and, especially, how health care resources are to be allocated and provided. Requiring authorization before ordering tests and X rays is just one example of how these changes have impacted health care. Many doctors' offices now have more people handling insurance claims than they have nurses providing direct care to patients. Physicians will need to be increasingly accountable to outside agencies.

"Managed care" is one common term used to describe a coordinated effort by physicians, hospitals, and insurers—also called insurance payers—to create an optimum balance between incredibly sophisticated medical technology on the one hand and our inability as a society to afford paying for every possible treatment and diagnostic test for every person in every situation on the other hand. The practice guidelines now being developed by various insurance carriers will probably become increasingly important in how services are provided and covered.

Because the patterns of delivering and monitoring health care are complex and changing, and because new payment systems are being created, it is absolutely essential that you completely understand the provisions of your health insurance plan. With increasingly expensive tests and treatments and more and more controls over payment for medical care, your best insurance is knowledge of your own insurance.

In this rapidly changing medical world, there will have to be a greater effort and understanding by all the participants in medical care—the patient, the physician, the health care team, and the governmental/insurance payers—to provide cost-effective, state-of-the-art health care.

Managed Care and Oncology: The New Care Systems

Malin Dollinger, M.D.

Joel Pollack, C.P.A.

During the past fifty years, there has been a profound shift in patterns of payment for health care. Before World War II, sophisticated tests and treatments did not yet exist. There were no intensive care units, CT or MRI scans, fancy blood tests, or, for that matter, specialists. The cost of medical care was relatively inexpensive and predictable, and individuals simply paid for medical expenses out of pocket.

In 1933, surgeon Dr. Sidney Garfield set up a makeshift hospital in the Mojave Desert to treat workers building the Los Angeles Aqueduct. He provided comprehensive care at a fixed price—a nickel a day—deducted from workers' paychecks. That caught the eye of shipbuilder Henry Kaiser, one of the largest employers in the country. He set up a similar program for workers building the Grand Coulee Dam in Washington State and for workers at shipyards in California, Oregon, and Washington. After World War II, Kaiser opened enrollment to the public. Within a year, AFL and CIO members were joining at the rate of two thousand per month, sparking a revolution in health care.

Kaiser set up an all-inclusive health care system for his employees. For the first time, one plan owned and controlled the hospitals, employed the physicians and other health care providers, and managed the whole enterprise, including preventive medicine, all under one roof. One monthly payment by the consumer took care of all medical problems, at least as defined by the contract. This became the first and largest health maintenance organization (HMO) and the first example of "managed care."

Broadly defined, managed care is the application of business principles to the delivery of health care. More specifically, it is a system of health care delivery that provides services at a fair and reasonable price and measures performance outcomes and quality of care. In such a system, everyone involved with health care delivery— physicians, hospitals, laboratories—has to be concerned with efficiency, timeliness, satisfaction, accountability, and costs, as well as quality.

Health Care Payment Systems

Once the Kaiser model was successful, other HMOs began to appear. From 1960 to 1980, a number of health care systems existed, offering several combinations and variations. Consumers could choose among systems according to their preferences, tastes, and means.

Fee-for-service or indemnity insurance became the most common type of insurance plan during the 1960s and remained so through the 1980s. Health insurance companies issued policies (often, but not always, in association with employers) that allowed the consumers to choose a physician and, indirectly, a hospital. The physician and/or hospital would then bill the insurance company for services rendered.

A primitive form of "quality control" emerged from this process, chiefly related to the concept of "usual and customary fees," which inhibited practitioners from charging, or at least being paid, excessive fees. Consumers quickly learned to walk away from providers and services that were equivalent in quality but excessive in cost. Competitive market forces began to standardize the costs of hospitalization, laboratory tests, X-ray exams, physical therapy, nursing homes, prescriptions, and every other aspect of health care.

Market forces also began to create discounts for physicians' services. Doctors agreed to accept, for example, a 10–20 percent discount in their

(Continued from page 399)

usual fees. In return, they wanted to be given an "exclusive" for patients of a particular health plan. Physicians' overhead costs were the same regardless of how many patients were seen. Their margin, the difference between gross income and the cost of doing business, became lower unless they could ensure an adequate number of patients.

The creation of the Medicare and Medicaid programs in 1965 was a major event in American history—and a watershed event in the field of health care. Previously, health care expenditures had been kept under control with prudent spending by physicians and consumers, but federal spending on these new programs unleashed health care expenditures as never seen before. Health care turned into a growth industry. Now the consumer had *carte blanche* for medical care, with the bills paid through Uncle Sam. The impact of this change led health care providers to search for new ways to control costs. They turned to managed care.

The Development of Managed Care

In the late 1980s and early 1990s, the gradual evolution of health care payment systems entered a new era. Several forces radically changed our health care payment systems. Health care more and more came to be delivered by contract between the physician or a group of physicians and the insurance company, which came to be called the payer. New doctors in town not only announced their names, addresses, specialties, and training but, for the first time, needed to indicate which insurance plans they accepted by contract.

Employers began to be primary contractors as well as decision makers for health care. This eventually created the problem of people with chronic and/or preexisting health problems being unable to change jobs for fear of losing their health insurance and not being able to replace it. On the other hand, a large employer might be able to extend coverage to people with preexisting illnesses (a history of cancer, for example) because of the clout they had by having a large number of employees enrolled.

Health care provider relationships changed dramatically. Physicians were more restricted in their referrals. They could only send their patients to physicians and consultants under contract with the same company or plan, unless their patients were willing to pay significantly more for treatments by physicians of their own choosing. Each health plan contracted with a certain hospital or hospitals for guaranteed—and often lower—rates. This tended to promote efficiency and drive inefficient or poorly organized hospitals out of business.

The contractual needs linking physicians and health plans made solo or small practices undesirable. Limited groups of physicians could not deliver services to large numbers of potential patients (now called "covered lives") nor offer the breadth of skills and specialties and geographic availability that came to be standard requirements of health care providers (the new term for doctors). Just as hospitals merged, so did physicians. Small groups became large ones and solo practitioners became rarities.

Cost and Control

Issues of cost and control became dominant in the 1990s. Each segment of the health care system realized its piece of the pie was in jeopardy and tried to increase its control. Hospitals either acquired the practices of generalist physicians and internists or formed joint ventures with primary care physicians, thereby capturing their patients and the income derived from their care.

As hospitals and physicians joined forces, practicing medicine became a business as well as a profession. While physicians had always had bills and taxes to pay and records to keep, in the past they had mostly taken care of patients and kept whatever was left over after expenses. Now, their livelihoods were determined by nonphysicians who controlled which patients they would see, how many patients there would be, which consultants and hospitals could be used, and where laboratory tests and X rays could be done. This new cost control was having an impact on patients as well as physicians. Behind the scenes in managed care,

(Continued from page 400)

organizations and administrators started requiring members to obtain "precertification" before a patient could visit a specialist or have X-ray or laboratory tests done.

In the old days, value was defined as "quality work done by the physician." Now value has another definition, borrowed from business, where value is equal to quality divided by cost. Given equal quality, the one who provides services at a lower cost now provides the greater value.

Managed Care Today

Managed care is becoming the dominant force in the health industry and participation is increasing at a rapid rate, especially among Medicare patients. As of 2000, at least half of the U.S. population participates in some system in which the health care providers furnish care based on an integrated economic, contractual, business, and professional program, with mutual contracts between all participants and management. California, Florida, and Minnesota are leading this trend, but new systems of managed care are quickly gaining predominance in other parts of the country.

There are different types of health care delivery systems under managed care, including Health Maintenance Organizations (HMO), Preferred Provider Organizations (PPO), Exclusive Provider Organizations (EPO), and Point of Service Plans (POS). In addition to PPOs, other physician provider groups that contract with various payer organizations are Independent Practice Associations (IPA) and Independent Physician Organizations (IPO).

HMO (Health Maintenance Organization). A health care delivery model in which beneficiaries are restricted to seeking health care services from a very specific network of health care providers. HMOs generally deny benefits when enrollees or members seek nonemergency services from non-network providers. An HMO integrates under one management system the entire health care program, including physicians, hospitals, outpatient services, and other services such

as prevention. Physicians are under contract, often on a full-time, salaried basis, although the HMO may also contract with PPOs and IPAs to provide contracted services at standard rates.

PPO (Preferred Provider Organization). A network of health care providers who agree to provide services at contracted rates and seek to direct patient volume to their contracted facilities by offering discounts to payers. PPOs generally offer patients an incentive for using network providers and penalize patients, but do not totally deny benefits, when they use non-network providers.

EPO (Exclusive Provider Organization). A plan which limits coverage of nonemergency care to contracted health care providers. An EPO operates similarly to an HMO plan, but it is usually offered as a self-insured or self-funded product.

POS (Point Of Service Plan). A managed care plan where those who go outside of the plan must pay more out-of-pocket expenses but are not denied access to non-network providers.

The Primary Care Physician

The dominance of the primary care physician (PCP) is one of the fundamental concepts of HMOs. All members of an HMO managed care plan select or are assigned to a primary care physician, who has complete control over patient care. The PCP determines which doctors the patient will see. If a patient has a lump in her breast, the PCP determines if she should see an oncologist, usually one within the HMO system. The primary care physician is usually referred to as the "gatekeeper." It is the gatekeeper's responsibility to refer patients to cancer specialists and to arrange for special testing when necessary.

Managing Risk

Not only is health care delivery moving toward managed care, but the financial risk of providing health care is being shifted from insurance companies and managed care organizations to physicians. The major types of risk-sharing are risk pools, capitation, and package-price plans.

(Continued from page 401)

Several versions of risk pools are common in HMOs. The physician may be paid a salary or a modified salary based on work time and patient allocation. Some of these earnings, however, are placed in a fund to be divided at the end of each year according to a formula based on factors such as productivity and/or cost cutting, including avoiding the inappropriate or unnecessary use of services, such as laboratory tests, X-ray examinations, or hospitalization. Because allocating medical care in HMOs is generally controlled by primary care physicians, the set-aside fund also is used to pay specialists if a member needs specialty care. There is, therefore, an incentive to be thrifty in effort and expense.

The hotly debated question nationally is whether care suffers by such methods of physician reimbursement. Federal legislation now requires physicians to disclose valid treatment options not covered by their health plan.

In capitation, the health care provider is paid a fixed amount each month to take care of anyone in a plan who becomes ill and needs the specified services. There is no charge for any specific illness or event. An oncology group, for example, might contract on a capitated basis to take care of 100,000 covered lives for a certain sum per member per month. A check for the full amount would arrive each month for any and all care required for those covered persons.

Using various calculations (and not simple ones), the physician group can estimate how many people out of 100,000 would get cancer each month, how much it would cost to see them, what services would be required, and how many years of care would be needed. If the estimate proves to be fairly accurate, the physician group might come out OK. If fewer people get cancer that month, money would be left over. If lots of people get cancer, particularly types that are expensive to treat, the physicians would operate at a loss.

In a capitated plan, then, the health care provider takes all the risk. If one person, ten people, or one thousand people show up for cancer care, the payment is still the same, so enough people have to be covered to make sure that an unusual number of people who need expensive care will not overwhelm the technical and financial ability of the health care provider.

This is analogous to automobile insurance. The insurance company, for a monthly fee, agrees to take care of whatever losses the car owner suffers. The company knows that each month there will be a certain number of car thefts and accidents and is willing to take the risk that the average number will remain roughly the same. The company needs to insure a lot of people to make the risk safer.

Physicians with capitated contracts usually protect themselves by obtaining "reinsurance" ("stop-loss" insurance) to cover the unusual patient or patients who require very expensive care. The reinsurance company needs proof ahead of time that the care given is "standard, reasonable, efficient, and cost-effective" to minimize the need to use the reinsurance.

Capitated medical plans are becoming more prevalent, and doctors are finding they need to understand business principles as well as they understand medical ones. Some physicians choose to concentrate on the business side of things.

In package-price plans or "carve outs," there is a fixed price for the defined "episode" of care. In a "carve out," the physician and/or organization agrees to provide all the care required for a certain illness, ailment, or procedure for a fixed price determined before care is begun. Again, the physician takes all the risk. If it costs less to deliver the care, the physician comes out ahead; if it costs more, the physician loses money.

It's difficult to create such plans in the cancer field because of the complexity and expense of care, rapid changes in technology and treatments, the length of time that care and follow-up are required (years), and the fact that many facilities and professionals are involved, not just the primary doctor (usually an oncologist). A complex and coordinated effort is required to discover and predict the costs of all the components of care for many different kinds of cancer accurately and reliably, as well as to place under contract (and under

(Continued from page 402)

risk) the many providers and health care facilities. One area of uncertainty is how to continue to pay for the vital clinical research trials that test promising new methods of treatment. Insurance companies may not wish to pay for trials of treatments whose role is not yet defined or proven.

While "carve outs" present an excellent opportunity to both control cost and coordinate all elements of cancer care, market acceptance of this innovative concept is lacking and benefits of this approach may not be realized for many years to come—if ever.

Managed Care Issues

Before managed care, there was no wish or need for anyone to coordinate the patterns of care or costs in all of the places where health care is provided, including doctors' offices, hospitals, pharmacies, and outpatient care facilities. Inevitably, there was some duplication and excessive use of services, not by intention, but because of the way the system developed.

Different physicians might order the same blood tests or X rays for the same patient, because the first results were not available to them. No standard care plan defined which type of physician took care of certain types of problems. It was often unclear which professional was in charge of medical care decisions. A cancer patient, for example, could easily be followed by four physicians: a primary generalist or internist, a surgeon, a radiation oncologist, and the medical oncologist. While patients may find it reassuring to have all these professionals watching over them, such a system does produce major increases in the cost of care.

Under managed care guidelines, a single practitioner determines the location and types of care. While this is often a generalist for most areas of medicine, with referral to specialists as needed, in the cancer field the medical oncologist usually becomes the case manager or "quarterback" who calls on other consultants. Thus, the medical oncologist now has to be concerned with cost factors as well as quality and efficiency.

Cost Control

In this era of managed care, cancer continues to be an expensive disease. A primary reason for spiraling costs is innovation in treatments and biotechnology, both resulting from advances in research and clinical trials. Other reasons include the reluctance to stop curative treatment and enter palliative care when uncertainty about treatment benefits exist. Further, cancer patients often require extensive diagnostic testing and complex costly treatments delivered by specialists and sub-specialists.

For all these reasons, managed care organizations—particularly HMOs—have found it difficult to control costs, and they have resorted to strict controls of their members in an effort to keep expenditures from exceeding budgeted levels and necessitating increases in member premiums.

Feedback

Effective managed care requires attention to several other factors besides quality and cost. There must be feedback to all parties—physicians, insurance carrier, and payer—about the quality of care, the efficiency of delivery, the results, and the satisfaction of patients with the care they receive. Such information must be integrated into the daily care plan and package, often with the aid of computers.

There is also a need for feedback among all participants so that inefficiencies and inappropriate or unnecessary care pathways can be discovered and improved. That is why the package-price plan or "carve out" has such potential for improving the cancer care system. It puts all the treatment, care management, cost management, and communication into one package to achieve the maximum value in quality and cost.

Prevention and Early Detection

Under managed care, a concerted effort is being made by the various plans to promote prevention and early detection of cancer. Primary care physicians familiar with their patients and dedicated to early detection and prevention can make a significant difference in cancer outcomes by insisting on

(Continued from page 403)

regular screenings and by educating patients about important lifestyle changes. When cancer is detected, prompt referral to a specialist and aggressive treatment can often make the difference between life and death.

Total Health Care

For the first time in the history of our health care system, the need for total cooperation exceeds the need for autonomy or total control. Doctors, hospitals, and other health care suppliers and facilities will need to consider the role of all other "players" in the system. We need to look at the entire health care picture as a single activity. If a service is done better, more efficiently, or less expensively at a hospital compared with a physician's office, that needs to be determined and mandated.

Under such a system, physicians' preferences will not determine how things are done, and some hospitals will be permitted to perform certain procedures. Laboratory tests, X rays, and other tests and procedures will be done at a designated facility or will not be paid for or reimbursed. In many managed care markets, the physician already has limited choices in these matters and frequently his or her choice of consultants is limited to those on the same plan or contract as the patient.

Managed care will develop and reward those systems and plans that are able to look at the entire spectrum of providers and facilities and distill an efficient health care package that provides high-quality and cost-effective care. This goal requires total management of every aspect of care.

Such care packages are developing at breakneck speed by the action of—and in response to—the providers, payers, and consumers of health care rather than by the government. In the cancer field, as in other areas of medicine, we are not sure how the final package will look. But a hint may be found in the not-so-accidental fact that one author of this article is a physician and the other is an accountant.

44

Decisions for Life:
Advance Directives

Ernest H. Rosenbaum, M.D.
Isadora R. Rosenbaum, M.A.
Thomas Addison, M.D.
Joanna Beam, J.D.
Meryl Brod, Ph.D.
David Claman, M.D.
Alan J. Coleman, M.D.
Malin Dollinger, M.D.
Michael Glover
Nancy Lambert, R.N., B.S.N.
Elmo Petterle
Patricia Sparacino, R.N., M.S.
Rabbi Jeffery Silberman, D.Min.
Kenneth A. Woeber, M.D.

We are all aware that at some point we must face death, but at the same time, most Americans avoid discussions about life and death as much as possible.

Although the Patient Self-Determination Act was passed in 1990, less than 10–15 percent of the U.S. population has prepared an advance directive. Advance directives are legal documents which convey instructions about your future health care should you be unable to speak for yourself. There are two basic types of advance directives, a living will and a medical power of attorney, although all fifty states have different laws regarding them. Advance directives are valuable to patients, their families, and doctors. Why, then, do so few of us complete these important documents?

In part, it's a result of the fact that many physicians do not bring up the subject because they don't want to increase the fear of death in their patients; and in part, it's because many people do not wish to make the kinds of difficult and cumbersome decisions required in completing an advance directive. Yet, because of major advances in medical care, such discussions are becoming more important.

Physicians often go to heroic lengths to keep terminal patients alive—often against the patient's wishes. Most people assume that when the time arrives for making life-and-death decisions, their physicians and family will make the same choices they would make. But the family's and the physician's views and decisions may not coincide with the patient's—or even with each other's. We should all assess our own values regarding quality of life and make decisions about how we wish to live and the type of care we desire at the end of our lives. This can be accomplished through advance directives and through filling out other forms that document your wishes about your future.

Experts advise that each person should organize the final details concerning his or her possible illness and death. By completing an advance directive and the forms provided at the end of Chapter 45, you will make life easier for your eventual survivors.

This chapter will help guide you through the maze of issues that are important for you to consider. It will offer suggestions about how to make decisions before or during a hospitalization. It will also offer a way in which

Three Case Histories

Case One

A twenty-four-year-old man has been in an automobile accident resulting in massive injuries. If he is to survive, CPR (cardiopulmonary resuscitation) is needed. Should it be administered?

Yes, you might say: this is an obvious choice. But let's carry the situation a step further. Suppose that the CPR is successful and the man's life is saved. But due to his injuries and unsuccessful treatment, he goes into a coma from which he is unlikely to recover. He now can be kept alive only by having a tracheal breathing (windpipe) tube inserted, being connected to a respirator, and by being fed intravenously through a tube. Again, should these measures be taken? Unless the man has made his wishes known, his doctors will keep him alive no matter what the effort, cost, or pain.

Case Two

A sixty-seven-year-old man has a medical history dating back fifteen years that includes undergoing lung surgery for low-grade cancer, with no recurrence. He also survived a heart attack and a successful heart angioplasty (coronary artery dilation). Recently, this man was admitted to the hospital with severe pneumonia and lung failure. His condition required that he be placed on a respirator in the intensive care unit. As part of his wishes for his emergency health care, he had already signed a medical emergency wallet card requesting that no CPR be performed on him and that he not be placed on a respirator. However, when advised that a pulmonary respirator might save his life, he verbally canceled his advance directive request that no respirator be used. After fourteen days in the ICU, he recovered from the pneumonia. His life and vitality have been restored, and he has returned to work.

Case Three

A fifty-four-year-old woman's health has been failing rapidly. She has advanced metastatic breast cancer and has been admitted to the hospital with acute gastrointestinal bleeding, jaundice, and progressive liver metastases. Despite having had many therapies, including a toxic course of chemotherapy, she is dying.

Her physician believes that her condition will not improve and that in her present state of ill health, her quality of life is minimal. He recommends a comfort care program to control pain and suffering and to afford her maximum comfort, rather than continuing active treatment to prolong life with inevitable suffering. She previously signed an advance directive designating her family as her "agent" in her medical power of attorney. Now her family is responsible for ensuring that her wishes are carried out.

These are a few examples that illustrate the issues faced by patients, families, and health care professionals. For those you love, a clear advance directive can be a legacy of your thoughts and wishes, and it will help alleviate the confusion that often occurs both before and after the death of a loved one. It is your choice: act now or leave these decisions to others later.

you can help your family and significant others deal with important details should your illness become terminal.

These topics may, by their very nature, be difficult issues for you. However, they are important decisions about how you may want to be treated and how you want your wishes to be carried out, at a later time, if you cannot make these decisions for yourself. Some of the necessary documents that will help ensure that your health care wishes are recognized and included.

Preparing for Your Decisions

Death is a part of life. We all know that we must die sometime, we just don't know when. Despite this reality, we often think of death as something that happens to other people. Most of us have a difficult time accepting our own mortality, and typically we avoid thinking about it until a crisis forces us to do so. Even then, we may fight and bargain to gain more time. Accepting death is an issue for doctors as well as for patients. Many doctors fight to preserve life at almost any cost in time, money, or effort—but most also know that there are circumstances in which it is right to let a person suffer no more and die a peaceful death.

Factors that May Influence Your Decision

How we live our lives and plan our deaths are personal choices. Society also influences us as we observe the attitudes, ceremonies, and rituals that surround death and dying in our culture. For guidance in these important decisions, many of us seek religious or spiritual advice. With the constant changes in medical technology, science may influence our decisions as well.

Since the late 1950s, advances in medical technology and medical practice have changed how patients, lawmakers, physicians, ethicists, and society in general think about and define life, death, and dying. Many of these changes have resulted in serious ethical dilemmas for the medical profession, causing doctors to reassess their roles in caring for patients. Patients and their loved ones, faced with the possibility of prolonged suffering and delayed death, have been asking for the power to make their own decisions and to die naturally and with dignity. Patients and their families should know about their choices for discontinuing aggressive treatment.

Each of us faces serious decisions about how we view the quality of our lives in terms of illness and death. Many of us would like to have some control over our medical care toward the end of our lives. To help us make our decisions known when we're unable to do so, documents called advance directives have been developed. Such documents give us some measure of control over our medical treatment when death threatens our survival. Through them, we can provide clear instructions should we be unable to state our wishes because a serious medical condition impairs our ability to communicate. With such documents, we also can ease the burden of responsibility left to our survivors by putting our business, legal, and personal affairs in order. In these ways, we can help make things easier for our loved ones.

Choosing Life: Living Your Life While Planning For Mortality

Despite the inevitability of death and the importance of planning for tomorrow, the purpose of life is to live. The diagnosis of an acute or chronic illness doesn't need to be experienced as an automatic death sentence. A medical diagnosis can be viewed as an important reminder to "live each day as if it were the last."

Not all people are able to cope successfully following the diagnosis of an illness. Some diseases may not respond to treatment, even if the patient has a strong will to live. When this occurs, many find the heartbreak and frustration very hard to bear. Other people say that the uncertainties of living with an illness can make life more meaningful. The smallest pleasures—flowers, the sky, sunshine—are intensified. It is a time to do things you have always wanted to do and to make peace with your family or friends.

Death eventually comes to us all, but we can choose the way we live our lives—and, to some extent, the way we die. One remarkable example of a "good" death is that of the national hero, Charles Lindbergh, who died in 1974. After being diagnosed with a lymphoma in 1972, he continued to live actively while undergoing radiotherapy and chemotherapy. He hoped that his life and death would reflect his simple birth and that they would serve as a memorial for his children and grandchildren. When he was informed that he had only a short time to live, he returned to his home on Maui in Hawaii. One of his doctors (Milton M. Howell, M.D., in "The Lone Eagle's Last Flight," *Journal of the AMA*, May 1975) noted the following:

In time, he made appropriate legal arrangements for his burial there and selected the site of his grave. Systematically, he arranged his personal affairs, and yet he maintained a sense of the past and an interest in the present. He planned for the next major event in his life, but it did not become an obsession.

He planned...[the] construction of his grave with a simple coffin. He planned his funeral services along with his family and requested that people attend in their working clothes. There was time for reminiscing, time for discussion and time for laughter. When he lapsed into coma he wanted no respirator, defibrillator (for electric shock), or other complicated paraphernalia. He received excellent, prompt responsive nursing care, oxygen when needed, a minimum of analgesia (for pain), and a great deal of love and consideration from his family and the medical staff (at home).

Lindbergh stated that he wished his death to be a constructive act in itself. His example of simplicity, his careful planning, his unfailing politeness and consideration for those around him, his public refusal of medical heroics, and his humble funeral are evidence of that wish. Death was another event in his life, as natural as his birth had been in Minnesota more than seventy-two years before.

Making Choices about Medical Treatment

Most of us have difficulty coping with the idea of our own deaths and, therefore, with the preparations that would be best for us and our loved ones. Yet, when we buy life insurance, draw up a will, or make a decision about organ donation, we're acknowledging that we will die someday. The decisions you make about your health care, including the parameters you set regarding the use of life-saving treatments, will protect your wishes as well as ease the burden of difficult decisions for your family. Remember, unless you have completed an advance directive, your doctors may feel obligated to do whatever is necessary to keep you alive. Sometimes these treatments may result in considerable pain and suffering for you, as well as emotional suffering for your family and your close friends. At other times, these procedures only result in delaying death.

Decisions about advance directives are not simple and may depend on the type of medical condition you have. Many people clearly do not want extraordinary treatment in hopeless situations, but they may accept such treatment in acute but potentially reversible situations. For example, using a mechanical breathing machine to treat pneumonia after an operation is usually temporary and may help recovery. The potential risks and benefits of various treatments depend on many factors, including the patient's age, type of illness, or other chronic medical problems.

"Standard" advance directives can sometimes cause confusion and should be discussed with your family and doctor. Advance directives should also be re-evaluated after each new illness. An acute disease (such as a heart attack) may be reversed, whereas advanced incurable diseases (such as terminal cancer, severe refractory heart disease, resistant infections, emphysema, or kidney failure) may be best treated with comfort care (care that is aimed at keeping a person comfortable, but does not treat the illness). Comfort care includes bathing, nutrition, fluids, massage, and pain medications. Including different types of general statements in your advance directive are useful with different types of illnesses—especially with regard to the reversibility of a condition. One example might be the following: "I will accept life-supportive treatments for acute, potentially reversible conditions that are very likely to be treated successfully and that are likely to result in full recovery and a return to independent life." A more conservative statement would be: "I prefer that all care be directed at comfort and that life-supportive treatments not be used." These directives are often very helpful to physicians and families charged with your care.

At times, individuals who have made rational plans when they were healthy change their minds when faced with a new illness and possible death: they then may change their previous directives to allow for aggressive treatment, including CPR or the use of a respirator. When writing an advance directive, it is important to remember that:

- any change in one's health can raise new questions
- talking with your physician and the members of the medical team who are treating your illness will help you make decisions about treatment choices
- a copy of your completed advance directive should be given to your doctor, lawyer, your hospital's medical records department, your family members, and any institution where you receive medical treatments

NOTE: You, a family member, your guardian, or your agent (the authorized person in your medical power of attorney) can reverse or cancel your advance directive verbally by telling your doctor that you have changed your mind.

It's important to realize that even if you don't make a decision, *that* is a decision!

What to Consider When Writing an Advance Directive

Each of us has the legal right to decide what life-sustaining treatments are acceptable to us. In some circumstances, depending on physical condition, age, and personal philosophy, we may choose to refuse certain measures. Part of this decision should be based on whether the illness can be reversed. In the case of a chronic illness, it is vital to consider the pain and suffering, the length of time likely remaining, and the likelihood of being able to reverse or improve the disease process or symptoms. To prepare for this kind of serious decision making, it's important to have full medical information, to consider your personal beliefs, and to understand what's involved in different types of life-saving measures.

Your decisions about what medical treatment you want may differ depending on the type of medical situation you are considering:

- an acute illness that will respond to treatment
- a chronic (incurable) illness that may respond to treatments for a period of time
- an irreversible coma
- an accident resulting in massive, irreversible injuries
- a sudden, catastrophic event—such as a heart attack—that cannot be cured by CPR, medicines, or an operation
- progressive failure of body organs (heart, lung, liver, kidney) when transplants are not feasible

Remember, if no information about your medical treatment decisions is available, your doctors may be obligated to take extraordinary measures to keep you alive. Before you make your decisions, you'll want to discuss all of the potential alternatives and the consequences of those choices with your doctor, agent, lawyer, and family. Make sure you understand what's involved and that your doctor and family will understand your wishes.

Here are some of the issues you may want to discuss with your physician:

- the quantity of medicines, procedures, or other treatments you would want if you were faced with a chronic or a potentially fatal illness;
- whether you would want to know what "extraordinary" measures to prolong your life are available to you;
- whether a cure would be possible;
- whether treatment could restore you to a level of activity acceptable to you or whether it would simply delay death; and
- whether, if you had a progressively incurable disease, you would want to reject medical or surgical treatment and simply choose relief of pain and "comfort care."

Types of Life-Saving Measures

If you are in the process of writing an advance directive, it may be helpful to review the many life-saving measures that can be used, so that you can evaluate which are acceptable or unacceptable to you.

Cardiopulmonary Resuscitation (CPR)

When a person's heart stops beating, several kinds of measures may be taken to start it again. These include chest compression (pushing against the breastbone), which in turn compresses the heart so that it will pump blood and thereby maintain circulation; electric shock to keep the heart beating; artificial breathing (see below); and the administration of drugs. The patient's chances for survival depend on what other medical problems are present and on how soon CPR is started. If you are already ill, your chances of recovery may be reduced. When the heart stops beating, circulation stops and the brain begins to die within four minutes. After ten minutes, brain damage is usually extensive, even if the person can be revived. If a person's chances of recovery are low, extreme measures are usually not successful.

Artificial Breathing (Use of a Ventilator)

A ventilator is a machine that helps a person breathe. A tube through the person's mouth or nose directs the air from the ventilator into the lungs. Sometimes the tube must go through an opening in the person's neck (a tracheostomy). Breathing with the help of a ventilator is often a temporary situation that can be discontinued once other medical treatment reduces or eliminates the breathing problem. A person with severe lung or brain problems may continue to need the machine to breathe for a long time. You are unable to speak with the tube in place, but you may be able to communicate your wishes through non-verbal signals or by writing them down. Pneumonia and other infections are possible complications.

Emergency Surgical Procedures

Emergency surgical procedures include head surgery (craniotomy) for bleeding, spine surgery (laminectomy) to reduce spinal nerve pressure that may cause paralysis, and chest or abdominal surgery for an acute infection (appendicitis) or for acute bleeding. Such procedures can sometimes be life-saving, but at other times may be futile and painful.

Artificial Feeding

When you cannot eat or drink enough to keep your body going, food and fluids may need to be given in different ways. A small tube can be inserted through the nose, leading down into the stomach. This may be a temporary measure if your condition improves, or it may be permanent. There is a risk that liquid food, instead of going into the stomach, may enter the lungs by mistake and cause pneumonia. Although this type of pneumonia is usually easy to treat, it can become life-threatening. Fluids and liquid feeding solutions can also be given through a tiny plastic tube directly into the veins, using an intravenous (IV) apparatus. Being fed this way is called hyperalimentation. Infection can occur where the tube enters the skin, causing either minor symptoms, such as pain and swelling, or more severe complications, including a blood infection.

Kidney Dialysis

Dialysis, the treatment used when a person experiences kidney failure, offers a chance to prolong life by clearing waste or toxins from the blood, but it does not cure the kidney failure. A kidney transplant is the only way to correct irreversible kidney failure.

Chemotherapy

Drugs used in cancer treatment may have many side effects, many of which can be controlled. In some cases, the drugs may actually cure the cancer; in others, they may produce temporary remissions or prolong life.

Pain Medications

These medicines are used to control pain and keep patients comfortable.

Antibiotics

Antibiotics are usually, but not always, effective in treating infections. If a serious infection is present and antibiotics are not taken, the patient may die of the infection. Possible side effects of antibiotics include lack of appetite, nausea, diarrhea, and allergic reactions.

Diagnostic Tests

Diagnostic tests might include such exams as a CT (computerized tomography) scan, MRI (magnetic resonance imaging), X rays, a spinal tap, a bone marrow aspiration, an endoscopy (the use of a flexible fiber-optic scope to examine the intestines, stomach, or colon), or a bronchoscopy (the use of a scope to examine bronchi, the large breathing passages of the lungs). Many of these tests require that a tube be inserted into the patient's body; pain medication also is usually given. Such tests may be necessary to find out what is wrong or to help the medical team decide whether or not further medical treatment is appropriate. Each test has risks associated with it, which can be mild to severe.

Hospital "Codes"

An area of information that's important to understand before making your decisions about life-and-death medical treatment is the hospital "codes" that specify what level of resuscitation (CPR) will be provided by your health care team when you are hospitalized.

Full Code. A patient with full-code status will receive all of the treatments needed to keep the heart beating and lungs breathing: chest compression, assisted breathing (breathing tubes and respirators), heart electrical shock (defibrillation), and/or special medications.

Modified Code. This involves less aggressive treatment, including a selection of some of the full-code measures listed above. The choice of treatment measures depends on your condition and on your expressed wishes.

Chemical Code (Pharmacologic Code). This restricts treatment to the use of special medicines given into your veins—usually for heart, lung, or kidney failure. No aggressive attempts (e.g., CPR) will be made to restart breathing or the heartbeat should they stop.

No Code (DNR—Do Not Resuscitate). This status means that no attempts will made to restart breathing or the heartbeat should they stop. Full efforts for comfort care will be given.

How to Safeguard Your Decisions

Several kinds of documents can be used to specify your treatment wishes to your doctors and family members. It's important to know that you can change or cancel any of these documents at any time as long as you can communicate your wishes.

Unless you or your surrogate signs an advance directive stating otherwise, if you have a sudden medical catastrophe, such as a heart attack, you will receive full resuscitative procedures, including cardiac resuscitation, heart electrical shock, assisted breathing (respirator), and drug therapy with life-sustaining drugs given intravenously.

A medical emergency wallet card is an easy way to specify your decisions in a simple format. It's important to carry information concerning medical treatment and code status requests on a card that you keep with you at all times, preferably near your driver's license. On this card, you can indicate which medical directives you have signed and where they can be found.

Types of Advance Directives

Several kinds of advance directives can be used to inform care providers of your treatment wishes, including a living will and a medical power of attorney. The relevant legislation for your state should be available through your local public library or through a lawyer. You can also obtain information and forms from a not-for-profit organization called Partnership for Caring. These forms can be downloaded for free from their website at www.partnershipforcaring.org, or you can order them by telephone (800) 989-9455 for $5.00 each.

After completing your advance directive, remember to give a copy to each of your doctors and to the person you name as your agent (if this is applicable). Also, take a copy with you whenever you go to a hospital or other treatment facility. Be sure that a copy of your advance directive is on file in your hospital's medical records department. MedicAlert (www.medicalert.org) also offers a national repository service.

Medical Power of Attorney

A medical power of attorney is the most complete and most effective document for ensuring that your desires regarding health care treatment are followed. With this document, you designate someone as your "agent" or "proxy" (attorney-in-fact), authorizing him or her to make decisions about your medical care, including withdrawal of life support, when you are unable to make decisions for yourself. Your agent may make all decisions about your health care, subject to any restrictions on that person's authority that you specify, as well as any restrictions imposed by law that are stated within the document.

When naming your agent, choose someone who knows your values, with whom you feel comfortable talking, who you can trust, who is likely to be there if you become seriously ill, and who can carry out the decisions you've made. You will want to discuss your specific wishes with the agent you select. (Even if you do not want to name someone specific to act as your agent, you can still use this document to spell out your intentions.)

Your document might include a statement of your specific preferences about treatment (a codicil) to give to your agent and doctor, or you might want to select one of the general statements below to reflect your wishes:

"I do not want efforts made to prolong my life and I do not want life-sustaining treatment to be provided or continued:
1. if I am in an irreversible coma or persistent vegetative state; or
2. if I am terminally ill and the application of life-sustaining procedures would serve only to artificially delay the moment of my death; or
3. under any circumstances where the burdens of the treatment outweigh the expected benefits. I want my agent to consider the relief of suffering and the quality as well as the extent of the possible extension of my life in making decisions concerning life-sustaining treatments."

(or)

"I want efforts to be made to prolong my life and I want life-sustaining treatment to be provided unless I am in a coma or persistent vegetative state which my doctor reasonably believes to be irreversible. Once my doctor has concluded that I will remain unconscious for the rest of my life, I do not want life-sustaining treatment to be provided or continued."

For specific information about completing a medical power of attorney in your state, ask your doctor, a reference librarian, or a lawyer, or contact Partnership for Caring at (800) 989-9455, or visit their website at www.partnershipforcaring.org.

To get more information about advance directives, you may call the American Medical Association at (800) 621-8335 to order the brochure *Advance Medical Directives for Patients*, or write to Pritchett & Hull Associates, Inc., Suite 110, 3440 Oakcliff Road NE, Atlanta, Georgia 30340-3079 to order the book *Decide for Yourself*.

A Special Directive—The Prehospital Do Not Resuscitate (DNR) Form

This document is for people who are at home, in a health care facility, in a hospice, or being transported from one such facility to another. It instructs emergency medical services (EMS) personnel not to perform resuscitation procedures, including chest compression, assisted breathing, cardiac drugs, and other extraordinary measures. The document is signed by the patient or an appropriate surrogate (the patient's legal representative—e.g., a medical power of attorney agent) and by the patient's physician. Consult your doctor to see if your state has legislation regarding such DNR forms. To make sure that EMS personnel honor your wishes, you can get a special instructive DNR wallet card and/or a DNR wrist or neck medallion from the Medic Alert Foundation.

If you don't want to draw up a formal document, you can simply inform your doctor of your wishes so that he or she can write them into your medical record, or you can talk with your family and friends. However, a written document signed by you and by the appropriate witnesses, or notarized, is the best way to make sure your intentions are carried out.

Forms are found in Chapter 45, "Your Legacy of Love." Information about advance directives and forms are also available from Partnership for Caring (800) 989-9455 and may be available locally from your public library or health care provider.

45

Your Legacy of Love

Ernest H. Rosenbaum, M.D.
Isadora R. Rosenbaum, M.A.
Thomas Addison, M.D.
Joanna Bean, J.D.
Meryl Brod, Ph.D.
David Claman, M.D.
Alan J. Coleman, M.D.
Malin Dollinger, M.D.
Michael Glover
Nancy Lambert, R.N., B.S.N.
Elmo Peterle
Patricia Sparacino, R.N., M.S.
Jeffery Silberman, D.Min.
Kenneth A. Woeber, M.D.

Life is full of unplanned events. Perhaps one of the most challenging events to cope with is the death of a loved one. It's been estimated that 93 percent of all families are not prepared when a relative dies. Important documents need to be located, funeral arrangements need to be made, and vital matters need to be decided.

It's important to realize that death is actually a shared experience. Although each of us must face our own death, our survivors are also affected by and suffer because of our dying. They are left to cope with both the emotional adjustment of losing a loved one and the responsibility of dealing with someone else's affairs.

How You Can Help Your Survivors

Your legacy of love for your survivors can, with careful thought and compassion, be one of clear decisions and planned arrangements—a house swept clean of personal, financial, and business cobwebs. By sorting out your affairs now, you can spare your survivors an inheritance of scattered papers and countless details to be waded through. Instead, you can bequeath to them the gifts of clear direction, rich memories, and unique insights.

The processes of dying and death dictate many decisions that must be carried out by your survivors, typically at a time of great stress. They often have to come up with answers to troubling questions—such as what last-minute medical treatments to accept or reject on your behalf, whom to notify if you die, what arrangements to make to tend to your body and pay tribute to your life, which resources to use to settle liabilities and disperse assets, and what memories to embrace in order to best remember you.

By taking time and care now to attend to each of the following areas of importance, you'll be providing benefits to yourself and those you love. In the short term, you'll reap the benefit of the peace of mind that comes from organizing your affairs, and in the long term you'll know that what will be done is what you would have wanted.

Before considering the areas listed below, first plan where you are going to store this information file so that those who will need it will be able to find it easily. Then, be sure to tell those who need to know where it is located. You might consider putting the most important legal documents in a safe-deposit box, but be sure to tell those who need to know that this box exists, where to find the key, and how to gain access to the box.

Advance Directives

By completing an advance directive, you are providing both your family and your health care team with guidance about your decisions. A copy of this directive should be given to a family member and to your doctor for inclusion in your medical record. It also should be included in your hospital record if you are hospitalized. Be sure to update your advance directive periodically so that it accurately reflects your wishes and any applicable new state legislation.

Be sure to include the name, address, and phone number of your primary care doctor and any other specialists in this medical information file.

Legal Will

Preparing a will is one of the most important responsibilities you have. Make this a priority. Should you die without a will (called "dying intestate") or leave an invalid will, state laws will govern the distribution of your estate. Your estate might wind up being administered by a total stranger appointed by the court. Should both parents of a child or children die without a will, a court-appointed guardian takes custody of any minor children and of the parents' estate.

Preparing a will encourages you to assess your financial situation and to ensure that your property, savings, benefits, and assets will be managed according to your wishes. The laws concerning wills are complex and vary by state. In most cases, you will need a lawyer to guide you and protect your estate. Writing your own will, though, is better than leaving none at all. An entirely handwritten (holographic) will, signed and dated by you, can be binding and enforceable. Not all states accept holographic wills.

Be sure to review your will periodically to keep your information up to date. If you divorce, separate, or remarry, or if the status of your named heirs changes, be sure to revise your will appropriately.

In considering your will's contents, be prepared to include information about an executor (the person you name to carry out the terms of your will), your children, anyone you wish to "disinherit," your assets, tax implications, gifts, trusts, revocable living trust (talk to a knowledgeable person about the advantages and disadvantages of this technique to avoid probate), life insurance, and charitable contributions.

Persons to Notify

Include the names, addresses, and phone numbers of doctors, attorneys, employers, relatives, friends, business associates, the executor or trustee of your estate, religious and social organizations, and anyone else who should be notified of your death.

Arrangements for Your Body

It is important to make decisions regarding organ donation, burial, cremation, and donation of your body for scientific research, and then make appropriate plans based on those decisions. You might want to compose your own inscription to appear on a headstone. It is wise to select and designate the plot and its location, and the mortuary of your choice in advance.

Note: If you wish to donate your organs, fill out the appropriate places on your driver's license and the medical emergency wallet card.

Obituary

What would you like your local newspaper to say about you? You can help your family by providing information about your place of birth, career background, education, special achievements, military service, membership in organizations, hobbies, and memorial contribution preferences.

Memorial Service

Your clergy can help provide guidelines regarding mourning or burial rituals. If you know the type of service you want (for instance, public or private), where the service should be held, what music should be played, who should officiate, and so on, this is the time to spell out your preferences in writing. Be sure to notify the appropriate family member or friend who would need to know this information.

Benefit Information

Survivors may be entitled to benefits you've either earned or provided for. These may include benefits from life insurance, pension, and profit-sharing plans, including Keogh plans, IRAs, Social Security,

Medicare, supplemental medical insurance, Veterans' benefits, or Workers' Compensation benefits. Assemble this information and mark it clearly. Provide account numbers, contact names, and addresses and phone numbers, if possible.

Assets and Liabilities

This section of the file should include information about savings and loan accounts (including T-bills and CDs); investments (stocks, bonds, and investment funds, including money market accounts, mutual funds, government securities, limited partnerships, and annuities); real estate (your home, investment properties, and other assets); notes, first or second mortgages (that you owe or that are owed to you); other liabilities (including home mortgage, investment properties, and business, auto, and personal loans); and any recommendations about investments for your survivors.

Insurance Information

Provide information on insurance policies for your home (whether you own or rent it) and automobiles. (Life insurance is listed under "Benefit Information.") Record the addresses of all insured properties and the license numbers of all insured cars. Provide the documentation for each insurance policy as well as contact names, addresses, and phone numbers.

Home and Personal Property Inventory

An inventory is a practical way of listing your belongings, identifying each item, specifying its location, estimating its value, and naming the heir to whom you're giving it.

Use this opportunity to give away items you're not interested in keeping—donate usable items to charity or have a garage sale. You may want to give away some of your belongings now to your family or friends and take advantage of the opportunity to see them enjoying your former possessions.

Your Personal or "Ethical" Will

This is a rare opportunity to take the time to express your innermost thoughts. You might want to write a personal note to your loved ones or specific personal messages to each of them. You might want to record your thoughts on audiotape or videotape. This is your most meaningful legacy—it can express who you are,

record your autobiography, and reflect your life philosophy. The thoughts you share here will provide a lasting and precious memory for your survivors. Include anecdotes, favorite quotations, and philosophies. You might also want to include any diaries, pictures, or journals you'd like to pass on.

You may wish to make a log booklet or a tape recording of your life history. Talk in depth about your early life experiences, beginning with your youth. Recount memories of parents, grandparents, aunts, uncles, siblings, children, friends, neighbors, colleagues, and pets.

Leave a rich family history by providing a family tree. This is also a good time to map out a family medical tree. Write down any medical conditions that you or your relatives may have had—this can be valuable information for your family now and for generations to come.

Checklist of Forms and Worksheets

The time to act is now: ninety-three percent of families are unprepared when a death occurs. Collecting the following information and putting it in one place will help you ensure that your loved ones are cared for after your death. Once you have gathered this information, be sure to tell several key people where it will be kept. Do not keep this information in a safe-deposit box (it will be sealed upon your death): give it to your doctor, family, lawyer, agent (as designated by your medical power of attorney), and hospital medical records department.

- ❑ Advance directives (see Chapter 44, "Decisions for Life")
- ❑ Additional Considerations for Advance directives (see form, p. 414)
- ❑ Prehospital Do Not Resuscitate (DNR) Order
- ❑ Medical Emergency Wallet Card (see form, p. 415)
- ❑ Copy of MedicAlert Service Form (see form, p. 416)
- ❑ Family Information (see form, p. 417)
- ❑ Location of Records (see form, p. 418)
- ❑ Legal Will
- ❑ Persons to Notify after Death (see form, p. 421)
- ❑ Arrangements for Your Funeral/Memorial Service (see form, p. 423)
- ❑ Obituary (see form, p. 422)

- ❏ Benefit Information
- ❏ Review of Assets and Liabilities (see form, p. 419)
- ❏ Insurance Information
- ❏ Home and Personal Property Inventory
- ❏ Your Personal or "Ethical" Will
- ❏ Your Legacy of Love

ADDITIONAL CONSIDERATIONS FOR THE ADVANCE DIRECTIVES
MY SPECIFIC PREFERENCES FOR LIFE SUPPORT (HEROIC MEASURES)

People's preferences for use or non-use of life sustaining measures may vary depending upon the specific life sustaining measure being considered. In addition, preferences are influenced by different health conditions. Below are several health situations you may encounter. Please check which life sustaining measures you want, do not want, or are undecided about for each of these different situations. In situation 5, you may put your own situation if it has not been covered. If you would like a limited trial only, place a T in the "I want" column.

NAME _____

DATE _____

WITNESS _____

WITNESS _____

(Please use the same witnesses as on Durable Powers Form)

Situation 1: I do not have a terminal illness and I can care for myself. However, everything takes much effort and I am in constant pain (as in arthritis). If I suddenly require medical help (as in a heart attack or pneumonia), treatment for this emergency can return me to my usual level of functioning. If not treated, I will most likely die. In such a case, my preferences are:

Situation 2: I have a chronic and terminal disease. I cannot accomplish my own self-care such as eating, toileting, dressing, walking, but I do recognize everyone around me. (This could be the case in advanced cancer, lung disease, paralysis from stroke.) If an emergency arises, my preferences are:

Situation 3: I have a disease from which I will become progressively confused and incapacitated, such as in Alzheimer's Disease. I may not always be able to take care of myself or recognize people. In an emergency occurs my preferences are:

Situation 4: I am in a persistent state of vegetation (coma). I cannot eat, dress, toilet myself or recognize people. (This could occur in the stages of Alzheimer's disease or severe stroke.) If an emergency occurs, my preferences are:

Situation 5: Please write in any other scenario which is important to you:

LIFE SUSTAINING MEASURES	Situation 1			Situation 2			Situation 3			Situation 4			Situation 5		
	I WANT	I DO NOT WANT	UNDECIDED	I WANT	I DO NOT WANT	UNDECIDED	I WANT	I DO NOT WANT	UNDECIDED	I WANT	I DO NOT WANT	UNDECIDED	I WANT	I DO NOT WANT	UNDECIDED
1. Cardiopulmonary Resuscitation															
2. Mechanical Breathing															
3. Artificial Food & Fluids															
4. Painful or Potentially Harmful Diagnostic Tests															
5. Antibotics															
6. Include here any other directives important to you															

TO SEAL YOUR CARD AT HOME —WRAP IN SCOTCH TAPE

MEDICAL EMERGENCY WALLET CARD©

NAME   SS NO.

                                        DOB   /   /

ADDRESS

                                        TEL.   /

NEAREST RELATIVE   TEL.   /   CITY

PHYSICIAN   TEL.   /   CITY

CLERGY   TEL.   /   CITY

DIAGNOSIS

MEDICATIONS

LEGAL WILL YES ☐ / NO ☐   LOCATION OF DOCUMENTS

Advance Directives Location_____
Durable Power of Attorney for Health Care   YES ☐ NO ☐
Desig. Agent   Tel. /   City
Prehospital Do Not Resuscitate (DNR) (Declaration to Physician) YES ☐ NO ☐
Resuscitation: Chest   Mechanical   Drugs
                            Compression   Ventilation   Therapy
Acute (Reversible)   YES ☐ NO ☐   YES ☐ NO ☐   YES ☐ NO ☐
Chronic (incurable)   YES ☐ NO ☐   YES ☐ NO ☐   YES ☐ NO ☐

Organ Donation: Cornea Y ☐ N ☐ Liver Y ☐ N ☐   Bones Y ☐ N ☐
                       Heart Y ☐ N ☐ Skin   Y ☐ N ☐
                       Kidney Y ☐ N ☐ Middle Ear Y ☐ N ☐

Signature   Date   /   /

Witness   Relationship

MEDIC ALERT® SERVICE FORM

TO ENROLL BY PHONE Call 1-800-432-5378 anytime. Have the following information ready: 1) Credit card number and expiration date; 2) Medical information; 3) Name, telephone number and address of persons and physician(s) to contact in an emergency; 4) Bracelet size (when ordering bracelet)

TO ENROLL BY MAIL Complete form and mail with payment to Medic Alert®, 2323 Colorado Ave, Turlock, CA 95382 Please photocopy form for other enrollees.

1. **ARE YOU OR HAVE YOU BEEN A MEDIC ALERT MEMBER?** Yes ☐ No ☐ If yes, Enter Member Number

2. **PERSONAL INFORMATION:** Print or type clearly.   Sex   Social Security Number

Last name   First   Middle

Mailing address   Phone Area Code ( )   Date of Birth Mo. Day Year

City   State   Zip

EMERGENCY CONTACTS: As a free service, Medic Alert will advise your physician of your enrollment, and emergency information.

Person 1   Phone ( )   Person 2   Phone ( )

Physician 1   Phone ( )   Physician 2   Phone ( )

Address   Address

3. **MEDICAL INFORMATION TO BE ENGRAVED ON EMBLEM:** (will also appear on computer record and wallet card). Dosage data not needed. Engraving space is limited. Small bracelet emblem: limit: 60 spaces. Large bracelet emblem and necklace emblems: limit 90 spaces. Allow one space between words.

4. **OTHER EMERGENCY MEDICAL INFORMATION:** For your computer record and wallet card. Dosage data not needed.

5. **STYLE AND SIZE OF EMBLEM:** *Select your emblem below by checking box:*

Metal Type	Necklace	Large Bracelet	Small Bracelet	Fee**
Stainless Steel	☐	☐	☐	$35
Sterling Silver (Raised)	☐	☐	☐	$50
Gold Filled (Raised design, 10 KT)	☐	☐	☐	$75
Designer Silver (Recessed Design)		☐	☐	$115

(Fees & Terms as of 10/93, subject to change without notice.)

*Bracelet Size: ☐ ☐ ☐ ☐ ☐ ☐ ☐
6" 6½" 7" 7½" 8" 8½" 9"

6. **PAYMENT CALCULATION**

REGISTRATION FEE: .... $_____
(Tax deductible medical expense.) Includes issuance of ID number, wallet card and one custom engraved emblem with chain.

ANNUAL MEMBERSHIP FEE: $15 (first year free) .... $_____
Covers 24 hour year round emergency hot line service and free updating of your computer record.

CONTRIBUTION: (tax deductible) .... $_____
Medic Alert, a non profit foundation, is partly supported by contributions for professional and public education programs.

TOTAL AMOUNT ENCLOSED: .... $_____

7. **METHOD OF PAYMENT:**
☐ Check ☐ MasterCard ☐ VISA ☐ Discover
☐ Money Order   *(no other cards accepted.)*

No CODs. Payment must accompany order. Send to:
Medic Alert, 2323 Colorado Ave., Turlock, CA 95382

Card Number
Expiration Date   _____ _____

LEGAL STATEMENT: IMPORTANT: The member agrees not to wear the emblem or carry the wallet card until the emergency record has been carefully checked by the member for correctness, and agrees to inform Medic Alert in writing of any error found. The member authorizes Medic Alert to relay information in response to emergency telephone calls. The member agrees to immediately notify Medic Alert Whenever his/her medical condition or address changes.

8. **I understand and accept the legal statement printed above.**

1643

FAMILY INFORMATION

Name	
Residence	
Telephone	
Birthdate and Place	
Social Security Number	
Military Service Serial Number	
Spouse or Next of Kin	
Children	Telephone
Special plans for children in event of parent's death	
Designated Guardian	
Mother	Telephone
Father	Telephone
Maternal Grandparents	
Paternal Grandparents	
Grandchildren	
Blood/Genetic Information	
VA Claim Number	
Date and Place of Discharge	
Significant Other Person	Telephone
Special plans for pets (name/type of/who will adopt)	
Additional significant information	

Signature	Date
Spouse/Partner	Date

LOCATION OF RECORDS

ITEM	LOCATION	
Wills		
Living Trust		
Legal Will		
Durable Power of Attorney		
Pre-nuptial Agreement		
Financial	Who has access	
Safe-deposit box	Key	Number
Banks/Account Nos:	Savings	Money Market Funds
	Checking	
*Stocks and Bonds		
*Deeds of Trust		
Loans	Loan Accounts	
Loans Owed to Us		
*T-bills, Cert. of Deposit		
Trusts	Attorney	
Address		
Business Records	Briefcase combination	
Limited Partnerships		
Real Estate Records		
Mortgage Documents		
Miscellaneous Contracts		
Pensions	IRA	Keough
Work/Company Pension Plan		
Workers Comp. Records		
Social Security Records		
Tax I.D. Number(s)		
Veterans Records		
*Insurance Policies		
*Auto Ownership Certificates		
Credit Cards		
Installment Payments		
Warranties		
Personal		
Passports		
*Birth Certificates		
Ministorage or Warehouse	Key/combination	
Charitable Gifts		
Church		
Individuals		
Organizations		

Signature	Date
Spouse/Partner	Date

*Recommend keeping in safe-deposit box

REVIEW OF ASSETS AND LIABILITIES
(Brief Review — To Be Expanded As Needed)

1. Stocks and Bonds (Broker)　　　　Location—To be given to

2. Properties (Name, Mortgage)　　　Location—To be given to

3. Bank Accounts (Account Numbers)　Location—To be given to

   Business

   Checking

4. Insurance Policies (Agent)　　　　Location—To be given to

5. Cars

6. Current Liabilities and Loans　　　Document Location

   Home Mortgage　　= $

   Business Loans　　= $

   Automobile Loans　= $

   Personal Loans　　= $

   IRS Income Tax　　= $

   Credit Union　　　= $

7. Home Assets Inventory

   Living Room　　　　　　　　　Designated Recipient

   　Furniture

   　Paintings

   　Rugs

   　Piano

   Dining Room

Furniture

Dishes

Miscellaneous

Silver

Crystal

Miscellaneous (Mirrors, lamps)

Antiques

Jewelry

Appliances

Televisions

Audio Equipment

Records/Audio- and Videotapes

Refrigerator/Stove

Washer/Dryer

Bedrooms

Stamp collection

Coin collection

Miscellaneous

It is worth making a home inventory list with an appraisal and designating the person(s) to whom you wish to will items. Dividing and distributing family pictures, heirlooms and special items can make decisions easier for those you love and can make a willed gift more appreciated.

Signature   Date

Spouse/Partner   Date

PERSONS TO NOTIFY AFTER DEATH
Directory of Officials, Relatives and Friends
Clergy
Telephone
Office Staff
Telephone Number(s)
Funeral Director
Telephone
For Organ Donation
Contact
Telephone
Attorney
Telephone
Accountant
Telephone
Executor/Executrix of Will
Telephone Number(s)
Life Insurance Agent
Telephone
Bank Trust Officer
Telephone
Social Security Admin
Veterans Administrator

ALSO NOTIFY

Other Relatives and Close Friends	Telephone Number(s)

Signature	Date
Spouse/Partner	Date

OBITUARY

Name

Notes about life and achievements

Birthplace

Career

Hobbies

Organizations

Names of Relatives

Achievements

College   Degree(s)

Military Service

Memorial Donations

Preferred Funeral Arrangements

Place of Funeral Service   Time

Additional Information or Instructions

Signature   Date

Spouse/Partner   Date

ARRANGEMENTS FOR YOUR FUNERAL/MEMORIAL SERVICE

Type of burial memorial
☐ Cremation   ☐ Casket
In church/temple
At funeral home
Open or closed casket
At the gravesite
The Committal should be   ☐ public   ☐ private
If cremation, instruction for ashes
Specific desires for the service, i.e., suggested readings/music
Viewing
Grave marker (tombstone)
Decoration
Flowers
Inscription
Casket: ☐ wood   ☐ metal
Burial: ☐ shroud   ☐ street clothes
Gravesite
Family plot located
Previously purchased gravesite location
Memorial gifts/donations to agencies or foundations
Other comments, instructions or wishes

Signature	Date
Spouse/Partner	Date

Forms adapted from *Getting Your Affairs in Order, Make Life Easier for Those You Leave Behind,* by Elmo Petterle, Robert C. Kahn and Marianne Rogoff, Bolinas, CA, Shelter Publications, 1993.

46

Choosing Life

Ernest H. Rosenbaum, M.D.
Isadora R. Rosenbaum, M.A.

Look to this day, for it is life,...
For yesterday is but a dream,
And tomorrow is only a vision.
But today, well lived,
Makes every yesterday a dream of happiness,
And every tomorrow a vision of hope.

—Sanskrit proverb

To the Patient

This book has presented concepts, information, and methods that can help give direction to your desire to rehabilitate yourself. Our concept of rehabilitation is one that requires a total approach to the person with cancer—one that addresses both the body and mind with exercise, nutrition, and supportive care, through your efforts as well as those of your health care team.

Only by acquiring specific knowledge can we begin to conceive possible solutions to our complex health problems. To achieve any level of success, you, the patient, must accept responsibility for the role you can play in your medical care. Having made the critical decision that you want to get well, you must believe that it is worth the effort and be willing to make sacrifices and give sufficient attention to the task.

Frequently, coping requires a compromise—to accept what cannot be changed and to proceed from there. A patient who copes can set new, realistic goals. He or she must leave anger and bitterness behind and free up energies to live in the present.

To live in the present, a patient must have hope, because hope is an essential part of the will to live. Hope can come from many sources: from the doctor who shares his or her therapeutic plans with the patient, or from the family members and friends who seek to help. But primarily, hope will come from the patient who is willing to help himself or herself.

The Mind

By knowing yourself, your goals in life, your limits, capacities, and how to compensate for the stresses and trials of daily life, you can accelerate your rehabilitation. Knowing how to keep your "cool," how to keep your frustration level low, and how to make appropriate use of support systems can make the difference between success and failure in treatment. Psychological and spiritual aids can help control the disturbances of external mental pressures.

The Body

When you have a disease, there is an accompanying chronic feeling of tiredness, often so subtle that you and your doctor may not recognize it for what it really is.

Expending energy appropriately is paramount, lest the tiredness be compounded and come to characterize daily life. An energy deficit manifests itself in how we feel, emotionally and physically. It can mean the difference between health or illness, misery or happiness. Fortunately, we have an energy reserve upon which to draw. Energy needs may be constant and predictable, yet vary in the ways they are met. The better our mental and physical states, the greater our vitality and energy reserves. The concepts and methods discussed in this book are designed to help you achieve the highest level of functioning possible within the limits of your disease.

Guidelines to Keep in Mind

Adequate Sleep. Your need for sleep will vary, depending in part on your activities and habits (not all people require eight hours of sleep nightly). Prolonged lack of sleep reduces efficiency and the ability to function. How you sleep is important, too. A good night's sleep is "as good as gold. " If sleeping pills or tranquilizers are helpful in obtaining an adequate night's rest, they should be used. Resolving any perplexing and annoying emotional problems helps immeasurably. The use of relaxing techniques, meditation, and biofeedback is often invaluable.

Nutrition. Fad nutritional notions and diets should be discouraged. Eating balanced meals, with adequate protein and calories, is vital in helping you to tolerate therapy, fight disease, and gain the strength to return to active life.

Physical Exercise. An active and organized exercise program—with appropriate rest periods—is absolutely essential for maintaining good physical status. Exercise provides a feeling of well-being, reduces stress, aids relaxation, increases reserve strength, and promotes better sleep. Graduated levels of exercise that add increasing variations as you improve will prevent fatigue and frustration. Nothing is more reassur-

ing than to see and feel self-improvement. Concurrent use of an occupational physical therapy program will help accelerate your recovery.

Sexuality. Your sexuality is still a part of your total being when you have a chronic illness, and it is an area of concern that should not be ignored. If adjustments in your patterns of sexual expression are necessary, communication between you and your partner may enable you to work these out alone. For those who need help, counseling is available.

Relaxation Time. Periods of "trained relaxation," two to three times a day, will help make life more enjoyable. We go through so many changes daily—from hectic stress periods to periods of diversion and relaxation—that we need a tool to help us cope with them. Meditation, biofeedback, and other techniques can relax the mind and reduce stress. Hobbies, sports, and various types of mental or physical games can help maintain energy resources. Allot specific time to "be good to yourself." These times should be private, personal, and inviolate. Don't use your relaxation time as a work period! To do so will only increase mental tension and physical exhaustion.

In short, a person needs to restructure his or her life to succeed in obtaining as full a rehabilitation as possible, no matter what the medical problem is. A person cannot change completely, but habitual daily patterns, even some of life-long duration, can be adjusted and altered by setting reasonable goals and personal priorities, so that time is used both efficiently and constructively. The self-help/self-support programs described in this guide are designed to help you formulate a better recovery program.

To the Family and Friends

There are many resources for patients with cancer, but probably the greatest allies to the physician are you, the close family and friends of the patient, who are available to help when the need arises; you offer a reserve that cannot be found in any other resource. Your continued love and compassion give hope and courage to the patient.

We all need love. The person who is ill is particularly vulnerable to the feelings of being alone and abandoned. Thus, the importance of your understanding of the patient cannot be overestimated. Without your support, the patient's recovery process may be improved and prolonged.

Illness, incapacity, and the threat of death are difficult subjects for a patient and his or her family and friends to discuss together. You may want to talk to each other but be hindered because you want to protect one another, or because you do not wish to face the truth yourselves. The inability to communicate can occur with all people at any time, but it is usually heightened under conditions of stress.

Families and friends faced with the life-threatening illness of a loved one have the dual problem of trying to control their own fears and anxieties while giving support to the patient. They may spend their time wondering how to ease the patient's emotional suffering, while the patient is busy worrying about the despair of those he or she loves. Each is searching for the most tactful way to deal with the other.

Our experience with patients has shown, however, that a deliberate policy of candor and openness will create an atmosphere that is beneficial to all concerned. It can remove the burden of secrecy and open the door for the alleviation of apprehensions. Candor may not be easily achieved, for often people are not in the habit of speaking about their deepest concerns. Even those who have established close relationships may become fainthearted in the presence of cancer and the threat of death. To achieve openness and to maintain it under stress is part of the challenge of living with cancer—for both the patient and the patient's family and friends.

Hearing what the others are experiencing is never as devastating as what the imagination can conjure up. Fears and frustrations should be talked about as they arise, rather than being left to fester until they become too frightening to mention, or until a habit of withholding evolves into inevitable isolation. Confronting each other's fears, therefore, becomes a means of keeping those fears under control. Candor will allow relationships to operate in a new realm, in which despair can be minimized or set aside and enjoyment and pleasure can resume their rightful places.

Candor between a patient and his or her family and friends includes recognizing one another's needs as well as one another's fears. Family and friends need to give, to feel they are doing something practical to hasten the patient's recovery, whether at home or in the hospital.

The separation caused by hospitalization is particularly traumatic to the family. They leave the hospital each evening and worry about whether their loved one will ever again lead a normal life, or whether he or she will even leave the hospital. Feeling powerless, they need to give of themselves. Fortunately there are many practical services a patient's family and friends can perform while the patient is in the hospital—services such as feeding, walking, turning, and massaging. These, along with the offer of special foods, a favorite pillow, or a comforting hand, become the routine of the daily hospital visit, giving solace to the family and friends as well as to the patient.

When the patient is critically ill, it is not unusual for at least one family member to be in attendance around the clock. This may mean sleeping in a chair beside the patient's bed. To obtain up-to-date information on the patient's condition, relatives may rearrange their schedules so as to be present when the doctor makes rounds or a particularly helpful nurse is on duty.

When the patient is at home, functioning well, there are still many opportunities for family and friends to give emotional and practical support. One need only consider what the cancer patient must sometimes be feeling: anxiety about a visit to the doctor, wondering whether a new problem will be discovered or a new treatment recommended, dreading the side effects from the day's treatment, and concern about lack of transportation to and from the doctor's office. A family member or friend can offer a ride or go with the patient on the bus. If everyone is working and cannot be with the patient during the day, there is still the evening, when the side effects of therapy may have to be endured. Patient, family, and friends all benefit from any means by which love and encouragement can be expressed.

To be realistic, however, not everyone is able to be open, loving, or supportive in crisis. Even stable relationships may be severely threatened by the pressures of long-term illness. Latent problems may emerge, and anger or guilt may surface in sudden attacks or recriminations, or in indifferent or overly solicitous behavior. The exhaustion and frustration of constant worry and care may break even the most loyal supporter. Family and friends must be reminded that they need time to themselves and moments of rest if they are to keep emotionally and physically fit. Calling on other friends or relatives for assistance can provide a respite from the responsibilities and worries of constant caring.

Children of cancer patients often need special understanding. Absence of a parent during hospitalization and the parent's fatigue following treatment may cause children to feel neglected and lost. Children may also feel they caused the illness; this misconception must be corrected quickly. Reassurance from other family members is important for children to realize they are still loved. Adolescents are particularly vulnerable to stress, as they may be asked to assume a supportive role, to approximate an adult partner or spouse. If this responsibility is beyond the adolescent's capabilities, he or she may rebel by not making hospital visits or by excessive drinking or drug use. Adolescents are adults—up to a point—but they still require the reassurance and comfort routinely given to younger children.

Lengthy illness can also break the most courageous of patients. When a person has fought long and hard against cancer, losing and regaining hope many times, and then realizes that the battle is not to be won, he or she may, at times, experience rage or depression that will focus on the nearest available person—the patient's spouse or significant other, child, parent, friend, or the nurse on duty. This anger usually manifests itself as irritation over trivial matters that normally would not even concern the patient. The person under attack needs to understand that this is not a rejection, but a cry of anguish.

In addition to anger and depression, a patient must also endure the endless boredom of being ill, as well as the fear of being a burden when he or she really wants and needs special attention. Ironically, the people from whom this attention is demanded may be suffering from the same tedium or from feelings of inadequacy and guilt for being unable to relieve the suffering. They may not be able to cope with the reality in which the patient is imprisoned. The result may be a gradual diminishing of attention and care by the family, and increased bitterness and fear of isolation for the patient.

No one should be blamed for the ways he or she responds to the crisis of a long-term illness or the threat of change and loss. Some people and some relationships grow stronger, experiencing new depths of love, respect, and understanding; some waver, yet hold together; and some collapse.

The most important thing that family and friends can do for a patient is to be supportive, give encouragement, and do everything possible to promote his or her recovery. However, it is vital that they do not err on the side of being overly solicitous, because this deprives the patient of the accomplishments that can give a sense of independence, purpose, and self-esteem, and concrete proof of progress in returning to a normal life.

The purpose of life is to live. The goal of the physician who treats cancer patients is not only to administer medical therapy but also to help them live as normally as possible while undergoing treatment. There is a widespread belief that a diagnosis of cancer is an automatic death sentence. This is not true. Today, 50 percent of all cancer patients are cured; the majority of those who are not cured are leading active, productive lives with the same odds and life expectancy as people who live with other chronic diseases.

Of course, a cure for cancer is not just around the corner. No single breakthrough will produce all the answers; the answers will come one by one, just as they have until now. Nevertheless, as of 1996, more than fourteen types of cancer were curable when diagnosed at an advanced stage. New forms of cancer will continue to be added to this list, because new discoveries are constantly being made and known techniques perfected. New methods of giving radiation therapy, new chemotherapeutic drugs and combinations of drugs, and the use of adjuvant chemotherapy, hormonal therapy, and experimental therapies—such as immunotherapy and hyperthermia—all give hope for the future.

In spite of the promise of these medical advances, though, living with cancer is an anxious, fearful time. Undergoing therapy and experiencing the side effects of treatment involve compromise. This compromise consists of accepting what has happened and at the same time being willing to fight for your life. But no matter how well informed you become about current therapies and available treatment alternatives, you will still feel a loss of control over your fate because you must trust the judgment of cancer specialists and pray for good luck. It is not unusual to be full of hope one day and full of gloom the next.

Sometimes we are able to survive a current crisis because of the way we coped with a crisis in the past. We acquire resilience; we learn how tough we really are and develop confidence in our ability to endure. By turning to these inner resources and to the resources offered by members of the medical team, a cancer patient will have the best chance of maintaining a good quality of life while living with cancer. Attention to nutrition and muscle strength can have marked physical and emotional benefits for the patient. Knowledgeable, sensitive nurses and physicians can assuage fear and offer reassurance as well as good medical care. Medical social workers can help with insurance problems, or arrange for home care or participation in a discussion group. Every patient should be aware of these services.

Thus, help is available from people in many professions who understand your needs. These needs can also be met by other cancer patients who have formed support groups. We are here to help each other. How you live with cancer is your choice.

All cancer patients must live with their disease. The decision of how to approach the problem is individual. With the proper support from family, friends, and the medical team, and with their own inner resources of courage and hope, cancer patients can continue to live a meaningful life.

Choose life—only that and always, and at whatever risk. To let life leak out, to let it wear away by the mere passage of time, to withhold giving it and spreading it, is to choose nothing.

—Sister Helen Kelley

Part VI

Resources

47

Supportive Care Resource Centers

Keren Stronach, M.Ph.,
Director,
Ida Friend Cancer
Resource Center,
USCF Comprehensive
Cancer Center

Resource centers that provide supportive care services for patients and their families are an essential part of cancer care. Effective centers serve an integrative function, bringing together information services, emotional support, and lifestyle programs so that the complex needs of the whole person are addressed. These programs offer multiple avenues for patients to get information, meet others, and links to community resources. Their overall aim is to improve quality of life and make it easier for patients to navigate the difficult periods of diagnosis, treatment, and recovery. As the importance of health information, support groups, and patient participation in decision making is recognized, numerous hospitals are developing such programs. Although there are many effective formats for providing supportive care services, the description below is modeled after the supportive care services offered at the Cancer Resource Center at the University of California at San Francisco (UCSF) Comprehensive Cancer Center. When receiving cancer treatment, make sure to inquire about supportive care services offered at your hospital.

Information Services

A good resource center provides information in a variety of formats, including written materials and educational audio and video tapes, so that individuals have multiple avenues to access information. Because researching can be stressful, it is helpful to have well-trained staff who can assist patients by providing individually tailored information packets on a particular diagnosis, treatment options, or clinical trials. Computers with access to the Internet, Medline, and other health data sources should also be available for patients to do their own research. Having instructions for using the Internet and for locating accurate and reliable sites at each computer allows novices to research independently.

An important component of information services is comprehensive and up-to-date information on community resources to help patients and their families access cancer-related and general services in their area, including hospice, home care, and transportation resources. Resource centers can also serve as clearinghouses for activities such as upcoming symposiums, conferences, and other cancer-related events. Monthly newsletters and community calendars, which list cancer events at the resource center and in the community, can be effective ways of informing patients of upcoming cancer activities.

Emotional Support

Support groups provide an important avenue for patients to meet each other, interact, and share feelings, stories, and information. Another beneficial service is a peer support program that allows patients to connect one-on-one, pairing veteran patients with newly diagnosed ones. In addition to serving as a source of support, speaking to a peer can provide a new patient with valuable tips and information.

Monthly discussion forums on different cancer-related topics can also be an effective way of bringing patients together in a supportive atmosphere. In addition to providing opportunities for patients to meet, such forums provide valuable information and teach important coping skills.

Lifestyle Programs

Exercise classes such as dance, yoga, and Qigong can combat depression, promote feelings of well-being, prevent muscle atrophy, and provide another way for patients to meet and interact. Nutrition counseling and cooking classes also encourage patients to adopt a healthier lifestyle by teaching them to eat more nutritious foods, thereby reducing the risk of malnutrition during treatment.

Meditation and visualization programs can be helpful in reducing stress and managing pain. As well, research has shown that creative expression can be an effective way to help patients cope. Programs such as Art for Recovery at UCSF encourage patients to paint, make quilts, and express themselves through writing. These are excellent ways to promote healthy coping.

Having fun, free activities, such as facials and tickets to the ballet, symphony, and other performances for people with cancer is another wonderful service to provide for patients and their families.

Medical Navigation Resources

Consultation planning programs provide patients with tools to communicate more effectively with their physicians. In these programs, patients can sit with a counselor and map out their main questions and concerns. A copy is then given to both the patient and the physician, serving as a road map to guide discussions and ensure that the patient's uncertainties are addressed.

Explanatory health insurance and benefits programs help patients navigate the coverage maze, take advantage of their benefits, prepare for disability, and inform them of viatication (the ability to sell your life insurance while still you're still alive).

Summation

Supportive services come in many variations and formats to accommodate the needs of different individuals. We hope that this description gives you a good starting point to seek the services that you need. If the program you are interested in is not provided through the resource center at your hospital, or if your hospital does not have a resource center, inquire to see if one can be developed. Or, if you believe that some of the services described above—such as the meditation, writing, or art—will provide an effective way of coping, find a way to incorporate them into your life.

For more information about the services described above, visit the webpage of the UCSF Cancer Resource Center at http://cc.ucsf.edu/crc.

48

Internet Resources

Alexandra Andrews, Webmaster,
The Cancer Supportive
Care Program

The Cancer Supportive Care website (www.cancersupportivecare.com) provides current and up-to-date resources. Here are a few sites to visit as you begin to navigate on the Internet.

American Cancer Society

www.cancer.org

The American Cancer Society is the nationwide community-based voluntary health organization. It is dedicated to eliminating cancer as a major health problem through prevention, treatment, and the diminishment of suffering from cancer through research, education-advocacy, and service. Assistance in English and Spanish is available. The hotline is 1-800-ACS-2345.

American Hospice Foundation

www.americanhospice.org

The American Hospice Foundation opens new doors to hospice care through public education programs focused on strategically selected audiences such as employers, schools, insurance companies, and religious organizations.

American Institute for Cancer Research—Online

www.aicr.org

The American Institute for Cancer Research is one of the nation's leading cancer charities, and is innovative in the field of cancer prevention and treatment through nutrition.

American Red Cross

www.redcross.org

The American Red Cross helps keep people safe every day as well as in emergencies.

American Society of Clinical Oncology (ASCO)

www.asco.org

The American Society of Clinical Oncology is an interactive resource for oncology professionals and cancer patients.

Association of Cancer Online Resources (ACOR)

www.acor.org

The ACOR.org cancer information system currently offers access to ninety-nine electronic mailing lists and a variety of unique websites.

Association of Oncology Social Work (AOSW) World Wide Web Site

www.aosw.org

Oncology social work is the primary professional discipline providing psychosocial services to patients, families, and caregivers facing the impact of cancer diagnosis and treatment.

R.A. Bloch Cancer Foundation, Inc

www.blochcancer.org

The Richard Bloch Cancer Foundation's website offers encouragement to newly diagnosed patients and provides information for them and their supporters.

The Cancer Answer

www.thecanceranswer.org

Cancer Answer second opinions by Malin Dollinger, M.D., F.A.C.P., coauthor of *Everyone's Guide to Cancer Therapy*, Clinical Professor, University of Southern California.

Cancer Care

www.cancercare.org

Since 1944, Cancer Care has been dedicated to providing emotional support, information, and practical help to people with cancer and their loved ones. The toll free number is: 800-813-HOPE (4673).

Cancer Links

www.cancerlinks.com

Cancer Links provides a complete source and guide to cancer information. Choose from hundreds of links with more added daily for your cancer needs.

Cancerlinks.org

www.cancerlinks.org

Cancerlinks.org contains links providing comprehensive information about cancer, its effects, and its treatment. It has many links to international cancer information.

Cancerlinks Hospital do Cancer—AC Camargo, Sao Paulo, Brasil

www.hcanc.org.br

This site provides cancer information in English, Spanish, and Portuguese.

Cancer Lynx—We Prowl the Net

www.cancerlynx.com

Advocating for cancer patients and their families. Your source for news, information, and very human stories about cancer.

CancerNet

www.cancernet.gov

This site contains credible, current, comprehensive cancer information from the National Cancer Institute, including types of cancer, cancer treatment options, clinical trials, cancer literature, cancer genetics, risk factors, prevention, testing, and more.

Cancer Supportive Care

www.cancersupportivecare.com

The Cancer Supportive Care Program by Earnest H. Rosenbaum, M.D., and David Spiegel, M.D., complements surgery, radiation therapy, chemotherapy, and immunotherapy for total supportive care.

CancerTrials: A Service of the National Cancer Institute

cancertrials.nci.nih.gov

A guide for patients with cancer to clinical trials that offers details on informed consent, risks, side effects, and medication trials.

Candlelighters Childhood Cancer Foundation (CCCF)

www.candlelighters.org

Candlelighters Childhood Cancer Foundation (CCCF) was founded in 1970 by concerned parents of children with cancer.

Children's Hospice International (CHI)

www.chionline.org

CHI is committed to the concept of hospice care. It recognizes the right and need for children and their families to choose health care and support whether in their own home, a hospital, or a hospice.

Choice in Dying, Inc.

www.choices.org

Choice in Dying, the inventor of living wills in 1967, is dedicated to fostering communication about complex end-of-life decisions.

Diseases, Disorders and Related Topics from the Karolinksa Institute

www.mic.ki.se/Diseases

Classified resources for the general public, health care professionals, and researchers from the Karolinksa Institute.

Food and Drug Administration Home Page

www.fda.gov

This is the site for the nation's foremost consumer protection agency.

Hardin MD—Hardin Meta Directory of Internet Health Sources

www.lib.uiowa.edu/hardin/md/index.html

This site is a list of lists providing comprehensive resource information in health-related subjects.

Healthfinder

www.healthfinder.gov

Healthfinder, developed by the U.S. Department of Health and Human Services, is a free guide to reliable health information.

Healthlinks On-Line Medical Resource Center—Health/Medical

www.healthlinks.com

An international health-related resource center, this site offers information for people in or dealing with the medical profession.

Hospice Foundation of America

www.hospicefoundation.org

The Hospice Foundation of America is a not-for-profit organization that provides leadership in the development and application of hospice and its philosophy of care.

International Federation of Red Cross and Red Crescent Societies

www.ifrc.org

The International Federation of Red Cross and Red Crescent Societies is the world's largest humanitarian organization, providing assistance without discrimination as to nationality, race, religious beliefs, class, or political opinions.

International Association for the Study of Pain

www.halcyon.com/iasp

This is an international, multidisciplinary, nonprofit professional association dedicated to furthering research on pain and improving the care of patients with pain.

International Union Against Cancer

www.uicc.orgdirectory/index.html

This is an international directory of cancer institutes and organizations.

Komen.org

www.komen.org

The Susan G. Komen Breast Cancer Foundation is dedicated to education and research on breast cancer causes, treatment, and the search for a cure.

Melanoma Patient Educator and Counselor

www.melanomasupport.com

Melanoma patient educator and counselor at the UCSF Melanoma Center, one of the country's leading melanoma treatment and research centers, Andrew W. Kneier, Ph.D., is available for telephone consultations.

MASCC—Multinational Association of Supportive Care in Cancer

www.mascc.org

The Multinational Association of Supportive Care in Cancer (MASCC) is a fully private, nonprofit-oriented professional and research-oriented association of physicians, nurses, and other healthcare professionals, aimed at optimizing all rational forms and aspects of supportive care in cancer patients, regardless of the stage of the disease.

Metastatic Cancer Index

www.cancerlynx.com/metastatic_index.html

This site provides advocate information for metastatic cancer patients and their families. It is a source for news, information, and personal stories about metastatic cancer.

National Center for Complementary and Alternative Medicine (NCCAM)

www.nccam.nih.gov

The National Center for Complementary and Alternative Medicine (NCCAM) at the National Institutes of Health (NIH) (www.nih.gov) is dedicated to exploring complementary and alternative healing practices in the context of rigorous science, training CAM researchers, and disseminating authoritative information.

National Cancer Institute

www.nci.nih.gov

This is the home page of the National Cancer Institute. It provides complete information on all aspects of cancer. A Spanish version is available.

National Cancer Survivors Day Foundation, Inc

www.ncsdf.org

The nonprofit National Cancer Survivors Day Foundation supports hundreds of local hospitals, support groups, and other cancer-related organizations throughout North America that hold National Cancer Survivors Day events. It provides guidance, education, and networking. In the beginning, cancer survivor Richard Bloch (cofounder of H&R Block) and his wife, Annette, held their first Cancer Survivor Rally in Kansas City. The idea soon caught on and has come to be known as National Cancer Survivors Day.

National Cancer Survivors Day—Northern California

www.survivorsday.com

On National Cancer Survivors Day, people from San Francisco and the Greater Bay Area gather to honor cancer survivors and join over seven hundred other communities throughout the United States and Canada in a celebration of life. It is also a day to recognize the medical professionals who are helping fight the battle against cancer.

National Institutes of Health (NIH)

www.nih.gov

This is the official website of the National Institutes of Health (NIH). The National Institutes of Health is one of the world's foremost medical research centers. An agency of the U.S. Department of Health and Human Services, the NIH is the federal focal point for health research. The NIH is the steward of biomedical and behavioral research for the nation. Its mission is science in pursuit of fundamental knowledge about the nature and behavior of living systems, the application of that knowledge to extend healthy life, and the reduction of the burdens of illness and disability.

National Library of Medicine—Home Page

www.nlm.nih.gov

The National Library of Medicine (NLM), on the campus of NIH in Bethesda, Maryland, is the world's largest medical library. It collects materials in all major areas of the health sciences, and to a lesser degree in such areas as chemistry, physics, botany, and zoology. The NLM has one of the world's finest medical history collections of old (pre-1914) and rare medical texts, manuscripts, and incunabula.

OncoLink: A University of Pennsylvania Cancer Center Resource

www.oncolink.com

This is a resource of the University of Pennsylvania Cancer Center. It offers in-depth information about cancer.

Oncology Nursing Society (ONS) Online
www.ons.org
This is the official Web service of the Oncology Nursing Society.

Additional Foreign Resources

American Cancer Society, Chinese Unit
www.cancer-chinese.org
Information in Chinese and English

Deutsches Krebsforschungszentrum
(German Cancer Research Center)
mbi.dkfz-heidelberg.de
DKFZ Heidelberg—Div. Medical and Biological Informatics
Information in German and English

Hebrew University Faculty of Medicine
www.md.huji.ac.il
Information in Hebrew and English

Institut Gustave-Roussy
www.igr.fr
Information in French and English

Karolinska Institutet
www.mic.ki.se/Diseases/
Information in Danish, English, Norwegian, and Swedish

King Faisal Specialist Hospital & Research Centre
www.kfshrc.edu.sa
Information in Arabic and English

National Cancer Center—Japan
www.ncc.go.jp
Information in Japanese and English

National Cancer Institute of Canada Website
(Site Web de l'Institut national du cancer du Canada)
www.ncic.cancer.ca
Information in French and English

49

A Web Tutorial

Alexandra Andrews
Teddy Andrews
Annamarie Baldessari
David Bradley
Bob Gill
Larry Hengl
Michael McMillan

First Things to Know about Websites, Web Addresses, and Security

Examples used here are based on the latest version of the Netscape Communicator. Other browsers may rearrange the features described below, but will usually include them in similar ways.

The term URL means Uniform Resource Locator. When you see HYPERLINK http://www.cancersupportivecare.com, it means (http:// = Hypertext Transfer Protocol) + (www = World Wide Web) + (domain = cancersupportivecare) + (.com = commercial).

If you type the Web address http://www.cancersupportivecare.com into the window and press Enter, you will see the following image.

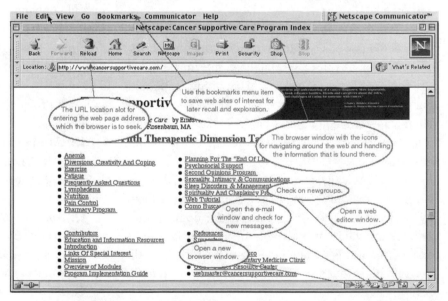

Type the address http://www.cancersupportivecare.com/links.html into the window and press Enter. This will take you to a page named links.html. (HTML means hypertext markup language.) Always type website addresses as shown. Never substitute capital letters for lower case, or vice versa. In general, copy the exact spacing of all letters, words, etc. Be sure to look closely: what may appear to a blank space may in fact be an underscore, and this, too, must be written as shown.

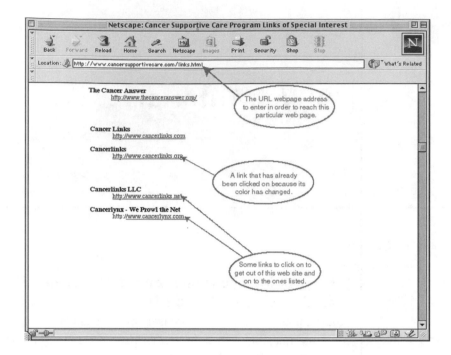

Keep in mind that many sites are not secure. Never use your normal login and password. Create a unique login and password for sites that ask for personal information. This will help protect you from unscrupulous Web pirates seeking your private data.

Cookies

Q: *What are cookies?*

A cookie is a piece of information stored in the visitor's browser. It might be database information, custom page settings, or just about anything. A popular analogy is to the receipt you get from a dry cleaner. When you return for your clothes, the dry cleaner matches tickets to ensure that the correct items are returned.

More technically, a cookie is an HTTP header consisting of a text-only string to be entered into the memory of a browser. This string contains the domain, path, lifetime, and value of a variable that a website sets. If the lifetime of this variable is longer than the time the user spends at that site, then this string is saved to file for future reference.

Users need to know that a website can only read the cookie it places on your browser. If the domain and path attributes match those of the host document (the default), cookies can be stored and retrieved. There is a common perception that someone can read everything in the cookie file. This is false. A website can only read what it puts there—nothing else.

Q: *Are they dangerous to my computer or my privacy?*

No. A cookie is a simple piece of text. It is not a program or a plug-in, and thus, it cannot access your hard drive. It cannot be used as a virus. Your browser (not a programmer) can save cookies to its memory (RAM) or a file on your hard disk if necessary, but that is the limit of its effects on your system. A cookie cannot read your hard drive to find out who you are, where you live, what your income is, or other personal information. The only way that information could end up in a cookie is if you provide it to a site and that site saves it to a cookie.

Q: *Can cookies fill my hard drive?*

No. Most major browsers (Netscape & Microsoft Internet Explorer) limit the number and size of cookies.

Q: *Am I at the mercy of the website when it comes to cookie control?*

No. You have the power to set your browser preferences to reject cookies.

Q: *Why do we need cookies?*

Cookies are very useful for identifying users of the Web. Unless something special is done, Web servers are only aware of users when a transaction such as sending or receiving information is in process. The moment the transaction is complete, the server forgets about the user. Only with cookies can transactions be correlated with previous exchanges. An HTTP connection and transaction can be distilled into the following steps:

1. The browser contacts the server at the address specified in the URL and requests a page. While open, the browser awaits the reply.
2. The server sends the state of the transaction back to the browser with the requested data or an error code.
3. The connection is closed. The server retains no memory of the transaction.

A few advertising companies use controversial cookie tactics. They have cleverly discovered ways to track users and access information without violating any laws. Advertisers can collect your personal information without you ever entering it on their sites. When you click on their graphics or banners, your cookies and data are transmitted to their sites that contain databases and store information about you. Such sites carrying this kind of advertising could be compromising your privacy. This usage of cookies has polarized opinions on cookies, privacy, and the Internet. Regulatory committees are currently working on proposals to ban or limit this kind of cookie usage.

Cookies have obvious appeal for corporate webmasters because they make it possible for users to customize their interaction with large, complex websites, and to customize the way they view a website.

For some situations, cookies offer the best and most practical business solution. One example is an online shopping site. The site's webmaster can use cookies to implement a "shopping cart," allowing you to spread a single shopping session across several visits to the site. Nominal customer information and shopping cart items can be stored in the cookie file, and recalled whenever the user revisits the online mall. In most cases, websites store minimal information in the persistent cookie on the user's system as an index of details, such as customer profiles and shopping cart items.

Temporary vs. Persistent Cookies

Netscape Communications and Amazon.com use temporary or session cookies to store information for shoppers. Temporary cookies can be used in conjunction with data stored in a login database to regulate participation in a website's service. When the user closes the browser or surfs to a new site, the cookie is either dropped or is written by the browser to the hard drive for later reference. They enable sites to spread products and information over multiple pages or to put order and entry forms on a separate page.

Persistent cookies—those stored on a user's file system—are used each time the user visits a website. They can prevent duplicate user identifications from being generated. Each time an established user logs into a restricted site, the server and database compare the browser cookie against the database record. Each connection attempt is logged, together with a variety of tidbits, such as browser type, Internet Protocol address, and operating system. If the browser cookie and the cookie stored in the server database match, access is granted and the cookie is replaced with a new unique identifier. This prevents others from using your login name and password.

Netscape uses persistent cookies to enable users to set preferences for viewing the site, for example with or without frames. Many sites use persistent cookies to customize what kind of information the user prefers to see when he or she logs onto the site. These cookies can also be used to store registration information so that users do not have to enter a login and password each time they visit a site. Websites store the information necessary for entrance in a persistent cookie. If a user loses or discards the cookie, he or she simply needs to repeat the manual login process, which establishes a new cookie.

If cookies are not used, there are still other methods for maintaining a user specific record. Information can be collected through forms and pasted between pages within the URL, as well as between pages in hidden HTML fields, which are actually passed in the HTTP header. Both methods have limitations. Both expose data during transmission (unless used in a secured session using something like secure sockets layer, or SSL).

Reminders

Users have the power to reject cookies, so if the Web industry wants to use them, it is going to have to use them responsibly. Privacy policies should be developed that give users proper notice, choices, and security regarding whatever information is being put into cookies and how those cookies are used.

You can choose your cookie options when you set up your preferences through your browser. You may

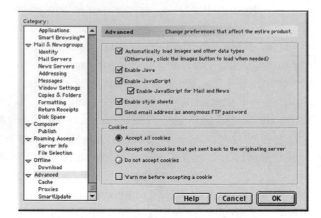

want to periodically erase the information in your cookie file. Go to the help file on your browser for more information.

To protect your privacy, be thoughtful when providing information that seems unrelated to the purpose of your visit, particularly if you encounter statements like the following:

> This information may be shared with our business partners on an aggregate basis only. The purpose of sharing this information is to help our business partners understand our customers.

> We also provide personal information to our vendors and suppliers where it is necessary for them to provide us with products and services related to better operation and maintenance of our website ("Vendors"). We will attempt to require that each of these Vendors not further use or disclose your personal information for any purpose other than providing us or you with products and services. Of course, we cannot guarantee their compliance with these restrictions.

Searches on the Internet
Internet Search Tips

1. Put in the search words—dog, cat. Then change the order of the words—cat, dog—to find other different sites that your first search might not have generated.
2. Add other keywords if you do not get many hits from your initial search.
3. You can chain the words together by adding a + sign (dog+cat+leash).
4. To do a narrower search, add quotation marks ("cat dog leash").
5. You can use the advanced search available on different search engines, but most people prefer to use open searches to get the most information possible.

Advanced Searches

If you want to find something really specific, an expert or power search can be really helpful. With power searching, you can specify exactly what you want, and more importantly, you can specify what you don't want. Power searches give you the ability to seek out and discover new civilizations—instead of just stumbling upon them.

Usually, the first search that you do on any given topic is a general search to get a sense of how many results will be returned. Then, to narrow your search, try an expert search. The following ideas apply to expert searches on most search engines:

- *keyword:* cats
- *case sensitivity* (capital and lower case type): Dogs will not match dogs
- *and:* dogs and cats
- *or:* dogs or cats
- *not:* dogs not cats, or dogs and not cats
- *phrase:* "dogs and cats" will not find cats and dogs
- *nested parentheses:* (small cell and lung cancer) and not (non small cell)

Every search engine also has its own features. You can learn more about the search engine that you are using by going to the help files on the site. The three following search engines are particularly useful:

1. **www.hotbot.com:** This engine allows you to use the advanced search, or there is a menu under "all the words" where you can select

phrases such as "small cell" and "lung cancer."

2. **www.northernlight.com:** This site has several searches listed at the bottom of the page. Try the power search.

3. **www.google.com:** Google has two types of searches. The open search is "google search" and the narrow search is "I'm feeling lucky."

When you are looking for information on a particular topic, sometimes distracting sites will pop up. It is easy to lose focus and become lost in a jungle of websites. Our suggestion is to bookmark the interesting sites as you search, and return to them later. Remember the phrase from Star Wars, "Stay on target, Luke!" To bookmark a site, pull down "bookmarks" or "favorites" at the top of your screen next to the location bar. Just click on Add and continue with your search. There is usually an "edit bookmarks" feature—or something similar—which will enable you to delete unwanted bookmarks.

Helpful Search Engines

www.aol.com

www.go.com

www.lycos.com

www.netscape.com

www.webcrawler.com

www.yahoo.com

www.dmoz.org

www.altavista.com

www.excite.com

www.looksmart.com

www.askjeeves.com

www.metacrawler.com

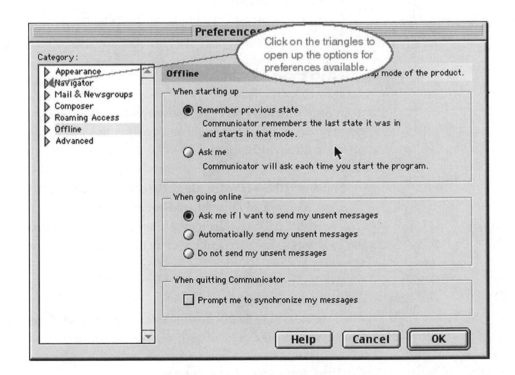

50

Directory of Resources and Support Groups

Meta-Search Engines for Cancer Information

If you are looking for specific cancer information, use one of these large cancer search engines. For more information or referrals, please contact the Cancer Resource Center at (415) 885-3693.

Cancer Links

www.cancerlinks.com

Over two thousand links to cancer information. A complete source and guide.

Cancerlinks.org

www.cancerlinks.org

A comprehensive and exhaustive listing of informative cancer URLs for twenty-four different types of cancers. Has links to cancer information in eighteen different languages.

Hardin M.D.—Hardin Meta-Directory of Internet Health Sources

www.lib.uiowa.edu/hardin/md/index.html

The entry page to Hardin M.D. from the University of Iowa. Provides the best lists of links in health and medicine.

Healthfinder

www.healthfinder.gov

A guide to reliable health information. Developed by the U.S. Department of Health and Human Services.

Online Cancer Resources

Here are some sites you may wish to visit as you begin your Internet research of supportive care centers.

American Cancer Society

www.cancer.org

The American Cancer Society is the nationwide community-based voluntary health organization dedicated to eliminating cancer as a major health problem by preventing cancer, saving lives, and diminishing suffering from cancer through research, education, advocacy, and service. Its services are available in English and Spanish. 1-800-ACS-2345 (hotline)

American Hospice Foundation

www.americanhospice.org

This organization teaches about hospice care through public education programs focused on strategically selected audiences such as employers, schools, insurance companies, and religious organizations.

American Institute for Cancer Research

www.aicr.org

The American Institute for Cancer Research is the nation's leading charity in the field of diet, nutrition, and cancer prevention.

American Red Cross

www.redcross.org

Provides emergency services.

American Society of Clinical Oncology: ASCO OnLine

www.asco.org

The American Society of Clinical Oncology is an interactive resource for oncology professionals and cancer patients.

Association of Oncology Social Work (AOSW)

www.aosw.org

Oncology social work is the primary professional discipline providing psychosocial services to patients, families, and caregivers facing the impact of cancer diagnosis and treatment.

Cancer Care

www.cancercare.org

Cancer Care provides emotional support, information, and practical help to people with cancer and their loved ones. 1-800-813-HOPE

Cancer Links Bone Marrow Transplants and Registries

www.cancerlinks.com/marrow.html

Cancer Supportive Care

www.cancersupportivecare.com

This site provides current and up-to-date resources to complement surgery, radiation, chemotherapy, and immunotherapy for total supportive care.

Candlelighters Childhood Cancer Foundation (CCCF)

www.candlelighters.org

Founded in 1970 by concerned parents of children with cancer.

Cancer Net from the National Cancer Institute

www.cancernet.nci.nih.gov

Credible, current, and comprehensive cancer information from the National Cancer Institute. 1-800-4-CANCER

Children's Hospice International

www.chionline.org

CHI recognizes the right and need for children and their families to choose the kind of health care and support they need, whether it is in their own home, hospital, or hospice.

Choice In Dying, Inc.

www.choices.org

Choice In Dying, Inc., the inventor of living wills in 1967, is dedicated to fostering communication about complex, end-of-life decisions. The nonprofit organization provides advance directives, counsels patients and families, trains professionals, advocates for improved laws, and offers a range of publications and services.

Hospice Foundation of America

www.hospicefoundation.org

A not-for-profit organization that provides leadership in the development and application of hospice and its philosophy of care.

Hospice HotLinks

www.teleport.com/~hospice/links.htm

Provides many links to hospices in the United States and around the world.

International Federation of Red Cross and Red Crescent Societies

www.ifrc.org

The International Federation of Red Cross and Red Crescent Societies is the world's largest humanitarian organization, providing assistance without discrimination as to nationality, race, religious beliefs, class, or political opinions.

International Association for the Study of Pain

www.halcyon.com/iasp

An international, multidisciplinary, nonprofit professional association dedicated to furthering research on pain and improving the care of patients with pain.

International Union Against Cancer

www.uicc.org/directory/index.html

An international directory of cancer institutes and organizations.

ONS Online

www.ons.org

The official Web service of the Oncology Nursing Society.

Resource Center Websites

On-Line Medical Resource Center—Health/Medical

www.healthlinks.com

Health-Related Resource Center, worldwide information for people in or dealing with the medical profession.

Hospital do Cancer—AC Camargo—Sao Paulo, Brazil

www.hcanc.org.br

A cancer reference hospital site in Sao Paulo, Brazil. The institution deals with treatment, prevention, research, and education in cancer-related topics. Information in English, Spanish, and Portuguese.

Mexican MedLine

www.medline.com.mx

Medical online information from Mexico.

National Institutes of Health (NIH)

www.nih.gov/health

The Consumer Health Page for the National Institutes of Health (NIH); administered by the NIH Office of Communications and Public Liaison.

National Library of Medicine

www.nlm.nih.gov

The National Library of Medicine (NLM), on the campus of NIH in Bethesda, Maryland, is the world's largest medical library. It collects materials in all major areas that health sciences offers. PubMed and Internet Grateful Med are two free systems to search MEDLINE.

OncoLink

www.oncolink.com

A University of Pennsylvania Cancer Center resource. Here you will find in-depth information about cancer.

Online Support Groups

Association of Cancer Online Resources (ACOR)

www.acor.org

ACOR.org cancer information system currently offers access to ninety-nine electronic mailing lists and a variety of unique websites. The mailing lists are specifically designed to be public, online support groups providing information and community.

CataList

www.lsoft.com/lists/listref.html

A catalog of LISTSERV lists. From this page, you can browse any of the 33,330 public LISTSERV lists on the Internet, search for mailing lists of interest, and find information about LISTSERV host sites.

Liszt

www.liszt.com

A large directory of mailing lists and newsgroups. You're bound to find something you're interested in.

Cancer Advocacy Groups

Komen.org

www.komen.org

The Susan G. Komen Breast Cancer Foundation's website. Information is provided in English and Spanish.

R.A. Bloch Cancer Foundation, Inc

www.blochcancer.org

Richard Bloch Cancer Foundation's website.

Additional Support Resources

American Cancer Society
1599 Clifton Road, NE
Atlanta, GA 30329
1-800-227-2345

American Cancer Society
235 Montgomery Street, Suite 320
San Francisco, CA 94104
(415) 394-7100
ACS is a nationwide organization dedicated to research, education, and service. Provides information on support groups, educational materials, financial aid, loans, and medical equipment.

American Foundation for Urologic Disease
300 W. Pratt Street, Suite 401
Baltimore, MD 21201
1-800-828-7866
Provides information on support groups for people with prostate cancer and their families, and information on other urologic disorders.

Cancer Care, Inc.
1180 Avenue of the Americas, 2nd Floor
New York, NY 10036
1-800-813-HOPE
Cancer Care is dedicated to providing psychological support and information to people with cancer and their families. Provides telephone and online support groups, a counseling line and free teleconferences for patients, families, and friends.

Cancer Hope Network
2 North Road, Suite A
Chester, NJ 07930
(877) HOPENET
www.cancerhopenetwork.org
Matches cancer patients to survivors. Also has a small database of family members and caregivers of cancer patients.

Ida and Joseph Friend Cancer Resource Center
University of California at San Francisco
Comprehensive Cancer Center
2356 Sutter Street, First Floor
San Francisco, CA 94143-1725
http://cc.ucsf.edu/crc
Provides health information on treatment options and clinical trials, health insurance and benefits counseling, nutrition counseling, support groups, peer support program, classes and workshops, and information and referral services in the San Francisco Bay Area. The Cancer Resource Center also has a library of books, audiotapes and videotapes, support groups, yoga, exercise, dance and movement classes, lectures, educational materials, and community referrals.

Candlelighters Childhood Foundation
7910 Woodmont Avenue, Suite 460
Bethesda, MD 20814
1-800-366-CCCF
The CCCF is an organization formed by parents of young cancer patients. An important goal of the organization is to help families cope with the emotional stresses of their experiences.

Center for Attitudinal Healing
33 Buchanan Drive
Sausalito, CA 94965
(415) 331-6161
Provides nonsectarian spiritual and emotional support. Services include: counseling and support groups, an information and referral service, and a speaker's bureau. Provides information, education, and referrals.

Choice in Dying, Inc.
200 Varick Street, 10th Floor, Room 1001
New York, NY 10014
1-800-989-9455
www.choices.org
Provides information that can help people prepare for "end of life" decisions. Services include legal assistance, pain management, and a speakers' bureau. Also has a twenty-four-hour counseling/crisis hotline for families concerned about treatments and refusal of treatment situations.

Commonweal
P.O. Box 316
Bolinas, CA 94924
(415) 868-0970
A center for service and research in health and human ecology. The program helps people seek physical, emotional, and spiritual healing. Offers workshops for people with cancer and for health care providers working with cancer patients.

Helpline
50 California Street, Suite 200
San Francisco, CA 94111-4696
(415) 772-HELP
General information and referral services for health and human service agencies in San Francisco and Marin Counties.

Hospice Education Institute
190 Westbrook Road
Essex, CT 06426
1-800-331-1620
Provides information to the public and professionals about hospice and palliative care. Services include a toll-free information and referral service (Hospice Link), regional seminars, professional education, advice, and assistance.

Leukemia and Lymphoma Society Northern California Chapter
832 Folsom Street, 9th Floor
San Francisco, CA 94105
(415) 543-9821
Provides information and referral, support groups, financial help with transportation, and a quarterly newsletter for people with leukemia, lymphoma, multiple myeloma, and Hodgkin's disease.

Lymphoma Research Foundation
8800 Venice Boulevard, #207
Los Angeles, CA 90034
(310) 204-7040
www.lymphoma.org
A nonprofit organization that funds research grants, provides educational materials, an information line, free support groups, a buddy program called "Cell Mates," and a quarterly newsletter.

National Alliance of Breast Cancer Organizations
9 East 37th Street
New York, NY 10016
A nonprofit central resource for education and information about breast cancer. Information for a network of three hundred seventy-five organizations providing detection, treatment, and care.

National Cancer Institute
Building 31, Room 10A16
Bethesda, MD 20892
1-800-4CANCER
NCI provides information on cancer treatments, clinical trials, and services for patients and their families. Also provides free publications.

National Chronic Pain Outreach Association
7979 Old Georgetown Road, Suite 100
Bethesda, MD 20814
(301) 652-4948
NCPOA works to lessen the suffering of people with chronic pain by educating pain sufferers, health care professionals, and the public about chronic pain and its management.

National Hospice Organization
1901 N Moore Street, Suite 901
Arlington, VA 22209
1-800-658-8898
Provides information and referrals to local hospice programs via a toll-free number. Other services include patient advocacy and professional education.

Planetree Health Resource Center
California Pacific Medical Center
2040 Webster Street
San Francisco, CA 94115
(415) 923-3680
Planetree has a library of books and resources. People can research topics at the library free of charge. Provides

in-depth research on any medical diagnosis for a fee, has a lecture series, and has a guide to community referrals.

RA Bloch Cancer Foundation, Inc.

4400 Main Street

Kansas City, MO 64111

1-800-433-0464

Matches cancer patients with survivors. Provides a list of institutions that provide multidisciplinary second opinions for patients if requested within three weeks of diagnosis or recurrence.

RESOLVE, Inc.

1310 Broadway

Somerville, MA 02144

(617) 623-0744

www.ihr.com/resolve

A national organization helping infertile people and the medical infertility community. Services include sexual therapy, support groups, a newsletter, a help-line, a physician referral service, medical call-in hours, a member-to-member contact system, and support services through local chapters.

The Wellness Community

1777 N. California Boulevard, Suite 200

Walnut Creek, CA

(925) 933-0107

Offers yoga, tai chi chuan, Qigong, relaxation, visualization, and support groups.

Women's Cancer Resource Center

3023 Shattuck Avenue

Berkeley, CA 94705

(510) 548-9272 or (510) 548-9286

Provides information and referral services, support groups, peer referral, library services, and educational materials.

51

Books and Tapes

Alexandra Andrews, Webmaster,
Cancer Supportive Care

Cancer: Diagnosis Information and Treatment

Understanding Cancer: What It Is and How It Is Treated

The Activist Cancer Patient: How to Take Charge of Your Treatment by Beverly Zakarian, introduction by Ezra M. Greenspan, M.D. John Wiley & Sons, 1996.

Be Prepared: The Complete Financial, Legal and Practical Guide for Living with a Life-Challenging Condition by David S. Landay. St. Martin's Press, 1998.

Biological Approaches to Cancer Treatment: Biomodulation by Malcolm S. Mitchell. Health Professions, 1992.

Cancer: 50 Essential Things to Do by Greg Anderson, introduction by O. Carl Simonton. Plume, 1999.

Cancer Clinical Trials: Experimental Treatments and How They Can Help You by Robert Finn. O'Reilly & Associates, 1999.

Cancer Treatment by Charles M. Haskell. W.B. Saunders Co., 1995.

The Complete Cancer Survival Guide: Everything You Must Know and Where to Go for State-of-the-Art Treatment of the 25 Most Common Forms of Cancer by Peter Teeley and Philip Bashe. Main Street Books, 2000.

Diagnosis Cancer: Your Guide to the First Few Months, 2nd ed. by Wendy Harpham. W.W. Norton & Co., 1997.

Everyone's Guide to Cancer Therapy by Malin Dollinger, Ernest H Rosenbaum, Margeret Tempero, and Sean J. Mulvihill. Andrews McMeel, 2001.

Informed Decisions: The Complete Book of Cancer Diagnosis, Treatment and Recovery by Gerald P. Murphy, Lois B. Morris, and Dianne Lange. Viking, 1997.

Making Informed Medical Decisions by Nancy Oster, Lucy Thomas, and Darol Joseff. O'Reilly & Associates, 2000.

One Renegade Cell: How Cancer Begins by Robert A. Weinberg. Basic Books, 1999.

The Wellness Community Guide to Fighting for Recovery from Cancer by Harold H. Benjamin and Susan M. Love. J. P. Tarcher, 1995.

What to Do When They Say "It's Cancer": A Survivor's Guide by Joel Nathan. Allen & Unwin, 1999.

When Bad Things Happen to Good People, rev. ed. by Harold Kushner. G.K. Hall, 1997.

When Your Friend Gets Cancer: How You Can Help by Amy Harwell, Kristine Tomasik et al. Harold Shaw Publishers, 1987.

Women's Bodies, Women's Wisdom: Creating Physical and Emotional Health and Healing by Christiane Northrup. Bantam Doubleday Dell Publishing Group, 1998.

Caregiving

American College of Physicians Home Care Guide for Cancer: How to Care for Family and Friends at Home by Peter S. Houts. American College of Physicians, 1996.

The Comfort of Home: An Illustrated Step-by-Step Guide for Caregivers by Maria M. Meyer and Paula Derr. CareTrust Publications, 1998.

Caregiver's Handbook by Visiting Nurses Association, Deni Bown. D.K. Publishing, 1998.

Helping Yourself Help Others: A Book for Caregivers by Rosalynn Carter. Times Books, 1996.

Share the Care: How to Organize a Group to Care for Someone Who Is Seriously Ill by Cappy Caposella and Sheila Warnock. Fireside, 1995.

Chemotherapy and Bone Marrow Transplantation

Autologous Stem Cell Transplants: A Handbook for Patients by Susan Stewart. The Blood & Marrow Information Network, 1999. To order call 1-888 597-7674.

Bone Marrow Transplants: A Book of Basics for Patients by Susan Stewart. The Blood & Marrow Information Network, 1992. To order call 1-888 597-7674.

Cancer Chemotherapy: Concepts, Clinical Investigations and Therapeutic Advances in Cancer Treatment and Research edited by F.M. Muggia. Kluwer Academic Publishers, 1989.

The Chemotherapy and Radiation Therapy Survival Guide by Judith McKay and Nancee Hirano. Harbinger, 1998.

Survivor's Guide to a Bone Marrow Transplant and Bone Marrow Transplant Resource Guide by Keren Stronach. The Blood & Marrow Information Network, 2000. To order, call 1-888-597-7674.

Clinical Trials

Cancer Clinical Trials: Experimental Treatments and How They Can Help You by Robert K. Finn, Linda Lamb. O'Reilly & Associates, 1999.

Children and Parents

How to Help Children Through a Parent's Serious Illness by Kathleen McCue, Ron Bonn. St. Martin's Press, 1996.

Moms Don't Get Sick by Pat Brack and Ben Brack. Melius Publishing Company, 1990.

Doctor Patient Relationship

The Activist Cancer Patient: How to Take Charge of Your Treatment by Beverly Zakarian, introduction by Ezra M. Greenspan, M.D. John Wiley & Sons, 1996.

Getting the Best from Your Doctor: An Insider's Guide to the Health Care You Deserve by Alan N. Schwartz. HarperCollins, 1999.

The Healing Touch: Keeping the Doctor-Patient Relationship Alive Under Managed Care by David L. Cram, Pamela A. Baj, edited by Rod Colvin. Addicus Books, 1997.

Take This Book to the Hospital with You: A Consumer Guide to Surviving Your Hospital Stay by Charles B. Inlander, contribution by Ed Weiner. St. Martin's Mass Market Paper, 1997.

What to Do When They Say "It's Cancer": A Survivor's Guide by Joel Nathan. Allen & Unwin, 1999.

When Your Friend Gets Cancer: How You Can Help by Amy Harwell, Kristine Tomasik et al. Harold Shaw Publishers, 1987.

Working with Your Doctor: Getting the Healthcare You Deserve by Nancy Keene. O'Reilly & Associates, 1998.

Lymphedema

Lymphedema: A Breast Cancer Patient's Guide to Prevention and Healing by Jeannie Burt, Gwen White, and Judith R. Casley-Smith. Hunter House, 1999.

Textbook of Dr. Vodder's Manual Lymph Drainage by Ingrid Kurz. Medicina Biologica, 1997.

Ostomy

The Ostomy Book: Living Comfortably with Colostomies, Ileostomies and Urostomies by Barbara Dorr Mullen and Kerry McGinn. Bull Publishing, 1991.

Pain

Cancer Pain edited by Richard B. Patt. Lippincott Raven, 1993.

A Child In Pain: How to Help, What to Do by Leora Kuttner. Hartley & Marks, 1996.

Managing Pain Before It Manages You by Margaret A. Caudill. Guilford Press, 1994.

Second Opinions
Second Opinions: Stories of Intuition and Choice in a Changing World of Medicine by Jerome Groopman. Viking, 2000.

The Role of the Mind, Alternative and Complementary Medicine

The Alternative Medicine Handbook: The Complete Reference Guide to Alternative and Complementary Therapies by Barrie R. Cassileth. W.W. Norton, 1998.

American Cancer Society's Guide to Complementary and Alternative Cancer Methods foreword by David S. Rosentha. The American Cancer Society, 2000.

Cancer as a Turning Point: A Handbook for People with Cancer, Their Families and Health Professionals by Lawrence LeShan. Plume, 1999.

Choices in Healing: Integrating the Best of Conventional and Alternative Approaches to Cancer by Michael Lerner. MIT Press, 1996.

Close to the Bone: Life-Threatening Illness and the Search for Meaning by Jean Shinoda-Bolen. Simon & Schuster,1998.

Full Catastrophe Living: Using the Wisdom of Your Body and Mind to Face Stress, Pain and Illness by Jon Kabat-Zinn, preface by Thich Nhat Hanh, and Joan Borysenko. Delta, 1991.

The Healer Within: The Four Essential Self-Care Techniques for Optimal Health by Roger O. Jahnke. Harper, 1999.

The Human Side of Cancer: Living With Hope, Coping With Uncertainty by Jimmie C. Holland and Sheldon Lewis. HarperCollins, 2000.

Inner Fire: Your Will to Live by Ernest H. Rosenbaum and Isadora Rosenbaum. Plexus, 1999.

Chicken Soup for the Surviving Soul: 101 Stories to Comfort Cancer Patients and Their Loved Ones edited by Jack Canfield, Bernie S. Siegel, and Patty Aubrey. Health Communications, 1996.

The Honest Herbal: A Sensible Guide to the Use of Herbs and Related Remedies by Steven Foster and Varro E. Tyler. Haworth, 1999.

The Relaxation Response by Herbert Benson. Wholecare, 2000.

Peace, Love and Healing: Bodymind Communication and the Path to Self-Healing: An Exploration by Bernie S. Siegel. HarperPerennial Library; 1990.

Self-Nurture: Learning to Care for Yourself As Effectively As You Care for Everyone Else by Alice D. Domar. Viking Penguin, 1999.

Guided Imagery for Groups: Fifty Visualizations That Promote Relaxation, Problem-Solving, Creativity and Well-Being by Andrew E. Schwartz. Whole Person Associates, 1995.

Love Just Screws Everything Up: A for Better or for Worse Collection by Lynn Johnston, Malin Dollinger, contribution by Greg Cable and Ernest H. Rosenbaum. Andrews McMeel, 1996.

For Poetry References
Finding What You Didn't Lose: Expressing your Truth and Creativity Through Poem-Making by John Fox and Jeremy P. Tarcher, 1995.

Poetic Medicine: The Healing Art of Poem-Making, John Fox and Jeremy P. Tarcher, 1997.

Group Support
Group Therapy for Cancer Patients: A Research-Based Handbook of Psychosocial Care by David Spiegel and Catherine Classen, 2000.

Massage Therapy
Compassionate Touch: Hands-On Caregiving for the Elderly, the Ill and the Dying by Dawn Nelson. Talman Company, 1993.

Medicine Hands: Massage Therapy for People with Cancer by Gayle MacDonald. Findhorn Press, 1999.

Care of the Body
The Essential Guide to Nutrition and the Foods We Eat: Everything You Need to Know about the Foods You Eat edited by the American Dietetic Association and Jean A. Thompson Pennington. HarperCollins, 1999.

The Hormone of Desire: The Truth About Sexuality, Menopause and Testosterone by Susan Rako. Three Rivers Press, 1999.

Sexuality and Fertility After Cancer by Leslie Schover. John Wiley & Sons, 1997.

Supportive and Social Services For Life and Death Issues
End of Life–Dying
Before I Say Goodbye: Recollections and Observations from One Woman's Final Year by Ruth Picardie. Henry Holt & Company, 2000.

The Dying Time: Practical Wisdom for the Dying and Their Caregivers by Joan Furman and David McNabb. Crown Publishing, 1997.

Dying Well: Peace and Possibilities at the End of Life by Ira Byock. Berkley Publishing Group, 1998.

The Fall of Freddie the Leaf: Story of Life for All Ages by Leo Buscaglia. Henry Holt & Co., 1982.

Final Gifts: Understanding the Special Awareness, Needs and Communications of the Dying by Maggie Callanan and Patricia Kelley. Poseidon Press, 1992.

The Handbook of Hospice Care by Robert W. Buckingham and forward by Rosemary Johnson Hurzeler. Prometheus Books, 1996.

Bereavement for Adults
How Do We Tell the Children?: A Step-by-Step Guide for Helping Children Two to Teen Cope When Someone Dies by

Dan Schaefer and Christine Lyons. Newmarket Press, 1993.

Mourning and Mitzvah: A Guided Journal for Walking the Mourner's Path Through Grief to Healing by Anne Brener. Jewish Lights Publishing, 1993.

Bereavement for Children

Straight Talk about Death for Teenagers: How to Cope with Losing Someone You Love by Earl Grollman. Beacon Press, 1993.

Talking About Death: A Dialogue Between Parent and Child by Earl Grollman. Beacon Press, 1990.

Planning For The Future

Cancer Survivors

After Cancer: A Guide to Your New Life by Wendy S. Harpham. HarperPerennial, 1995.

Be Prepared: The Complete Financial, Legal and Practical Guide for Living with a Life-Challenging Condition by David S. Landay. St. Martin's Press, 1998.

A Cancer Survivor's Almanac: Charting the Journey, 2nd ed. edited by Barbara Hoffman. Chronimed Publishing, 1998.

Childhood Cancer Survivors: A Practical Guide to Your Future by Nancy Keene, Wendy Hobbie, and Kathy Ruccione. O'Reilly & Associates, 2000.

Getting Your Affairs in Order by Elmo A. Petterle. Shelter Publications, 1993.

Living Beyond Breast Cancer: A Survivor's Guide for When Treatment Ends and the Rest of Your Life Begins by Maris C. Weiss, contribution by Ellen Weiss. Times Books, 1998.

Medicare Made Easy, 1999 by Charles B. Inlander and Michael A. Donio. Fine Communications, 1999.

The Savvy Medical Consumer by Charles B. Inlander. People's Medical Society, 1997.

The Road Back to Health: Coping with the Emotional Aspects of Cancer, rev. ed. by Neil A. Fiore. Celestial Arts, 1995.

Audiotapes

Coping with Cancer by Malin Dollinger, 1991.
   To order: 4305 Torrance Blvd #409
   Torrance, CA 90503

Understanding Cancer. Malin Dollinger. 1990.
   To order: 4305 Torrance Blvd #409
   Torrance, CA 90503

Body Relaxed—Mind at Ease by Harriett Sanders Karis. New Harbinger, 1994.

Cancers

The ABC's of Advanced Prostate Cancer by Mark A. Moyad and Kenneth J. Pienta. Sleeping Bear Press, 2000.

Advice to Doctors and Other Big People from Kids by the Center for Attitudinal Healing. Celestial Arts, 1991.

American Cancer Society: Women and Cancer: A Thorough and Compassionate Resource for Patients and Their Families by Carolyn D. Runowicz, Jeanne A. Petrek, Ted S. Gansler, Carolyn Runowitz, and Jeanne Petrick. Villard Books, 1999.

Assess Your True Risk of Breast Cancer by Patricia Kelly. Owl Books, 2000.

Breast Cancer: The Complete Guide by Y. Hirshaut and P. Pressman. Bantam, 1993.

The Breast Cancer Survival Manual: A Step-By-Step Guide for the Woman With Newly Diagnosed Cancer by John Link. Owl Books, 2000.

Cancer and Self-Help: Bridging the Troubled Waters of Childhood Illness by Mark A. Chesler and Barbara Chesney. The University of Wisconsin Press, 1995.

Cancers of the Mouth and Throat: A Patient's Guide to Treatment by William Lydiatt and Perry Johnson. Addicus Books, 2000.

The C-Word: Teenagers and Their Families Living with Cancer, rev. ed. by Elena Dorfman. New Sage Press, 1998.

Childhood Cancer: A Parent's Guide to Solid Tumor Cancers by Honna Janes-Hodder and Nancy Keene. O'Reilly & Associates, 1999.

Childhood Cancer Survivors: A Practical Guide to Your Future by Nancy Keene, Wendy Hobbie, and Kathy Ruccione. O'Reilly & Associates, 2000.

Colon and Rectal Cancer: A Comprehensive Guide for Patients and Families by Lorraine Johnston. O'Reilly & Associates, 2000.

The Cure of Childhood Leukemia: Into the Age of Miracles by John Lazlo. Rutgers University Press, 1996.

Dr. Susan Love's Breast Book, 3rd rev. ed. by Susan Love. Perseus Book Group, 2000.

Entre Mujeres: Su Recuperacion Fisica y Emocional Depues de la Mastectomia by Rosalind D. Benedet and illustrated by Shannon Abbey, Casa Hispana. Benedet Publishing, 1999. Breast cancer treatment information in Spanish. Also available at www.cancerlinks.com/Mujeres/index.html.

First Aid Yourself: Essential Breast Cancer Websites by Betsy Dance. Hope Springs Press, 2000. Also at www.firstaidyourself.org.

Gilda's Disease: Sharing Personal Experience and Medical Perspective on Ovarian Cancer by M. Steven Piver, with Gene Wilder. Prometheus Books, 1996.

The Gliomas edited by Mitchel S. Berger and Charles B. Wilson. W.B. Saunders, 1998.

The Guide to Living with Bladder Cancer by Mark P. Schoenberg. The Johns Hopkins University Press, 2000.

Living with Lung Cancer: A Guide for Patients and Their Families, 4th ed. by Barbara G. Cox et al. Triad Publishing Company, 1998.

The Lung Cancer Manual by the Alliance for Lung Cancer Advocacy, Support and Education (ALCASE). ALCASE, 1999. Can be ordered spiral-bound from ALCASE. Alliance for Lung Cancer, P.O. Box 849 Vancouver, WA, 98666 1(800) 298-2436 (US only), 360-696-2436, info@alcase.org.

Melanoma: Prevention, Detection and Treatment by Catherine M. Poole with DuPont Guerry, IV. Yale University Press, 1998.

Men, Women and Prostate Cancer: A Medical and Psychological Guide for Women and the Men They Love by Barbara Rubin Wainrib, et al. New Harbinger Publications, 2000.

Myths & Facts about Lung Cancer: What You Need to Know by John C. Ruckdeschel. PRR, Inc., 1999.

Neuro-Oncology: The Essentials by Mark Bernstein and Mitchel S. Berger. Thieme Medical Publishers, 1999.

Non-Hodgkin's Lymphoma: Making Sense of Diagnosis, Treatment and Options by Lorraine Johnston, 1999.

The Prostate Cancer Answer Book: An Unbiased Guide to Treatment Choices by Marion Morra, Eve Potts, and Vincent DeVita. Avon Books, 1996.

Saving Your Skin: Early Detection and Treatment of Melanoma and Other Skin Cancers, 2nd ed. by Barney J. Kenet and Patricia Lawler. Four Walls Eight Windows, 1998.

Additional References

1999 Oncology Nursing Drug Handbook by Gail M. Wilkes, Karen Ingwersen, and Margaret Barton Burke. Jones & Bartlett, 1998.

The American Cancer Society Cancer Book: Prevention, Detection, Diagnosis, Treatment, Rehabilitation, and Cure by Arthur I. Holleb et al. Doubleday, 1993.

The Cancer Dictionary by Robert Altman and Michael Sarg. Facts on File, 1994.

Cancer Nursing: Principles and Practice, 3rd ed. by Susan L. Groenwald et al. Jones and Bartlett, 1993.

Cancer: Principles and Practice of Oncology, 6th ed. by Vincent T. DeVita Jr. et al. Lippincott, 2000.

Cancer Chemotherapy Handbook, 4th ed. by David S. Fischer and M. Tish Knobf. Year Book Medical Publishers, 1993.

Cancer Chemotherapy: Principles and Practice by Bruce A. Chabner et al. Lippincott, 1990.

Cancer Medicine, 5th ed. by James F. Holland et al. Lea & Febiger, 2000.

Clinical Oncology, 2nd ed. edited by Martin D. Abeloff, James O. Armitage, and Allen S. Lichter. Churchill-Livingstone, 2000.

Comprehensive Textbook of Oncology, 2nd ed. by A.R. Moosa et al. Williams & Wilkins, 1991.

Consumers Guide to Cancer Drugs by The American Cancer Society. Jones & Bartlett, 2000.

The Encyclopedia of Medical Tests by Michael B. Brodin. Mass Market Paperback, 1997.

Everything You Need to Know about Medical Tests by Marcia Andrews. Springhouse Publishing Company, 1997.

Handbook of Pediatric Oncology by Roberta A. Gottlieb and Donald Pinkel. Little, Brown & Co., 1989.

Handbook of Psychooncology: Psychological Care of the Patient with Cancer by Jimmie C. Holland and Julia Rowland. Oxford University Press, 1989.

Manual of Clinical Oncology, 3rd ed. by Dennis Albert Casciato. Little, Brown & Co., 1995.

Manual of Oncologic Therapeutics, 3rd ed. by John S. MacDonald. Lippincott Raven, 1995.

The Merck Manual of Medical Information: Home Edition edited by Robert Berkow, Mark H. Beers, and Andrew J. Fletcher. Pocket Books, 1999.

Neoplastic Diseases of the Blood, 3rd ed. by P.H. Wiernik, G.P. Canellos, R.A. Kyle, and C.A. Schiffer. Churchill Livingstone, 1996.

Physicians' Desk Reference 2001, (PDR Series) by Medical Economics Staff, 2000.

PDR for Herbal Medicines Physician's Desk Reference for Herbal Medicines, 2nd ed. by Medical Economics Data, 2000.

The PDR Family Guide to Natural Medicines and Healing Therapies edited by David W. Sifton. Ballantine Books, 2000.

Principles and Practice of Radiation Oncology, 2nd ed. by Carlos A. Perez and Luther W. Brady. Lippincott Raven, 1992.

Authors and Contributors

Ernest H. Rosenbaum, M.D.

Clinical Professor of Medicine, University of California–San Francisco Comprehensive Cancer Center; Medical Director, Better Health Foundation, San Francisco; Clinical Professor, Department of Medicine, Stanford University Medical Center; Director, Cancer Supportive Care Program, Stanford Complementary Medicine Clinic, Stanford University Medical Center.

Ernest H. Rosenbaum's career has included a fellowship at the Blood Research Laboratory of Tufts University School of Medicine (New England Center Hospital) and MIT. He teaches at the University of California–San Francisco Comprehensive Cancer Center. He was the cofounder of the Northern California Academy of Clinical Oncology and founded the Better Health Foundation and the Cancer Supportive Care Program at the Stanford Complementary Medicine Clinic Stanford University Medical School.

His passionate interest in clinical research and developing ways to improve patient care and communications with patients and colleagues has resulted in more than fifty articles on cancer and hematology in various medical journals. He also has participated in many radio and television programs and frequently lectures to medical and public groups.

He has written numerous books, including *Living with Cancer: A Home Care Training Program for Cancer Patients; Decisions for Life: You Can Live 10 Years Longer with Better Health; The Comprehensive Guide for Cancer Patients and Their Families* and *Everyone's Guide to Cancer Therapy*. For the latter two works, Ernest and Isadora Rosenbaum, Malin Dollinger, M.D., and Greg Cable received Honorable Mention for Excellence in Medical Publications in 1980 and 1991 from the American Medical Writers Association. Dr. Rosenbaum also coauthored *Nutrition for the Cancer Patient*.

Isadora Rosenbaum, M.A.

Isadora Rosenbaum is a medical assistant who worked in immunology research and is currently at an oncology practice at the UCSF Comprehensive Cancer Center offering advice and psychosocial support. She coauthored *Nutrition for the Cancer Patient* and *The Comprehensive*

Guide for Cancer Patients and Their Families. She has written chapters in *Everyone's Guide to Cancer Therapy, Living with Cancer,* and *You Can Live 10 Years Longer with Better Health.*

Gary M. Abrams, M.D.
 Associate Professor of Clinical Neurology, University of California School of Medicine, San Francisco, CA

Mark Abramson, D.D.S.
 TMD, Orofacial Pain Management, Mindfulness-Based Stress Reduction Programs, Stanford Complementary Medicine Clinic, Health Improvement Program, Stanford University School of Medicine.

Thomas Addison, M.D.
 Clinical Professor of Medicine, UCSF, Kaiser Permanente, San Francisco, CA

Alexandra Andrews.
 Webmaster, The Cancer Supportive Care Program, cancerlinks.com or cancerlynx.com

Rabbi Joseph Asher (deceased)
 Temple Emanuel, San Francisco, CA

Joseph S. Bailes, M.D.
 Director, Executive Vice President and Medical Director, Physician Reliance Network, Inc., Dallas, Texas; Past President and Member, Board of Directors, and Chairman, Clinical Practice Committee, American Society of Clinical Oncology; Clinical Associate Professor of Medicine, University of Texas Health Science Center, San Antonio, TX

Joanna Beam, J.D.
 University Counsel, University of California

Christopher Benz, M.D.
 Associate Professor of Medicine, Cancer Research Institute and Division of Hematology-Oncology, University of California School of Medicine, San Francisco, CA

Sharya Vaughn Bourdet, Pharm.D.
 Pharmacology, UCSF

Judy Bray, O.C.
 Formerly Chief, Occupational Therapy, UCSF/ Mt. Zion Hospital

David G. Bullard, Ph.D.
 Associate Clinical Professor of Medicine and of Medical Psychology (Psychiatry), University of California School of Medicine, San Francisco, CA

Jean M. Bullard, R.N., M.S.
 Utilization Management, Veterans Administration Medical Center, San Francisco, CA; Formerly counselor for Patients' Sexual Issues, Veterans Administration Medical Center, San Francisco, CA; Lecturer, Department of Nursing, San Francisco State University, CA

Barrie R. Cassileth, Ph.D.
 Chief, Integrative Medicine, Department of Medicine, Memorial Sloan-Kettering, New York, NY

Paula Chung
 Office Oncology Practice, UCSF Comprehensive Cancer Center, San Francisco, CA

Catherine Coleman, R.N.
 Coleman Breast Cancer Center Consultation Services, Tiburon, CA

John P. Cooke, M.D., Ph.D.
 Division of Cardiovascular Medicine, Falk Cardiovascular Research Center, Stanford University School of Medicine, Stanford, CA

Diane Craig, R.N. Onc, B.S.H.S.
 Ida Friend Infusion Center, UCSF Comprehensive Cancer Center, San Francisco, CA

Janet Amber Damon, M.S.W.
 Private Practice, Sausalito, CA

Dominique Davis, M.A.
 Oncology Practice, UCSF Comprehensive Cancer Center, San Francisco, CA

Susan Diamond, L.C.S.W.
 Senior Group Psychotherapist, Psychosocial Therapy Laboratory, Psychiatry and Behavioral

Sciences, Stanford University School of Medicine, Stanford, CA

Michael C. Dohan, M.D.
Private practice, Boston, MA

Malin R. Dollinger, M.D.
Clinical Professor of Medicine, University of Southern California School of Medicine, Los Angeles, CA

Mark J. Doolittle, Ph.D.
Professor of Psychology, Sonoma State University, Rohnert Park, CA

Eric Durak, M.Sc.
Director of Medical Health and Fitness, Santa Barbara, CA

Kathleen Dzubur, M.S.
Kinesiologist, Exercise Program, Cancer Supportive Care Program, Stanford Complementary Medicine Clinic, Stanford, CA; Private Practice, San Francisco, CA

Lee Daniel Erman, NCTMB
Stanford Complementary Medicine Clinic, Stanford, CA; Private Practice, Mountain View, CA

Bernadette Festa, M.S., R.D.
Dietitian, Ida Friend, Cancer Resource Center, UCSF Comprehensive Cancer Center, San Francisco, CA; Nutritional Consultant, Cancer Supportive Care Program, Stanford Complementary Medicine Clinic, Stanford, CA

Pat Fobair, L.C.S.W., M.Ph.
Program Coordinator, Cancer Supportive Care Program, Stanford Complementary Medicine Clinic, Stanford, CA

David A. Foster, Ph.D.
Professor, Department of Biological Sciences, Hunter College of The City University of New York

John Fox, C.P.T.
Associate Professor California Institute of Integral Studies, San Francisco, CA; Adjunct Professor John F. Kennedy University, Orinda, CA; Institute for Transpersonal Psychology, Palo Alto, CA

Alan B. Glassberg, M.D.
Clinical Professor of Medicine, UCSF; Associate Director for Clinical Care, UCSF Comprehensive Cancer Center, San Francisco, CA

Mary Godfrey, O.T.
Private Practice, San Francisco Bay Area

Brenda Golianu, M.D.
Attending Physician, Department of Complementary Medicine; Assistant Professor of Anesthesia and Pain Management, Stanford University, Stanford, CA

Irene Harrison, L.C.S.W. (Retired)
Hospice Care, Kaiser Permanente Hospital, Hayward, CA

Daphne Haas-Kogan, M.D.
Assistant Professor of Radiation Oncology, UCSF Comprehensive Cancer Center, San Francisco, CA

Margaret Hawn, R.N.
Nurse Coordinator/Assistant Director, Cancer Supportive Care Program, Stanford Complementary Medicine Clinic, Stanford, CA

Susan Molloy Hubbard B.S., R.N., M.P.A.
Director, International Cancer Information Center, National Cancer Institute, Bethesda, MD

Robert Ignoffo, Pharm.D.
Clinical Professor of Pharmacology, UCSF School of Pharmacy, San Francisco, CA

Patricia T. Kelly, Ph.D.
Medical Geneticist, Catholic Healthcare West, Bay Area Region, Private Practice, Genetic Counseling, Berkeley, CA

Andrew Kneier, Ph.D.
Clinical Psychologist, UCSF Comprehensive Cancer Center, San Francisco, CA

Pat Kramer, M.S.N., R.N., A.O.C.N.
Fatigue Program, Cancer Supportive Care

Program, Stanford Complementary Medicine Clinic, Stanford, CA

Jack LaLanne
National physical fitness and nutrition expert

Nancy Lambert, R.N., B.S.N.
Risk Assessment Coordinator, Department of Quality Management, UCSF, San Francisco, CA

Reverend Elmer Laursen, D.Min.
Chaplain and Supervisor, Clinical Pastoral Education, UCSF, San Francisco, CA

Britt-Marie Ljung, M.D.
Professor of Pathology, UCSF Comprehensive Cancer Center, San Francisco, CA

Regina Linetskaya, M.A.
Oncology Practice, UCSF Comprehensive Cancer Center, San Francisco, CA

Betty Lopez, C.M.A.
Office Oncology Practice, UCSF Comprehensive Cancer Center, San Francisco, CA

Frederic Luskin, Ph.D.
Director of the Stanford Forgiveness Project, Stanford University, Stanford, CA

Francine Manuel, R.P.T.
Exercise Program, Cancer Supportive Care Program, Stanford Complementary Medicine Clinic, Stanford, CA; Rehabilitation specialist, Private Practice, San Francisco Bay Area

Eugenie Marek, R.N.
Discharge Coordinator, Stanford University Medical School, Stanford, CA

Lawrence Margolis, M.D.
Professor of Radiation Oncology, UCSF Comprehensive Cancer Center, San Francisco, CA

T. Stanley Meyler, M.D.
Professor of Radiation Oncology (Retired), UCSF Comprehensive Cancer Center, San Francisco, CA

Larry Mintz, M.D.
Associate Professor of Medicine, Infectious Disease, UCSF

Jim Murdoch
Art for Recovery, UCSF Comprehensive Cancer Center, and the Lorna Barati Music for Recovery Program, Mount Zion Health Systems, Inc., San Francisco, CA

John Park, M.D.
Assistant Professor of Medicine, UCSF Comprehensive Cancer Center, San Francisco, CA

Cynthia Perlis, B.A.
Director, Art for Recovery, UCSF Comprehensive Cancer Center; Director, the Lorna Barati Music Program, Mount Zion Health Systems, Inc., San Francisco, CA

Elmo Petterle
Author, San Rafael, CA

Barbara F. Piper, R.N., A.O.C.N., F.A.A.N.
Associate Professor of Nursing, University of Nebraska–Omaha

J. Jerill Plunkett, M.D.
Associate Professor of Anesthesiology, UCSF/Fresno; Private Practice, Fresno, CA

Joel Pollack, C.P.A.
Administrative Director, President's Office, John Wayne Cancer Institute, Saint John's Health Center, Santa Monica, CA

Lee L. Pollak, L.C.S.W.
Private Practice, Jewish Family and Children's Services, and Coordinator of the Bereavement Center

Barbara Quinn
Manager, Billing and Collection Supervisor, Private Practice, Los Angeles, CA

Wendye R. Robbins, M.D.
Chief Medical Officer and President of Neuroges X, Inc., San Francisco, CA

Sabrina Selim, B.A.

Formerly Clinical Research Associate, UCSF Comprehensive Cancer Center, San Francisco, CA; currently a medical student at Dartmouth Medical School.

Reverend John D. Shanahan (deceased)

Formerly Roman Catholic Chaplain, UCSF, San Francisco, CA and Pastor, Star of the Sea Church, Sausalito, CA

Rabbi Jeffrey Silberman, D.Min.

Director, Pastoral Care and Education, Beth Israel Medical Center, New York City, NY

Sol Silverman, M.A., D.D.S.

Professor of Oral Medicine, University of California School of Dentistry, San Francisco, CA

Stu Silverstein, M.D.

Private Practice, Stamford, CT

Patricia Sparacino, R.N., M.S.

Quality Improvement Clinical Coordinator, Institute for Aging, San Francisco, CA

David Spiegel, M.D.

Professor and Associate Chair of Psychiatry and Behavioral Sciences, Stanford University School of Medicine, Stanford, CA

Keren Stronach, M.Ph.

Coordinator, Cancer Resource Center, UCSF Comprehensive Cancer Center, San Francisco, CA

Andrzej Szuba, M.D.

Division of Cardiovascular Medicine, Falk Cardiovascular Research Center, Stanford University School of Medicine, Stanford, CA

Carol S. Viele, R.N., M.S.

Clinical Nurse Specialist, Hematology/Oncology and Bone Marrow Transplant, UCSF, San Francisco, CA

Ian E. Wickramasekera, Ph.D., A.B.Ph., A.B.P.P.A

Clinical Professor of Psychiatry and Behavioral Sciences, Saybrook Institute and Stanford Medical School, Stanford, CA

Chris Wilhite

Director, Friend to Friend Gift Shop, UCSF Comprehensive Cancer Center, San Francisco, CA

Kenneth A. Woeber, M.D.

Chief of Medicine, UCSF, San Francisco, CA

William Wong, M.A.

Oncology Practice, UCSF Comprehensive Cancer Center, San Francisco, CA

Glossary of Medical Terms

Malin Dollinger, M.D.

A

absolute neutrophil count (ANC). The actual count of the white blood cells (also called polys or granulocytes) that engulf and destroy bacteria. There is some concern about infection if the count is less than one thousand.

acupressure. The use of finger pressure over various points on the body (the same points used in acupuncture) to treat symptoms or disease.

adenocarcinoma. Cancer that arises from glandular tissues. Examples include cancers of the breast, lung, thyroid, colon, and pancreas.

adenoma. A benign (nonmalignant) tumor that arises from glandular tissues, such as the breast, lung, thyroid, colon, and pancreas.

adjuvant chemotherapy. Chemotherapy used along with surgery or radiation therapy. It is usually given after all visible and known cancer has been removed by surgery or radiotherapy, but is sometimes given before surgery. (*See* **neoadjuvant chemotherapy**.) Adjuvant chemotherapy is usually used in cases where there is a high risk of hidden cancer cells remaining, and may increase the likelihood of cure by destroying small amounts of undetectable cancer.

advance directives. Legal documents that specify the type of medical care a person wants or does not want.

alkaline phosphatase. A blood enzyme commonly used in medical diagnosis. It is elevated in cases of bile obstruction (liver disease or cancer involving the liver) and in various bone diseases, including cancer involving bone. A variation of this test can distinguish between elevations due to bone and liver disease.

alkylating agents. A family of anticancer drugs that combine with a cancer cell's DNA to prevent normal cell division.

allogeneic transplant. A form of transplantation or transfer of a tissue—bone marrow, for example—from one individual to another. It is preferable that the tissue types match, but this is not always possible.

alopecia. Partial or complete loss of hair. This may result from radiotherapy to the head (hair may not completely return after therapy) or from certain chemotherapeutic agents (hair always returns).

alpha-fetoprotein. A protein that is elevated in the blood of patients with certain forms of cancer, such as liver or testis.

ambulatory care. The use of outpatient facilities—doctors' offices, home care, outpatient hospital clinics, and adult daycare facilities—to provide modern medical care without the need for hospitalization.

ambulatory infusion. The administration of chemotherapy by a small pump device usually worn under the clothes. The pump delivers anticancer drugs slowly and gradually twenty-four hours a day, with minimal or no side effects. Because there is no need to remain in the hospital or even at home, this method allows patients to work and carry on with their normal activities.

amenorrhea. The temporary or permanent lack of menstrual periods. This may be a normal part of the menopause or is sometimes brought on by severe physical or emotional stresses. Some anticancer drugs can produce amenorrhea, especially if the woman is near the age when menopause would normally begin.

amino acids. The building blocks of proteins, analogous to the freight cars making up a train.

analgesic. A drug that relieves pain. Analgesics may be mild (aspirin or acetaminophen), stronger (codeine), or very strong (morphine). There are also a large number of mild, moderate, or strong synthetic analgesics.

anaplastic. A tumor that appears "wild" under a microscope, having no resemblance to the normal tissue of the organ involved. It is possible to tell where anaplastic tumors originate by knowing where the biopsy was taken, knowing the area of involvement, or by inference.

anastomosis. The point where two organs are joined together. In cancer therapy, it usually refers to joining two portions of the bowel after a segment containing cancer has been removed.

androgens. Male sex hormones. Testosterone is produced naturally, and several synthetic ones are used in treatment.

anemia. Having less than the normal amount of hemoglobin or red cells in the blood. This may be due to bleeding, lack of blood production by the bone marrow, or to the brief survival of blood already manufactured. Symptoms include tiredness, shortness of breath, and weakness.

aneuploid. Tumor cells that do not have the normal number (forty-six) of chromosomes in a human cell. Tumor cells that have forty-six chromosomes are called euploid. Aneuploid tumors often have a worse prognosis than euploid tumors. *See also* **chromosomes**.

angiogenesis. The growth of new blood vessels. This may be stimulated by certain chemicals produced by cancers, and may be a requirement for cancers to spread. New treatments are being investigated to prevent this new blood vessel formation.

angiography. The taking of X-ray pictures of blood vessels by injecting a "dye" into the blood vessel. Angiograms may be taken to determine a tumor's blood supply before surgery, to place a catheter or infusion pump, or to determine the site for other procedures in the blood vessels.

antibody. A protein (gamma globulin) made by the body in response to a specific foreign protein, or antigen. The antigen may result from an infection, a cancer, or some other source. If the same alien substance attacks again, the white blood cells are able to recognize it and reproduce the specific antibody to fight it.

antiemetics. Drugs given to prevent or minimize nausea and/or vomiting.

antigens. Substances that cause activation of the immune system.

antimetabolites. A family of antitumor drugs that resemble normal vitamins or building blocks of metabolism. They bind to the tumor's enzymes and chemical pathways. The tumor cells "think" they are

getting the real vitamin or building block and starve to the point where they can't grow or multiply.

apoptosis. The programming of cells in the body to become old and die at the correct time. This vital feature of healthy human cells allows for replacement of tissues as needed. Cancer cells may persist because they may escape apoptosis. Some new methods of therapy are being studied to reprogram cancer cells to relearn to die.

asbestosis. Scarring of the lungs and the lining of the chest cavity from the inhalation of asbestos dust. This increases the risk of lung cancer and cancer of the chest cavity lining (mesothelioma).

ascites. An abnormal fluid collection in the abdomen from cancer or other causes.

aspiration. Removal of fluid or tissue, usually with a needle or tube, from a specific area of the body. This procedure may be done to obtain a diagnosis or to relieve symptoms.

atrophy. A withering or reduction in size of a tissue or a part of the body. This may result from lack of use during immobilization or prolonged bed rest or from pressure from an adjacent tumor.

atypical. Not usual or ordinary. For example, cancer is the result of atypical cell division.

autoimmunity. A condition in which the body's immune system fights and rejects its own tissues.

autologous transplant. Removal of a patient's own tissue, especially bone marrow, and its return to the same patient after chemotherapy. This might more correctly be called bone marrow reinfusion, or protection, rather than transplantation.

autolymphocyte therapy. A form of outpatient immunotherapy being tested, especially in kidney cancer, that involves readministering a patient's lymphocytes after they have been stimulated by a lymphokine (substances that stimulate immunity) mixture. This is a form of "adoptive immunotherapy," in which the aim is to transfer to patients their own stimulated antitumor effector cells.

autosomal. A non-sex-linked method of inheritance. The inherited characteristic does not depend on whether the person is male or female because the gene in question is not found on the sex (X or Y) chromosomes.

axilla. The armpit. Lymph glands in the armpit are called the axillary nodes.

B

bacteremia. *See* **sepsis**.

barium enema. An X-ray study of the colon (large bowel) in which the patient is given an enema of a liquid barium mixture before the X rays are taken. Laxatives and/or regular enemas are usually required beforehand.

barium swallow. An X-ray study of the portion of the digestive canal between the throat and stomach (esophagus) in which the patient swallows a barium mixture while the radiologist watches for signs of narrowing, irregularity, or blockage. No preparation is required except fasting. Sometimes, in a procedure called an upper gastrointestinal (UGI) series, the barium also is observed after it enters the stomach to check for stomach problems or ulcers.

basal cell carcinoma. A form of skin cancer that grows very slowly and is curable in almost all cases by surgery or other local treatment. The growth may be so slow that malignancy is not at first suspected.

B cell. Lymphocytes are the cells in the body that are intimately involved in the immune response. They occur in the blood, in lymph nodes, and in various organs. The two types of lymphocytes are B cells and T cells. Special techniques are needed to tell them apart because they look the same when viewed by ordinary methods under a microscope. It is essential to make this distinction in cases of lymphomas, because the treatment and prognosis of B cell lymphomas are very different from that of T cell lymphomas.

BCG. A material prepared from killed bird tuberculosis bacteria. This has been widely used, especially in Europe, to vaccinate health care workers who work closely with tuberculosis patients. It also has been used in cancer treatment to stimulate the immune system.

bench surgery. Complete removal of a selected organ or tissue from the body during surgery in order to perform a separate, often delicate or complex, surgical procedure on it. The organ is then replaced into the body (usually in its original site, although sometimes the location is changed). Bench surgery can allow: (1) better control for removal of a tumor, particularly in a vital organ that cannot or does not have to be totally sacrificed, (2) delicate surgery that requires a microscope, (3) delineation of margins of resection to assure tumor is fully excised or to lessen spilling of cancer cells into the surrounding tissue or cavity, such as the peritoneum, and (4) cooling the organ to permit more time for surgery. A good example of bench surgery is in the treatment of kidney cancer, especially when it occurs in a patient with only one kidney or with borderline renal failure, and when the tumor is located in the center of the kidney. Blood vessels are disconnected temporarily; the kidney is completely removed to a separate operating table (bench); the tumor is removed, with repair to the kidney; and then the kidney is replaced into the body.

benign. A tumor that has no tendency to grow into surrounding tissues or spread to other parts of the body. In other words, it is not malignant. Under a microscope, a benign tumor does not resemble cancer.

bilateral. Occurring on both sides of the body.

biologic response modifiers. Substances and agents that may have a direct antitumor effect, and also affect tumors indirectly by stimulating or triggering the immune system to fight cancer. Examples include interferon, IL-2, and LAK cells.

biological therapy. Certain complex substances produced within the body regulate cell growth and immunity. Biological therapy, which includes immunotherapy, is the use of these same substances to treat cancer. They may be produced in the laboratory or a production facility, or the person with cancer may be given drugs that stimulate the production of these substances.

biopsy. The surgical removal of a small portion of tissue for diagnosis. In almost all cases, a biopsy diagnosis of cancer is required before appropriate and correct treatment planning can take place. In some cases, a needle biopsy may be enough for diagnosis, but in others, the removal of a pea-sized wedge of tissue is needed. In many cases, the biopsy may be the first step of the definitive surgical procedure that not only proves the diagnosis but also attempts to cure the cancer by completely removing the tumor.

blastic. A bone lesion that appears on an X ray to have more calcium (density) than normal.

bleeding disorders. Blood clotting is a complex process involving the interaction of many substances in the blood that promote coagulation. A deficiency of any of these substances results in a bleeding disorder. Some disorders are inherited (hemophilia, for example) and some are acquired (such as liver disease). A common disorder associated with cancer is a low platelet count (thrombocytopenia), which sometimes results from chemotherapy or radiotherapy and may make platelet transfusions necessary. Sophisticated tests are often needed to diagnose bleeding disorders.

blood-brain barrier. A microscopic structure in the brain that separates blood capillaries from nerve cells. This prevents some substances from entering the brain. Many cancer chemotherapeutic agents, for example, cannot be used to treat brain tumors because they cannot pass through the barrier. Some others (CCNU, BCNU) are designed to penetrate it. There are techniques that can eliminate the barrier temporarily to allow the use of other antitumor drugs. *See also* **nitrosoureas.**

blood cells. The red cells, white cells, and platelets that make up the blood. They are made in the bone marrow.

blood chemistry panel. Multiple chemical analyses prepared by an automatic apparatus from a single blood sample. These panels often include measurements of electrolytes (minerals) and proteins as well as tests of liver, kidney, and thyroid function. The advantages of panels include less cost and greater accuracy and speed, with results often available the same or the following day.

bolus (or "push") chemotherapy. Administration of intravenous chemotherapy over a short time, usually five minutes or less. The other method is called infusion chemotherapy, which may last from fifteen minutes to several hours or days.

bone marrow. A soft substance found within bone cavities. Marrow is composed of developing red cells, white cells, platelets, and fat. Some forms of cancer can be diagnosed by examining bone marrow.

bone marrow examination. The process of removing bone marrow by withdrawing it through a needle for pathological examination. It usually is withdrawn from the breastbone (sternum) or the hipbone. Both these bones are just under the skin, making the removal of marrow easy, safe, and only momentarily uncomfortable with a local anesthetic. The procedure takes about ten minutes—nine and a half minutes for the anesthetic to take effect and thirty seconds for the extraction.

bone marrow suppression. A decrease in one or more of the blood counts. This condition can be caused by chemotherapy, radiation, disease, or various medications.

bone scan. A picture of all of the bones in the body taken about two hours after injection of a radioactive tracer. "Hot spots" indicate areas of bone abnormality that may indicate tumors, although they can also be due to other causes, such as arthritis. No preparation is required and the test is easy. The main problem is lying still on a hard table for fifteen minutes. This test can help determine if cancer has spread to the bones, if therapy is working, and/or if damaged bony areas are healing.

brachytherapy. The use of a radioactive "seed" implanted directly into a tumor. This allows a very high but sharply localized dose of radiation to be given to a tumor while sparing surrounding tissues from significant radiation exposure.

brain scan. A picture of the brain taken after the intravenous injection of a radioactive tracer. CT and MRI scans have, in most cases, replaced such brain scans, because CT and MRI tend to discover smaller lesions and are more useful for following up the effects of therapy.

bronchogenic carcinoma. Carcinoma of the lung.

bronchoscopy. Inspection—and often biopsy—of the breathing tubes (bronchi) going to the lungs by means of a long tube inserted through the mouth or nose. The instrument usually used is a fiberoptic bronchoscope that is flexible and allows excellent visualization around corners. The procedure is often done on an outpatient basis after local anesthesia and sedation.

bypass. A surgical procedure to "go around" an organ or area affected by cancer and allow normal flow or drainage to continue. In cancer of the pancreas, for example, the bile ducts may be blocked. A bypass procedure will allow the bile to drain directly into the small bowel, as it normally would after passing through the gallbladder.

C

cachexia. The wasting away of the body, often due to malnutrition, disease, or cancer.

calcium. An important body mineral that is a vital component of bone. The calcium level may be elevated if tumors involve bone.

candidiasis. A common fungal infection often seen as white patches on the tongue or the inside of the mouth. *See also* **moniliasis.**

carcinogenesis. The development or production of cancer.

carcinoma. A form of cancer that develops in the tissues covering or lining organs of the body such as the skin, uterus, lung, or breast (epithelial tissues). Eighty to ninety percent of all cancers are carcinomas.

carcinoma in situ. The earliest stage of cancer, in which the tumor is still confined to the local area, before it has grown to a significant size or has spread. In situ carcinomas are highly curable.

cardiomyopathy. A condition in which the heart muscle is diseased. It may develop because of the toxic effect of a few anticancer drugs.

cardiopulmonary resuscitation (CPR). The use of chest compressions, drugs, and electric shock to restart the heart and/or a breathing tube and ventilator (respirator) to maintain lung function.

CAT scan. *See* **CT scan.**

catheter. A tube made of rubber, plastic, or metal that can be inserted into a body cavity such as the bladder to drain fluid or to deliver fluids or medication.

catheterization. The process of introducing a catheter. The term is also used when a tube is placed into an artery or a vein to take X rays.

CEA (carcinoembryonic antigen). A tumor marker in the blood that may indicate the presence of cancer. It may be elevated in some cancers, especially of the breast, bowel, and lung. By monitoring the amount of CEA, doctors can detect the presence of these cancers and/or assess the progress of treatment.

cell cycle. Each cell in the body, including a cancer cell, goes through several stages every time it divides. Various anticancer drugs affect the cell at certain stages of this cell cycle.

cell-cycle-specific. Chemotherapeutic drugs that kill only cells that are dividing rather than resting.

cell surface markers. Special proteins on the surface or edge of cells that can be used to identify them or their characteristics.

cells. The fundamental units, or building blocks, of human tissues.

cellular immunity. Immunity brought about by the action of immune cells such as lymphocytes.

cellulitis. Inflammation of the skin and underlying tissues.

centigray (cGy). A unit of measurement of radiation therapy that is replacing the older term RADS. *See* **RADS.**

cervical dysplasia. The presence of abnormal—and possibly precancerous—cells in the mouth of the uterus (cervix).

cervical (lymph) nodes. The lymph nodes in the neck.

cervix. The lower portion of the uterus, which protrudes into the vagina and forms a portion of the birth canal during delivery. The Pap smear test is designed to check this area for cancer.

chemoprevention. Attempting to prevent cancer through drugs, chemicals, vitamins, or minerals.

chemotherapy. The treatment of cancer by chemicals (drugs) designed to kill cancer cells or stop them from growing.

choriocarcinoma. A carcinoma composed of cells arising in the placenta or the testes.

chromosomes. The fundamental strands of genetic material (DNA) that carry all of our genes. There are twenty-three pairs of chromosomes in each cell. Tumor cells sometimes have more or fewer than twenty-three pairs. *See* **aneuploid.**

clinical. Refers to the treatment of humans, as opposed to animals or laboratory studies. Also refers to the general use of a treatment by a practicing physician, as opposed to research done in cancer research centers ("preclinical").

clinical trials. The procedure in which new cancer treatments are tested in humans. Clinical trials are conducted after experiments in animals and preliminary studies in humans have shown that a new treatment method might be effective.

clone. A strain of cells—whether normal or malignant—derived from a single original cell.

clonigenic assay. A test done by growing tumor cells in the laboratory and identifying which chemotherapy agents will prevent their growth. This information is sometimes useful in deciding which drugs to use or not to use in treatment.

cobalt treatment. A radiotherapy machine using gamma rays generated from the radioisotope cobalt 60.

coin lesion. A spot on a chest X ray that may be a tumor, infection or other lesion. Given this name because it resembles the shadow of a coin.

colonoscopy. A procedure to inspect the rectum and colon by means of a long, fiber-optic telescope that is lighted and flexible. Biopsy specimens of suspicious tissue also can be obtained. *See also* **proctoscopy; sigmoidoscopy.**

colony-stimulating factor (CSF). A substance that stimulates the growth of bone marrow cells. Current clinical trials are using CSF to try to increase the dosage of chemotherapy that can be given safely.

colostomy. An artificial opening in the abdominal wall created so that feces drain from the colon into a bag. A colostomy is sometimes necessary after the removal of a diseased section of the large intestine, and can be either temporary or permanent. *See also* **ileostomy; ostomy; stoma.**

colposcopy. A way to detect small lesions by inspecting the cervix with special binocular magnifying instruments after applying a solution to stain cancer tissue.

combination chemotherapy. The use of several anticancer drugs at the same time. Most chemotherapy is now given this way because it is a much more effective method.

combined modality therapy. Treatment with two or more types of therapy—surgery, radiotherapy, chemotherapy, and biological therapy. These may be used at the same time or one after the other. Surgery, for example, is often followed by chemotherapy to destroy random cancer cells that may have spread from the original site.

comfort care. Care that helps keep a person comfortable but does not treat an illness. Such measures can include bathing, nutrition, fluids, massage, and pain medications (narcotics and sedatives).

computerized tomography. *See* **CT scan.**

cone biopsy. Removal of a ring of tissue from the opening of the cervix.

congestive heart failure. Weakness of the heart muscle usually due to heart disease, but sometimes due to other causes, resulting in a buildup of fluid in body tissues.

consolidation. A second round of chemotherapy to further reduce the number of cancer cells.

contralateral. On the opposite side of the body. In cancer therapy, it refers to a tumor or a site of disease. *See also* **ipsilateral.**

convulsion. *See* **seizure.**

cooperative groups. Clinical trials of new cancer treatments require many patients, generally more than any single physician or hospital can see. A number of physicians and/or hospitals form a cooperative group to treat a large number of patients in the same way so that the effectiveness of a new treatment can be evaluated quickly.

cortisone. A natural hormone produced by the adrenal glands. The term is also loosely used to designate synthetic forms of the hormone (such as prednisone) that are used to treat inflammatory conditions and diseases, including certain cancers.

cranial irradiation. The delivery of radiation to the brain to treat brain tumors.

creatinine clearance. A sensitive test of kidney function that requires a twenty-four-hour urine sample and a blood sample. The test is often required to make sure it is safe to give anticancer drugs that may be toxic to the kidneys.

cruciferous vegetables. Vegetables such as cauliflower and brussels sprouts that are high in beta-carotene and are thought to help protect against colon cancer.

cryotherapy or cryosurgery. The use of an extremely cold probe as a surgical instrument to freeze areas of cancer, killing the cancer cells. The process usually involves several episodes of freezing and thawing, and is carefully controlled with temperature probes to avoid damage to surrounding healthy tissue.

CT scan. A CT (computerized tomography) scan creates cross-section images of the body which may show cancer or metastases earlier and more accurately than other imaging methods. This type of X-ray machine has revolutionized the diagnosis of cancer and other diseases.

Cushing's syndrome. A condition characterized by swelling of the face and the back of the neck with purple lines over the abdomen. It results from an excess of cortisone or hydrocortisone caused either by disease or by the administration of these substances or their synthetic derivatives.

cyst. A fluid-filled sac of tissue that is usually benign but which can be malignant. Cysts are sometimes removed just to be sure they are benign. Lumps in the breast are often found to be harmless cysts rather than cancer.

cystitis. An inflammation and irritation of the bladder caused by bacterial infection, chemotherapy, or radiation treatments. Symptoms include a burning sensation when urinating or a frequent urgent need to urinate.

cystoscopy. Inspection of the inside of the bladder by means of a telescope. During the procedure, a catheter also may be placed, biopsies taken, or tissue removed.

cytogenetics. Laboratory study or analysis of the chromosome pattern of a cell.

cytokine. A substance secreted by immune system cells, usually to send messages to other immune cells.

cytology. The study under a microscope of cells that have been cast off or scraped off of organs such as the uterus, lungs, bladder, or stomach. Also called exfoliative cytology.

D

debulking. A procedure that removes a significant part or most of a tumor in cases where it is not possible to remove all of it. This may make subsequent radiotherapy or chemotherapy easier and more effective.

differentiation. The process of maturation of a cell line of cancer cells. When they are fully differentiated or well differentiated, they more closely resemble the normal cells in the tissue of origin.

diuretics. Drugs that increase the elimination of water and salts in the urine.

DNA (deoxyribonucleic acid). The building block of our genetic material. DNA is responsible for passing on hereditary characteristics and information on cell growth, division, and function.

dose limiting. A side effect, complication, or risk that makes it impossible or unwise to exceed a specific dose of a chemotherapeutic agent. A total dosage of bleomycin of more than 400 units, for example, may produce severe lung scarring. Lung toxicity is, therefore, dose limiting.

drug resistance. The development of resistance in cancer cells to a specific drug or drugs. If resistance develops, a patient in remission from chemotherapy may relapse despite continued administration of anticancer drugs.

dysphagia. Difficulty in swallowing; a sensation of food sticking in the throat.

dysplasia. Abnormal developments or changes in cells, which are sometimes an indication that cancer may develop.

dyspnea. Shortness of breath.

dysuria. Difficult or painful urination; burning on urination.

E

edema. The accumulation of fluid within tissues.

effusion. A collection of fluid inside a body cavity, such as around the lungs (pleural), intestines (peritoneal), or heart (pericardial). This can be caused by cancer invading the cavity.

electrolytes. Certain chemicals—including sodium, potassium, chloride, and bicarbonate—found in the tissues and blood. They often are measured as an aid to patient care.

electron beam. A form of radiotherapy in which the beam does not penetrate completely through the body as ordinary X rays do. It is used for treating the skin or lesions beneath the skin.

electrophoresis. *See* **serum protein electrophoresis**.

emboli. Pieces of tissue, usually blood clots but sometimes tumor cells, that travel in the circulatory system until they lodge in a small artery or capillary, often in the lungs.

embolization. A method of treating tumors in a localized area by blocking the blood vessels to that area. This is done by inserting a thin tube (catheter) into an artery and injecting tiny pellets or other materials, which then block the smaller arteries. The pellets also may carry chemotherapeutic agents for release in the area (chemoembolization).

emesis. Vomiting.

endemic. Refers to a disease that is common in a particular community or population.

endocrine glands. Glands—such as the pituitary, thyroid, ovaries, and testes—that secrete hormones to control digestion, reproduction, growth, metabolism, or other body functions.

endometrial carcinoma. A cancer of the inner lining (endometrium) of the uterus.

endoscope. An instrument (telescope) for examining hollow organs or body cavities. There are many specialized types such as the cystoscope for the bladder, colonoscope for the colon, gastroscope for the stomach, and bronchoscope for the lungs.

endoscopy. Examination of interior body structures with an endoscope. The physician is able to take photographs, obtain small samples of tissue, or remove small growths during the procedure.

enteral feeding. Administration of liquid food (nutrients) through a tube inserted into the stomach or intestine.

enteroclysis. A method of taking X rays of the small bowel using a contrast agent administered through a tube inserted into the bowel.

enterostomal therapist. A medical professional specializing in the care of artificial openings in the abdominal wall and elsewhere—ileostomies, gastrostomies, or colostomies, for example.

enterostomy. The opening used for enteral feeding or for drainage if the bowel is obstructed.

enzymes. Proteins that play a part in specific chemical reactions. The level of enzymes in the blood is often measured because abnormal levels may be a sign of various diseases.

epidermoid carcinoma. A cancer arising from surface cells in an organ and resembling skin (epidermis) when viewed under a microscope.

epidural. The space just outside the spinal cord. Plastic catheters may be inserted in the space to deliver anesthetics or morphine for pain control.

Epstein-Barr (EB) virus. A virus known to cause infectious mononucleosis and associated with Burkitt's lymphoma and certain cancers of the head and neck.

ERCP (endoscopic retrograde cholangiopancreatography). A procedure in which a catheter is introduced through a gastroscope into the internal bile ducts.

esophageal speech. A way of speaking used by people who have had their larynx (voice box) removed. As air is expelled from the esophagus, the walls of the pharynx and esophagus vibrate to produce sound.

esophagitis. Soreness and inflammation of the esophagus due to infection, toxicity from radiotherapy or chemotherapy, or some physical injury.

estrogen. The female sex hormone produced by the ovaries. Estrogen controls the development of physical sexual characteristics, menstruation, and pregnancy. Synthetic forms are used in oral contraceptives and in various therapies.

estrogen-receptor (ER) assay. A test that determines whether the breast cancer in a particular patient is stimulated by estrogen.

excision. Surgical removal of tissue.

extravasation. Leakage into the surrounding tissues of intravenous fluids or drugs—especially cancer chemotherapeutic agents—from the vein being used for injection. Extravasation may damage tissues. *See* **infiltration**.

F

familial polyposis. A hereditary condition in which members of the same family develop intestinal polyps. Also called Gardner's syndrome, it is considered a risk factor for colorectal cancer.

fiber-optics. Flexible tubes that transmit light by means of glass fibers. They are used to inspect and treat internal parts of the body. Various types of endoscopes use fiber-optic technology.

fibrocystic breasts. A condition, which may come and go in relation to the menstrual cycle, in which fluids normally absorbed by breast tissue become trapped and form cysts. There may be difficulty distinguishing between cysts and breast cancer.

fine needle aspiration (FNA). A simple and painless way to obtain small bits of tissue for diagnosis. After local anesthesia, a small needle is inserted through the skin directly into a tumor and a sample of tissue is drawn up inside the needle. In some cases—thyroid cancer, for example—FNA has become an integral part of the early diagnostic process. But the amount of tissue obtained this way may not be enough to diagnose lymphomas and some other cancers. *See* **needle biopsy**.

fissures. Cracks or a splitting in the skin or an internal membrane.

fistula. An abnormal opening between the inside of the body and the skin or between two areas inside the body.

frozen section. A procedure done by the pathologist during surgery to give the surgeon an immediate answer as to whether a tissue is benign or malignant. Tissue is removed by biopsy, frozen, cut into thin slices, stained, and examined under a microscope. This information is vital in helping the surgeon decide the most appropriate course of action.

G

gamma globulin. Proteins in the blood that contain antibodies, part of the body's defense against infection.

gamma rays. The form of electromagnetic radiation produced by certain radioactive sources. They are similar to X rays but have a shorter wavelength.

gene. A biological unit of DNA capable of transmitting a single characteristic from parent to offspring.

grade of tumor. A way of describing tumors by their appearance under a microscope. Low-grade tumors are slow to grow and spread, whereas high-grade tumors grow and spread rapidly.

graft-versus-host (GVH) disease. After bone marrow transplantation, immune cells in the donated (grafted) material may identify the patient's tissues (the host) as foreign and try to destroy them. This can be a serious problem, and drugs are available to combat it. However, in some cases, a GVH reaction actually helps control the cancer.

granulocyte. The most common type of white blood cell. Its function is to kill bacteria. Also called neutrophil, poly, PMN.

guaiac test. A test to see if there is hidden blood in the stool. A positive result may be a sign of cancer, but many benign conditions also cause bleeding. *See* **stool for occult blood.**

gynecomastia. Swelling of the breast tissues in men. Although this can be caused by medications and other diseases, in the cancer field it is caused by certain cancers of the testis or by female hormones used to treat prostate cancer.

H

helicobacter pylori (H. pylori). Previously, it was believed that peptic ulcers were caused by too much stomach acid and/or stress. A specific bacteria has now been found to be an important cause. This bacteria, H. pylori, can be cited as a cause of certain cancers of the stomach.

hematocrit. A way of measuring the red cell content of the blood. The normal level is from forty to forty-five in men and from thirty-seven to forty-two in women. A low hematocrit is a sign of anemia.

hematologist. A physician (internist) who specializes in blood diseases.

hematoma. A blood lump under the skin that appears as a bruise.

hematopoietic. Pertaining to the blood-forming organs such as the bone marrow.

hematuria. Blood in the urine. This may be obvious (gross hematuria) or hidden (microscopic hematuria).

hemoglobin. A way of measuring the red cell content of the blood. The normal value in men is about 13 to 15 grams, in women from 12.5 to 14 grams.

hemolytic anemia. Anemia resulting from the breakdown of red blood cells in the bloodstream before the end of their usual life span of 120 days.

hemorrhagic cystitis. A bladder irritation, which may be caused by the anticancer drugs cyclophosphamide (Cytoxan) or ifosfamide.

hepatic. Pertaining to the liver.

hepatotoxicity. Adverse effects of drugs on the liver indicated by abnormal blood tests of liver function. It is also sometimes associated with jaundice. *See* **jaundice.**

herpes simplex. A common acute viral inflammation of the skin or mucous membranes characterized by the development of blisters. This infection around the mouth is commonly called a cold sore.

herpes zoster or shingles. A painful eruption in the skin caused by a virus infection that affects nerves. The same virus that causes shingles causes chicken pox.

histology. The appearance of tissues, including cancers, under a microscope.

hormonal anticancer therapy. A form of therapy that takes advantage of the tendency of some cancers—especially breast and prostate cancers—to stabilize or shrink if certain hormones are administered.

hormones. Naturally occurring substances that are released by the endocrine organs and circulate in the blood. Hormones control growth, metabolism, reproduction, and other functions, and can stimulate or turn off the growth or activity of specific target cells. Some hormones are used after surgery to treat breast, ovarian, prostate, uterine, and other cancers.

hospice. A facility and a philosophy of care that stress comfort, peace of mind, and the control of symptoms. Hospice care, provided on either an outpatient or inpatient basis, is generally invoked when no further anticancer therapy is available and life expectancy is very short. Hospice also helps family and friends to care for and cope with the loss of a dying loved one.

humoral immunity. Immunity mediated by substances such as proteins (gamma globulins) produced by the immune system.

hyperalimentation. Artificial feeding—temporary or permanent—by means of concentrated protein and fat solutions delivered intravenously. A special catheter is usually needed. *See also* **parenteral nutrition; TPN.**

hypercalcemia. High levels of calcium in the blood. It is a sign of some forms of cancer or of cancer spreading to bone and also occurs in some benign conditions.

hyperplasia. The overgrowth of healthy cells; not a precursor of cancer.

hyperthermia. Increased body temperature. Often caused by the use of special devices to raise body temperature as a way of treating cancer. It is usually used along with radiation therapy.

hypoechoic. An ultrasound examination produces a picture of the area being examined. Hypoechoic areas "bounce" or echo the sound waves less than surrounding tissues (e.g., by a benign cyst in the breast).

hypothermia. Excessively low body temperature.

hysterectomy. Surgical removal of the uterus.

I

IL-2. *See* **interleukins.**

ileostomy. An artificial opening in the skin of the abdomen, leading to the small bowel (ileum). *See also* **colostomy; ostomy; stoma.**

iliac. The part of the lower abdomen just above the hip bone on each side of the body. Also refers to the iliac bone just above the hip joint.

immune or immunity. A state of adequate defense against infections or foreign substances. Some cancers are believed to produce immune responses.

immune system. The body mechanisms that resist and fight disease. The main defenders are white blood cells and antibodies, which, along with other specialized defenders, react to the presence of foreign substances in the body and try to destroy them.

immunoelectrophoresis. A way to separate serum gamma globulins—called IgA, IgG, and IgM—into groups according to their immunologic qualities.

immunosuppression. The state of having decreased immunity, and thus, being less able to fight infections and disease.

immunosuppressive drug. A drug that modifies the natural immune response so that it will not react to foreign substances. This type of drug is most commonly given after organ transplants so that the new organ will not be rejected.

immunotherapy. A method of cancer therapy that stimulates the body's defense mechanisms to attack cancer cells or combat a specific disease.

incontinence. Inadvertent loss of urine or feces, usually due to loss of nerve or muscle control.

induction. The initial treatment—usually with chemotherapy—to eliminate or control cancer. Usually applied to leukemia or lymphoma.

induration. Firmness or hardness of tissues.

inferior vena cava. The large vein draining the blood from the legs and abdomen back into the heart.

infiltration. The leaking of fluid or medicines into tissues from a tube or needle. This can cause irritation or swelling. *See* **extravasation.**

inflammation. The triggering of local body defenses causing defensive white blood cells (leukocytes) to pour into the tissues from the circulatory system. It is characterized by redness, heat, pain, and swelling.

informed consent. A legal standard defining how much a patient must know about the potential benefits and risks of therapy before agreeing to receive it.

infusion. Administration of fluids and/or medications into a vein or artery over a period of time.

infusion pumps. Small, preloaded mechanical devices used to continuously administer intravenous chemotherapy over a designated time.

infusion chemotherapy. Intravenous therapy given in sessions ranging from ten minutes to many hours.

inguinal. Pertaining to the groin, the common site for hernias and the location of the inguinal lymph nodes, an area where cancer may spread.

in situ. A very early stage of cancer in which the tumor is localized to one area. *See also* **localized cancer.**

interferons. Natural substances produced in response to infections. They have been created artificially by recombinant DNA technology in an attempt to control cancer.

interleukins. A group of cytokines produced by body cells that convey molecular messages between cells of the immune system. Interleukin-2 (IL-2), the best known of these, acts primarily on T lymphocytes; it is being used in the treatment of cancer.

intra-arterial. Drugs directed into an artery through a catheter.

intracavitary therapy. Treatment directed into a body cavity via a catheter.

intramuscular (IM). The injection of a drug into a muscle; from there it is absorbed into the circulation.

intraperitoneal. Delivery of drugs and fluids into the abdominal cavity.

intrapleural. Delivery of drugs and fluids into the space around the lung. Often employed when fluid collects there as a result of cancer.

intrathecal. Administration of drugs into the spinal fluid.

intravenous (IV). Administration of drugs or fluids directly into a vein.

intravenous pyelogram (IVP). An X ray of the kidneys taken after the intravenous administration of a radio-opaque dye that is concentrated and excreted by the kidneys. This technique makes the kidneys and drainage system visible on an X ray.

invasive cancer. Cancer that spreads to the healthy tissue surrounding the original tumor site. This contrasts with in situ and localized cancers, which have not yet begun to spread.

ipsilateral. On the same side of the body. *See also* **contralateral.**

IU. international unit or standard amount of a biologic.

J

jaundice. The accumulation of bilirubin, a breakdown product of hemoglobin, which results in a yellow discoloration of the skin and the whites of the eyes. Jaundice is a sign of liver disease or blockage of the major bile ducts.

K

kidney failure. Malfunction of the kidneys due to disease or the toxic effects of drugs or chemicals. Urine volume may or may not be diminished. Also called renal failure.

L

laparotomy. An operation in which the abdominal cavity is opened.

large cell carcinoma. A type of cancer of the lung, although large cell cancers may occur in other organs.

laryngectomy. The surgical removal of the larynx (voice box) resulting in the loss of normal speech. A laryngectomee is someone who has undergone this operation.

laryngoscopy. Inspection of the lower throat, pharynx, and larynx by means of a small mirror placed in the back of the throat (indirect laryngoscopy) or by direct examination under anesthesia (direct laryngoscopy).

leukocyte. White blood cell.

leukocytosis. An increase in the number of leukocytes (white blood cells) in the blood.

leukopenia. A decreased white blood cell count (below five thousand).

leukopheresis. A washing procedure that removes white blood cells from the blood.

leukoplakia. White plaque on the mucous membranes of the mouth and gums. This may be precancerous.

linear accelerator. A radiation therapy machine that produces a high-energy beam.

liver function tests. A group (panel) of blood tests to check if the liver is healthy.

lobectomy. Removal of one lobe of a lung; the right lung contains three lobes, the left lung contains two.

localized cancer. A cancer confined to the site of origin without evidence of spread. *See also* **in situ**.

lumbar puncture. Removal of spinal fluid for examination. This simple procedure—also called a spinal tap—involves numbing the skin of the back with a local anesthetic and placing a needle into the numbed area to remove the spinal fluid.

lumpectomy. The removal of a breast cancer (lump) and the surrounding tissue without removing the entire breast. It is a less-radical procedure than mastectomy and usually is followed by radiation treatment.

L.V.N. (licensed vocational nurse). A nurse trained to do some, but not all, tasks performed by a registered nurse (R.N.).

lymph nodes. Oval-shaped organs, often the size of peas or beans, which are located throughout the body and contain clusters of cells called lymphocytes. These cells produce infection-fighting lymphocytes and also filter out and destroy bacteria, foreign substances, and cancer cells. Small vessels called lymphatics connect them. Lymph nodes act as our first line of defense against infections and the spread of cancer.

lymphangiogram. An X-ray picture of the abdominal lymph nodes obtained by injecting a contrast substance under the skin on the feet, which then travels to the abdomen. This test helps to determine if cancer has spread to the abdominal lymph nodes.

lymphatic system. The system of lymph nodes and the lymphatic vessels that connect them.

lymphedema. Swelling, usually of an arm or leg, caused by obstructed lymphatic vessels. It can develop because of a tumor or as an unusual post-surgery or post-radiotherapy effect.

lymphocytes. A family of white blood cells responsible for the production of antibodies and for the direct destruction of invading organisms or cancer cells.

lymphokine. A specific protein (cytokine) created by lymphocytes.

lytic. A bone lesion that has less calcium than normal. On a scan, it may appear to be a "hole" in the bone.

M

macrophages. White blood cells that destroy invading organisms by ingesting them.

malaise. Tiredness or lack of drive.

malabsorption. The body's failure to absorb sufficient available calories and nutrients through the intestines.

malignant. An adjective meaning cancerous. Two important qualities of malignancies are the tendency to sink roots into surrounding tissues and to break off and spread elsewhere (metastasize).

markers. Chemicals in the blood that are produced by certain cancers. Measuring the markers is useful for diagnosis, but especially useful for following the course of treatment. Also called

tumor markers. *See* **CEA**.

mediastinum. The central portion of the chest, comprising the heart, large blood vessels, esophagus, trachea, and surrounding tissues.

metaplasia. Cells that appear abnormal under a microscope and do not yet show signs of malignancy.

metastasis. The spread of cancer from one part of the body to another by way of the lymph system or bloodstream. Cells in the new cancer are like those in the original tumor.

methadone. A synthetic narcotic pain reliever related to morphine.

milligrams/meter squared (mg/m2). A formula for calculating dosages of chemotherapy drugs according to the surface area of the body. Since the amount of skin is hard to determine exactly, it is closely estimated from height and weight. An average person might have 1.7 square meters of body surface area. If the standard drug dosage was 650 mg/m2, then 650 x 1.7 = 1105 mg of drug to be given.

mitosis. The process of cell reproduction or division. Cancer cells usually have higher rates of mitosis than normal cells. The number of divisions seen under a microscope reflects how aggressive the cancer is.

modality. A general class or method of treatment. The basic modalities of cancer therapy include surgery, radiation therapy, chemotherapy, and immunotherapy.

moniliasis. A common fungal infection often seen as white patches on the tongue or the inside of the mouth. *See also* **candidiasis**.

monoclonal antibodies (MAbs). Highly specific antibodies, usually manufactured in a laboratory, that react to a specific cancer antigen or are directed against a specific type of cancer. Current research is studying their role in therapy. One potential use is to deliver chemotherapy and radiotherapy directly to a tumor, thus killing the cancer cells and sparing healthy tissue. Studies also are trying to find out if monoclonal antibodies can be produced to detect and diagnose cancer cells at a very early and curable stage.

monoclonal gammopathy. An elevation in gamma globulin in the blood caused by a single clone of plasma cells or lymphocytes. Such a protein pattern may be associated with multiple myeloma.

morbidity. Sickness, illness, symptoms, and signs of disease. Not to be confused with mortality.

mortality. Death.

MRI (magnetic resonance imaging). A method of creating images of the body using a magnetic field and radio waves rather than X rays. Although the images are similar to those of CT scans, they can be taken in all three directions (planes) rather than just in cross-sections. There is no X-ray exposure. *See also* **nuclear magnetic resonance**.

mucosa or mucous membrane. The inner lining of the gastrointestinal tract or other structures such as the vagina and nose.

mucositis. Inflammation of the mucous membranes. Soreness—like cold sores—can develop in the mouth as a side effect of chemotherapy.

multicentricity. A tumor that appears to start growing in several places at once.

multimodality. Using a combination of two or more types of therapy—for example, radiotherapy plus chemotherapy, radiation plus surgery, or chemotherapy plus surgery.

mutation. A permanent change in a cell's DNA that alters its genetic potential. It may be a response to a chemical substance (mutagen) or result from a physical effect such as radiation. Sometimes the daughter cells may be cancerous.

myelogram. An X ray of the spinal cord after the introduction of radio-opaque dye into the sac surrounding it. Used to see if a tumor involves the spinal cord or nerve roots.

myeloma. A cancer of the protein-producing plasma cells of the bone marrow. Multiple bone lesions are common.

myelosuppression. A fall in the blood counts caused by therapy, especially chemotherapy and radiotherapy.

N

nadir. The lowest point to which white blood cell or platelet counts fall after chemotherapy.

narcotics. Pain-relieving (analgesic) substances whose use is closely regulated by government. There are natural and synthetic types.

nasopharynx. The part of the nasal cavity behind the nose and above the part of the throat that we can see.

National Cancer Institute. A highly regarded research center in Bethesda, Maryland, that conducts basic and clinical research on new cancer treatments and supervises clinical trials of new treatments throughout the United States.

National Surgical Adjuvant Breast/Bowel Project (NSABP). A group of dedicated research and clinical physicians who have formed a large cooperative group to study new treatments. Many major advances in treatment are attributed to this group.

natural killer (NK) cells. Large, granular lymphocyte cells, normally present in the body, whose normal function is to kill virally infected cells. Some methods of cancer treatment take advantage of this ability of NK cells.

necrosis. The disintegration of tissues caused by some physical or chemical agent or by lack of blood supply. Cancers treated effectively by chemotherapy, radiotherapy, heat, or biological agents undergo necrosis.

needle biopsy. Removing a tiny bit of tissue for diagnosis by placing a needle into a tumor. The procedure is usually done under local anesthesia. *See* **fine needle aspiration.**

neoadjuvant chemotherapy. Chemotherapy given before the primary treatment—either surgery or radiation therapy—to improve the effectiveness of treatment. *See* **adjuvant chemotherapy.**

neoplasm. A new abnormal growth. Neoplasms may be benign or malignant.

nephrotoxic. Toxic to the kidneys. The term is generally used to refer to a drug's effect.

nerve block. Removing pain by numbing a nerve temporarily (with a local anesthetic) or permanently (with an alcohol injection).

neuropathy. Malfunction of a nerve, often causing numbness (sensory nerve) or weakness (motor nerve). It is sometimes a side effect of anticancer drugs.

neutropenia. Reduced (low) white blood cell count, usually from chemotheraphy of radiotherapy.

neurotoxicity. Toxic effects (usually of drugs) on the nervous system.

neutrophils. One of the white blood cells that fights infection. Also called granulocytes, polys, or PMNs.

nitrosoureas. A class of chemical compounds that can enter the brain through the blood-brain barrier. The anticancer drugs BCNU, CCNU, and methyl-CCNU are nitrosoureas. *See* **blood-brain barrier.**

NK cell. *See* **natural killer cells.**

no code. An order written in a hospital chart after careful and considered discussions, to not attempt to resuscitate a patient if breathing and/or the heartbeat should stop. This is usually considered if the patient, after all reasonable therapeutic efforts have been made and have failed, is suffering greatly and rapidly failing from a far-advanced malignancy. Also called a Do Not Resuscitate or DNR order.

nodes. *See* **lymph nodes.**

nodule. A small lump or tumor that can be benign or malignant.

non-cell-cycle specific. Chemotherapeutic drugs capable of destroying cells that are not actively dividing.

nuclear magnetic resonance (NMR). An old term for MRI.

O

oncogenes. Specific stretches of cellular DNA that, when activated in the wrong way, contribute to the transformation of normal cells into malignant ones.

oncologist. A physician who specializes in cancer therapy. There are surgical, radiation, pediatric, gynecologic, and medical oncologists. The term oncologist generally refers to medical oncologists who are internists with expertise in chemotherapy and handling the general medical problems that arise during the disease.

oncology. The medical specialty that deals with the diagnosis, treatment, and study of cancer.

oophorectomy. The surgical removal of one or both ovaries.

opportunistic infections. Many common fungi and bacteria and a few microscopic parasites do not ordinarily cause infections in healthy people. But such ordinarily harmless organisms can produce severe, life-threatening, and hard-to-control infections in cancer patients by taking advantage of the reduced immune response resulting from the disease or therapy.

organ donation. The authorized giving of one or more organs (such as a heart, kidney, or liver) to another person.

ostomy. A surgically created opening in the skin, leading to an internal organ, for purposes of drainage. *See also* **colostomy; ileostomy; stoma.**

ototoxicity. Toxic effects on the ears, generally resulting in a ringing in the ears or hearing loss.

P

palate. The roof of the mouth. The hard palate is in front, the soft palate just behind.

palliative. Treatment that aims to improve well being, relieve symptoms, or control the growth of cancer but not primarily intended or expected to produce a remission or cure.

palpation. Examination by feeling an area of the body—such as the breast or prostate—with the fingers to detect abnormalities. A palpable mass is one that can be felt.

paracentesis. Removing fluid from the abdomen by inserting a small needle through the skin. This is usually done under local anesthesia.

paraneoplastic syndromes. Various symptoms and signs—changes in body minerals, nerve function, or water balance, for example—that indicate the presence of a tumor in the body but that are not related to direct pressure by the tumor.

parenteral nutrition. Artificial feeding by the intravenous administration of concentrated amino acid, sugar, and fat solutions. *See also* **hyperalimentation; TPN.**

pathologic fracture. A fracture (break) in a bone through an area weakened by cancer. Usually little or no injury or trauma precedes the fracture, unlike the usual fracture of healthy bones.

pathologist. A physician skilled in the performance and interpretation of laboratory tests and in the examination of tissues to provide a diagnosis.

pathology. Study of disease through the examination of body tissues, organs, and materials. Any tumor suspected of being cancerous must be diagnosed by pathologic examination. The physician who does this is called a pathologist.

PDQ (Physician Data Query). A comprehensive, up-to-date information service on state-of-the-art cancer treatment provided by the National Cancer Institute via computer and fax.

percutaneous endoscopic gastrostomy. Placement of a feeding tube through the skin directly into the stomach. This employs a technique of shining a light inside the stomach by means of a gastroscope to identify the exact location to safely pass the feeding tube through the skin, using a small incision under local anesthesia.

performance status. A measurement of how well a cancer patient is functioning. Index numbers from 0 to 100—increasing in steps of 10—document and record functional status, as opposed to other measurements that indicate the size of a tumor. A person with a performance status of 80 functions better than one with a score of 50. Also called Karnofsky score.

perineum. The part of the body between the anus and the genitals.

perioperative. Occurring at or around the time of surgery. Often used with reference to chemotherapy or radiotherapy treatments.

peritonoscopy. Inspection of the inside of the abdominal cavity by means of a telescope inserted under anesthesia through a tiny opening in the skin.

persistent vegetative state. The condition of a person who is in a coma and has no hope of regaining consciousness even with medical treatment.

PET (positron emission tomography). A new type of scan that detects areas of cells that are living and growing more rapidly than others. It may find areas of cancer by detecting their growth, rather than the space they occupy as in CT and MRI scans.

petechiae. Tiny areas of bleeding under the skin usually caused by a low platelet count.

phlebitis. Inflammation of the veins, often causing pain and tenderness. *See also* **pulmonary embolism; thrombophlebitis.**

photodynamic therapy. The injection of a light-sensitizing chemical or dye and the subsequent application of light, usually laser, to a tumor. The chemical improves the effect of the laser treatment and thus minimizes or prevents damage to normal tissues.

photosensitivity. Extreme sensitivity to the sun. Some medications—including a few anticancer drugs as well as tetracycline antibiotics—produce photosensitivity as a side effect, leaving the patient prone to sunburn.

placebo. An inactive substance, used in a research study or clinical trial, that looks like the medication being tested in the trial. It is used to isolate the improvement that may result from the belief that a medication is being given, rather than the actual effect of the medication.

plasmapheresis. The replacement or washing of a patient's plasma by donor plasma or saline.

platelet. One of the three kinds of circulating blood cells. The normal platelet count is about 150,000 to 300,000. Platelets are responsible for creating the first part of a blood clot. Platelet transfusions are used in cancer patients to prevent or control bleeding when the number of platelets has significantly decreased.

plateletpheresis. Collection of platelets in a machine for transfusion into another person.

pneumonectomy. Surgical removal of a lung.

polycythemia. An excessively high red blood cell count. This may be caused by a primary blood disease or as a response to another type of disease.

polyp. A growth that protrudes from mucous membranes, often looking like a tiny mushroom. Polyps may be found in the nose, ears, mouth, lungs, vocal cords, uterus, cervix, rectum, bladder, and intestine. Some polyps occurring in the cervix, intestine, stomach, or colon can eventually become malignant and should be removed.

poorly differentiated. A tumor that, under a microscope, has little or only a slight resemblance to the normal tissue from the same organ. *See also* **anaplastic; undifferentiated; well differentiated.**

port (infusion). A small disk with a soft center (about the size of a quarter) that is surgically placed just below the skin in the chest or abdomen. A tube coming out of the side is connected to a large vein. Fluids, drugs, or blood products can be delivered directly to the bloodstream without worrying about finding an adequate (healthy) vein, making multiple venipunctures, or causing leakage of the fluids into surrounding tissues by passing a small needle through the skin into the disk. *See also* **port-a-cath.**

port-a-cath. One type of infusion port, a venous (vein) access device that has nothing protruding from the skin. Injections are made into a chamber implanted just under the skin. *See* **port.**

potassium. An important mineral in the body that is often lost during illness, especially with diarrhea. Low potassium levels can cause weakness.

precancerous. Abnormal cellular changes or conditions—intestinal polyps, for example—that tend to become malignant. Also called premalignant.

primary tumor. The place where a cancer first starts to grow. Even if it spreads elsewhere, it is still known by the place of origin. For example, breast cancer that has spread to the bone is still breast cancer, not bone cancer.

proctoscopy. *See also* **colonoscopy; sigmoidoscopy.**

progesterone. One of the female hormones (the other is estrogen). It causes the buildup of the uterine lining in preparation for conception and performs other functions before and during pregnancy. Certain synthetic forms of the hormone are used in cancer treatment.

progesterone-receptor (PR) assay. A test that determines if breast cancer is stimulated by progesterone.

prognosis. A statement about the likely outcome of disease—the prospect of recovery—in a particular patient. In cancer, it is based on all available information about the type of tumor, staging, therapeutic possibilities, expected results, and other personal or medical factors. For example, breast cancer patients who are diagnosed early usually have a good prognosis.

progression. The growth or advancement of cancer indicating a worsening of the disease. A progression may be slow or fast, and its rate may increase or decrease.

prophylactic. Treatment designed to prevent a disease or complication that is likely to develop but has not yet appeared. Also may be called adjuvant treatment.

prostate-specific antigen (PSA). A substance in the blood derived from the prostate gland. Its level may rise in prostatic cancer and is useful as a marker to monitor the effects of treatment.

prosthesis. An artificial replacement or approximation of a body part—such as a leg, breast or eye—that is missing because of disease or surgery.

protocol. A carefully designed and written description of a cancer treatment program. It includes dosages and formulas for any drugs to be administered.

proto-oncogene. A class of genes that encourages cell growth. Mutation of these genes produces a carcinogenic oncogene, one that can cause cancer.

pulmonary embolism. A life-threatening condition in which a blood clot travels to the lungs from veins in the legs or pelvis, often from thrombophlebitis. The clots are diagnosed with a lung scan and treated with anticoagulants. *See also* **phlebitis; thrombophlebitis.**

R

radiation oncologist or **radiotherapist.** A physician who specializes in the use of radiation to treat cancer.

radiation therapy. *See also* **radiotherapy.**

radical mastectomy. Removal of the entire breast along with underlying muscle and the lymph nodes of the armpit (axilla). In a modified radical mastectomy, the underlying (pectoral) muscles are left in place.

radical neck dissection. An extensive surgical operation to remove all of the lymph glands on one side of the neck, usually in association with surgery to remove a primary tumor that may have spread to the lymph glands in the neck.

radical surgery. An extensive operation to remove the cancer and the adjacent structures and lymph nodes.

radioactive implant. A source of high-dose radiation that is placed directly into and around a cancer to kill the cancer cells.

radioactive isotope. A radioactive substance used for diagnosis (tracer dose used for scans) or treatment (therapeutic dose).

radiologist. A doctor who specializes in the use of X rays as well as other imaging techniques such as ultrasound, MRI, and radioactive tracers to diagnose and investigate disease. New radiology techniques are also used for treatment in some cases (interventional radiology).

radiosensitive. A cancer that usually responds to radiation therapy. The opposite is radioresistant.

radiosensitizer. A drug or biological agent that is given together with radiation therapy to increase the therapy's effect.

radiotherapy. The use of high-energy radiation from X-ray machines, cobalt, radium, or other sources for control or cure of cancer. It may reduce the size of a cancer before surgery or be used to destroy any remaining cancer cells after surgery. Radiotherapy can be helpful in treating recurrent cancers or relieving symptoms. *See also* **radiation therapy.**

RADS. An obsolete unit measuring radiation dosage, now replaced by the centigray (cGy).

recurrence. The reappearance of a disease after treatment had caused it to apparently disappear.

red blood cells. Cells in the blood that bring oxygen to tissues and take carbon dioxide from them.

refractory tumors. Tumors that do not respond to chemotherapy.

regional involvement. The spread of cancer from its original site to nearby surrounding areas. Regional cancers are confined to one general location in the body.

regression. The shrinkage of a cancer, usually as the result of therapy. In a complete regression, all tumors disappear. In a partial regression, some tumor remains.

rehabilitation. Programs that help patients adjust and return to a full productive life. Rehabilitation may involve physical measures such as physical therapy and prostheses, as well as counseling and emotional support.

REM. Rapid eye movement, one of the stages of sleep.

remission. The partial or complete shrinkage of cancer, usually occurring as the result of therapy. Also the period when the disease is under control (not growing). A remission is not necessarily a cure.

renal. Pertaining to the kidney. *See also* **kidney failure.**

resection. The surgical removal of tissue.

residual disease or **residual tumor.** Cancer left behind after surgery or other treatment.

resistance. Failure of a tumor to respond to radiotherapy or chemotherapy. The resistance may be evident during the first treatment (primary), or during a subsequent treatment (secondary).

retroperitoneum. The area of the abdomen near the back, behind all the organs, including the bowel.

reverse isolation. Isolation to prevent visitors or hospital staff from carrying an infection into a patient's room. This usually means that everyone coming into the patient's room must wear a gown, mask, and gloves.

ribonucleic acid (RNA). A nucleic acid present in all cells and similar to DNA. It is the biochemical blueprint for the formation of protein by the cells.

risk factors. The habits or conditions that promote the development of many cancers. Cigarette smoking, for example, is a major risk factor for lung cancer. The major risk factor for skin cancer is overexposure to the sun.

risk reduction. Techniques used to reduce the chances of developing cancer. High-fiber diets, for example, may help reduce the risk of colon cancer.

RNA. *See* **ribonucleic acid.**

S

salvage. The attempt to cure a patient by a second, third, or later alternative treatment program after the first-line treatment has failed to produce a cure.

sampling. Removal of a portion of a tissue for diagnostic tests.

sarcoma. A cancer of supporting or connective tissue such as cartilage, bone, muscle, or fat. Sarcomas are often highly malignant but account for only 2 percent of all human cancers.

scans (radioisotope). Diagnostic procedures for assessing organs such as the liver, bone, or brain. Radioactive tracers are introduced intravenously and if a malignant tumor or other foreign material is present, pictures of the organ will show abnormalities that may indicate the presence of a tumor. There is no significant risk with this small, brief radiation exposure.

screening. The search for cancer in apparently healthy people who have no cancer symptoms. Screening may also refer to coordinated programs in large populations.

second-look surgery. Sometimes the only way to determine if aggressive therapy has worked is to explore the patient surgically some time after initial therapy. Second-look surgery can discover if there is any residual or recurrent cancer, which may help decide whether treatment is complete or if more radiotherapy or chemotherapy is needed. Residual tumors may also be removed during this operation.

segmentectomy. Surgical removal of a portion (segment) of the breast or lung.

seizure or convulsion. Shaking of a part or all of the body, often with loss of consciousness. This can be caused by an injury, a benign condition (such as idiopathic epilepsy), or a brain tumor.

selective angiography. X-ray pictures of an organ taken after a catheter is passed through the artery to the organ and a dye, which shows on X rays, is injected.

sepsis or **septicemia** or **bacteremia.** Bacterial growth within the bloodstream. This very serious situation usually requires hospitalization for intravenous antibiotics.

serum protein electrophoresis (SPEP). A laboratory testing method that separates serum proteins into different groups—albumin, alpha globulin, beta globulin, and gamma globulin. The different patterns produced are characteristic of various diseases.

shingles. *See* **herpes zoster.**

sigmoidoscopy. An examination of the rectum and lower colon with a hollow lighted tube called a sigmoidoscope. It is used to detect colon polyps and cancer, to find the cause of bleeding, and to evalu-ate other bowel diseases. A newer instrument using fiber-optics—the flexible sigmoidoscope—permits easier, safer, and more extensive examination. *See also* **colonoscopy; proctoscopy.**

sodium. An important mineral in the body that helps to maintain fluid balance. It is measured as part of an electrolyte panel.

sonography. The use of ultrasound pictures in diagnosis.

sphincter. A circular muscle that tightens around an organ or cavity to close it, and to regulate the flow of material. If the sphincter around the rectum and the mouth of the bladder isn't functioning properly, for example, urine and stool might be lost involuntarily.

spleen. An organ adjacent to the stomach, composed mainly of lymphocytes, that removes worn-out blood cells and foreign materials from the bloodstream.

sputum. Material coughed up from the lungs. Also called phlegm.

squamous cell (epidermoid) carcinoma. Cancer arising from the skin or the surfaces of other structures, such as the mouth, cervix, or lungs.

staging. An organized process of determining how far a cancer has spread. Staging involves a physical exam, blood tests, X rays, scans, and sometimes surgery. Knowing the stage helps determine the most appropriate treatment and the prognosis.

stem cells. Primitive or early cells found in bone marrow and blood vessels that give rise to all of our blood cells. To protect patients from low blood counts and the resulting complications after high-dose chemotherapy, a complex device is used to remove stem cells from a vein in the arm and give them back intravenously a few days later. They find their way back into the bone marrow and replace the marrow that was depressed by chemotherapy. The use of peripheral stem cell transplants has made the need to collect bone marrow itself much less important. This procedure should really be called peripheral stem cell protection rather than transplantation because patients get their own cells back.

stereotaxic needle biopsy. A procedure often used in the diagnosis of brain tumors. A specialized frame is used to hold a patient's head or other body part stationary while the biopsy needle is directed to exactly the right spot. Usually, a CT scanner or other computer-associated equipment is used to find the correct position. This method has also been applied recently to very small breast cancers.

steroids. A class of fat-soluble chemicals—including cortisone and male and female sex hormones—that are vital to many functions within the body. Some steroid derivatives are used in cancer treatment.

stoma. A surgically created opening in the skin for elimination of body wastes. A stoma is made in the abdominal wall for elimination of wastes, for example, when the colon and/or rectum no longer can perform this function. *See also* **colostomy; ileostomy; ostomy.**

stomatitis. Inflammation and soreness of the mouth. This is sometimes a side effect of chemotherapy or radiotherapy.

stool. Feces or bowel movement.

stool for occult blood. A test to determine if bleeding has occurred. This may show signs of bleeding that are too mild to see with the naked eye. *See* **guaiac test.**

superior vena cava. The large vein draining the blood from the head, neck, and arms back into the heart.

suppository. A way to administer medications by absorbing the drug into a wax preparation, then inserting it into the rectum or vagina. Suppositories are used to treat local conditions such as vaginitis or hemorrhoids, and are also used when pills cannot be swallowed or kept down because of nausea, sore mouth or narrowing of the esophagus. Antinausea suppositories such as Compazine and Tigan are often used to combat this side effect of chemotherapy.

systemic disease. Disease that involves the entire body rather than just one area.

T

T cell. *See* **B cell.**

telangiectasia. Prominent or dilated small veins in the skin. This can occur without known cause as part of certain medical conditions, and sometimes as a result of radiation therapy.

TENS (transcutaneous electrical nerve stimulation). The use of a small device that is connected to the skin and sends small, harmless amounts of electricity into the pain fibers so that they are "too busy" to recognize the real pain.

teratogenic. A drug or toxin that, if taken during pregnancy, can cause the fetus to be malformed.

terminal. This term has a number of definitions. Some people use it when cure is not possible, even if treatment can add years to the patient's life. Others say a patient is terminal when he or she has a specific short life expectancy, perhaps six months or less. Still others mean that no other treatment can be given and "nature will take its course." If this term comes up, discuss with your doctor exactly what is meant by it.

thoracentesis. Insertion of a needle or tube between the ribs and into the chest cavity to remove fluid. The procedure is done for diagnostic or treatment reasons and is performed under local anesthesia.

thoracic. Pertaining to the thorax or chest.

thoracotomy. A surgically created opening into the chest.

thrombocytopenia. Having an abnormally low number of platelets (thrombocytes)—fewer than 150,000—due to disease, reaction to a drug, or toxic reaction to treatments. Bleeding can occur if there are too few platelets, especially if the count falls to less than 20,000.

thrombophlebitis. Inflammation of veins with blood clots inside the veins. Usually associated with pain, swelling, and tenderness. *See also* **phlebitis; pulmonary embolism.**

thrombosis. Formation of a blood clot within a blood vessel.

tissue. A collection of cells of the same type. There are four basic types of tissues in the body: epithelial, connective, muscle, and nerve.

TNM classification. A complex and exact system for describing the stage of development of most kinds of cancer. This system is not used for lymphomas, leukemias, or Hodgkin's disease.

TPN (total parenteral nutrition). The use of complex protein and fat solutions to supply enough calories and nutrients to sustain life. The solutions are delivered intravenously. *See also* **hyperalimentation; parenteral nutrition.**

tracheostomy. An artificial opening in the neck leading to the windpipe (trachea). The opening is created surgically to allow breathing when the trachea is blocked.

tumor. A lump, mass, or swelling. A tumor can be either benign or malignant.

tumor markers. *See also* **CEA; markers.**

tumor necrosis factor. A natural protein substance produced by the body that may make tumors shrink.

tumor-suppressor gene. A class of genes that suppresses cell growth.

U

ulcer. A sore resulting from corrosion of normal tissue by some irritating process or substance such as stomach acid, chemicals, infections, impaired circulation, or cancerous involvement.

ultrasound. The use of high-frequency sound waves to create an image of the inside of the body. Also called ultrasonography.

undifferentiated. A tumor that appears "wild" under a microscope, not resembling the tissue of origin. These tumors tend to grow and spread faster than well-differentiated tumors, which do resemble the normal tissue they come from. *See also* **anaplastic; poorly differentiated; well differentiated.**

unilateral. On one side of the body.

urethra. The tube that leads from the bladder to the outside of the body to allow elimination of urine. Cancers rarely begin there.

urostomy. A surgical procedure in which the ureters, which carry urine from the kidneys to the bladder, are cut and connected to an opening on the skin outside the abdomen. This allows urine to flow into a collection bag. *See* **stoma.**

uterus. The female reproductive organ, located in the pelvis; the womb in which a fetus develops until birth.

V

venipuncture. Inserting a needle into a vein in order to obtain blood samples, start an intravenous infusion, or give a medication.

ventricles. Four fluid-filled cavities in the brain, all connected with each other. There are two lateral ventricles in the top part of the brain—one on each side, with the third and fourth ventricles in the center of the brain. Obstruction of the connections or the outflow tract leads to swelling (hydrocephalus). Also refers to the chambers in the heart.

vesicant drugs. Chemotherapeutic agents that can cause significant tissue irritation and soreness if they leak outside the vein after injection.

virus. A tiny infectious agent that is smaller than bacteria. Viruses cause many common infections such as colds and hepatitis. Viruses invade cells, alter the cells' chemistry, and cause them to produce more of the virus. Several viruses produce cancers in animals. Their role in the development of human cancers is now being studied.

W

well differentiated. A tumor that under a microscope resembles normal tissue from the same organ. *Also see* **anaplastic; poorly differentiated; undifferentiated.**

white blood cells. Cells in the blood that fight infection. These are composed of monocytes, lymphocytes, neutrophils, eosinophils, and basophils. The normal count is 5,000 to 10,000. It may be elevated or depressed in a wide variety of diseases. Chemotherapy and radiotherapy usually cause low white counts.

Index